Quantitative Cancer Modeling and Risk Assessment

Charles D. Holland

President, Texas Institute for Advancement of Chemical Technology
and
Professor Emeritus, Texas A&M University

Robert L. Sielken Jr.

President, Sielken, Inc.

P T R Prentice Hall, Englewood Cliffs, New Jersey 07632

Library of Congress Cataloging-in-Publication Data

Holland, Charles Donald.
Quantitative cancer modeling and risk assessment / Charles D. Holland and Robert L. Sielken, Jr
p. cm.
Includes bibliographical references and index.
ISBN 0–13–117110–0
1. Carcinogens is—Mathematical models. 2. Carcinogens—Dose-response relationships. 3. Cancer—Risk facts. 4. Cancer—Environmental aspects. 5. Health risk assessment—Mathematical models. 6. Health risk assessment—Statistical methods.
I. Sielken, Robert L. II. Title.
[DNLM: 1. Dose-Response Relationship, Drug. 2. Models, Theoretical. 3. Neoplasms—prevention & control. 4. Risk. QZ 200 H734q 1993]
RC268.5.H64 1993
616.99'4071'015118—dc20
DNLM/DLC 92-48367
for Library of Congress CIP

Dedicated to the Members of the
Texas Institute for Advancement of
Chemical Technology, Inc.

Acquisitions Editor: Mike Hays
Production Editors: Fred Dahl and Rose Kernan
Copy Editor: Rose Kernan
Cover Designer: Eloise Starkweather
Prepress & Manufacturing Buyer: Mary McCartney

Printed in the United States of America
10 9 8 7 6 5 4 3 2 1

ISBN 0-13-117110-0

Prentice-Hall International (UK) Limited, *London*
Prentice-Hall of Australia Pty. Limited, *Sydney*
Prentice-Hall Canada Inc., *Toronto*
Prentice-Hall Hispanoamericana, S.A., *Mexico*
Prentice-Hall of India Private Limited, *New Delhi*
Prentice-Hall of Japan, Inc., *Tokyo*
Simon & Schuster Asia Pte. Ltd., *Singapore*
Editora Prentice-Hall do Brasil, Ltda., *Rio de Janeiro*

Contents

Foreword

At current mortality rates, a baby born today in the United States has roughly one chance in four of dying from cancer in his or her lifetime. As America continues to make progress against heart disease and accidents, cancer may emerge as the dominant cause of premature death in this country. Even among developing countries, the incidence of cancer rises as infectious diseases and the ills of stark poverty are conquered. These actuarial facts, combined with the public's understandable fears about this painful and debilitating cause of death, have caused cancer prevention to emerge as a major public health priority.

Much has been made of the promise of clinical treatment of cancer and the search for vaccines and medical cures. President Nixon's highly touted "War on Cancer" has not yet produced the clinical advances that were envisioned. While important advances in cancer treatment have been discovered, the emerging consensus is that more emphasis should be placed on the primary prevention of cancer through changes in diet, lifestyle, and environmental conditions.

Early thinking about cancer prevention is reflected in the concept of a "carcinogen," a physical or chemical agent that, following human exposure, has the capability to cause cancer. Radiation and cigarette smoke are perhaps the prototypical examples of carcinogens. The traditional viewpoint is that only a small fraction of chemical and physical agents are carcinogens and rudimentary scientific tools, such as epidemiological studies or long-term laboratory animal tests, can be employed to distinguish carcinogens from noncarcinogens.

The traditional viewpoint is reflected in the Delaney Clause of the 1958 Federal Food, Drug, and Cosmetic Act and related laws. Congress mandated that any "cancer-causing" additive that concentrates in food should be prohibited. By ridding the food supply of man-made "carcinogens," Congress believed that they might prevent an important cause of human cancer. More recently, the International Agency for Research on Cancer of the World Health Organization has begun to classify chemicals and mixtures with regard to evidence of carcinogenic activity in human and experimental systems. Building on the IARC approach, the U.S. Environmental Protection Agency has designed a carcinogen classification system that is used by regulatory agencies, legislatures, and the public to distinguish carcinogens from noncarcinogens. Typifying this approach is a continual request from Congress to the U.S. Department of Health and Human Services to publish each year a list of chemicals that are known to be or are reasonably anticipated to be "carcinogens."

Although the alleged distinction between carcinogens and noncarcinogens is quite seductive, a growing number of scientists have come to the conclusion that the distinction is not very meaningful or useful. The "carcinogen" concept is becoming outdated because a majority of the chemicals examined for carcinogenicity in high-dose animal tests are testing positive. Many more chemicals may have tested "positive" if the number of animals or species tested had been larger, if the tests of statistical significance had been relaxed slightly, if the doses had been slightly higher, or if the exposure conditions had been subtly altered. Since it is now apparent that we live in a sea of "carcinogens" produced by nature and man, it is no longer feasible to entertain the idea that we will simply prohibit all carcinogenic exposures.

Scientists are also beginning to question whether all carcinogens were created equal. Since some chemicals exert much more potent carcinogenic activity than others, the suggestion has been made that the public should focus cancer prevention resources on the largest carcinogenic risks. The wisdom of this position is underscored by the fact that human exposure to some carcinogens is much more widespread than is exposure to others. Since we cannot possibly eliminate carcinogenic exposures, we desperately need analytical procedures to quantify the biggest causes of human cancer.

At the same time that scientist have discovered many more rodent carcinogens than were anticipated, they have also learned that not all animal carcinogens are relevant to humans. While this insight is quite distressing to scientists who have built careers around animal testing, the developing sciences of comparative pharmacokinetics and pharmacodynamics are calling into question some of the basic assumptions of the high-dose animal tests. It is too early to tell how many animal carcinogens do not endanger people, but it is already apparent that our risk assessment procedures must allow for this distinct possibility.

In *Quantitative Cancer Modeling and Risk Assessment*, Charles D. Holland and Robert L. Sielken, Jr. have responded to the public's demand for analytical procedures to make sense out of the sea of carcinogens that may endanger us. The analytic procedures in this book will help the public distinguish the serious causes of human cancer from the trivial speculation. The book is a highly rigorous yet accessible treatment of the biology of human cancer, the mathematical models of carcinogenesis, the emergence of risk assessment tools, key concepts in statistical analysis of cancer data, improved models that account for pharmacokinetics and pharmacodynamics, and decision-analytic procedures for characterizing the magnitude of cancer risks and associated uncertainties.

This book is essential reading for anyone who aspires to be a knowledgeable participant in technical and public discussions about the primary prevention of human cancer. It will also prove to be a useful textbook and reference book for college professors, students, regulatory scientists, and risk assessors in industry, government, labor unions and environmental advocacy groups. More than any other publication, this book illustrates that scientists can do and must do more than tell the public whether or not a chemical is a "carcinogen."

John D. Graham
Professor of Policy and
Decision Sciences,
Harvard School of Public Health

Director,
Harvard Center for
Risk Analysis

Preface

This book was written for the purpose of providing engineers and scientists with a fundamental understanding of the various models that have been proposed for cancer formation and their use in risk assessment. The developments begin with first principles and assume that the reader has a fundamental understanding of mathematics, but not of probability and statistics. Some of the simpler concepts of probability and statistics are introduced with the development of the subject matter while the more complex concepts are presented in Chapter 4, thereby making it unnecessary for the student to refer to standard texts on this topic.

The material on cancer modeling and its use in risk assessment is scattered throughout the scientific literature. This book brings the material on these two topics together in a logical and detailed manner that makes it possible for someone without prior knowledge to follow without referring to other books or the scientific literature. Chapter 1 is an overview of the basic concepts of the scientific fields of biology, biochemistry, and epidemiology which are needed in subsequent chapters. The developments of the most widely used classical models for cancer formation are presented in Chapter 2. These developments draw heavily on the concepts of probability and statistics.

In Chapter 3, the models developed in Chapter 2 are used in the quantification of virtually safe doses and risk assessment. Three different types of methods are presented for the characterization of virtually safe doses: the Mantel-Bryan method, the EPA method, and the nonparametric bootstrap method. Numerical examples are used to demonstrate both the application of the methods and some of their properties. This chapter is concluded by demonstrating the use of fitted models in the estimation of the risk of a population from a given exposure.

Recent advances in the modeling and analysis of dose-response experiments are presented in Chapter 5. A kinetic development is given for a two-stage dose-response model including cell birth, death, and mutation processes. The subject of Physiologically Based Pharmacokinetics (PBPK) Modeling is introduced, and some results obtained by the use of these models are discussed. Chapter 6 provides a treatment of biologically based dose scales for dose-response modeling. The dose scale selected strongly affects the dose-response model which in turn has a significant impact on the risk assessment.

A weight-of-evidence approach to quantitative cancer risk assessment is presented in Chapter 7. In this approach all relevant infomation of the cancer risk is incorporated into the cancer risk assessment. Because the different sources of information have differing levels of scientific support and relevance, the sources are weighted. In contrast to this approach which reflects all available, relevant information, the "conservative" or "worst case" approach is the most widely used today. In the conservative approach, the analysis having the largest risk is selected as the risk assessment, and all other information discarded. The true utility and economic soundness of the conservative approach is presently the subject of considerable controversy.

The authors gratefully acknowledge and appreciate the time and effort devoted to the reviewing of Chapter 1 by Claudia L. Barton, D.V.M. (Professor of Veterinary Small Animal Medicine and Surgery, Texas A&M University; Diplomate, American College of Veterinary Internal Medicine, Specialties of Internal Medicine, Oncology); Sally R. Cowles, M.D., Dr.P.H. (Medical Director Health Surveillance—Epidemiology, Shell Oil Company), and Donald E. Stevenson, Ph.D., M.R., C.V.S., F.R.C. Pathology (Toxicology Director, Health, Safety, & Environment, Shell Oil Company). Their many suggestions and significant contributions are reflected throughout this chapter. The authors are deeply indebted to Dr. Paul F. Deisler, Jr. (Private Consultant and Past President of the Society for Risk Analysis) for not only reviewing the book and providing many excellent suggestions, but also for his continued encouragement.

Also, the authors acknowledge the many contributions of the staffs of the Texas Institute for Advancement of Chemical Technology (TIACT) and of Sielken, Inc. The extensive collaboration by Dr. Ciriaco Valdez-Flores (Quantitative Risk Assessment Consultant, Sielken, Inc.) in the preparation of Chapters 6 and 7 was particularly helpful and is greatly appreciated. The preparation of several figures for Chapters 6 and 7 by Mrs. Becky Pankratz (Assistant, Sielken, Inc.) is also appreciated. The efforts of Ms. Janice Mitchell (Staff Assistant, TIACT) and Mr. Robert E. Holthus (Graduate Assistant, Texas A&M University) in the preparation of the manuscript are appreciated. The editorial contributions of Mrs. Wanda K. Greer (Secretary, TIACT, and Assistant to the President) are gratefully acknowledged and appreciated.

Charles D. Holland and Robert L. Sielken Jr.

Introduction

With the technology age has come not only the highest standard of living ever experienced by mankind and the longest expected lifetimes, but also technology-related risks. Among these risks, environmental risks have received the most intense focus because of the possible link between industrial chemicals and and some cancer.[1] In response to these technology related environmental health risks, a staggering number of state and federal laws have been enacted and regulations promulgated that pertain to the assessment and management of these risks.

As a result of the emphasis on the assessment and management of risks, this general area of knowledge has grown at an ever increasing rate. Subject matter now ranges from the most scientific areas, such as the behavior of chemicals at the molecular level in body chemistry, to sociopolitical, ethical, and judicial concerns.

Risk assessment is generally used to mean the characterization of potential adverse health effects from human exposures [as suggested by the National Academy of Science[2]], and it can be divided into the four major steps which are discussed below. Although this book focuses on *human* health effects, ecotoxicity and other environmental impacts not directly affecting human health are sometimes also considered to be part of a risk assessment.

Risk management is the process of evaluating alternative actions and selecting the most beneficial method for avoiding or reducing an unacceptable risk. Risk management begins with the results of a risk assessment and takes into account all applicable and relevant state and federal laws and regulations as well as political, social, economic, and engineering information and perceptions.

In order to prevent the scientific findings and technical activities embodied in risk assessment from being influenced by political and economic considerations as well as the consequences of regulatory action or the consequences of risk management decisions in general, the consensus of opinion is that the two activities, risk assessment and risk management, should be carried out independently.[1,2,3] The independence of risk assessment, a scientific and technical activity, from risk management, a policy- and value-oriented activity, is not intended to prevent the communication of information, explanations, clarifications, or needs. The independence is intended to keep risk assessments free from the wishes and policy judgements of risk assessors as well as the feelings of risk assessors about the merits of different risk management options. The independence is also intended to prevent risk managers from making judgements on scientific matters outside their areas of expertise.

Although no attempt is made to treat the topic of risk management in this book, it was introduced because of its role relative to risk assessment. Also, because of the diversity of scientific disciplines involved in the different components of risk assessment as it is currently defined, only parts of the risk assessment field are covered in a detailed quantitative manner. Furthermore, the emphasis in this book on chemical carcinogenicity as opposed to ionizing and nonionizing radiation carcinogenicity or non-cancer endpoints. As described below, all four parts of risk assessment enter into the qualitative and quantitative discussions in the book but the primary focus of the book is on dose-response assessment. Risk assessment is a rapidly evolving and developing field, and there is more to risk assessment than what is covered in this book.

By present consensus, risk assessment is now divided into four areas:

1. *Hazard identification*
2. *Dose-response assessment*
3. *Exposure assessment*
4. *Risk characterization*

as illustrated in the following diagram.

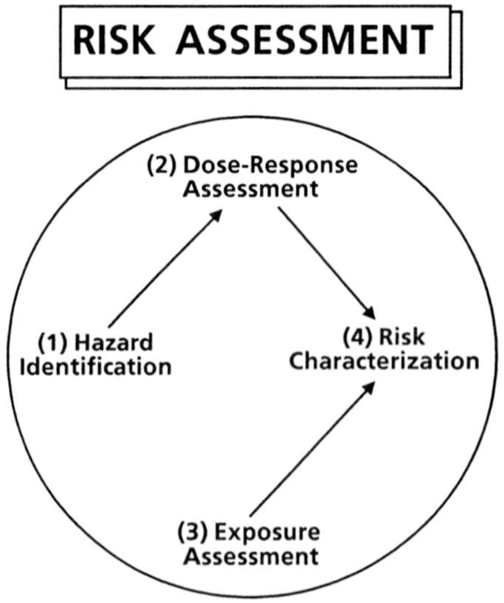

Dose-response assessment (2) is the primary focus of this book and the quantitative aspects of dose-response assessment are given an in-depth treatment. Hazard identification (1) determines the need for dose-response assessment (2) and the responses of special interest. Exposure assessment (3) combines with dose-response assessment (2) to produce risk characterization (4).

A brief description of these areas follows. Hazard identification may be defined as the process of determining whether exposure to a given substance can cause an increase in the incidence of a health condition (cancer, birth defect, neurotoxicity, etc.) in humans.[2] Hazard identification involves characterizing the quality, nature, and strength of evidence of causation. This evaluation often results in a weight-of-evidence or strength-of-evidence qualitative classification scheme.[4] As described briefly in Chapter 1, information for hazard evaluation is obtained from epidemiological studies, clinical evidence, animal studies, and various types of other tests. Hazard identification is the first step in the risk assessment process. The information obtained in hazard identification determines to a large extent the necessity for performing the remaining steps in risk assessment and, if they are necessary, focuses attention on responses of potential concern.

Dose-response assessment is the determination of the relationship between the doses of an administered substance and the incidence of an adverse health effect in humans. In an exposed population, the exposure leads to a dose, and the dose-response assessment characterizes the impact of that dose on the incidence of a specified response. The specified response is defined in terms of the site and severity of one or more adverse health effects. Dose-response assessment incorporates information on the extrapolation of results from high to low doses and from animals to humans. As indicated above, the quantitative portion of dose-response assessment is the book's primary focus.

Exposure assessment is the process of measuring or estimating the levels, frequency, duration, schedule, and route of human exposures to a substance currently present in the environment as well as estimating potential exposures that might arise from the future release of substances into the environment.[2] Exposure assessment incorporates field measurements, estimated exposures, and characterizations of populations potentially at risk including their behaviors, sizes, and natures. For the most part exposure assessment is independent of hazard identification and dose-response assessment. However, hazard identification indicates the need for an exposure assessment and, sometimes, indicates populations, routes, and temporal dose patterns of particular concern. Also, exposure assessment may suggest dose levels of special interest in the dose-response assessment. Although exposure assessment is not treated in depth in this book, the quantitative results of exposure assessments are used in the demonstration of the combination of dose-response and exposure assessments in risk characterization, particularly in Chapter 7.

Risk characterization is the process of describing the likelihood of an adverse health effect in a given human population by combining the dose-response and exposure assessments.[2] Risk characterizations can include different types of quantitative descriptions of risk such as most likely values, bounds, and probability distributions and should reflect uncertainty, variability, and sensitivity. Risk characterization is the concluding step in risk assessment and an important input to risk management. Some of the past, present, and future aspects of risk characterization are discussed and illustrated in Chapter 7.

Because of the importance of the role played by cancer modeling in both dose-response assessment and risk characterization and because of the extensive quantitative treatment of this topic in this book, cancer modeling is specifically identified in the book's title. Nevertheless, many of the quantitative methods and qualitative discussions are also applicable to non-cancer endpoints.

REFERENCES

1. Deisler, P. F., Jr. "The Risk Management-Risk Assessment Interface," *Environmental Science & Technology*, **22**, 15 (1988).
2. National Research Council, "Risk Assessment in the Federal Government: Managing the Process," National Academy Press: Washington, D.C. (1983).
3. *Federal Register*, **50**; 10372 (1985).
4. U.S. Environmental Protection Agency, "Guidelines for Carcinogen Risk Assessment," *Federal Register*, **51**; 33992 (1986).

1

A Review of the Science of Cancer Formation

Mathematical modeling is the name given to the attempt to quantify the theories and understanding of any type of process. To provide a background for cancer modeling, a brief review of the status of the science of cancer formation from both the molecular and epidemiological points of view are given. The molecular basis for cancer formation is an emerging field of science and all of the answers are not yet in. Potential advances in this field hold the key to the preventions and cures of the diseases called cancer.

Over the past decade, significant advances in the understanding of cancer formation at the molecular level have been made. If our knowledge at the molecular level were complete, neither animal nor epidemiological studies would be required for cancer. It is far from complete, however. Thus, to provide an overview of the status of the cancer problem at this time requires not only a review of the status of our understanding of cancer formation at the molecular level but, also a review of the causes of cancer as deduced by classical epidemiological and animal studies.

In Section 1.1 of this chapter, an abbreviated review of cellular replication is presented, while in Section 1.2 the present status of the causes of cancer as deduced by epidemiological studies is presented. This chapter is concluded with Section 1.3, which consists of a brief review of some of the recent research on cancer formation at the molecular level, trends in cancer therapies, individual risk identification, and cancer prevention.

1.1 AN ABBREVIATED REVIEW OF CELLULAR REPLICATION

The following discussion of *cells*, *chromosomes*, and *genes* is not intended to be a definitive treatise on these topics, but instead an abbreviated one with enough detail to aid in the subsequent discussions of the general field of cancer formation, research, and therapies. Excellent overviews of the literature concerning the topics, cells, chromosomes, genes, and mutations are given in a number of texts, such as those by Ham,[1] Bailey and Ollis,[2] Aiba et al.,[3] Gardner and Snustad.[4] These sources were very helpful in the preparation of the following summary of cellular structure and replication.

According to Ham,[1] a cell may be defined as the smallest unit of living material which is capable of existing independently in a nonliving environment by synthesizing substances which it needs from nutrients absorbed from the environment. Most cells also have the capacity to reproduce themselves. The condition of a nonliving environment rules out the classification of *viruses* as cells because viruses require a living environment.

Cells have also been defined in terms of their structure; namely, as a minute body of *protoplasm* surrounded by a limiting *membrane* and containing a *nucleus*. Protoplasm was defined by Huxley as the physical basis of life. It is now generally accepted that the manifestations of life are dependent upon the continuance of a vast number of chemical reactions occurring in and also involving the protoplasm. The total amount of protoplasm present in the mature body remains essentially constant because it is consumed and produced at approximately the same rates. Protoplasm is produced within the cell by chemical reactions involving the surrounding nutrients.

The complete set of all chemical reactions occurring in a cell is called its *metabolism.* Most chemical reactions occurring within a cell are catalyzed by *enzymes,* which consist of proteins that have been synthesized from amino acids. After the principal parts of a cell have been identified, some of the chemical constituents of a cell as well as some of the chemical reactions that occur within a cell are presented.

Cells in mature individuals may be divided into three fundamental classes; namely

1. those which never reproduce themselves such as nerve cells,
2. those which constantly reproduce themselves to replace those that are lost, such as intestine and bone marrow cells, and
3. those which have the capacity to reproduce themselves but do not ordinarily do so or do so very slowly, such as liver cells.

The *germ cells* of an organism are those cells whose function it is to produce all the cells of the entire organism. The germ cells are also called the *sexual* cells. By the process called *differentiation*, germ cells produce cells which are *different* or *specialized.* These cells are responsible for the development of the body as well as the performance of body functions, and are thus called *somatic* or body cells. As a consequence of differentiation, *cell families* are formed. Not all cells of a family can reproduce themselves. Only *stem* cells have the capacity to reproduce themselves. Furthermore, stem cells belonging to one family can produce only cells which belong to its family and not to some other family. Cells of a given

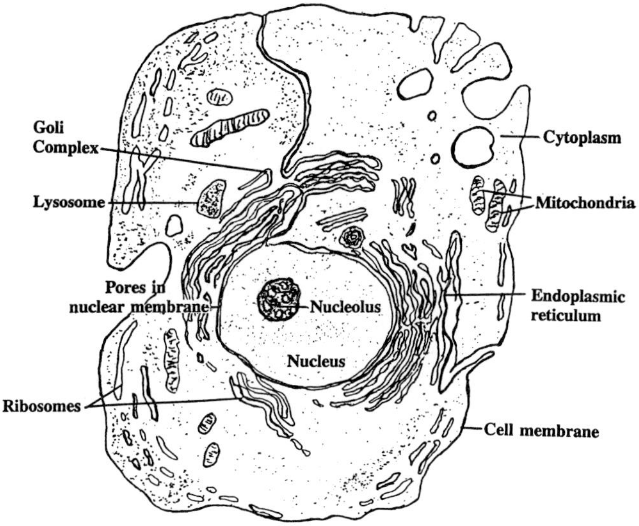

Figure 1.1 Principal Components of a Typical Animal Cell.

family may further differentiate to the point where they can no longer reproduce themselves. The supply of cells capable of reproducing themselves is maintained essentially constant by the stem cells of the given family.

1.1.1 Cellular Structure

Cells of humans and all higher organisms belong to the class of cells known as *eukaryotic cells* or *eukaryotes*. Although the various types of human cells differ in many respects, they all have many of the same characteristics. A sketch of a cell and some of its component parts is shown in Figure 1.1.

Eukaryotic cells have diameters that range from 5 μm to 50 μm* and are enclosed by an outer membrane. The two principal parts of the cell are (1) the *nucleus* and (2) the material called *cytoplasm* that fills the space between the nucleus and the outer *membrane* of the cell. The nucleus, also enclosed by a *nuclear membrane*, controls the chemical reactions that occur in the cytoplasm. The nucleus contains the chromosomes, the chromosomes contain the *deoxyribonucleic acid (DNA)*, and the DNA contains the genes. Characteristics of heredity among other things are controlled by the chromosomes, and the genes control the production of their associated *enzymes* from the amino acids. The enzymes catalyze or cause selected chemical reactions to take place. In addition to the nucleus, several other elements in the cytoplasm called *organelles* are enclosed by membranes. Some of

* 1 m (meter) $= 10^6$ μm (micrometer, formally known as a micron) $= 10^9$ nm (nanometer) $= 10^{10}$ Å(angstrom units).

the organelles shown in Figure 1.1 are: *endoplasmic reticulum*, *mitochondria*, *ribosomes*, *lysosomes*, and *Golgi complex*. The endoplasmic reticulum consists of a membrane system that leads from the cell membrane to the nucleus. Mitochondria are organelles that utilize oxygen in chemical reactions that produce energy. They are also the sites for other important chemical reactions. *Ribosomes* are organelles which serve as sites for chemical reactions. The remaining organelles perform various functions associated with the production of the chemical constituents of new cells, and they also isolate the unique chemical reactions that occur within them from the cytoplasm.

1.1.2 Nucleus

The *nucleus* of a cell is enclosed by an outer membrane, and at or near its center is a membrane-enclosed *nucleolus*. The space between the nucleolus and the outer membrane of the nucleus is filled with *chromatin*. The chromatin is also referred to as *chromatin granules* because in one phase of the cell division process the chromatin takes on the appearance of granules. The name chromatin comes from the *chrome* color that the granules exhibit in a staining procedure used for identification. In the latter stages of cell division, some of the chromatin takes on the form of "crooked" cylinders which are the chromosomes, and they contain the DNA and associated genes. Other constituents of the chromatin consist of the various types of proteins, which are classified as *histones* and *nonhistones*. Also, *ribonucleic acid (RNA)* has been identified as a constituent of the chromatin. RNA is similar to DNA, though differing in important details, and is also involved in cell division as discussed in a subsequent section.

When the chromatin of the nucleus is examined by use of an electron microscope, among the types of structures found are the *nucleosomes*, which consist of beads joined by DNA threads. As discussed in detail below, a DNA molecule consists of two strands of chemically bonded sugars which are crosslinked by nitrogen bases. Each pair of nitrogen bases that form a crosslinkage is called a *nucleotide pair*. Chemical analysis and X-ray diffraction studies have shown that these beads consist of 140-nucleotide pairs which are wound around a core composed of 4 pairs of proteins called *histones*, *H2a*, *H2b*, *H3*, and *H4*. According to Gardner and Snustad,[4] over 50 percent of the nucleus is chromatin and the remaining major constituent is *nonchromatin*. The chromatin consists of about equal amounts of DNA, *histone proteins*, *nonhistone proteins*, and a smaller amount of RNA.

1.1.3 Nucleolus

Chromatin in the nucleolus consists primarily of the RNA ribosomes and proteins. Since the ribosomes of the nucleolus are thought to be the precursors of the ribosomes found in the cytoplasm, the chief role of the nucleolus appears to be the production of *ribosomal RNA*. After formation, the ribosomal RNA subsequently migrates to the cytoplasm where it serves as a site for protein synthesis.

1.1.4 Human Chromosomes

There are a total of 46 human chromosomes, and two of these are the sex chromosomes. For the female, the sex hormones are denoted by XX and for the male by XY. The remaining 22 identical pairs of chromosomes are called the *autosomes*. It is now generally accepted that there is one DNA molecule per chromosome. The length of the DNA molecule in the largest human chromosome is 85 mm.[4] However, when a cell is in the process of division it is about 0.5 μm in diameter and 10 μm long.[4]

The chromosomes have been divided into groups. Group A contains 6 chromosomes, or the first three pairs (1, 2, 3), and is denoted by A(1-3). Similarly the remaining 22 chromosome pairs are classified and grouped as follows: B(4-5), C(6-12), D(13-15), E(16-18), F(19-20), G(21-22). The 23rd pair consist of two X chromosomes for a female, and an X and a Y chromosome for a male. The complete set of genes in the chromosomes is called the *nucleotides genome*, and the human genome is said to contain an estimated 3×10^9 nucleotide pairs.[4]

1.1.5 Blood Cells and Their Functions

The chemical reactions in the cells throughout the body are fueled by oxygen supplied by the blood, a fluid in which whole cells and fragments of cytoplasmic are suspended. The fluid is called *plasma* and the cytoplasmic fragments, produced by special cells in the bone marrow, are called *platelets* because they are shaped like disks.

There are two main types of blood cells, *red cells* and *white cells*. The red cells are called *erythrocytes* and the white cells are called *leukocytes*. The red cells perform their function of supplying oxygen to other body cells while in the bloodstream. Leukocytes perform their functions when they leave the blood stream and enter the loose connective tissue. The blood is used by the leukocytes as a means of transport to the locations where they perform their functions.

About 20 to 30 percent of the leukocytes in the blood are *lymphocytes*. This group of cells is responsible for the immunological reactions. They perform their function as they circulate from the blood stream through the *lymphatic tissue* and back to the blood. Lymphocytes are formed in the lymphatic tissue and the bone marrow. They have the ability to recognize and be affected by *antigens* which are usually proteins and carbohydrates. More generally, antigens may be defined as any substance capable of provoking a response by the lymphocytes.

When activated by an antigen, the small lymphocytes begin macromolecular synthesis to form large lymphocytes which proliferate and differentiate into B cells and T cells. The B cells direct the synthesis of antibodies to react with antigens, thereby performing their immune function.

The *T lymphocytes* differentiate further forming *killer T cells* or T lymphocytes that can recognize viral protein fragments displayed on the surface of the infected cell by a class *I major histocompatibility complex (MHC)* protein. The killer *T* cell performs its immunological function by binding to the infected cell.

1.1.6 Some of the Basic Chemicals Involved in Body Chemistry

In addition to the chemicals discussed below in connection with the structures of DNA and RNA, there follows an enumeration of some other basic chemicals involved in body chemistry.

The name *lipids* is given to the group of compounds which are soluble in nonpolar solvents (such as benzene, chloroform, and ether) and which are insoluble in water. Lipids are found in the plasma and organelle membranes. *Fats* serve as biological food storage, and they belong to the lipid class of compounds.

Saturated fatty acids have the following general chemical structure.

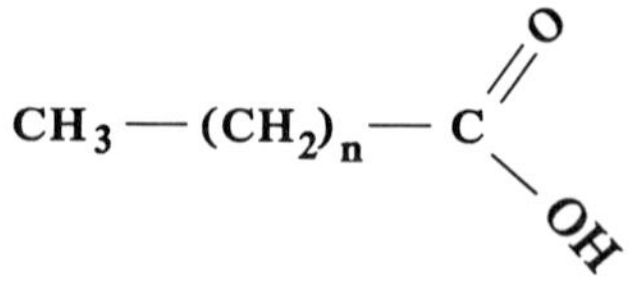

The number n is even in biological systems and ranges between 12 and 20. Saturated fatty acids consist of two types of chemical groups, the polymer group

$$CH_3-(CH_2)_n\bullet$$

and a terminal carboxylic group

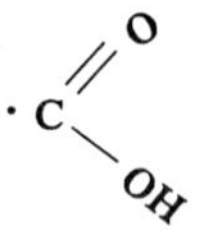

In *unsaturated fatty acids*, the central pair of carbon atoms of the polymer form are connected by a double bond rather than a single bond. For example,

$CH_3-(CH_2)_{16}-COOH$	$CH_3-(CH_2)_7-HC=CH-(CH_2)_7-COOH$
Stearic Acid	*Oleic Acid*
(Saturated fatty acid)	(Unsaturated fatty acid)

Steroids are biochemical lipids, and *hormones* are steroids which are very sensitive controllers of biochemical reactions. Two of the best-known hormones are *estrogen* and *testosterone*, which are the female and male sex hormones. Their structures are shown in Figure 1.2 as well as those of two well-known steroids, *cholesterol* and *cortisone*, which have structures roughly similar to those of estrogen and testosterone.

Other chemicals involved in body chemistry consist of vitamins and the cations H^+, K^+, Na^+, Ca^{++}, and the anions OH^-, CO_3^{--}. Also, the sugars, nitrogen bases, amino

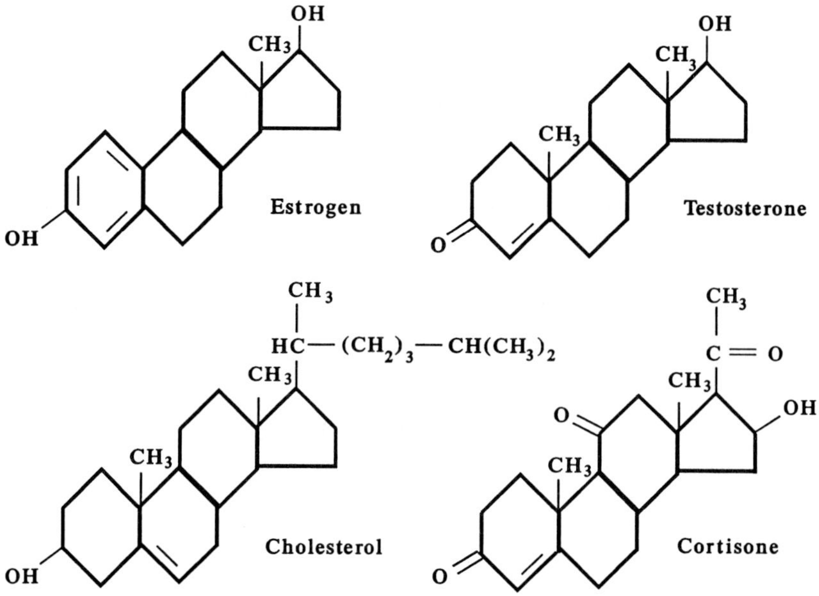

Figure 1.2 Structures of Estrogen, Testosterone, Cholesterol, and Cortisone.

acids, and proteins which are involved in body chemistry are presented in the following discussion of DNA and RNA.

1.1.7 Structures of DNA and RNA

A benchmark in the understanding of cell behavior was provided by the structural concept for DNA (*deoxyribonucleic acid*) proposed in 1953 by Watson and Crick.[5] The *biopolymer DNA* contains all of the cell's hereditary information. The DNA molecule is composed of three components:

1. *phosphoric acid*,
2. *deoxyribose sugar*, and
3. the *nitrogen bases*, *thymine* (*T*), *cytosine* (*C*), *adenine* (*A*), or *guanine* (*G*).

The *biopolymer RNA* has a structure similar to DNA, and it assists in the replication of DNA. Instead of deoxyribose sugar and thymine, RNA contains *d-ribose sugar* and the nitrogen base *uracil*. The strands of the DNA molecule consist of the sugar *deoxyribose* connected by the *phosphatediester bonds*, and the strands are crosslinked by the nitrogenous bases (*adenine*, *thymine*, *cytosine*, and *guanine*). A diagram of a portion of the double helix DNA molecule is shown in Figure 1.3.

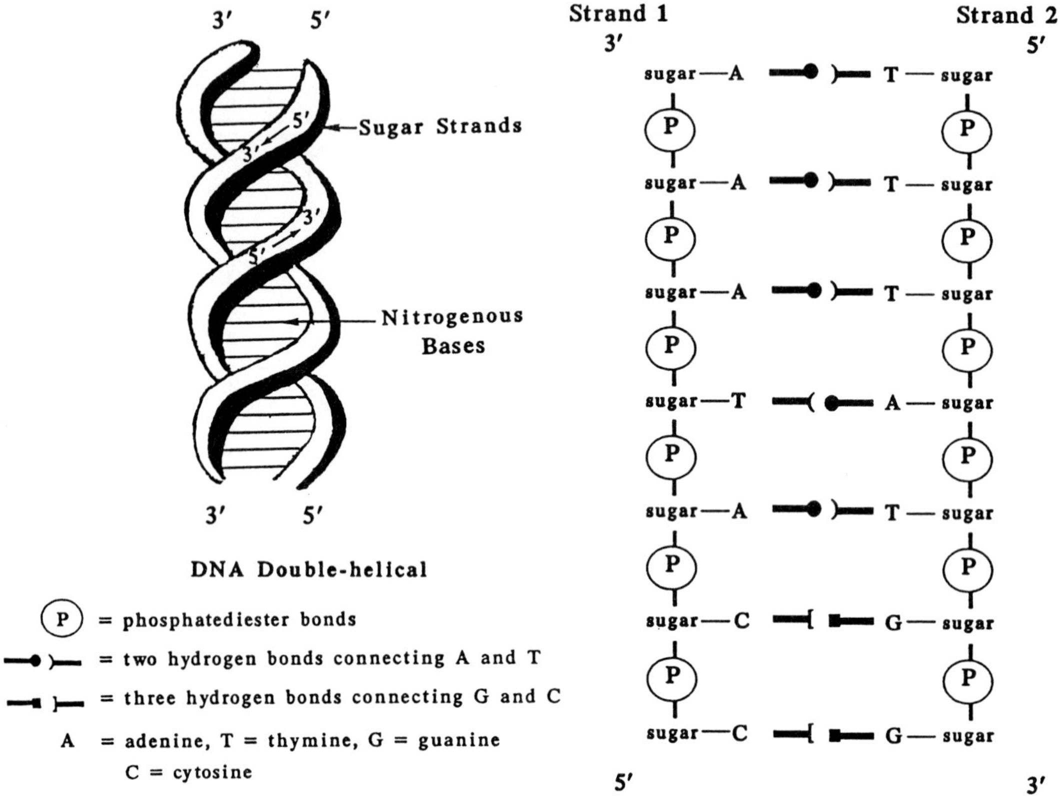

Figure 1.3 Sketch of the DNA Double-Helix, the Deoxyribose Sugar Strands, the Phosphatediester Bonds, and the Nitrogen Bases.

Structures of the sugars, deoxyribose and d-ribose which make up the nucleotides of the strands of DNA and RNA, respectively, are shown in Figure 1.4. These respective sugars are formed in strands by reacting with phosphoric acid to form the connecting phosphatediester bonds, and the *crosslinks* are formed by adding the nitrogen bases at the number 1 positions of the sugars. A typical strand of DNA is shown in Figure 1.5. Note that the 5′*end* of a DNA strand has a CH_2OH group and the 3′*end* has an OH group. The deoxyribose of the DNA and the d-ribose of the RNA are usually derived from either *purine* or *pyrimidine* which have the structures shown in Figure 1.6.

The nitrogenous bases are shown in Figure 1.7. The crosslinkages of the DNA consist of pairs of nitrogenous bases which are attached to each other by hydrogen bonds as shown in Figures 1.8 and 1.9. According to Spencer,[6] adenine and thymine are connected by two hydrogen bonds as shown in Figure 1.8. Also as indicated in Figure 1.9, thymine is always paired with adenine, and cytosine is always paired with guanine.

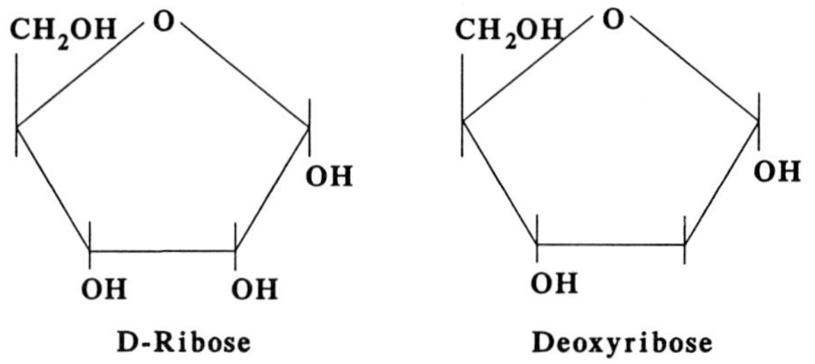

Figure 1.4 Structures of the Sugars Deoxyribose and D-Ribose.

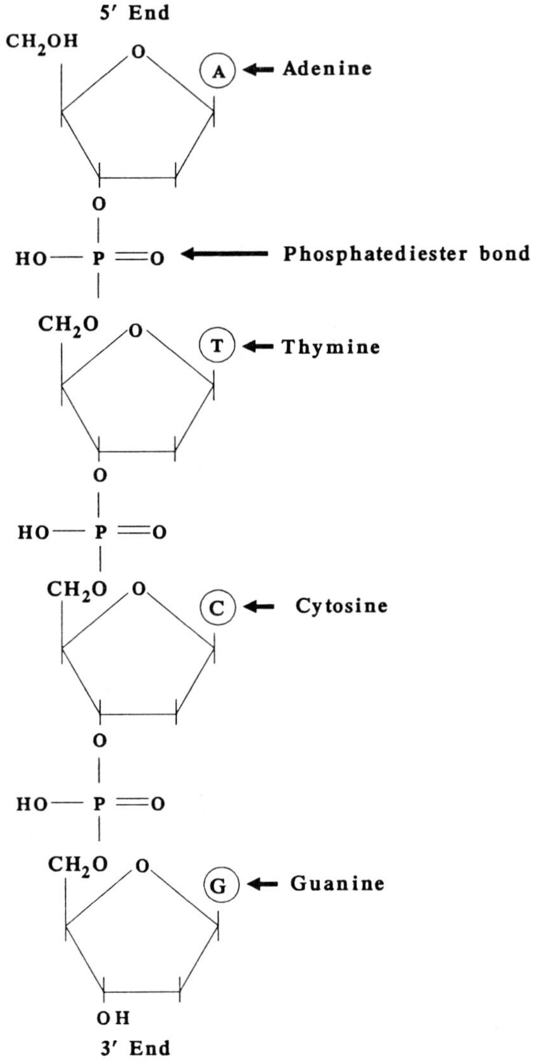

Figure 1.5 A Single Strand of DNA Showing the Deoxyribose Sugars Connected by the Phosphatediester Bond.

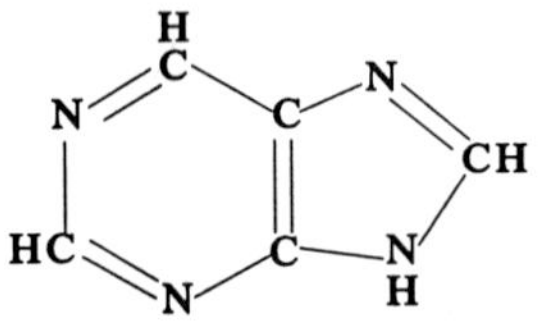

Purine

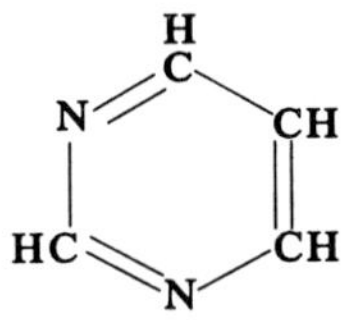

Pyrimidine

Figure 1.6 Structures of Purine and Pyrimidine.

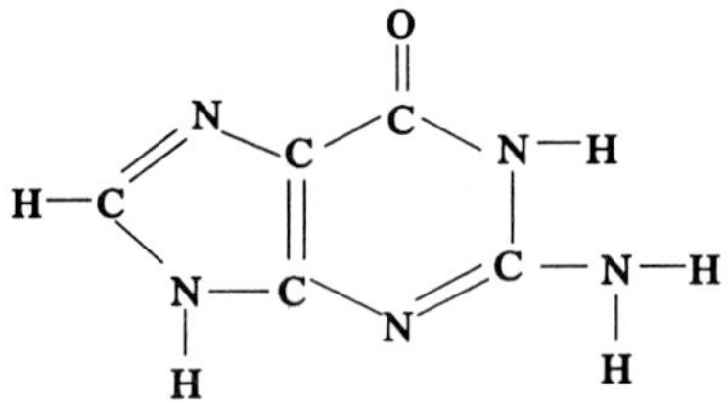

Guanine
(in both DNA and RNA)

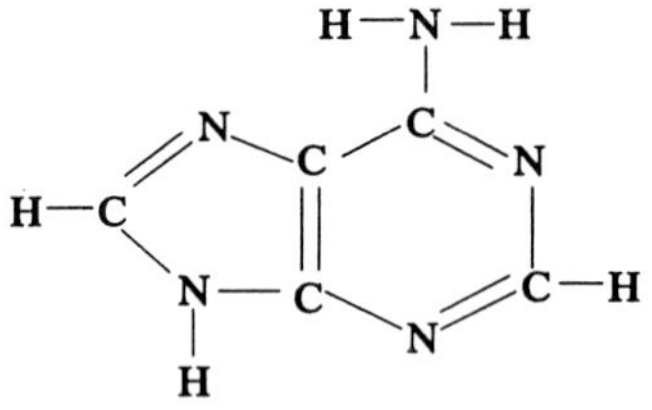

Adenine
(in both DNA and RNA)

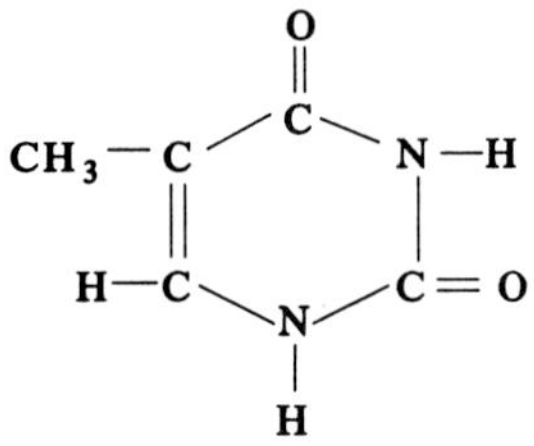

Thymine
(in DNA only)

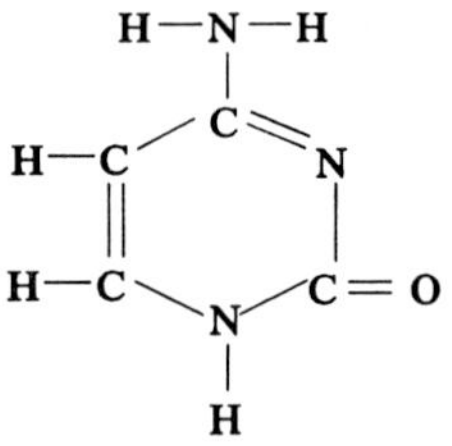

Cytosine
(in both DNA and RNA)

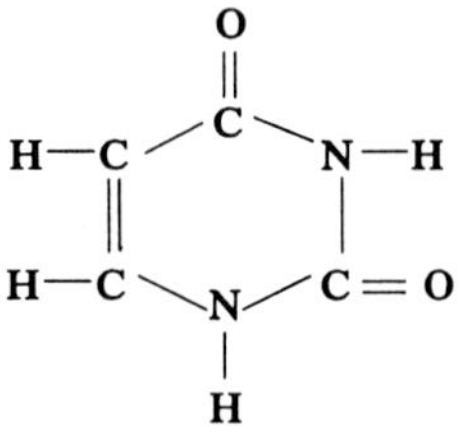

Uracil
(in RNA only)

Figure 1.7 The Nitrogen Bases in DNA and RNA.

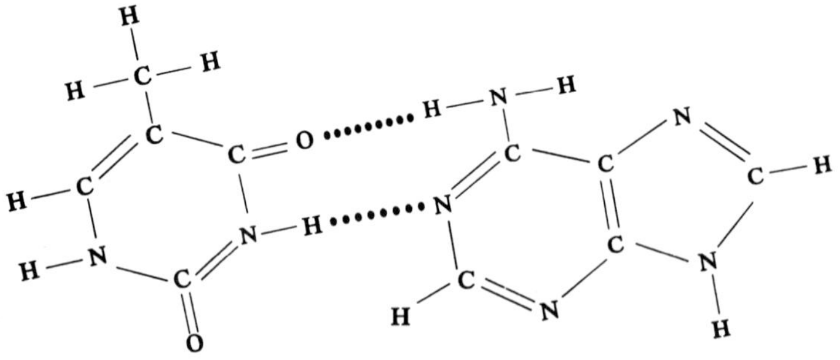

Adenine

Thymine

Figure 1.8 Hydrogen Bonding of the Adenine and Thymine in the DNA Crosslinks.

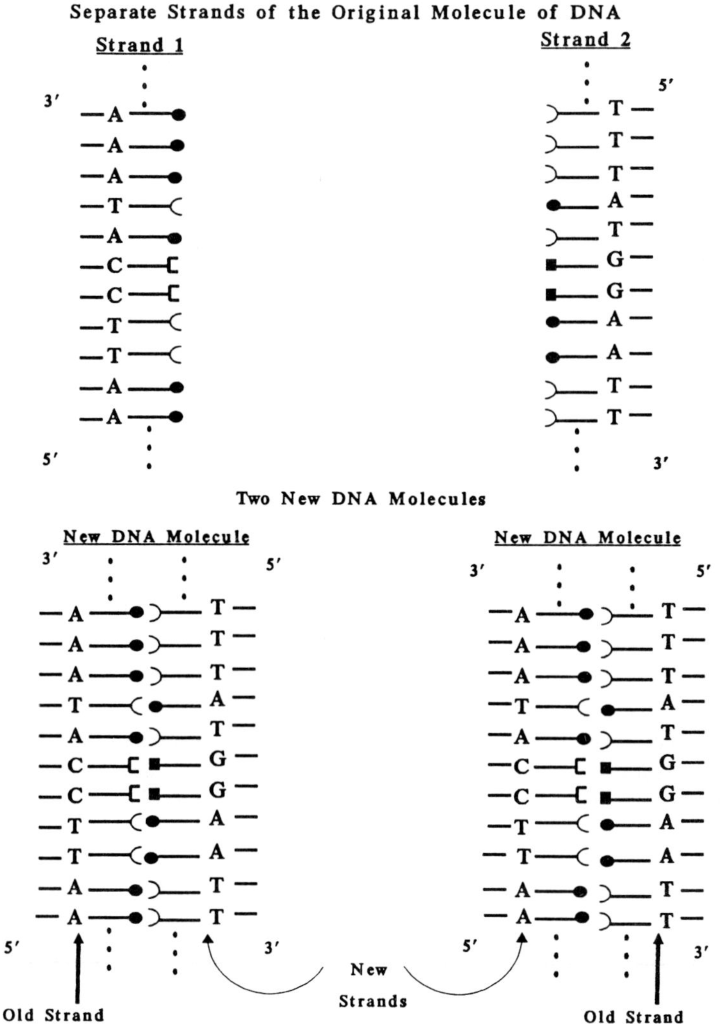

Figure 1.9 Division of the DNA Molecule Followed by Duplication.

The first step in the duplication of a DNA molecule is the separation of the two strands by the breaking of the weak hydrogen bonds connecting the nitrogenous bases as shown in Figure 1.9. After the two strands have been separated, a new strand is synthesized beside each of the original strands, and the two new molecules of DNA formed are exact replicas of the original DNA molecule.

Table 1.1 The Amino Acids Involved in the Synthesis of Protein Enzymes.

Name	Abbreviation	Name	Abbreviation
Alanine	Ala	Leucine	Leu
Arginine	Arg	Lysine	Lys
Asparagine	Asn	Methionine	Met
Aspartic acid	Asp	Phenylalanine	Phe
Cysteine	Cys	Proline	Pro
Glutamic acid	Glu	Serine	Ser
Glutamine	Gln	Threonine	Thr
Glycine	Gly	Tryptophan	Trp
Histidine	His	Tyrosine	Tyr
Isoleucine	Ile	Valine	Val

1.1.8 Biological Implication of the DNA Duplication Process

During the process of cell division, the DNA molecule of each chromosome in the nucleus of the cell duplicates itself in the manner illustrated in Figure 1.9. Prior to cell division, the nucleus appears as a well-defined mass in the cell. During the division process, known as *mitosis*, the *nuclear membrane* dissolves and the chromosomes of the nucleus become rodlike in form. The chromosomes consist of DNA molecules and proteins, which had been identified by use of a microscope long before the structure of DNA was proposed by Watson and Crick[5] in 1953. The chromosomes carry all of the hereditary information in the form of genes. Although much effort had gone into the visual identification of the genes prior to the proposed structure of DNA, it met with no success because it has now been established that genes are not physical entities, but consist merely of the ordering of the nitrogenous bases connecting the sugar strands of the DNA. This sequencing of the bases controls the synthesis of proteins. In particular, the genes consist of the sequences of "three letter words" selected from the four letters T, A, C, and G corresponding to the four nitrogenous bases. Only code words of three letters each are needed to specify the 22 amino acids required for synthesis of the appropriate proteins. The amino acids listed in Table 1.1 are those which are involved in the formation of protein enzymes by condensation. As an example, consider the formation of a simple protein polymer by condensation of two amino acids (containing two alkyl groups denoted by R_1 and R_2) as follows in Figure 1.10.

The dashed-box region containing the six atoms shown constitutes the *peptide bond*. In a similar manner, another amino acid may be added to this protein by a peptide bond.

1.1.9 Roles of RNA

There are at least three types of RNA and all three types are involved in the mechanism whereby information stored in the DNA chromosomes participates in the DNA duplication process at the sites of protein synthesis. The three types of RNA are called:

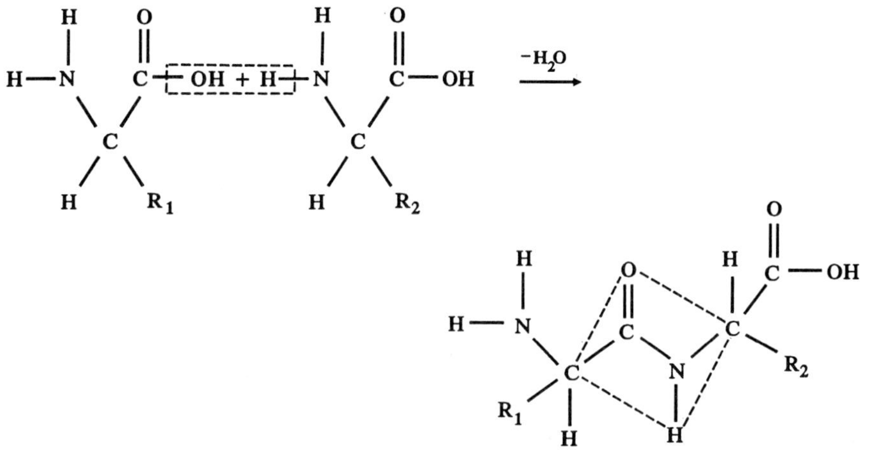

Figure 1.10 Formation of a Protein Polymer by the Condensation of Two Amino Acids.

1. *messenger RNA*,
2. *ribosomal RNA*, and
3. *transfer RNA*, and they are denoted by *mRNA*, *rRNA*, and *tRNA*, respectively.

All of these are formed in the nucleus. The constituents of RNA are the same as those of DNA except as noted above; namely, RNA has the base uracil instead of thymine, and the sugar d-ribose instead of deoxyribose. Also, most kinds of RNA are single-stranded, although some may be double-stranded.

As the strands of DNA begin to separate, the synthesis process for the production of two new DNA strands for pairing with the original strands begins. In the first step of gene expression, which is called *transcription*, an enzyme known as *RNA polymerase* catalyzes the synthesis of messenger RNA (mRNA) in an order specified by the template (the 3′ to 5′ strand of DNA) as shown in Figure 1.11.

The synthesis of messenger RNA is called *transcription* because the mRNA carries the inscription of the 3 letter words formed from *A*, *C*, *G*, and *U*. The molecular weights of mRNA range from 25,000 to 1,000,000 according to Bailey and Ollis.[2]

Perhaps the most amazing aspect of the protein production process depicted above is the fact that the code for the specification of each amino acid by a 3 letter word of the mRNA (*codons*) has been broken. This code is presented in Table 1.2 which was taken from Bailey and Ollis.[2] Observe that from this table, the codon *AUG* of the mRNA has two functions: the first is to start the process of condensation of the amino acids and the second is to specify that the first acid in the protein chain is to be methionine (*Met*). The next codon *GAA* specifies that the second amino acid is to be glutamic acid (*Glu*). Finally, the last codon *UAA* has the single function of stopping the process.

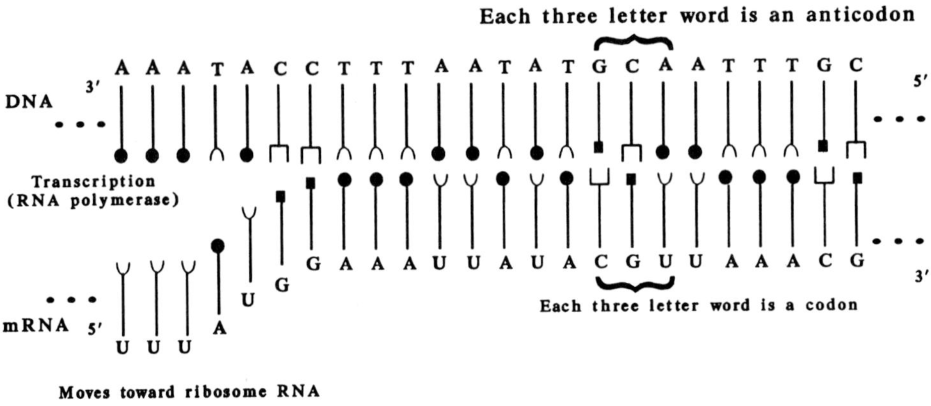

Figure 1.11 Synthesis and Transcription of mRNA.

Table 1.2 Code of the Codons of mRNA. [Taken from Bailey, J.E., and D.F. Ollis, *Biochemical Fundamentals*, 2nd Ed., McGraw-Hill Book Company, New York, NY (1986).]

first	second				third
	U	C	A	G	
U	Phe	Ser	Tyr	Cys	U
	Phe	Ser	Tyr	Cys	C
	Leu	Ser	Stop	Stop	A
	Leu	Ser	Stop	Trp	G
C	Leu	Pro	His	Arg	U
	Leu	Pro	His	Arg	C
	Leu	Pro	Gln	Arg	A
	Leu	Pro	Gln	Arg	G
A	Ile	Thr	Asn	Ser	U
	Ile	Thr	Asn	Ser	C
	Ile	Thr	Lys	Arg	A
	Met	Thr	Lys	Arg	G
G	Val	Ala	Asp	Gly	U
	Val	Ala	Asp	Gly	C
	Val	Ala	Glu	Gly	A
	Val	Ala	Glu	Gly	G

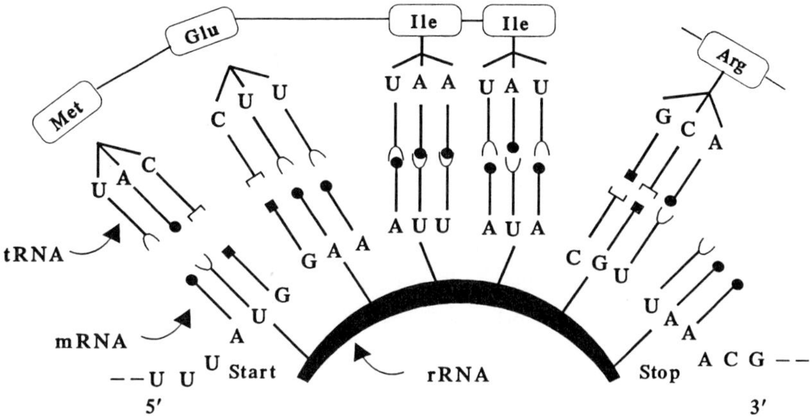

Figure 1.12 Formation of Protein Enzymes.

As the mRNA is formed it begins to move away from the DNA strand in the direction of the ribosome RNA (rRNA). The ribosome RNA and transfer RNA are synthesized in a manner similar to that shown for mRNA, by using a portion of a DNA strand as a template.

The sequencing of the bases attached to tRNA is the same as that of the bases attached to the 3′ and to the 5′ DNA strands where, of course, uracil replaces thymine. Each three letter word of tRNA attaches itself to one specific amino acid from among the 20 different types of amino acids in the neighborhood of the messenger RNA (mRNA) and the ribosome RNA (rRNA). The rRNA acts as a site for the mRNA as it participates in the formation of the protein enzymes. This process may be visualized as shown in Figure 1.12.

1.1.10 Some Mechanisms of DNA Damage and Repair

From the foregoing discussion of the roles of DNA and RNA in cell replication, it is evident that the most critical step in the utilization of the information carried by the genes of the DNA is the formation of protein enzymes from the amino acids. Since these enzymes catalyze the chemical reactions required to produce the compounds utilized in cell replication, the production of the unique enzymes is of primary importance in the true replication of cells. In view of the complexity of this process, spontaneous errors in the replication of DNA do occur.

A mutation consists of a change in the genetic material which in turn causes a change in the proteins formed from the amino acids. *Point mutations* consist of changes in the genetic material involving the substitution of one pair of nitrogen bases for another or the duplication or deletion of a single pair of nitrogen bases. Mutation is the source of all genetic variation, and it can allow organisms to adapt to new environments.

Mutations which occur without a known cause are called *spontaneous mutations*. Two examples of spontaneous mutations consist of mistakes in DNA replication and of the reaction of mutagenic agents in the environment with the nitrogen bases or the DNA strands. Actually, most of the spontaneous mutations are induced by errors in cell replication, and they are commonly referred to as *induced mutations*. These mutations occur due to physical agents such as ultraviolet rays from the sun and chemical agents, particularly oxygen. Spontaneous mutations occur infrequently and vary from gene to gene. For eukaryotes the detectable mutations per nucleotide pair per generation ranges from 10^{-7} to 10^{-9}, which according to Gardner and Snustad[4] is based on extensive data. Since the average gene is assumed to contain 1000 nucleotide pairs, there are from

$$10^{-9} \times 10^{3} = 10^{-6} \text{ mutations per gene per generation}$$

to

$$10^{-7} \times 10^{3} = 10^{-4} \text{ mutations per gene per generation.}$$

Thus, the spontaneous errors in the replication of the DNA are relatively low, of the order of one error for every 10^4 to 10^6 gene replications.

In order for a mutation to be detected it is generally necessary for the mutation to cause a *phenotypic* change in the organism or host. Phenotypic changes range from very minor alterations of the host which are detectable only by very special genetic and biochemical devices to modifications which are so gross that they can lead to death. Mutations that occur in somatic cells are called *somatic mutations*. Such mutations can produce cells like those of the family in which the mutation occurred. If the mutation occurs in a germ cell, it is called a *germinal mutation*. These mutations may be expressed in the cells of the immediate offspring or may lead to the death of the offspring. Mutations in which more than one trait is altered are referred to as *pleiotropy mutations*. Such mutations may occur in either somatic cells or germ cells.

As pointed out by Watson and Crick, some of the spontaneous mutations can be attributed to *tautomeric shifts* of the nitrogen bases connecting the DNA strands. Thymine and guanine may alternate between their *keto* and *enol* forms; whereas, cytosine and adenine may alternate between their *amino* and *imino* forms. As shown in Figure 1.13 for thymine and cystosine, the two forms of the nitrogen bases result from a shift of a hydrogen atom from the 1 to the 6 position.

Similar shifts of hydrogen occur in the tautomeric forms of adenine and guanine. These bases can be expected to exist in their *rare* tautomeric forms only for short periods of time. However, if replication happens to occur while a base is in a rare tautomeric form, a mutation can result. Errors in transcription can also result from the incorporation of analogs of the correct bases in the DNA crosslinks. Since base analogs have structures similar to the normal nitrogenous bases, they may replace one of the nitrogen bases in the DNA replication. An example is 5-*bromouracil*, which is a thymine analog and has the following structure.

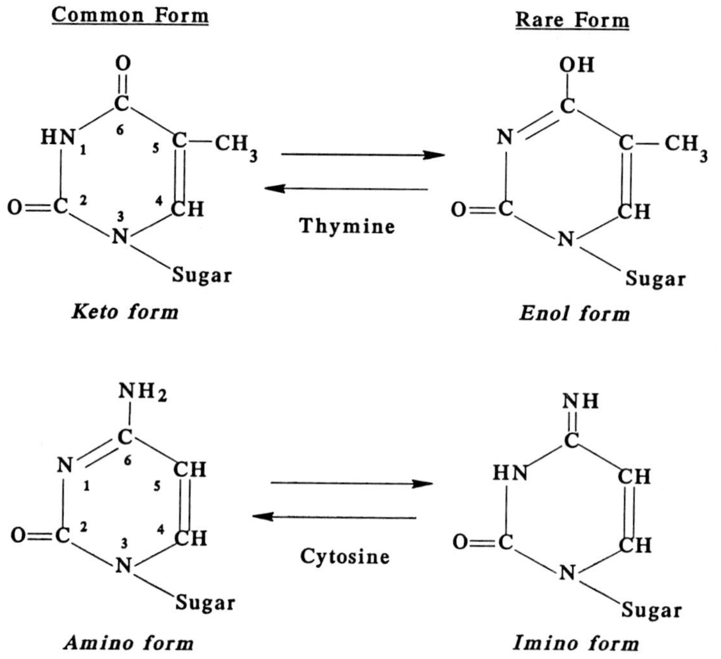

Figure 1.13 Tautomeric Forms of Thymine and Cytosine.

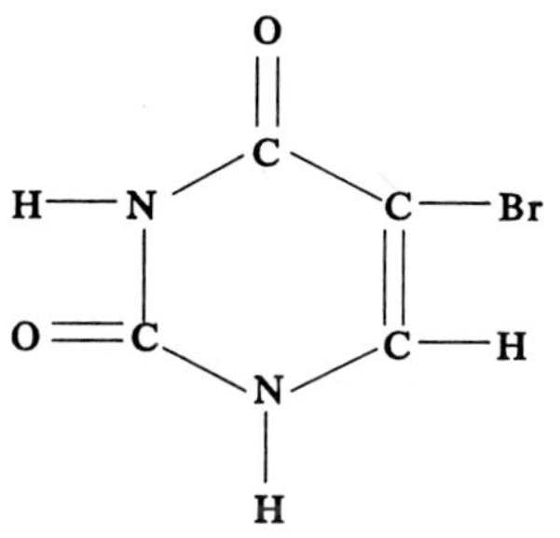

5 - bromouracil

The bromine (Br) in the ring is similar in some respects to the methyl group (CH_3) in thymine. However, after 5-bromouracil has been incorporated in the DNA, it tends to increase the probability of tautomeric shifts and thus increases the chance of a mutation.

Mutations can also be induced by chemicals. The first known chemical mutagen, *mustard gas*, was discovered by C. Auerback and her associates during World War II. This compound has the structure:

$$Cl–CH_2–CH_2–S–CH_2–CH_2–Cl$$

Mustard gas
(dichloroethyl sulfide)

Mustard gas and some of its related compounds as well as other alkylating agents cause mutations in both replicating and nonreplicating DNA. These alkylating agents transfer alkyl groups (CH_3, CH_3CH_2, etc.) to the nitrogen bases in DNA.

Another mutagen is nitric acid which can induce mutations in either replicating or nonreplicating DNA by *oxidative deamination* of the nitrogenous bases that contain the amino group; namely, adenine, guanine, and cytosine. For example, adenine is deaminated to hypoxanthine which forms a base pair with cytosine rather than thymine thereby producing a direct mutation. In contrast to the above types of induced mutations by a variety of chemicals, the hydroxylating agent *hydroxylamine*, NH_2OH, induces only GC to AC transitions.

Damage of DNA bases can be induced by a host of classical chemical reactions such as alkylation. These chemical reactions can lead to a number of different types of damage to DNA such as:

1. single and double breaks of the DNA strands,
2. base alterations and strand alterations,
3. intra-strand crosslinks of DNA,
4. crosslinks of the proteins, and
5. crosslinks between proteins and a DNA strand.

An extensive research effort has been made in the identification of these mechanisms of damage, and the literature is voluminous. For example, the books by Spencer,[6] Simic,[7] Hygaard and Simic,[8] and Floyd[9] contain hundreds of references to other publications in this area.

Of all the possible mechanisms for DNA damage, the free radical mechanism is generally conceded to be the one which contributes the greatest variety of DNA damage. Many biological reactions occur by the free radical mechanism in a manner analogous to petrochemical polymerization reactions. Free radicals may be formed in a number of ways. For example, ionizing radiation such as X-rays and γ-rays generates ions which generally lead to free radical formation.

As demonstrated by H.J. Muller in 1927, mutations can be induced by X-ray irradiation. High energy radiations such as X-rays can cause ionization of chemicals within the body, and ionizations can cause gross changes in chromosome structure such as breaks, deletions, duplications, inversions, and translocations. Low levels of irradiation over long periods of time have been found to be as effective in inducing mutations as the same total dose at high intensity levels over short periods of time.[4]

In view of all the possible mechanisms for damaging DNA, the situation might appear hopeless, but the bio-systems have a remarkable capacity for the repair of damage. Wilson (see pg. 1, Ref. 7) attributes the survival of the species to the inhibitory, scavenging and the biochemical repair systems. In the event that free radicals are formed, they are generally scavenged immediately by nearby organic material. If, however, some do reach vital molecules and oxidize them, there is still the opportunity for repair.

Almost all classes of chemical carcinogens are capable of generating free radicals by enzymatic reactions. On the other hand, noncarcinogenic compounds are relatively stable and difficult to convert to free radicals under the same conditions. As pointed out by Nagata (see pg. 58, Ref. 8), these results suggest a role of free radicals in chemical carcinogenesis. In fact, one of the general theories of cancer formation asserts that it is caused by uncontrolled free radical reactions. An extension of this theory is that the active forms of most chemical carcinogens are free radicals. Most of the studies support these concepts but do not constitute a proof that free radicals initiate the reactions which cause malignant transformations.[9] Also, experimental evidence points to a role of free radicals in the rate of cell division.

In summary, chemicals (and other agents) can contribute to cancer incidence in two ways. First, the agent may react directly with DNA, increasing the number of damaged DNA molecules and thereby increasing the probability that a damaged DNA molecule will escape repair before cell division. Second, the agent may react with some other component in the cell which causes an increase in cell division or the agent may kill the cell. If it kills the cell, there follows a temporary increase in the rate of cell division such as is observed in the formation of scar tissue, which in turn contributes to cancer formation by increasing the probability of occurrence of mutations resulting from uncontrollable events such as those enumerated above. Thus, the concept of accelerated cell division provides an explanation for the causation of cancer by agents such as viruses which may not react directly with DNA but which do cause damage and chronic irritation.

By increasing the rate of cell division, the probability that damaged DNA will undergo division before it can be repaired is increased. Thus, the mutation becomes fixed irreversibly in all future cells. Increased rates of cell division also increase the probability of the occurrence of mutation from uncontrollable events such as those resulting from errors in DNA transcription, cosmic radiation, and natural mutagens. Normally all or nearly all damaged DNA macromolecules are repaired. However, any damaged DNA which is not repaired before cell division leads to a genetic change or mutation that becomes fixed in future cells.

The role of intercellular communication in the uncontrolled division and replication of cancer cells has been addressed recently by Trosko and Chang[10] and by Yamasaki.[11] Tests for the degree of intercellular communication between cells show that cancer cells neglect to communicate with their neighboring cells and grow autonomously over surrounding cells. That is, communication between cancerous cells appears to be blocked. This communication phenomenon is referred to as *gap junction intercellular communication*. It appears that cells communicate with each other through electrical transport of ions such as calcium and hydrogen and mass transport of other compounds which can affect chemical reactions occurring within the cells.

At the present time there is a difference of opinion pertaining to the relative importance of *mitogenesis* (induced cell division) in carcinogenesis between Ames and Gold[12] and others including Perera,[13] Rall,[14] and Weinstein.[15] Ames and Gold attribute a dominant role of mitogenesis in carcinogenesis to two factors. First, a cell in the process of division is in its most active state. Second, the supply of *endogenous oxidants* (oxidants produced within the body), as estimated by Ames and Gold, is sufficient to cause a significant number of mutations. Ames and Gold pointed out that *nongenotoxic agents* [substances that do not cause mutations in the DNA, for example saccharin] can be a carcinogen at high doses in animal tests just by causing chronic mitogenesis and inflammation. Such observations led them to question the utility and meaning of routine animal tests. Perera,[13] Rall,[14] and Weinstein[15] presented counter arguments in favor of animal tests, and agreed with the suggestion of Ames and Gold[12] that research for the identification of major cancer risks should be increased and that more mechanistic studies should be performed.

At a conference on chemically induced cell proliferation, Cohen and Ellwein[16] presented one of a series of papers on various aspects of cell proliferation. Cell proliferation is caused by two classes of chemicals called *genotoxic* and *nongenotoxic*. Genotoxic chemicals react with the DNA causing proliferation and subsequent malignant tumors. Examples of such chemicals discussed by Cohen and Ellwein[16] are N–[4–(5–Nitro–2–furyl)–2–thiazolyl] formamide, denoted by FANFT and 2–Aceytlaminofluorene, denoted by AAF.

Nongenotoxic chemicals do not react with DNA but when administered at sufficiently high doses they cause cell proliferation. When the doses are administered over long periods of time, malignant tumors may result as a consequence of genomic errors in DNA replication. Also, some of these nongenotoxic chemicals cause cell proliferation because they are cytotoxic, they kill cells. Again, malignant tumors may be produced from errors because of the increased DNA replication.

Another theory of cancer formation is based on many studies involving the exposure of different animal species to a variety of substances. The results of these studies suggest that the carcinogenic process can be described in terms of three stages: *initiation, promotion*, and *progression*. According to Boutwell,[17] the initiation step consists of an exposure of an animal to a substance from which no tumor results. However, current evidence indicates that a heritable change does occur, but one in which no detectable change in the rate of DNA synthesis, cell division, or enzyme activity is observed.

On the other hand, promoters cause a phenotypic response. The term *phenotype* pertains to the observable features in the physical, biochemical, and physiological makeup of an individual as determined genetically and environmentally. Generally, promoters are not carcinogenic when applied alone, but when applied sometime after an initiator has been applied to an animal, many benign and some malignant tumors appear. After a sufficient exposure to a promoting agent, the changes in the initiated cells become irreversible and progress to the malignant stage.

1.2 CANCER MORTALITIES AND CAUSES

Since the causes of cancer are not fully understood on a molecular basis, clinical observations, exposure studies, and classical epidemiological studies have been used in the past and will continue to be used in the foreseeable future for the determination of the causes of the various types of cancer. In general causative agents have been found because clinical observations have raised the suspicion, and subsequent epidemiological studies have confirmed the suspicion. Our inability to find cures for all of the dreaded set of diseases known collectively as cancer makes cancer an emotional issue. Out of confusion, the general public has become an easy prey for those who claim to know all of the answers. Exaggerated claims in the 1970s by a number of people, including some with scientific training, that almost all cancer was caused by industrial pollution have been discredited by the careful studies of Doll and Peto[18*], Higginson,[19] Higginson and Muir,[20] Cole,[21] and Wynder and Gori[22] in which the major causes of cancer have been identified. The work of Doll and Peto,[18] published in 1981, is the most detailed analysis of the causes of cancer that has been published up to this time, and parts of it are presented in subsequent sections.

1.2.1 Comparison of Cancer Mortality with the Production of Chemicals

A cancer *epidemic* has been alleged and attributed to "man-made chemicals." As shown in Figure 1.14, the facts do not support this allegation.[23,24,25] A disease may be highly prevalent, but this fact alone does not make it an epidemic. If a disease is growing rapidly throughout a population at a rate clearly in excess of that normally expected, it is classified as an epidemic. Cancer is a prevalent disease but it is not an epidemic because the total mortality rate of cancer has increased only slightly from 1930 to 1987. As discussed below, the small increase is attributed mainly to lung cancer, which is caused primarily by the use of tobacco.[24] [To correct for yearly changes in population, all rates have been age-adjusted relative to the population for the year 1970.[26]] Over this period of time, the production

* The study of Doll and Peto is the most thorough and massive of those made to date, and it is heavily drawn from throughout the present analysis. At the time this study was published, Sir Richard Doll was Honorary Director, Imperial Cancer Research Fund, Cancer Epidemiology and Clinical Trials Unit and Warden of Green College, Oxford, United Kingdom, and Mr. Richard Peto was Imperial Cancer Research Fund Reader in Cancer Studies, Nuffield Department of Clinical Medicine, University of Oxford, Radcliffe Infirmary, Oxford, United Kingdom.

This study by Doll and Peto was commissioned by the Office of Technology Assessment, U.S. Congress, to provide background material for their Assessment of "Technologies for Determining Cancer Risks from the Environment" (OTA, 1981).

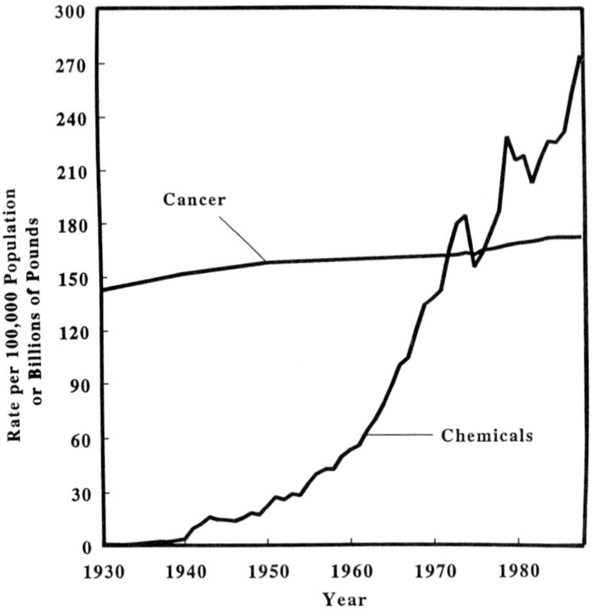

Figure 1.14 Comparison of the Total Cancer Mortality Rate with the Production Rate of Organic Chemicals. [Taken from United States International Trade Commission Synthetic Organic Chemicals. United States Production and Sales, 1930, 1931, . . . , 1988, and *Cancer Facts and Figures–1991*, American Cancer Society, Inc., Atlanta, Georgia (1991). Cancer rates age-adjusted to 1970 population.]

rate of chemicals increased over two hundred fold. Likewise emissions from automobiles and diesel-powered vehicles (which contain some carcinogenic material) have increased enormously, but the total cancer mortality rate has not. Even accounting for a latency period of 15 to 25 years for cancer to develop after exposure, the data do not demonstrate any detectable cancers from the exposures enumerated above.

The history of cancer deaths from 1930 through 1987 is displayed in Figure 1.15 for males and in Figure 1.16 for females.[27] The decrease in stomach, colon, uterus, and ovarian cancer rates is approximately equal to the increase in lung cancer rates. If it were not for lung cancer, the total cancer mortality rate would have declined. These figures demonstrate that there is no epidemic of cancer in the United States except possibly for lung cancer, which is known to be caused primarily from the use of tobacco. The perception that there is a significantly higher cancer rate today than there was in the past results in part from the following reasons. First, because of the discovery of preventions and cures for once fatal infectious diseases, cancer has become a more prevalent cause of death. Also, as illustrated by Figure 1.17, great strides have been made in the treatment of the major cardiovascular diseases.[24,25,28] Since everyone must die of something, the prolonging of life allows time for tumors and cancers to develop with the result that cancer will become

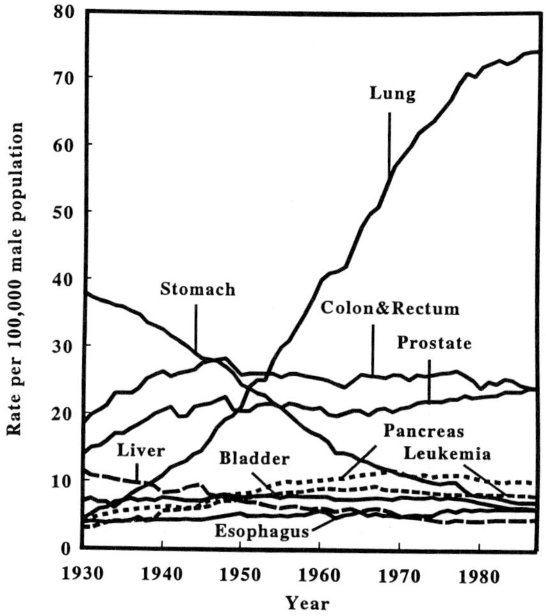

Figure 1.15 Age-adjusted Cancer Death Rates for Selected Sites, Males, United States. [Data taken from *Ca—A Cancer Journal for Clinicians*, **41** (No. 1) 1991, *Cancer Statistics*, 1988, The American Cancer Society, 1991, and U.S. Department of Health and Human Services, National Center for Health Statistics, Hattesville, Maryland, 1988. Cancer rates age-adjusted to the 1970 population.]

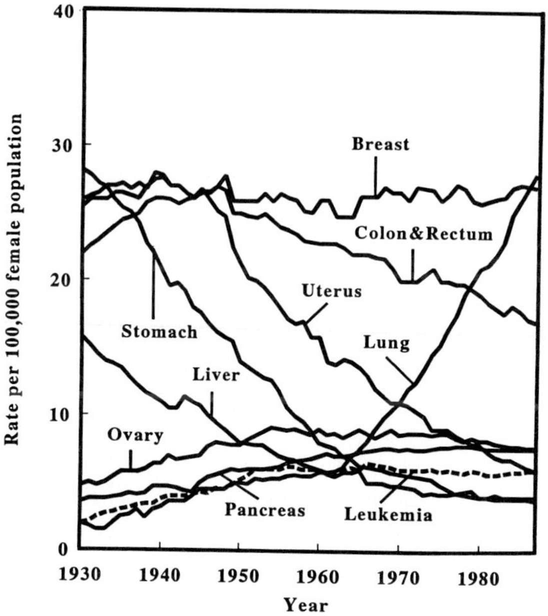

Figure 1.16 Age-adjusted Death Rates for Selected Sites, Females, United States. [Data taken from *Ca—A Cancer Journal for Clinicians*, **41** (No. 1) 1991, *Cancer Statistics*, 1988, The American Cancer Society, 1991, and U.S. Department of Health and Human Services, National Center for Health Statistics, Hattesville, Maryland, 1988. Cancer rates age-adjusted to the 1970 population.]

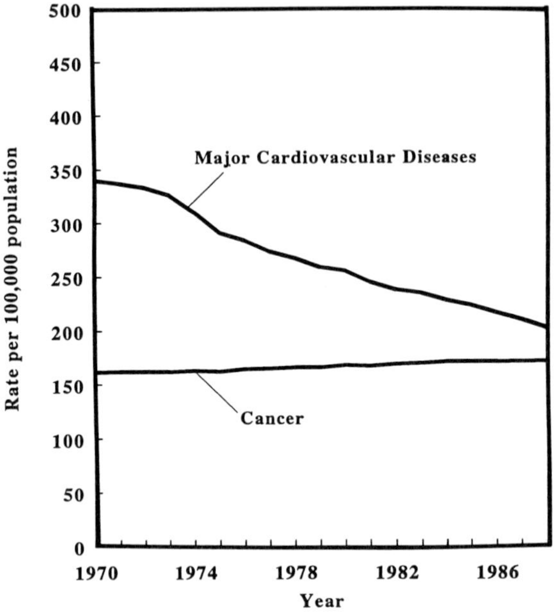

Figure 1.17 Age-adjusted Death Rates for Major Cardiovascular Diseases and Malignant Neoplasms. [Source: *Vital Statistics of United States, Volume II—Mortality, Part A—1985*. U.S. Department of Health and Human Services, National Center for Health Statistics, Hyattsville, Maryland, 1988, and *Cancer Facts and Figures–1991*, American Cancer Society, Inc., Atlanta, Georgia, 1991.]

even more prevalent than it is today as a "disease of old age." Figure 1.18 demonstrates that cancer is a disease of the aged. Our success in the treatment of other diseases has contributed to cancer becoming more and more a disease of the elderly; 60 percent of cancer deaths occur in persons 65 or older, 34 percent in persons 45 to 64, and 6 percent in persons under 45 years of age, according to Schottenfeld.[29] Also, many cancers were not diagnosed in the past, particularly in the elderly, whose deaths were frequently attributed to "natural causes" and "old age." Diagnostic methods have been and are continuing to be improved, leading to the identification and treatment of cancers which would have been missed in the past. Furthermore, people are more open today about the diagnosis of cancer and the subsequent treatments than they were in the past. There was a tendency to keep the diagnosis of cancer a secret and in many instances it was even withheld from the patient.

1.2.2 Leading Causes of Cancer

On the basis of an analysis of data compiled on various types of cancer mortality up until 1980, Doll and Peto[18] deduced the distribution of the causes of cancer mortality shown in Figure 1.19. According to their analysis, diet is the leading cause which accounts for 35 percent of the cancer mortalities. Doll and Peto point out that although the figure of 35 percent is a plausible total, the parts that contribute to it are uncertain in the extreme. The range of acceptable estimates is 10 to 70 percent, as shown in Table 1.3. Use of tobacco is second in the cause of cancer mortalities, and accounts for 30 percent with an acceptable

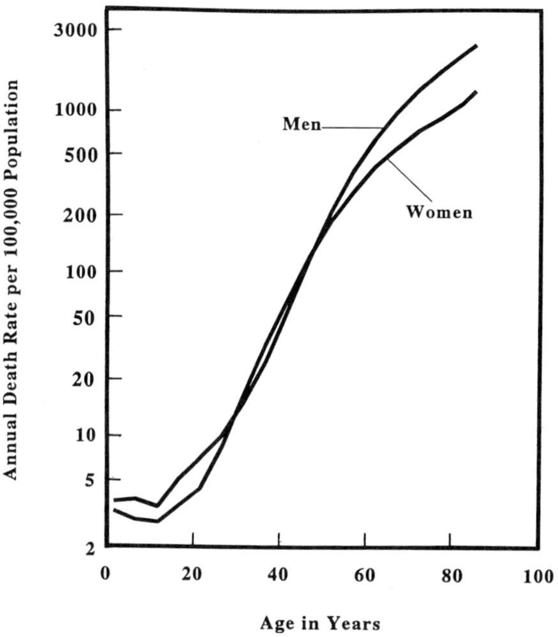

Figure 1.18 Cancer Death Rates by Age and Sex for 1984–1988. [Taken from *Cancer Statistics Review 1973–1988*. Editors, Ries, L.A. G., B.F. Hankey, B.A. Miller, A.M. Hartman, B.K. Edwards, National Cancer Institute, NIH Publication No. 91-2789, 1991.]

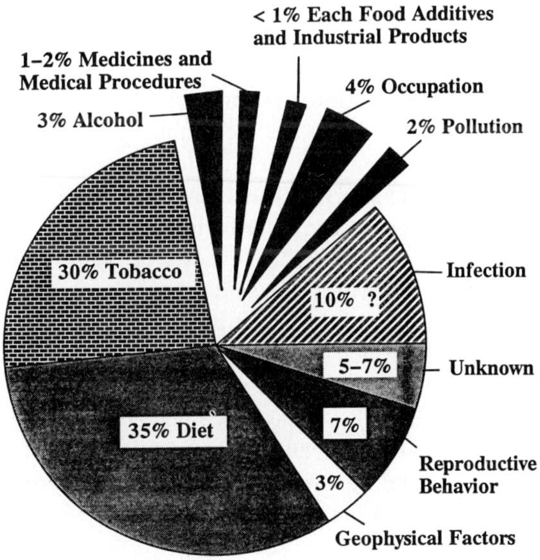

Figure 1.19 Distribution of Cancer Mortalities as Deduced by Doll and Peto. [Taken from Doll, R. and R. Peto, "The Causes of Cancer: Quantitative Estimates of Avoidable Risks of Cancer in the United States Today," *JNCI*, **60**, (No. 6); 1191 (1981).]

Table 1.3 Range of Best Estimate for the Cause of Cancer Shown in Figure 1.6. [Taken from Doll, R. and R. Peto, "The Causes of Cancer: Quantitative Estimates of Avoidable Risks of Cancer in the United States Today," *JNCI*, **66** (No. 6), 1191 (1981).]

	Percent of All Cancer Deaths	
Cause of Cancer	Best Estimate	Range of Acceptable Estimates
Tobacco	30	26 to 40
Alcohol	3	2 to 4
Diet	35	10 to 70
Food Additives	<1	<-5 to 2
Reproductive and Sexual Behavior	7	1 to 13
Occupation	4	2 to 8
Pollution	2	<1 to 5
Industrial Products	<1	<1 to 2
Medicines and Medical Procedures	1	0.5 to 3
Geophysical Factors	3	2 to 4
Infection	10 ?	1 to ?
Unknown	5 to 7*	?*

* The "?" used by Doll and Peto denotes their uncertainty, and it has been replaced by 5 to 7 percent so that the best estimates have a sum of approximately 100 percent.

range of estimates from 25 to 40 percent. A figure of less than 1 percent was attributed to food additives with a range of accepted estimates of -5 to 2 percent. The -5 percent allows for a possible protective effect of antioxidants and other preservatives which may behave as anticarcinogens.

The figure of 4 percent allocated for occupational hazards by Doll and Peto was thought to be accurate by a factor of about two, and thus the acceptable range of estimates was given as 2 to 8 percent. A token figure of 2 percent was assigned to pollution, due chiefly to the uncertain effect of the combustion products of fossil fuels in urban air. Because of the uncertainties involved in attempting to account for the effects of pollution, the best estimate for the distribution of industrial hazards of 4 percent is shown in Figure 1.20. The acceptable range of estimates of less than 1 to 5 percent was said to be rather arbitrary.

Although there is no cause for alarm from trends in cancer incidence, many industrial products have been so recently introduced that their effects would not yet be apparent. Even though less than 1 percent was attributed to cancer mortality caused by industrial products with a range of acceptable estimates of less than 1 to 2 percent, Doll and Peto cautioned that there is too much ignorance for complacency to be justified. The figure of 1 to 2 percent for medicines and medical procedures has a range of acceptable estimates of 0.5 to 3 percent. Geophysical factors such as radiation may account for about 3 percent with a range of acceptable estimates of 2 to 4 percent.

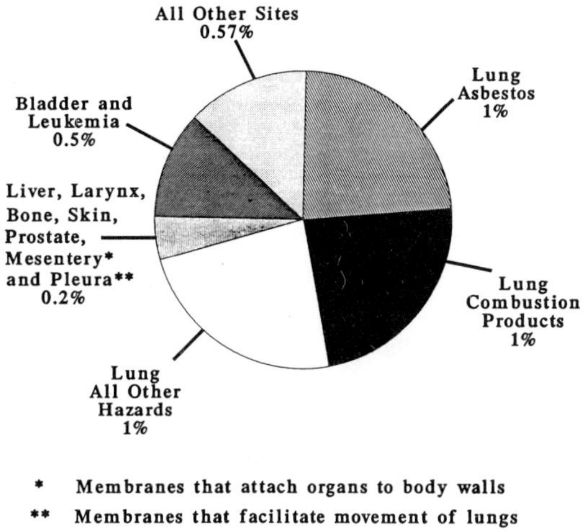

Figure 1.20 Distribution and Types of the 4 Percent Occupational Cancer Mortalities Estimated by Doll and Peto. [Taken from Doll, R. and R. Peto, "The Causes of Cancer: Quantitative Estimate of Avoidable Risks of Cancer in the United States Today," *JNCI*, **60**, (No. 6); 1191 (1981).]

The best estimate of 10 percent for cancer caused by infections contains a lot of uncertainty, and only the lower number of 1 percent was given for the range of acceptable estimates. In the case of unknown causes, Doll and Peto gave no numbers, and the number shown in Figure 1.19 was obtained by difference. Doll and Peto point out that the firmest estimates in Figure 1.19 are those for tobacco, alcohol, and geophysical factors. Tobacco and diet are seen to be by far the largest contributors to cancer mortality.

The estimates of Doll and Peto are supported by the fact that similar studies have been carried out by others and there is general agreement, although not exact, between the various studies. Those by Higginson and Muir[20] and Wynder and Gori[22] are shown in Table 1.4. Higginson and Muir refer to "lifestyle" rather than diet, meaning factors such as lack of dietary fiber, caloric intake, excess fat, and possibly hormone carcinogenesis.

The classifications used by Doll and Peto and others are quite general, and further classifications will be added as more is learned about the causes of cancer. For example, in a recent paper by zur Hausen,[30] approximately 15 percent of worldwide incidence of cancer is attributed to viruses, and with the outbreak of AIDS this figure can be expected to increase. Cancers caused by viral infections are included as contributions under other headings in Table 1.3, such as Reproductive and Sexual Behavior, Infection, and Unknown.

Hormones are another cause of cancer which is not listed as a separate classification in Table 1.3. According to a survey of the recent literature by Henderson et al.,[31] hormones were associated with almost one-third of the new cancer cases in 1990. Endometrial cancer and breast cancer are caused by the cumulative exposure to estrogen in the absence of progestogens. Also, ovarian cancer is related to ovulation, which is in turn related to

Table 1.4 Causes of Cancer as Deduced by Higginson and Muir and by Wynder and Gori. [Taken from Higginson, J., and C.S. Muir, "Environmental Carcinogenesis: Misconceptions and Limitations to Cancer Control," *JNCI*, **63**, 1291 (1979), and Wynder, E.L. and G.B. Gori, "Contributions of the Environment to Cancer Incidence. An Epidemiologic Exercise," *JNCI*, **58**, 825 (1977).]

Cause	Birmingham Region England Cancer Mortality in % Higginson and Muir[22]		United States Cancer Mortality in % Wynder and Gori[20]	
	Male	Female	Male	Female
Tobacco	30	7	28	8
Tobacco/alcohol	5	3	4	1
Diet			40	57
Lifestyle	30	63		
Occupation	6	2	4	2
Sunlight and Ionizing radiations	11	11	8	8
Iatrogenic	1	1		
Exogenous (external) hormones				4
Congenital (present at birth) and unknown	17	13	16	20

complex hormonal changes. Prostate cancer is thought to be related to the cumulative exposure to testosterone and perhaps estrogen.

1.3 IDENTIFICATION OF HUMAN CARCINOGENS

From the standpoint of the public, the definition of a *carcinogen* is taken to mean any substance which causes cancer in humans. Since substances which cause cancer in animals do not necessarily cause cancer in humans, carcinogens should be classified into two subgroups: *human carcinogens* and *animal carcinogens*, and further subdivided into mouse, rat, etc. Confusion in the general public exists because only the single designation, carcinogens, is used for both humans and animals.

Identification of human carcinogens has been through clinical observations of small populations with confirmation by epidemiological studies rather than experimental investigations of potential cancer causing substances. Epidemiological studies are studies of human populations in which the disease outcomes are examined. The populations may be defined in a variety of ways such as industrial cohorts and specific groups as discussed in a subsequent section on epidemiological studies. Case-control studies begin not with an experimental investigation of all possible pollutants in a given city which might have caused cancer deaths, but with all of the deaths which have occurred in the city over a

Table 1.5 Human Carcinogens—Industrial Processes and Chemicals. [Taken from IARC Monographs on the Evaluation of the Carcinogenic Risk of Chemicals to Humans, Supplement 7 (1987) and Volumes 43, 44, 1988; 45, 47, 1989; 49, 50, 1990; 54, 55, 1992.]

	Degree of evidence for carcinogenicity*	
1. Industrial Processes and Occupational Exposures	Human	Animal
Aluminum production	S	—
Auramine manufacture	S	—
Coal gasification	S	—
Coke production	S	—
Hematite underground mining with exposure to radon	S	—
Iron and steel founding	S	—
Isopropyl alcohol manufacture (strong-acid process)	S	—
Leather boot and shoe manufacture and repair	S	—
Magenta manufacture	S	—
Painter	S	—
Rubber industry	S	I
Strong-inorganic-acid mists containing sulfuric acid	S	—
Wood furniture and cabinet making	S	I

given period of time, and tries to determine the major causes of these actual deaths. By use of an analysis of death certificates, case histories and personal interviews, they attempt to establish the major cause of each death and the exposure and life style of the decedent.

This approach consisting of clinical observations followed by epidemiological confirmations has led to the discovery of most if not all of the presently known human carcinogens. Of the more than 600 chemicals and chemical mixtures evaluated by the International Agency for Research on Cancer (IARC) expert working groups, 44 chemicals and 13 processes have been associated with cancer in humans.[32] A tabulation of the industrial processes, chemicals, and groups of chemicals presently classified as human carcinogens is presented in Table 1.5. The evidence, both human and animal, supporting the classification of a substance as a human carcinogen is also presented in Table 1.5. Observe, however, that every entry classified as a human carcinogen is supported by sufficient human evidence and denoted by *S* under the heading *Human*. Human evidence is said by IARC to be sufficient evidence of carcinogenicity if it indicates that there is a causal relationship between the exposure and human cancer. Supporting evidence of the classification as a human carcinogen is provided by the results of studies of carcinogenicity in experimental animals and short-term tests. The ranking of the degree of this evidence is presented under the heading *Animal* in Table 1.5 and the ranking procedure is described in the Preamble to Supplement 7.[32]

In addition to the list of substances classified as human carcinogens by IARC, lists of substances classified as human carcinogens have also been issued by the Occupational Safety and Health Administration (OSHA), the Environmental Protection Agency (EPA), the National Toxicology Program (NTP), and the American Conference of Governmental

Table 1.5 (cont'd) Human Carcinogens—Industrial Processes and Chemicals. [Taken from IARC Monographs on the Evaluation of the Carcinogenic Risk of Chemicals to Humans, Supplement 7 (1987) and Volumes 43, 44, 1988; 45, 47, 1989; 49, 50, 1990; 54, 55, 1992.]

2. Chemicals and Groups of Chemicals	Degree of evidence for carcinogenicity* Human	Animal
Aflatoxins	S	S
Alcoholic beverages	S	I
4-Aminobiphenyl	S	S
Arsenic and arsenic compounds**	S	L
Asbestos	S	S
Azathioprine	S	L
Benzene	S	S
Benzidine	S	S
Betel quid with tobacco	S	L
N, N-Bis (2-chloroethyl)-2-naphthylamine (Chlornaphazine)	S	L
Bis (chloromethyl) ether and chloromethyl methyl ether (technical Grade)	S	S
1-4 Butanediol dimethanesulphonate (Myleran)	S	L
Chlorambucil	S	S
1-(2-Chloroethyl)-3-(4-methylcyclohexyl)-1-nitrosourea (Methyl-CCNU)	S	L
Hexavalent chromium compounds	S	S
Ciclosporin (Cyclosporin A)	S	S
Coal-tar pitches	S	S
Coal-tars	S	S
Cyclophosphamide	S	S
Erionite	S	S
Melphalan	S	S
8-Methoxypsoralen (Methoxsalen) plus ultraviolet radiation	S	S
Mineral oils, untreated and mildly treated oils	S	S
MOPP and other combined chemotherapy including alkylating agents	S	I
Mustard gas (sulphur mustard)	S	L
2-Naphthylamine	S	S
Nickel compounds	S	S
Nonsteroidal estrogens	S	—
Diethylstilbestrol	S	S
Steroidal estrogens	S	—
Estrogen replacement therapy	S	—
Sequential oral contraceptives	S	—
Combined oral contraceptives	S	—
Phenacetin analgesic mixtures	S	L
Shale-oils	S	S
Solar radiation	S	S
Soots	S	I
Talc containing asbestiform fibers	S	I
Tobacco products, smokeless	S	I
Tobacco smoke	S	S
Treosulphan	S	ND
Tris (1-aziridinyl) phosphine sulfide (Thiotepa)	S	S
Vinyl chloride	S	S

* I = inadequate evidence; L = limited evidence; ND = no adequate data; S = sufficient evidence; – = no information.

** This evaluation applies to the group of chemicals as a whole and not necessarily to all chemicals within the group.

Industrial Hygienists (ACGIH). There are differences in the criteria for evidences of carcinogenicity of a chemical, chemical mixture, or process used by the organizations as well as differences in the substances listed as human carcinogens.

In an evaluation of the relevance of the above human carcinogens to the chemical industry, Doll[33] recently pointed out that only 13 are of direct concern to the chemical industry. The remaining agents consist of medicines, fossil fuels and their combustion products, unidentified chemicals in certain manufacturing processes or trades, and materials in the natural environment or tobacco smoke and alcohol.

The above listing of the chemicals classified by IARC as human carcinogens in Table 1.5 tends to perhaps overemphasize the role of chemicals in the formation of human cancers. According to Henderson et al.[31] we are now in the threshold of an era when most of the prevalent human cancers can, to a significant extent, be prevented by lifestyle changes or medical intervention. In a reaffirmation of the Doll and Peto study, Henderson et al.[31] state that occupational exposures to specific carcinogenic agents are not likely to account for more than 4 percent of the cancers in the United States. Asbestos is the most important known occupational carcinogen and it seems to have passed its peak in the 1980s.

1.3.1 Animal Tests and Associated Problems

In order to avoid the possibility of introduction of chemicals into the environment which would cause cancer, an extensive effort has been under way to develop a laboratory test which would predict the carcinogenicity of a substance in humans. However, the best test to date consists of using animals as a surrogate for humans.

Although animal tests are used for the determination of the carcinogenicity of chemicals, this approach is fraught with difficulties because of the different responses exhibited by animals to chemicals. Responses may differ not only from one animal species to another, but from male to female of the same species, and also from animals to humans. For example, mice get cancer from perchloroethylene, but rats, rabbits, guinea pigs and monkeys do not.[34] Rats and humans develop cancer from Aflatoxin B_1, but mice and monkeys are relatively resistant[35] as described in Figure 1.21. Humans and dogs get cancer from β-naphthylamine, but most strains of rats[36] and hamsters do not.[37] Thus, the extrapolation of the results of tests made on animals to humans always has uncertainties. Just because a chemical is an animal carcinogen does not prove that it is a human carcinogen.

To further complicate the picture and add to the confusion is the fact that a given carcinogen can affect entirely different organs in different mammalian species. For example, benzidine is said to cause bladder tumors in man, liver tumors in the hamster, and acoustic tumors in the rat, while estrogen is reported to cause breast tumors in mice, uterine and abdominal tumors in the guinea pig, and kidney tumors in the hamster.[38]

Also, arguments have persisted in scientific circles concerning the number of animal species which are needed for a reliable extrapolation to humans. Some say three, others say two, and some including OSHA say one positive test in one animal species is sufficient to label a substance as a potential human carcinogen.

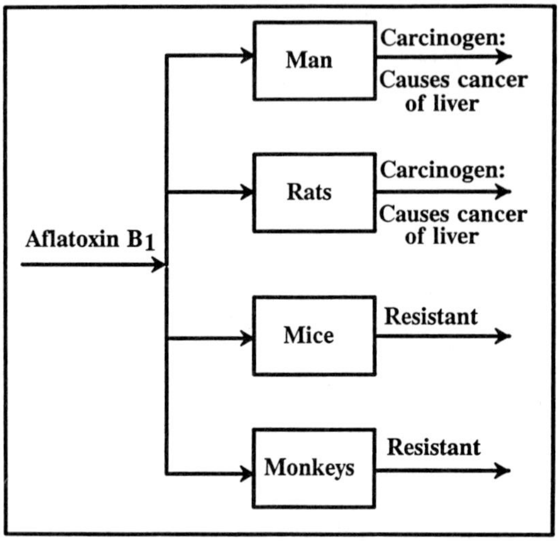

Figure 1.21 Aflatoxin B_1, a Natural Carcinogen Found in Grains and Peanuts, has a Different Effect on Different Animal Species.

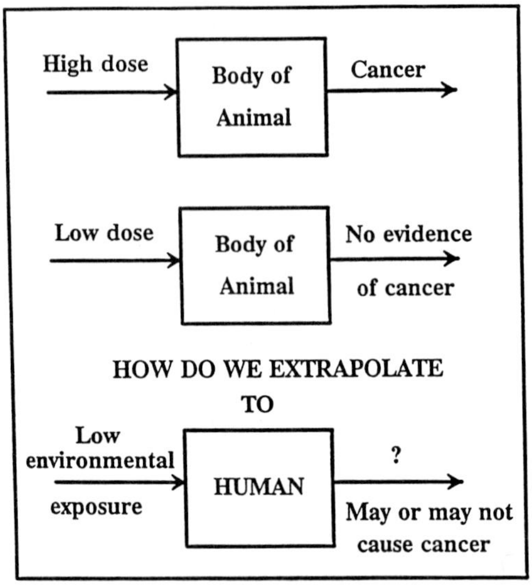

Figure 1.22 The Problem of Extrapolating from High Animal Doses to Low Human Exposures.

1.3.2 Problems in Extrapolation from High-Dose Animal Tests to Low-Level Human Exposure

Human exposure to chemicals ordinarily occurs at low-dose levels. For animal tests at these correspondingly low levels of exposure to be meaningful, a prohibitively large number (millions) of animals would be required. The alternative of obtaining a significant number of tumors in a relatively small population by use of high doses has become standard procedure in animal tests. However, this approach leads to further difficulties because many chemicals are carcinogenic at high doses but not at low doses. These difficulties are illustrated graphically in Figure 1.22.

Because of the above considerations and the observation that high dose tests tend to increase cell division which in turn promotes tumor formation, Ames and Gold[12] recommended rethinking the utility and meaning of routine animal tests. Their article was concluded with the statement that "the most important contribution that animal studies can offer is an insight into carcinogenesis mechanisms and into the complex natural world in which we live."

On the other hand, Perera,[13] Rall[14] and Weinstein[15] argue that animal tests represent the best method for evaluating the carcinogenicity of new chemicals being introduced into the public domain. At best, animal tests constitute a holding action until research provides a better understanding of the causes of the various types of cancer at the molecular level.

1.3.3 Epidemiological Studies

A number of epidemiological studies have been made and are continuing to be made both inside and outside of the chemical industry. Inside the industry, many studies have been made involving large groups of people over periods of 20 or more years, and the general finding is that their workers enjoy better health, live longer, and have fewer cancers than the general population. This finding is so frequent that it is referred to as the *healthy worker effect*, and can be attributed to several factors. The conditions for employment require that people entering the work force be in good health. The nature of the employment requires that people establish a healthier lifestyle (a regular routine for work, rest, and meals) than is followed by the general public. Workers also receive better medical care than does the general public. The healthy worker effect is the most prevalent result of the extensive industrial studies, but within any given study there could be an occasional small group of workers with a higher cancer mortality rate than that of the general public. The Texas Chemical Council[39,40] recently reported the results of a study involving 133, 000 chemical plant and refinery workers from six major companies. These employees were followed for 20 years or more over their lifetime, and it was found that they experienced 21 percent fewer cancer mortalities than the general public.[39,40]

Of the many studies that have been performed by professionals outside the chemical industry, only one is described. This particular study, called the *TEAM study,* was selected for presentation because it is suggestive of ways that people can improve their own personal safety. The TEAM study, described by Ember,[41] was an intensive five-year exposure study performed by the EPA, and the results were reported in 1985. The scientists concluded that, contrary to popular belief, people living in heavily industrialized areas containing petrochemical, paint and plastic processing plants are not subjected to greater exposures to the commonly identified toxic chemicals than are people living in less industrialized, or even in rural areas. This conclusion was based on studying 355 people in the highly industrialized cities of Bayonne and Elizabeth, New Jersey, 25 people in the urban city of Greensboro, North Carolina, and another 25 people in rural Devils Lake, North Dakota.

A further significant finding was that people are exposed to far greater concentrations of toxic chemicals indoors than they are outdoors, even in those cities where plants that manufacture or use these chemicals are located. This finding has also been confirmed by European studies. By use of both indoor and outdoor monitoring systems, the EPA investigators found indoor levels to be two to five times greater than outdoor levels for the commonly identified toxic chemicals. At highest exposures, the indoor levels were up to 70 times greater than outdoor levels.

Since people spend up to 95 percent of their time indoors where the pollution levels of toxic chemicals are far higher than they are outdoors, one comes to the obvious conclusion that our present method of basing exposure estimates on fixed-station monitors located outdoors does not accurately reflect the total human exposure.

1.4 TRENDS IN CANCER MORTALITIES AND SURVIVAL RATES

A summary of the trends in mortality for various types of cancers over the past 30 years was recently published by the American Cancer Society.[24] The changes in the number of mortalities recorded for the various types of cancers over the 30-year period from 1955 through 1987 are shown for males and females in Table 1.6. The corresponding mortalities for each type of cancer in 1991 are also shown in this table.

Overall, the mortality for all sites has increased by 21 percent for males while remaining essentially constant for females. As shown in this table, lung cancer mortalities for both males and females not only increased at the highest rates but also accounted for the largest number of cancer mortalities in 1991. Other major contributors to the cancer mortalities were colorectal cancers,

To reflect the progress in the diagnosis and treatment of the various types of cancer, the corresponding relative 5-year survival rates are given in Table 1.7. Although the relative 5-year survival rates for colon and colorectal cancers have improved since 1960, the rates for lung cancer have not. However, the survival rate for whites for all sites has increased from 39 percent for 1960–1963 to 52 percent for 1981–1986.

1.5 CANCER INCIDENCES AND CAUSES

The percentage of the total of 1,040,000 new cancer cases in 1990 attributed to the major cancer sites are listed in Table 1.8. This table is based on one prepared by Henderson et al.[31] The causes of the various types of cancer shown in this table were deduced by Henderson et al.[31] on the basis of what they regarded as sufficient and consistent evidence. The total number of incidences is generally about twice the total number of mortalities for a given year; see for example Table 1.6 of this chapter and Table I-1 of Reference 25.

Henderson et al.[31] concluded that we now have sufficient knowledge for the prevention of a significant proportion of human cancer. As shown in Table 1.7, the majority of the causes of cancer, such as tobacco, alcohol, animal fat, obesity, and ultraviolet light are associated with the personal choices of lifestyle and not with the environment. Henderson et al.[31] also pointed out that the widespread public perception that environmental pollution is a major cancer hazard is incorrect.

1.5.1 The Controversy Over the Interpretation of Cancer Data

Although the number of mortalities attributed to brain cancer amounted to only 2 percent of the total cancer mortalities in 1991, a controversy has arisen over the cause of the increase in these cancers over the past 15 years in people 65 years of age and older (see Table 1.11 of Problem 4). According to Marshall,[42] this controversy involves the interpretation of the cancer data and not the data itself.

Although according to the U.S. census,[26] there has been an increase in the number of people 65 and over since 1950 as shown in Table 1.9, it does not necessarily follow that an increase in the mortality rate from brain cancer for people 65 and over should be expected.

Table 1.6 Percent Changes in Age-Adjusted Cancer Death Rates for Males and Females Over the 30-Year Period 1955–57 to 1985–87. [Taken from *Cancer Facts and Figures—1991*, American Cancer Society, Inc., Atlanta, Georgia (1991).]

Site	Changes in Percent 1955–1957 to 1985–1987	Estimated Deaths 1991	Site	Changes in Percent 1955–1957 to 1985–1987	Estimated Deaths 1991
All sites			Cervix		
Male	+21	272,000	Female	-70	4,500
Female	*	242,000	Other Uterus		
Lung			Female	-50	5,500
Male	+131	92,000	Brain		
Female	+420	51,000	Male	+21	6,200
Colon			Female	+24	5,300
Male	+19	26,000	Kidney		
Female	-18	27,000	Male	+37	6,300
Rectum			Female	+18	4,300
Male	-58	4,000	Bladder		
Female	-37	3,500	Male	-20	6,400
Breast			Female	-43	3,100
Male	-11	300	Multiple Myeloma		
Female	*	44,500	Male	+100	4,600
Prostate			Female	+97	4,500
Male	+10	32,000	Melanoma		
Non-Hodgkin's			Male	+132	3,775
Lymphoma			Female	+45	2,725
Male	+53	9,600	Other Skin		
Female	+59	9,100	Male	-26	1,625
Leukemia			Female	-66	375
Male	*	9,800	Esophagus		
Female	-12	8,300	Male	+20	7,300
Stomach			Female	+22	2,500
Male	-63	8,100	Oral		
Female	-68	5,300	Male	-22	5,275
Pancreas			Female	+18	2,875
Male	*	12,000	Larynx		
Female	+18	13,200	Male	*	2,900
Ovary			Female	+150	750
Female	-10	12,500	Hodgkin's Disease		
Liver			Male	-66	1,000
Male	-18	6,300	Female	-63	600
Female	-49	5,800			

* Percent changes not listed because they are not meaningful.

The mortality rate is defined as the number of deaths due to a given type of cancer in a given age group divided by the total number of people in that age group. Thus, if over a given period of time, the proportional increase in the number of deaths from a given type of

Table 1.7 Trend in Relative 5-year Survival Rates for Cases Diagnosed in 1960-1963 and 1981-1986. [Taken from *Cancer Facts and Figures–1991*. American Chemical Society, Inc., Atlanta, Georgia (1991).]

	White Relative 5-Year Survival		Black Relative 5-Year Survival	
Site	1960–1963	1981–1986	1960–1963	1981–1986
All Sites	39%	52%	27%	38%
Lung & Bronchus	8	13	5	11
Colon	43	57	34	48
Rectum	38	54	27	41
Breast (female)	63	78	46	64
Prostate Gland	50	75	35	62
Non-Hodgkin's Lymphoma	31	51	–	45
Leukemia	14	36	–	29
Stomach	11	16	8	18
Pancreas	1	3	1	4
Ovary	32	39	32	38
Liver	2	5	–	4
Cervix Uteri	58	67	47	57
Corpus Uteri	73	84	31	55
Brain & Nervous System	18	24	19	32
Kidney & Renal Pelvis	37	53	38	51
Urinary	53	79	24	59
Multiple Myeloma	12	26	–	28
Melanoma of Skin	60	81	–	65
Larynx	53	69	–	52
Hodgkin's Disease	40	76	–	74
Thyroid Gland	83	94	–	96
Testis	63	92	–	92

cancer for people in a given age group is equal to the proportional increase in the number of people in the given age group, the cancer rate remains constant for that age group (see Problems 1, 2, and Appendix I).

However, the composition of the group of people 65 and older is constantly changing. Many of the members of this group have had life extended because they have avoided death from infectious diseases, cardiovascular diseases (heart attacks and strokes), changes in lifestyle, or because of cancer treatments as reflected by the increases in the 5-year survival rates. This change in the composition of the group of people 65 and over has quite probably contributed to the increased mortality rate due to brain cancer.

The determination of whether the increase in the brain cancer mortality rate for people 65 and over can be accounted for on the basis of the factors enumerated above or whether

Table 1.8 Estimated New Cancer Cases in the U.S. in 1990 by Site and Major Cause [Taken from Henderson, B.E., R .K. Ross, and M.C. Pike, "Toward the Primary Prevention of Cancer," *Science*, 254, 1131 (1991)]

Cancer Site	Percentage (Based on 1,040,000 Cases)	Major Cause or Causes Known or Probable	Possible
Lung	15	Tobacco	
Colon and rectum	15	Animal Fat, low fiber	Alcohol, sedentary life-style
Breast	15	Ovarian Hormones	
Prostate	10	Testosterone	Estrogen
Bladder	5	Tobacco	
Non-Hodgkin's lymphoma	3	(HIV,HTLV-I)†	
Uterus (endometrium)	3	Estrogen	
Oral cavity and pharynx	3	Tobacco, alcohol	
Pancreas	3	Tobacco	
Leukemia	3	X-rays	
Melanoma	3	Ultraviolet light (sunburning)	
Kidney	2	Tobacco	Analgesics, diuretics
Stomach	2	Salt, tobacco	*Helicobacter pylori*
Ovary	2	Ovulation	
Brain and other nervous system	2	Trauma, X-rays‡	
Cervix	1		Papillomaviruses
Liver	1	Hepatitis viruses, alcohol	Tobacco§
Larynx	1	Tobacco, alcohol	
Thyroid	1		Iodine excess
Multiple myeloma	1		
Esophagus	1	Alcohol, tobacco	
Hodgkin's disease	<1		
Testis	<1		In utero estrogen
All other sites¶	7	Multiple factors	
Total	100		

† Although HIV is an increasingly important cause of non-Hodgkin's lymphoma, it nonetheless currently accounts for only a small proportion of cases. HTLV-1 refers to human T cell lymphotrophic virus.

‡ Trauma and X-rays are causes of meningiomas and acoustic neuromas, which constitute about 35% of all brain and other nervous system tumors. The cause or causes of the other types of brain tumors, mainly gliomas, are unknown.

§ Aflatoxin contamination of nuts and grains may constitute a major cause of liver cancer worldwide but it is unimportant in the United States.

¶ The number of new cases of Kaposi's sarcoma has been increasing as a sequel of HIV infection. These nonepithelial cancers of the skin were not separately estimated in this report. However, the actual number of cases in 1990 may exceed the number of testis cancer cases. References are given for these statements by Henderson et al.

Table 1.9 Increase in the Percentage of People 65 and Older from 1950 through 1990 [Taken from *Census of the Population*, Volume I: Characteristics of the Population, Part I, United States Summary, United States Department of Commerce, Bureau of the Census (1950, 1960, 1970, 1980).]

Year	Total Population	65 and Over	Percentage of People 65 and Older
1950	$150.697,361 \times 10^6$	$12.269,537 \times 10^6$	8.14
1960	$179.979,462 \times 10^6$	$16.675,141 \times 10^6$	9.27
1970	$203.211,926 \times 10^6$	$20.065,502 \times 10^6$	10.11
1980	$226.245,805 \times 10^6$	$25.549,427 \times 10^6$	11.29
1990	$248.709,873 \times 10^6$	$31.241,831 \times 10^6$	12.56

there are some other factors that have been introduced into our lifestyle over the past 15 to 25 years must await further study and perhaps additional data.

The postponement of death because of all of the factors listed above and perhaps others has contributed to an increase in life expectancy. As pointed out by Cole,[43] the increase in life expectancy during the first half of the 20th century resulted from the reduction of infant mortality. During the last half of the 20th century, the increase in the life expectancy resulted from the postponement of death in the adult population.

1.6 ADVANCES IN CANCER RESEARCH AND TREATMENTS

To provide an insight into the forefront of the general field of cancer research, selected articles are reviewed for the purpose of providing a sense of direction that the research is taking. The articles reviewed were selected from a vast volume of literature, not necessarily because of their importance in the field, but because they were regarded as good examples of the type and direction of research efforts at the present time.

The search for the causes and cures of cancer has been a major motivating force for the understanding of cellular behavior at the molecular level. Over the past decade and a half, the field of molecular epidemiology has been growing at an increasing pace. The knowledge gained from this research is now being applied in the associated areas of:

1. cancer therapies,
2. testing for individual risks for selected types of cancer, and
3. cancer prevention or *chemoprevention*.

1.6.1 The Genome Project

A new program which is in its beginning is the *genome project*. The objective of this project is the mapping of the 100,000 or so genes of the human *genome* (the complete gene complement). The mapping of the human genome is an enormous task. Charles R. Cantor (a principal scientist in DOE's genome program) has been credited with the statement that just to write down the sequence of the human genome would fill 200 telephone directories.[44] When completed it will help scientists diagnose and ultimately treat hundreds of diseases caused by genetic defects. The genome mapping project could eventually provide a person with a list of all diseases or ailments imprinted in his or her genes. Many experts think that this knowledge will revolutionize how Americans pay for their medical care.

1.6.2 Genes and Associated Cancers

Research in the molecular level has implicated two types of genes in cancer formation, *oncogenes* and *tumor suppressor genes*.[45] The past decade saw a significant research effort at the molecular level in the identification of oncogenes associated with various types of cancer, and Weinberg[46] predicts that the next decade will see a shift of the research effort to the investigation of the role of suppressor genes in cancer formation. It is now generally believed that oncogenes are formed from certain cellular genes called *proto-oncogenes* by a variety of molecular events including point mutations and small insertions and deletions as well as juxtaposition to other chromosome sequences.[45]

Tumor suppressor genes, like proto-oncogenes are normal cellular genes. However, they contribute to cancer formation through their loss rather than their activation.[45] Although these two mechanisms are quite different physiologically, there is accumulating evidence which suggests that the progression of any tumors to full malignancy requires both types of changes in the tumor cell genome.[46]

The identification of defective or mutated genes associated with different types of cancer has been and continues to be a major research effort. The discovery of these genes should aid in screening of individuals for cancer risks as well as early detection of cancer and its treatment. To demonstrate the rapid pace at which these discoveries are being made, a few of the most recent findings are presented.

In the case of both *sporadic colorectal cancer* as well as *familial adenomatous polyposis* (FAP), a suppressor gene* of the 5q21 chromosome region appears to be involved in the early stages of both of these types of cancer as reported by Kinzler et al.[47] FAP is an inherited disease in which affected individuals develop hundreds to thousands of polyps

---

* The nomenclature of genes used in this section is complicated and an explanation of it is beyond the scope of this book. For a treatment of this topic; see for example, *Oncogenes* by Geoffrey M. Cooper, Jones and Bartlett Publishers, Boston, Massachusetts (1990), and *Cancer: Principles and Practice of Oncology*, Vincent de Vita, Samuel Hellman, Steven Rosenberg, Editors, J. B. Lippincott Company, Philadelphia, Pennsylvania (1989).

in the colon, and some of these can progress to malignancy. In the case of breast cancer, Hall et al.[48] recently reported that chromosome 17q21 appears to be the locale of a gene associated with the inherited susceptibility to breast cancers in families that carry this gene.

In another recent study, Malkin et al.[49] associated germ line p53 with the dominantly inherited *Li-Faumeni syndrome* (LFS). Included in this syndrome are a wide variety of cancers, such as breast carcinomas, soft tissue carcinomas, brain tumors, osteosarcoma, leukemia, and adrenocortical carcinoma. Family members characteristically develop these cancers at early ages and multiple primary tumors are frequent. Other publications in 1990 in this same general area were recently reviewed by Wright.[50]

The involvement of the tumor suppressor gene p53 in the formation of diverse human cancers [lung, breast, colon, esophagus, liver, bladder, ovary, sarcoma, brain, lymphomas and leukemias] was examined by Hollstein et al.[51] by a review of 280 reported base substitution mutations of the p53 gene. Ninety-eight percent of these mutations examined in the review fell within a 600 base-pair region of the p53 gene [codons 110 to 307]. As suggested by the authors, the differences in the mutations can lead to a better understanding of the exogenous and endogenous factors involved in human carcinogenesis.

Scientists have long known that every cell having a nucleus decorates its surface with bits of all of the different types of proteins that it is making. These peptides are held at the surface by a *Class I major histocompatibility complex* (MHC) protein. This phenomenon is known as *antigen presentation*. These fragments of proteins are recognized by the *killer T cells* of the immune system. If the peptides presented are foreign to the particular cell such as viral proteins, the T cells kill the infected cells. Scientists have been searching for years for the process by which the protein fragments are transported from the interior of the cell, where they are made in the chromosomal region, to the surface. Barinaga[52] recently described the research results presented in four papers which may provide the answer. It appears that *transporter proteins* are responsible for transporting the protein fragments. Candidates for the transporter proteins have been discovered and confirmation experiments are in progress.[52]

1.6.3 Recombinant DNA Technology

Recombinant DNA technology was initiated by experiments performed in 1973 by A. Chang and S. Cohen.[4] By the late 1970s, the technologies that made recombinant DNA possible had been developed. These technologies permit the insertion of a set of new genetic instructions in living cells. The key breakthrough consisted of the discovery of several enzymes which can be used to cut and join DNA molecules in a test tube. These enzymes are called *restriction endonucleases*. More than 100 of these restrictive enzymes have been discovered.[2] To illustrate the action of these enzymes, consider the restrictive enzyme *Eco*RI which recognizes the double-stranded six-nucleotide sequence,

$$\begin{array}{c} \downarrow \qquad\qquad\qquad\qquad \\ \cdots - G - A - A - T - T - C - \cdots \\ \cdots - C - T - T - A - A - G - \cdots \\ \qquad\qquad\qquad\qquad\quad \uparrow \end{array}$$

The cleavage points are denoted by the arrows. In the presence of *Eco*RI, separation of the DNA strands occurs at these cleavage points to give the following fragments.

$$\begin{array}{ll} \cdots - G & \qquad\qquad A - A - T - T - C - \cdots \\ \cdots - C - T - T - A - A & \qquad\qquad\qquad\qquad\qquad\; G - \cdots \end{array}$$

Techniques have been developed for inserting these fragments, called *restrictive sites*, into foreign DNA which has also been fragmented by the restrictive enzyme *Eco*RI.

The problem with the restrictive enzymes is that they cut the larger DNA molecules into too many fragments. Roberts[53] recently reported that Koob and Szybalski have described a procedure for cutting the DNA into fragments of more manageable sizes.

The techniques described above may be used to clone a segment of DNA referred to as *foreign DNA*. Through the use of these techniques, the foreign DNA segments may be joined in a test tube to certain bacterial DNAs, called *plasmids*. These plasmids containing the foreign DNA segments are referred to as *recombinant plasmids* or *recombinant DNA*. The recombinant DNA is then introduced into a bacterial cell which in turn reproduces a colony of genetically identical cells containing the foreign DNA segments of interest. These identical cells are called *clones*, and the process by which they were produced is called *cloning*.

1.6.4 Recent RNA and DNA Discoveries and Developments

In 1982, Thomas Ceck of the University of Colorado discovered that RNA could act as an enzyme. Up until that time, it was thought that only proteins could act as enzymes.[54] Ceck has more recently observed that *preribosomal RNA* (also know as *ribozymes*) can cut and splice itself, thereby removing sequences not needed in the biological function.[54] This discovery was complemented by the finding of Sidney Altman of Yale who showed that the transfer RNA could be cut by another separate piece of RNA and a protein. Furthermore, this process could be repeated over and over in a manner analogous to the participation of an enzyme or a catalyst in a chemical reaction.[54] The potential applications of these results could enable scientists to manipulate RNA in the same manner that they have learned to manipulate DNA. This technique has the potential of being used to snip the RNA of threatening viruses, bacteria, and fungi that cause diseases in humans and crops. RNA is at the heart of all viral diseases in man. Thus, the potential applications include therapies for almost all of the viral diseases.

Further elucidation of RNA editing, provided by a number of researchers, has been described by Hoffman.[55] These researchers have deduced from the results of recent research that the information needed for messenger RNA editing comes from the DNA in the minicircles of the mitochondria located inside the cell but outside the nucleus.

According to Moffat,[56] the most recently reported gene cutter is the *triple-stranded DNA* which was first produced in 1957 by David Davis and Gary Felsenfeld. Several research laboratories are exploring the potential use of triplex DNA as a new type of "molecular scissors" for cutting DNA. It is anticipated that the triplex DNA scissors will be able to cut the DNA at only one or a few sites thereby giving a much more manageable collection of large DNA pieces.[56]

Also, the role of viruses in human cancer is under intense investigation as described by zur Hausen.[30] He points out that viruses account for about 15 percent of the worldwide cancer incidence. Viruses are thought to contribute to the development of human tumors indirectly by inducing immunosuppression or directly by altering the host-cell proteins at the site where the viral DNA is inserted into the host-cell's DNA. Cancer of the cervix and hepatocellular carcinoma represent about 80 percent of the virus-associated cancers. Other viruses associated with human cancers are papillomavirus, hepatitus B virus, Epstein-Barr virus, human T cell leukemialymphoma virus (HTLV), and human immunodeficiency virus (HIV).

The above examples serve to illustrate the direction of cancer research in the area of molecular epidemiology. Although the understanding of the molecular basis for cancer is still far from complete, the research of the past decade and a half is beginning to pay off in terms of new cancer therapies.

1.6.5 Trends in Cancer Therapies

The research involving new cancer therapies makes use of the fundamental understanding gained from the research on oncogenesis over the past decade and a half. Marx[57] describes several variations of a novel type of a cancer therapy in which a direct attack is made on cancer cells that deprives them of the proteins they need to divide and grow. Marc Lippman's group at Georgetown University School of Medicine has shown that breast cancer cells produce a number of growth factors. It is believed that some of these agents may contribute to the ability of these cancer cells to grow and invade new tissues. Thus, blocking their activity might be one way of controlling cancer cell growth. In the case of breast cancer, one of the most promising targets for therapy is the oncogene known as *erb*B2, *HER*, or *neu*.

This oncogene encodes a protein which appears to be a growth factor that controls cell division and differentiation. Marx[57] describes the findings of Dennis Salmon and his colleagues, at the University of California School of Medicine in Los Angeles, who have shown that the growth of human breast and ovarian tumor cells that have been transplanted into nude mice can be inhibited by injecting the animals with a monoclonal antibody that binds to the *erb*B2 receptor protein. A clinical trial of the monoclonal antibody in patients with advanced cancer is planned. Antibodies are a member of a class of proteins called *immunoglobulins cells* which are cultured from a single *hybridoma cell* that produces one single type of antibody called a *monoclonal antibody*. A hybridoma cell consists of a hybrid cell formed by fusing an antibody-producing white blood cell to a rapidly growing mycloma cell. The monoclonal antibodies are highly specific with respect to antigens.

Also, Marx[57] describes the finding of Lippman's Georgetown group that discovered a number of other growth factors including *fibroblast growth factors* (FGF). The role of FGF in tumor growth is the stimulation of the formation of the blood vessels needed to nourish expanding tumors. Lippman et al. have shown that *pentosan polysulfate*, a carbohydrate related to the natural anticoagulant heparin, blocks the growth of mammary tumors in nude mice by binding to the FGF. Clinical trials of the drug in patients with advanced breast and other types of cancer are underway.

Other gene therapies have been reported in a survey article by Culliton.[58] These therapies are based on the fact that tumors cannot live without a blood supply. Steven Rosenberg, a surgeon with the National Cancer Institute, has found that when a potent natural tumor killer called *tumor necrosis factor* (TNF) is injected into the bloodstream of mice, tumors begin to shrink in a short period of time (hours). In the case of humans, it caused regression in surface tumors, but was unsatisfactory for deep-seated tumors because it could not be given in the bloodstream in sufficient quantities due to its toxicity. In order to get an effective quantity of TNF to the deep-seated tumors, Rosenberg uses a procedure known as *TNF/TIL*. In this procedure, *tumor infected lymphocytes* (TIL) are taken from surgically removed pieces of the tumor. Then they are grown in large numbers in a culture in the presence of *interleukin-2* (IL-2). To this culture is added a cloned gene for TNF which is attached to a retrovirus that has had its replicating genes removed. This engineered virus infects the TIL in the culture and deposits its genes in the TIL's own DNA. Then the lymphocytes which have been grown in this manner are injected into the blood stream. Thus, the debilitated retrovirus which has an affinity for the tumor is merely a vector or vehicle for transporting the TNF to the tumor. Tests using patients with malignant melanomas are planned. A similar experimental gene treatment has been proposed by R.M. Blaise and W.F. Anderson in collaboration with their NIH colleagues Kenneth Culver and Steven Rosenberg for the treatment of children who are born with the severe immunodeficiency called *enzyme adenosine deaminase* (*ADA*).

The experimental cancer therapies described above demonstrate the beginning of a new trend based on the understanding of cancer formation at the molecular level.

1.6.6 Testing for Individual Cancer Risk

Classical methods of epidemiology have worked well enough in the identification of groups of people who have a high risk of developing cancer, but provide no information pertaining to individual risks. For example, the results of classical epidemiology show that one cigarette smoker in ten will develop lung cancer. However, as pointed out by Marx,[59] classical epidemiology is unable to answer the question every individual wants to know, and that is: What is my risk of developing cancer?

Because of the advances made in the understanding of cancer at the molecular level, progress is being made in predicting individual risks. Markers are now being identified. For example, it has been found that 95 percent of the children carrying the *retinoblastoma gene* will develop eye cancer by age 5. This inherited gene can be detected by screening infants, and if those carrying the gene are treated, a survival rate of almost 100 percent can be achieved. In other cases, the utility of the test is open to question because the test may reveal a high susceptibility for a cancer for which there is no known cure.

The testing for individual cancer risks will play an ever-increasing role as more knowledge is accumulated about cancer at the molecular level. Although genetic screening appears to be an excellent scientific tool for risk assessment, it is fraught with difficulties. The practical application of this technique must take into account all of the social, financial, and legal implications from the Equal Opportunity Act.

All of the new information such as the genetic causes of cancer, the new incidence rates with the probable causes of cancer given by Henderson[31], and the incidence rate of cancer caused by viruses given by zur Hausen[30] suggests that a new study of the Doll-Peto[18] type could clarify questions such as the one raised by Nicholson.[60] In particular, Nicholson suggested that the studying of cancer mortalities of occupational groups instead of the population as a whole could provide some additional insight into the causes of cancer, and to illustrate this approach, an example was used that raised questions for which answers are needed. Nicholson's analysis begins with the finding of the Doll-Peto study[18] that 4 percent of all cancer mortalities can be attributed to exposures in the workplace. In their study, "workplace" is spoken of very broadly with the implication that it includes all members of society who were ever employed in any segment of industry, and not just the so-called "smokestack industries" or the industries regulated by OSHA.

To estimate the number of cancer mortalities for the workers in the OSHA industries, Nicholson begins with the Doll-Peto[18] number corresponding to 4 percent of all cancer mortalities. Next it is supposed that all of these cancer mortalities (4 percent of the total cancer mortalities) occurred in only those workers who were most likely to have been the heaviest exposed, the blue-collar male workers in the OSHA industries. On this basis, Nicholson[60] found that the corresponding cancer mortality attributable to workplace exposure for these workers could be as high as 30 percent of all cancers experienced by these workers.

However, this high figure has not been found in studies that have been made in the chemical or oil industries such as the one described by Phillips[40] nor is it suggested by new incidence data given by Henderson[31] and zur Hausen[30] or by all the new genetic causes that have been identified during the past decade. The fact that the 30 percent cancer mortalities for blue-collar male workers has not been observed, strongly suggests that Nicholson's assignment of *all* of the 4 percent cancer mortalities for the workplace to only the blue-collar male workers was inappropriate. And it once again emphasizes the need for redoing the Doll-Peto study with the new information available and with clearer definitions.

1.6.7 Cancer Prevention

Cancer prevention (*chemoprevention*) research aimed at the prevention of cancer is a new rapidly developing field. The need for a better understanding of cancer at the molecular level has served as a catalyst for this research. As described by Marx,[59] a number of trials are now in progress. Some selected agents in chemoprevention trials have been described by Marx.[59]

Retinoids such as vitamin A and its precursor *β-carotene* induce maturation and as a result inhibit cell proliferation. Cancers of the skin, lung, breast, and cervix are thought to be prevented by retinoids.[59]

Anti-oxidants, a class of substances which includes *vitamin E* may protect against gene mutation caused by free radicals. One test involving 19,000 subjects will determine whether vitamins C and E, when given with *β-carotene,* can prevent lung cancer in women who smoke.[59]

Nonsteroidal anti-inflammatory agents such as aspirin and ibuprofen (an active ingredient in Advil® and Nuprin®) may suppress cancer by inhibiting cell proliferation and also by reducing free radical formation. Tests have shown that these agents can cause the disappearance of polyps, which can cause colon cancer if not removed.[59]

Calcium carbonate and *calcium lactate* may prevent colon cancer by suppressing cell proliferation caused by the action of acids on the intestinal lining.[59]

Diet, a major contributor to cancer according to Doll and Peto,[18] can be expected to play a major role in chemoprevention as more is learned about cancer formation at the molecular level.

1.6.8 Summary

The abbreviated reviews provide an overview of the present status of the causes of cancer as reflected by epidemiological studies as well as the trends in cancer research, evolving cancer therapies, and cancer preventions. Also, the concepts of cancer formation presented serve as a basis for the development of quantitative models in the next chapter.

PROBLEMS

1. This problem and those that follow are based on the concepts presented in Appendix I on age-adjustment of cancer mortality rates to the 1970 population. Let the mortality rate for a given type of cancer for people in age category i be denoted by d_i and the number of people

in this age category by n_i. Further, let the proportionality factors relating these respective quantities for the years 1973 and 1987 be defined as follows:

$$d_{i,1987} = \alpha_i d_{i,1973}$$
$$n_{i,1987} = \beta_i n_{i,1973}$$

Also, let w_i be the weight factor for the age-adjustment to the 1970 population. Then, show that the necessary condition for there to be an increase in the percentage change in the age-adjusted cancer mortality rate from 1973 to 1987 is that $\alpha_i/\beta_i > 1$.

2. To demonstrate the effect of the changes in the number of mortalities as well as the number of people in two or more age groups on the age-adjusted cancer mortality rate, the following problem is posed. Let it be required to find the percentage change in the age-adjusted cancer mortality rates over the 15 year period from 1973 through 1987 for age groups i and $i+1$. The rates are age-adjusted to the 1970 population distribution.

(a) Develop the formula for making this calculation using the following notation.

$d_{i,k}$ = cancer mortalities for a given type of cancer for age group i and for years $k = 1973$ and $k = 1987$ per 100,000,000 population where the weight factor w_i is defined on this basis

$n_{i,k}$ = number of people in age group i for years $k = 1973$ and $k = 1987$.

w_i = weight factor = $\frac{n_{i,1970}}{n_{T,1970}} \times 10^8$, where n_T = total population in 1970.

$d_{i+1,k}, n_{i+1,k}, w_{i+1}$ = same definitions as above except for age group $i+1$.

(b) Let

$$d_{i,1987} = \alpha_i d_{i,1973}$$
$$n_{i,1987} = \beta_i n_{i,1973}$$
$$d_{i+1,1987} = \alpha_{i+1} d_{i+1,1973}$$
$$n_{i+1,1987} = \beta_{i+1} n_{i+1,1973}$$

Show that if $\alpha_i/\beta_i = \alpha_{i+1}/\beta_{i+1} = 1$, then the percentage change over the 15 year period is equal to zero.

(c) Show that if $\alpha_i/\beta_i = \alpha_{i+1}/\beta_{i+1} > 1$, an increase in the percentage change is obtained, and if $\alpha_i/\beta_i = \alpha_{i+1}/\beta_{i+1} < 1$, a decrease in the percentage is obtained.

(d) For $\alpha_i/\beta_i = 1+\epsilon$, $\alpha_{i+1}/\beta_{i+1} = 1-\epsilon$, $0 < \epsilon < 1$, show that the percentage change may be either plus or minus depending on the relative sizes of $(d_{i,1973}/n_{i,1973})w_i$ and $(d_{i+1,1973}/n_{i+1,1973})w_{i+1}$.

3. Use the data presented in Table A-1 of Appendix I for lung cancer deaths for U.S. males for 1977 and the male populations for 1970 and 1977 to compute the following rates:

(a) the age-standardized lung cancer death rate for 1977 (age-adjusted to the 1970 population per 100 million U.S. males) for U.S. males per 100 million U.S. males aged 65 and over.

Table 1.10 U.S. Population[23]

Age Group	1970	1980	1990
0–4	17,154,337	16,348,254	18,354,443
5–9	19,956,247	16,699,956	18,099,179
10–14	20,789,468	18,242,129	17,114,249
15–19	19,070,348	21,168,124	17,754,015
20–24	16,371,021	21,318,704	19,020,312
25–29	13,476,993	19,520,919	21,313,045
30–34	11,430,436	17,560,920	21,862,887
35–39	11,106,851	13,965,302	19,963,117
40–44	11,980,954	11,669,408	17,615,786
45–49	12,115,939	11,089,755	13,872,573
50–54	11,104,018	11,710,032	11,350,513
55–59	9,973,028	11,615,254	10,531,756
60–64	8,616,784	10,087,621	10,616,167
65–69	6,991,625	8,782,481	10,111,735
70–74	5,443,831	6,798,124	7,994,823
75–79	3,834,834	4,793,722	6,121,369
80–84	2,284,311	2,935,033	3,933,739
85 and over	1,510,901	2,240,067	3,080,165
	203,211,926	226,545,805	248,709,873

(b) the age-standardized lung cancer death rate for 1977 (age-adjusted to the 1970 population per 100 million U.S. males) for U.S. males per 100,000 U.S. males aged 65 and over.

4. The distributions of the total population for the U.S. for the years 1970, 1980, and 1990 follow as well as the brain cancer mortalities for the years 1971, 1972, 1973, and 1985, 1986, 1987 by age groups in Tables 1.10 and 1.11.

(a) Adjust the 1970 population distribution to the basis of 100 million U.S. population.

(b) Calculate the age-standardized brain cancer mortality rates for 1971, 1972, and 1973 (age-adjusted to the 1970 total U.S. population per 100 million) for people under 65 and for people 65 and over. To obtain the intermediate populations between 1970 and 1980, interpolate linearly for each age group.

The total brain cancer mortalities for both male and female in the U.S. for each age group are shown in Table 1.11[25]

5. (a) Calculate the age-standardized brain mortality cancer rates for 1985, 1986, and 1987 (age-adjusted to the 1970 total U.S. population per 100 million) for people under 65 and for people 65 and over. Use the data presented in Problem 4.

(b) Compute the averages of the years 1971, 1972 and 1973 of the age-standardized brain cancer mortality rates for people under 65 and for people 65 and over and for the years 1985, 1986, and 1987.

Table 1.11 U.S. Brain Tumor Mortalities[25]

Age Group	1971	1972	1973	1985	1986	1987
0–4	312	298	333	124	139	119
5–9	306	264	256	162	163	166
10–14	235	242	198	120	124	88
15–19	172	212	182	129	114	102
20–24	174	154	178	120	137	127
25–29	185	158	186	208	209	205
30–34	219	208	215	281	296	300
35–39	273	274	294	384	381	383
40–44	389	418	423	433	426	474
45–49	627	594	626	497	499	541
50–54	857	832	903	703	679	756
55–59	1,094	1,094	1,106	1,020	977	1,032
60–64	1,107	1,142	1,127	1,396	1,322	1,415
65–69	980	966	986	1,352	1,478	1,528
70–74	615	720	712	1,342	1,331	1,404
75–79	372	380	386	952	964	1,042
80–84	137	112	146	509	562	563
85 and over	40	38	53	269	266	328
	8,094	8,106	8,311	10,001	10,067	10,573

(c) What is the percentage change from the average of 1971, 1972, and 1973 and the average of 1985, 1986 and 1987 for people less than 65 and 65 and over.

Answer: 18.0 percent decrease for people under 65 and 53.4 percent increase for people over 65.

(d) Find the percentage change in the age-adjusted brain cancer rate for all age groups from 1971, 1972, and 1973 to 1985, 1986, and 1987.

Answer: 0.9 percent increase.

REFERENCES

1. Ham, A.W., *Histology*, 6th Ed., J.B. Lippencatt Company, Philadelphia, PA (1969).
2. Bailey, J.E., and D.F. Ollis, *Biochemical Fundamentals*, 2nd Ed., McGraw-Hill Book Company, New York, NY (1986).
3. Aiba, S., A.E. Humphrey, and N.F. Mills, *Biochemical Engineering*, 2nd Ed., Academic Press, Inc., New York, NY (1973).
4. Gardner, E.J., and D.P. Snustad, *Principles of Genetics*, 6th Edition, John Wiley & Sons, New York, NY (1981).

5. Watson, J.D., and F.H.C. Crick, *Nature, General Implications of the Structure of Deoxyribonucleic Acid*, **171**, 737 (1953).
6. Spencer, J.H., *The Physics and Chemistry of DNA and RNA*, W. B. Saunders Company, Philadelphia, PA (1972).
7. Simic, M.G., L. Mossman, and A.C. Upton, Editors, *Mechanisms of DNA Damage and Repair*, Plenum Press, New York, NY (1983).
8. Hygaard, O.F., and M.G. Simic, Editors, *Radioprotectors and Anticarcinogens*, Plenum Press, New York, NY (1983).
9. Floyd, R.A., Editor, *Free Radicals and Cancer*, Marcel Dekker, Inc., New York, NY (1982).
10. Trosko, J.E. and C. Chang, "Nongenotoxic Mechanisms in Carcinogenesis: Role of Intercellular Communication," *Banbury Report 31 Carcinogen Risk Assessment: New Directions in Qualitative and Quantitative Aspects*, Cold Spring Harbor Laboratory, O-87969-231-6/88.
11. Yamasaki, H., *Banbury Report 25: Nongenotoxic Mechanisms in Carcinogenesis*, Cold Spring Harbor Laboratory, 0-87969-225-1/87.
12. Ames, B.N., and L.S. Gold, "Too Many Rodent Carcinogens: Mitogenesis Increases Mutagenesis," *Science*, **249**, 970 (1990).
13. Perera, F.P., Letter to Editor, *Science*, **250**, 1644 (1990).
14. Rall, D.P., Letter to Editor, *Science*, **251**, 10 (1991).
15. Weinstein, "Mitogenesis is Only One Factor in Carcinogenesis," *Science*, **251**, 387 (1991).
16. Cohen, S.M. and L.B. Ellwein, "Cell Proliferation and Bladder Tumor Promotion," in *Chemical Induced Cell Proliferation—Implication for Risk Assessment*, Editors: B.E. Butterworth, T.J. Slaga, W. Farland, M. McClain, and Wiley-Liss, John Wiley & Sons, Inc., New York, N.Y. (1991).
17. Boutwell, R.K., "Model Systems for Defining Initiation, Promotion, and Progression of Skin Neoplasms," in *Skin Cancer Carcinogenesis and Mechanisms and Human Relevance*, Editors: T.J. Slaga, A.J.P. Klein-Szanto, R.K. Boutwell, D.E. Stevenson, H.L. Spitzer, and B. D'Motto, Alan R. Liss, Inc., New York, N.Y. (1989).
18. Doll, R., and R. Peto, "The Causes of Cancer: Quantitative Estimates of Avoidable Risks of Cancer in the United States Today," *JNCI*, **66**(6), 1191 (1981).
19. Higginson, J., "Perspectives and Future Developments in Research on Environmental Carcinogenesis," in *Carcinogens: Identification and Mechanisms of Action*, A.C. Griffing, Ed., Raven Press, New York, N.Y. (1979).
20. Higginson, J., and C.S. Muir, "Environmental Carcinogenesis: Misconceptions and Limitation to Cancer Control," *JNCI*, **63**, 1291 (1979).
21. Cole, P., "Cancer and Occupation: Status and Needs for Epidemiology Research," *Cancer*, **39**, 1788 (1977).
22. Wynder, E.L., and G.B. Gori, "Contributions of the Environment to Cancer Incidence. An Epidemiologic Exercise," *JNCI*, **58**, 825 (1977).
23. United States International Trade Commission. Synthetic Organic Chemicals U.S. Production and Sales, Washington, D.C. (1930, 1931, . . . , 1988).
24. *Cancer Facts and Figures—1991*, American Cancer Society, Inc., Atlanta, Georgia (1991).
25. *Cancer Statistics Review 1973–1988*, Editors: L.A. G. Ries, B.J. Hankey, B.A. Miller, A.M.

Harman, and B.K. Edwards, National Cancer Institute, NIH Pub. No. 91–2789 (1991).

26. *Census of the Population*, Volume I: Characteristics of the Population, Part I, United States Summary, United States Department of Commerce, Bureau of the Census (1950, 1960, 1970, 1980; 1990 Census, Personal Communication, 1991).
27. *Ca—A Cancer Journal for Clinicians*, **41** (No 1) Cancer Statistics, 1988, The American Cancer Society (1991).
28. *Vital Statistics of the United States—1985*, Volume 2—Mortality, Part A, U.S. Department of Health and Human Services, National Center for Health Statistics, Hyattsville, Maryland (1988).
29. Schottenfeld, D., "The Epidemiology of Cancer: An Overview," *Cancer*, **47**(5), 1095 (1981).
30. zur Hausen, H., "Viruses in Humans," *Science*, **254**, 1167 (1991).
31. Henderson, B.E., R.K. Ross, and M.C. Pike, "Toward the Primary Prevention of Cancer," *Science*, **254**, 1131 (1991).
32. International Agency for Research on Cancer (IARC), *IARC Monographs on the Evaluation of the Carcinogenic Risk of Chemicals to Humans*, IARC: Lyons, France, Supplement 7 (1987) and Volume 50 (1990).
33. Doll, R., The Leon Goldberg Memorial Lecture: "Hazards of Cancer in the Chemical Industry," *BIBRA Bull.* **30**, 183 (1991).
34. Environmental Protection Agency, "Potential Industrial Carcinogens and Mutagens," prepared for the Office of Toxic Substances by Lawrence Fishbein, Washington, D.C., May 5 (1977).
35. Hsieh, D.P.H., J.J. Wong, C. Michas, and B.H. Ruebner, "Hepatic Transformation of Aflatoxin and its Carcinogenicity," in *Origins of Human Cancer*, Hyatt, H.H., J.D. Watson and J.A. Winsten, Ed., Book B *Mechanisms of Carcinogenicity*, Cold Spring Harbor Laboratory, New York, N.Y. (1977).
36. Weisburger, J.H., "Bioassays and Tests for Chemical Carcinogens," *Chemical Carcinogens*, Ed. C.E. Searle, American Chemical Society, Washington, D.C. (1976).
37. Schneiderman, M.A., and C.C. Brown, "Estimating Cancer Risks to a Population," *Environmental Health Perspectives*, **22**, 117 (1978).
38. Efron, E., *The Apocalyptic Cancer and the Big Lie*, Simon and Schuster, New York, N.Y. (1984).
39. "Caring for Texas," The Texas Chemical Council, Austin, Texas (1990).
40. Phillips, G., *Personal Communication*, Texas Eastman Company, Longview, Texas (1991).
41. Ember, L., "Toxic Chemical Levels Higher Indoors than Out (Based on TEAM Study)," *C&EN*, **22**, June 24 (1985).
42. Marshall, E., "Experts Clash Over Cancer Data," *Science*, **250**, 900 (1990).
43. Cole, P., "Of Light Bulbs and Wine Glass: Risk Factors and Mortality Trends," *Unnatural Causes: The Three Leading Killer Diseases in America*. Editor: Russell C. Maulitz (1989).
44. Roberts, L., "DOE's Genome Project Comes of Age," *Science*, **252**, 498 (1991).
45. Solomon E., E.J. Borrow, and A.D. Goddard, "Chromosome Aberrations and Cancer," *Science*, **254**, 1153 (1991).

46. Weinberg, R.A. "Tumor Suppressor Genes," *Science*, **254**, 1138 (1991).

47. Kinzler, K.W., M.C. Nilbert, B. Bogelstein, T.M. Bryan, D. B. Levey, K.J. Smith, A.C. Preisinger, S.R. Hamilton, P. Hedge, A. Markham, M. Carlson, G. Goslyn, J. Groden, R. White, Y. Miki, Y. Miyoshi, I. Nishisho, and Y. Nakamura, "Identification of a Gene Located at Chromosome 5q21 that is Mutated in Colorectal Cancers," *Science*, **21**, 1366 (1991).

48. Hall, J.M., K.M. Lee, B. Newman, J.E. Morrow, L.A. Anderson, B. Huey, and M.C. King, "Linkage of Early-Onset Familial Breast Cancer to Chromosome 17q21," *Science*, **250**, 1684 (1990).

49. Malkin, D., F.P. Li, L.C. Strong, J.F. Fraumeni, Jr., C.E. Nelson, D.H. Kim, J. Kassel, M.A. Gryka, F.A. Bishoff, M.A. Tainsky, and S.H. Friend, "Germ Line p53 Mutations in a Familial Syndrome of Breast Cancer, Sarcomas, and Other Neoplasms," *Science*, **250**, 1233 (1990).

50. Wright, K., "Breast Cancer: Two Steps Closer to Understanding," *Science*, **250**, 1659 (1990).

51. Hollstein, M., D. Sidransky, B. Kogelstein, and C.C. Harris, "p53 Mutations in Human Cancers," *Science*, **253**, 49 (1991).

52. Barinaga, M., "Immune Mystery Revealed: How MHC Meets Antigen," *Science*, **250**, 1659 (1990).

53. Roberts, L., "New Scissors for Cutting Chromosomes," *Science*, **249**, 127 (1990).

54. Gibbons, A., "Molecular Scissors: RNA Enzymes Go Commercial," *Science*, **250**, 521 (1991).

55. Hoffman, M., "RNA Editing: What's in a Mechanism?" *Science*, **253**, 136 (1991).

56. Moffat, A., "Triplex DNA Finally Comes of Age," *Science*, **252**, 1374 (1991).

57. Marx, J., "Oncogenes Evoke New Cancer Therapies," *Science*, **249**, 1376 (1989).

58. Culliton, B.J., "One Step Closer for Gene Therapy," *Science*, **248**, 1182 (1989).

59. Marx, J., "Zeroing in on Individual Cancer Risk," *Science*, **253**, 612 (1991).

60. Nicholson, W.H., "Research Issues in Occupational and Environmental Cancer," Archives of Environ. Health, **39**, (No. 3), 190 (1984).

2

Development of Selected Classical Models for Cancer Formation

The fundamental concepts of probability and statistics play a significant role both in the development of proposed models for the formation of cancer and in the estimation of dose–response relationships in animals or humans that are exposed to carcinogenic substances. Some of the relatively simple concepts of probability and statistics are introduced in the development of the models while other concepts of a less obvious nature are presented in Chapter 4.

This chapter is divided into two parts. In Section 2.1, an introduction to the fundamental concepts of probability is presented. In Section 2.2, the classical models that have been proposed for the quantitative description of cancer formation are presented. In particular, expressions are developed for the probability of *one* cell of *one* animal developing a tumor as a result of having been exposed to a daily dose d over a given time period. Next, expressions are developed for the probability of developing at least *one* tumor in *one* animal having N cell lines. The expressions for the latter probabilities are used in estimating the probability that exactly r animals develop a tumor out of the n animals exposed to a daily dose d over a given time period.

2.1 INTRODUCTION OF THE CONCEPTS OF PROBABILITY

Probability may be defined in terms of an experiment such as the random drawing of a bean from a collection of black and white beans. The chance or probability of the bean drawn being black is equal to the fraction of the total number of beans that are black.

The basis for this definition rests on the results of experimentation. For example, consider the case in which a bean is drawn from a hat containing 10 identical beans except for color; 4 of which are black and 6 are white. Further suppose that after each draw, the color of the bean drawn is noted, and then the bean is returned to the hat (referred to as *sampling with replacement*). Suppose that the described sampling process is repeated 1000 times with the result that 430 black beans are drawn. Then the relative frequency of drawing a black bean is given by

$$\frac{430}{1000} = 0.43$$

Further suppose that the drawing process is repeated for another 1000 times with the result that 380 black beans are drawn with replacement. Thus, the relative frequency is given by

$$\frac{380}{1000} = 0.38$$

Then for the 2000 draws with replacement, the relative frequency of drawing a black bean is

$$\frac{430 + 380}{2000} = 0.405$$

As the number of draws with replacement is increased indefinitely, the relative frequency of drawing a black bean approaches the limit of 0.4. The limit, as the number of draws with replacement is increased indefinitely, is equal to the probability of drawing a black bean on a single draw. Thus the probability of drawing a black bean on a single draw is equal to the number of ways of success, 4, divided by the number of ways of success plus the number of ways of failure [$4 + 6 = 10$]. On the basis of this fundamental understanding of probability, further quantitative developments of this topic are presented in Chapter 4.

The concepts of probability are used in both the quantification of the theories of cancer formation and in the quantification of the dose–response relationships for situations where a fixed daily dose of a substance is administered to a group of animals over a fixed time period. For example, when a group of animals are exposed to a carcinogenic substance, some of them may develop tumors while others may not. Furthermore, when the experiments are repeated, the number of animals that develop tumors may vary from experiment to experiment—just as the number of black beans drawn from a hat in the above example varied from experiment to experiment.

The models developed in this chapter are an attempt to quantify the fundamental biological and chemical processes involved in cancer formation. An abbreviated presentation of the theories of cancer formation and the roles of DNA, genes, cell *mitosis*, and mutation is presented in Chapter 1.

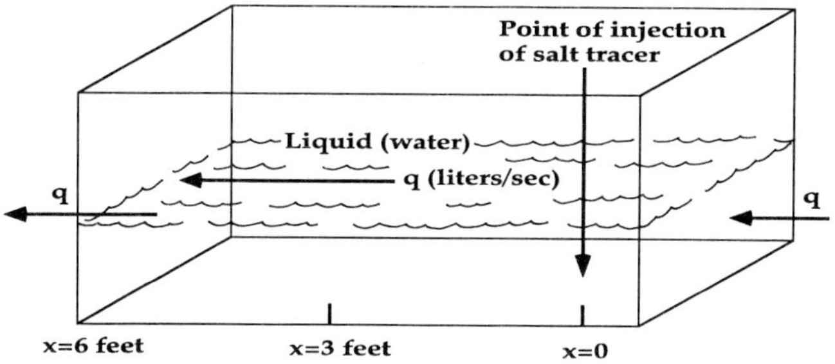

Figure 2.1 At Time $t = 0$, A Grams of a Salt Tracer Are Introduced Almost Instantaneously into the Flowing Stream of Water at $x = 0$.

2.1.1 The Probability Density Function and the Cumulative Distribution Function

A useful concept in the application of probability theory is the *probability density function*. As an example of this concept, some of the results of an experimental investigation by Welch et al.[1] on the mixing that occurs in a water stream as it flows across the plate of a distillation column are presented. A sketch of the system is shown in Figure 2.1. In this experiment, a solution containing A grams of salt was introduced almost instantaneously at time $t = 0$ into the water flowing past the plane at $x = 0$. The salt sample of A grams was so small that it did not change the flow rate q (*liters/sec*) of the water flowing across the plate to any detectable extent. The flow rate q was held constant throughout the course of the experiment. From time $t = 0$, the concentration of the salt was recorded continuously at two locations ($x = 3$ feet and $x = 6$ feet) downstream from $x = 0$. The random motion within the water stream as it flows across the plate causes the various parts of the salt sample to pass by points $x = 3$ feet and $x = 6$ feet at different times. The experimentally recorded concentration versus time profiles shown in Figure 2.2 were taken from Reference 2. The concentration in grams of salt per liter of solution at any x at time t is denoted by $\Psi(x, t)$. Observe that the salt tracer of A grams is added over a very small time interval of 0.3 seconds as shown in Figure 2.2. Further observe that as the distance from the point of injection of the salt sample or tracer increases, the dispersion of the salt increases as reflected by the flatter and more elongated concentration profile at $x = 6$ feet than the one at 3 feet.

Since all of the salt must eventually pass any plane, say the one at $x = 3$, it follows that

$$\int_0^\infty q\left(\frac{liters}{sec}\right)\Psi\left(\frac{grams\ salt}{liter}\right)dt(sec) = A(grams\ salt) \tag{2.1}$$

The rate (*grams salt/sec*) at which the salt flows past any plane x at time t is given by

$$\begin{pmatrix}Flow\ rate\ of\ salt\\ in\ grams/sec\end{pmatrix} = q\left(\frac{liters}{sec}\right)\Psi(x,t)\left(\frac{grams\ salt}{liter}\right)$$

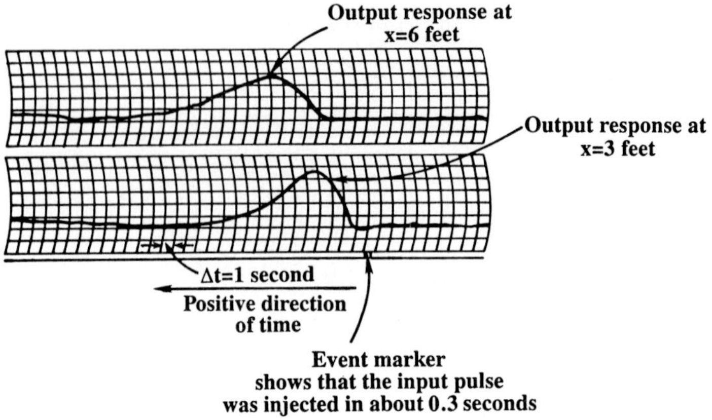

Figure 2.2 Typical Output Responses of the Concentrations of the Salt Tracer at the Positions $x = 3$ feet and $x = 6$ feet. [Taken from *Unsteady State Processes with Applications in Multicomponent Distillation*, Prentice–Hall Inc., Englewood Cliffs, N.J., 1966.]

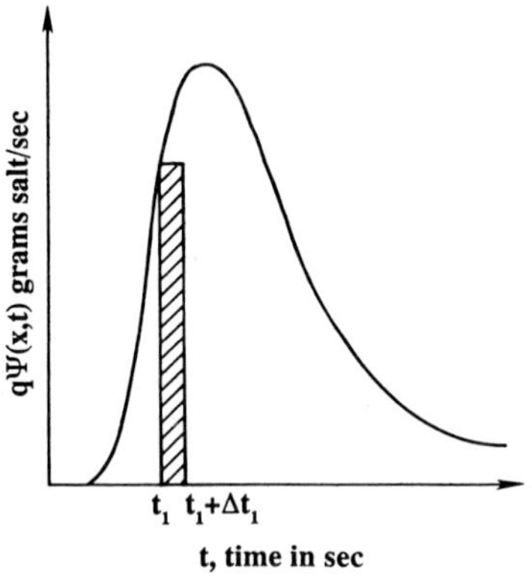

Figure 2.3 The Number of Molecules (or Grams of Salt) Flowing Past the Plane at $x = 3$ Feet at Time t_1 Is Approximated by the Shaded Area.

The integrand $q\Psi(x,t)$ represents the flow rate of the salt past any plane, say $x = 3$ feet at time t. [For definiteness it is supposed that $x = 3$ feet in the remainder of the discussion.] A graph of the flow rate of salt $q\Psi(x,t)$ versus time such as the one shown in Figure 2.3 may be constructed by use of the experimental results presented in Figure 2.2. Observe that over the time period Δt_1, from t_1 to $t_1 + \Delta t_1$, the grams of salt that pass plane $x = 3$ is equal to the area under the curve in Figure 2.3 from t_1 to $t_1 + \Delta t_1$, which is approximately equal to the area of the rectangle $[q\Psi(x,t_1)\Delta t_1]$. Furthermore, this salt sample $[q\Psi(x,t_1)\Delta t_1]$ resided in the system bounded by the planes $x = 0$ and $x = 3$ feet a period of time t_1, called its *residence time*, which lies between t_1 and $t_1 + \Delta t_1$. The language used in these statements may be placed in correspondence with that employed in probability and statistics by first dividing both sides of Equation (2.1) by the total amount of salt tracer A introduced at time

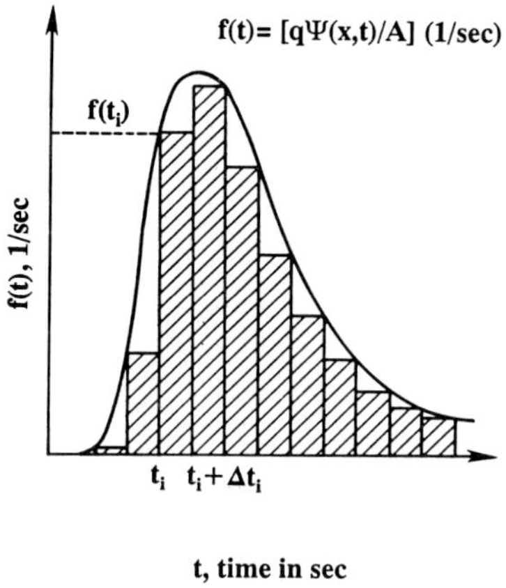

Figure 2.4 Distribution of Residence Times at the Fixed Position $x = 3$ Feet. [The fraction of the molecules (or grams) of salt introduced at time $t = 0$ at $x = 0$ that have a residence time lying between t_i and $t_i + \Delta t_i$, is equal to approximately $[[q\Psi(x, t_i)/A]\Delta t_i.]$

$t = 0$ at $x = 0$ to give

$$\int_0^\infty f(t)\,dt = 1 \tag{2.2}$$

where

$$f(t) = \frac{q\Psi(x,t)}{A}$$

A graph of the normalized integral equation is shown in Figure 2.4. Observe that since the elements of area with base Δt_i will be involved eventually in a limit, the construction of the rectangles is arbitrary and that shown in Figure 2.4 may be used. Further observe that the area represented by $f(t_i)\Delta t_i$ is equal to the fraction of molecules of salt introduced at time $t = 0$ that have a residence time lying between t_i and $t_i + \Delta t_i$. In probability analysis, the function $f(t)$ is called the *probability density function (p.d.f.).*

Further significance is attached to the name *probability density function* by observing that at a fixed x, say $x = 3$ feet, the magnitudes of the areas $f(t_i)\Delta t_i$ at fixed sizes of Δt_i depend on the density [or concentration] $\Psi(x, t_i)$, since q and A are constants. Thus, as the density increases, the areas $f(t_i)\Delta t_i$ increase, and the probabilities $f(t_i)\Delta t_i$ that each t_i lies between t_i and $t_i + \Delta t_i$ increases or becomes more *dense* as $f(t_i) = q\Psi(x, t_i)/A$ increases, and hence the name *probability density function.*

To generalize the definition of the probability density function given by Equation (2.1), the range of integration is extended to include the general case wherein the limits of integration range from $-\infty$ to $+\infty$. The most general definition of the probability density function is as follows. Let $f(x)$ be a non-negative function over all x $(-\infty < x < \infty)$ which has the property that the area under the curve $f(x)$ over all x is equal to unity; that is,

$$\int_{-\infty}^\infty f(x)\,dx = 1 \tag{2.3}$$

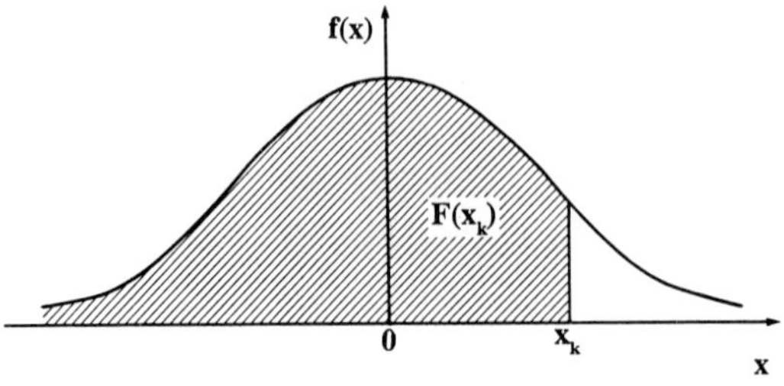

Figure 2.5 The Probability that X Have a Value between $-\infty$ and x_k Is Equal to the Shaded Area Under the Curve.

A function $f(x)$ having these properties is called the *probability density function (p.d.f.)*. The probability that a random variable X lies between x_i and $x_i + \Delta x_i$ is equal to approximately $f(x_i)\Delta x_i$ which is analogous to the shaded area $f(t_i)\Delta t_i$ shown in Figure 2.4, where the variable X has been replaced by the variable t.

The likelihood that X has the value x_0 is equal to $f(x_0)$. The probability that X has some value between $-\infty$ and x_k is equal to the area under the curve of $f(x)$ over the interval from $-\infty$ to x_k as shown in Figure 2.5. The area under the curve from $-\infty$ to a fixed value x_k is denoted by $F(x_k)$; that is,

$$F(x_k) = \int_{-\infty}^{x_k} f(x)\,dx \tag{2.4}$$

If instead of a constant x_k for the upper limit, suppose that the upper limit is a variable, say z, which may take on any value between $-\infty$ and $+\infty$. For this case Equation (2.4) becomes

$$F(z) = \int_{-\infty}^{z} f(x)\,dx \tag{2.5}$$

The function $F(z)$ defined by Equation (2.5) is called the *cumulative distribution function*. The definition of the cumulative distribution function permits a further elucidation of the probability density function. From Equation (2.5), it follows that the probability density function is the rate of change of the cumulative distribution function $F(z)$ with respect to z; that is,

$$\frac{dF(z)}{dz} = f(z) \tag{2.6}$$

For the space domain x, the name *probability density function* is suggested by the following considerations which are analogous to those presented for the time domain in the analysis of the salt example. Observe that at any x, the integrand $f(x)$ of Equation (2.5) represents the heights of the probability curve (see Figure 2.5). The higher the curve the greater the value of $f(x)$, and the greater is the contribution of the increment of area $f(x)\Delta x$ (or the probability that X lies between x and $x + \Delta x$) to the total area under the curve. That is at a fixed Δx, the probability $f(x)\Delta x$ increases as $f(x)$ increases. Thus, in the region where $f(x)$ takes on larger values, the corresponding probabilities $f(x)\Delta x$ are larger than those for other regions where the values of $f(x)$ are smaller. Since the region of higher values of $f(x)$ result in higher probabilities $[f(x)\Delta x]$, the probabilities per unit length $f(x)$ can be thought of as being more dense in this region, and hence the name *probability density function.*

A more physical interpretation of the probability density function is afforded by consideration of the analogy of a rod of mass $m(kg)$ with a constant cross section S (cm^2) whose density ρ (g/cm^3) increases uniformly as the length x of the rod increases. The fraction of the mass of material over a small fixed increment of length Δx is given approximately by $\rho(x) \cdot S \cdot \Delta x/m$. Let $\rho(x) \cdot S/m = f(x)$, which is the density expressed in the units of the fraction of mass per unit length of rod. Then the fraction of mass corresponding to the length Δx is equal to $f(x)\Delta x$. In this analogy, the fraction of mass plays the same role as probability, and the mass per unit length $f(x)$ plays the same role as the probability per unit length, which suggests the name *probability density function.*

2.2 DEVELOPMENT OF SELECTED CLASSICAL MODELS FOR CANCER FORMATION

This section begins with the development of the multistage models. First to be presented is the development of the one-stage model which is based on one of the earliest quantitative theories of cancer and is attributed to Iversen and Arley[3,4]. In the development of the one-stage model and other classical models for cancer formation, the review work of Whittmore and Keller[5] was very helpful.

2.2.1 The One-Stage Model

This model pertains to the behavior of *one* cell (or *one* cell line) of *one* animal. Each cell and its progression toward the formation of a tumor is commonly referred to as a *cell line*. In this development and those that follow, a *normal cell* is defined as one that can be transformed. In the case of the one-stage model, it is supposed that after a transformation has occurred, the transformed cell can generate a tumor. The *transformed cell* is the progenitor of a tumor, and not its descendent. That is, in the one-stage model, it is postulated that a cell can generate a tumor only after it has undergone one *transition*. (The transition of a cell is generally regarded as a mutation which can lead to tumor formation. An abbreviated review of the role of cell division and DNA replication and mutation in cancer formation is presented in Chapter 1.) Thus, in this model a cell can be in either one or two states, the normal state, denoted by 0 (zero), or the transformed state, denoted by 1 (one). Let $p_0(t)$ denote the probability that a cell is in state 0 at time t (that is, no transition has occurred between time = 0 and time = t), and $p_1(t)$ the probability that it is in state 1 at time t. A schematic representation of this model is shown in Figure 2.6.

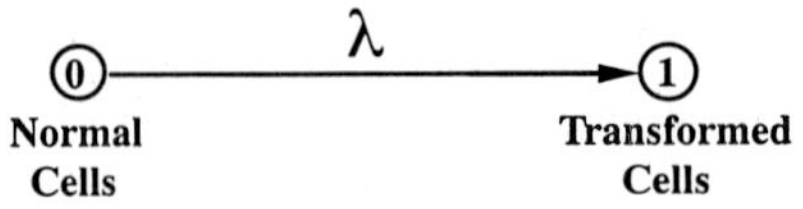

Figure 2.6 Schematic Representation of the One-Stage Model Proposed by Iversen and Arley.[3,4]

That a cell must be in either state 0 (normal cell) or state 1 (transformed cell) is a certainty. Consequently, for all t,

$$p_0(t) + p_1(t) = 1 \tag{2.7}$$

Since $p_0(t)$ and $p_1(t)$ must always have a sum equal to unity for all t, the probabilities $p_0(t)$ and $p_1(t)$ can be said to be conserved in the same sense that mass is conserved. In the formulation of the equations required to describe the process, the concept of conservation of probability is utilized. This approach makes the formulation analogous to that required to describe a set of consecutive chemical reactions occurring in a batch reactor.

Postulate that the rate of disappearance of $p_0(t)$, denoted by $r_0(t)$ or simply r_0, is equal to the product of $p_0(t)$ and $\lambda(t)$; that is,

$$r_0(t) = \lambda(t)\, p_0(t) \tag{2.8}$$

where $\lambda(t)$ is the *transition probability rate*. The integral-difference equation for the conservation of mass or any other entity which is conserved is given by

$$\int_{t_n}^{t_n+\Delta t} \left[\frac{\textit{Input to System}}{\textit{Time}} - \frac{\textit{Output from System}}{\textit{Time}} \right] dt = \left. \begin{matrix} \textit{Holdup} \\ \textit{in System} \end{matrix} \right|_{t_n+\Delta t} - \left. \begin{matrix} \textit{Holdup} \\ \textit{in System} \end{matrix} \right|_{t_n} \tag{2.9}$$

Thus, for the conservation of the probability $p_0(t)$, Equation (2.9) becomes

$$\int_{t_n}^{t_n+\Delta t} [0 - r_0]\, dt = p_0(t)|_{t_n+\Delta t} - p_0(t)|_{t_n} \tag{2.10}$$

By use of the *mean value theorem of integral calculus* (see Appendix II), it is possible to restate the left hand side of Equation (2.10) as follows:

$$\int_{t_n}^{t_n+\Delta t} [0 - r_0]\, dt = [-r_0]|_{t_n+\alpha\Delta t}\, \Delta t \tag{2.11}$$

where $0 \leq \alpha \leq 1$. The right-hand side of Equation (2.10) may be restated in the following form by use of the *mean value theorem of differential calculus* (see Appendix II).

$$p_0(t)|_{t_n+\Delta t} - p_0(t)|_{t_n} = \left. \frac{dp_0(t)}{dt} \right|_{t_n+\beta\Delta t} \Delta t \tag{2.12}$$

where $0 < \beta < 1$. After the results given by Equations (2.11) and (2.12) have been substituted into Equation (2.10), the following result is obtained upon division by Δt.

$$-r_0\big|_{t_n\alpha\Delta t} = \left.\frac{dp_0(t)}{dt}\right|_{t_n+\beta\Delta t} \tag{2.13}$$

In the limit as Δt is allowed to go to zero, Equation (2.13) reduces to

$$r_0\big|_{t_n} = -\left.\frac{dp_0(t)}{dt}\right|_{t_n} \tag{2.14}$$

Since t_n was arbitrarily selected, Equation (2.14) holds for all t in the time domain of interest which is implied by the restatement of Equation (2.14) in the form

$$r_0 = -\frac{dp_0(t)}{dt} \tag{2.15}$$

Elimination of r_0 from Equations (2.8) and (2.15) yields the first of the two differential equations required to describe the process.

$$-\frac{dp_0(t)}{dt} = \lambda(t)p_0(t) \tag{2.16}$$

Since the cell is taken to be normal at time $t = 0$, it follows that Equation (2.14) is subject to the following initial condition.

$$p_0(0) = 1 \tag{2.17}$$

The second differential equation describing the process may be obtained by making a balance on $p_1(t)$. In this case, $p_1(t)$ is being produced at the same rate at which $p_0(t)$ is disappearing; namely r_0. Thus Equation (2.9) becomes

$$\int_{t_n}^{t_n+\Delta t} [r_0 - 0]\, dt = p_1(t)\big|_{t_n+\Delta t} - p_1(t)\big|_{t_n} \tag{2.18}$$

By following the same procedure demonstrated above for Equation (2.10) in obtaining Equation (2.15), it is readily shown that

$$r_0 = \frac{dp_1(t)}{dt} \tag{2.19}$$

and in view of Equation (2.8), the second differential equation is obtained; namely,

$$\frac{dp_1(t)}{dt} = \lambda(t)p_0(t) \tag{2.20}$$

In this case the initial condition is

$$p_1(0) = 0 \tag{2.21}$$

[Alternately, Equation (2.20) could have been obtained by first differentiating Equation (2.7) termwise with respect to t and rearranging to obtain, $dp_0(t)/dt = -dp_1(t)/dt$. Replacement of the left hand side of Equation (2.16) by this result gives Equation (2.20).]

2.2.2 Solution of Equations (2.16) and (2.20)

Equation (2.16) may be solved by separation of variables. Rearrangement of this equation followed by integration yields

$$\int_{p_0(0)=1}^{p_0(t)} \frac{dp_0(\tau)}{p_0(\tau)} = -\int_0^t \lambda(\tau)d\tau \tag{2.22}$$

Integration followed by rearrangement yields

$$\log_e p_0(t) = -\int_0^t \lambda(\tau)d\tau \tag{2.23}$$

which is readily restated in exponential form to give

$$p_0(t) = \exp\left[-\int_0^t \lambda(\tau)d\tau\right] \tag{2.24}$$

After $p_0(t)$ in Equation (2.20) has been replaced by its equivalent as given by Equation (2.24), the resulting differential equation is readily solved for $p_1(t)$ by separation of variables in a manner similar to that demonstrated for Equation (2.16). Alternately, instead of solving the differential equation given by Equation (2.20) for $p_1(t)$, the desired solution may be obtained directly by use of Equations (2.7) and (2.24) as follows:

$$p_1(t) = 1 - p_0(t) = 1 - \exp\left[-\int_0^t \lambda(\tau)d\tau\right] \tag{2.25}$$

2.2.3 The Multistage Model

In the multistage theory of Muller[6] and Nordling,[7] it is postulated that a cell can develop a tumor only after it has undergone a certain number of irreversible changes or mutations, and these events must occur in a prescribed order. In the quantitative extension of this theory by Armitage and Doll,[8] it is assumed that the k changes occur at different transition rates $\lambda_i(t)$, $i = 0, 1, \ldots, k-1$. In the analysis of this model , let p_i(t), $i = 0, 1, \ldots, k$, be the probability that at time t a particular cell is in stage i; that is, the specified cell has undergone the first i changes. This model also includes the probability $p_D(t)$ of the death of a cell at time t at each of the stages $i = 0, 1, \ldots, k-1$ as represented by the death state D in Figure 2.7.

It is postulated that all cells begin in stage zero as normal cells, and that the transformations take place consecutively from stage $i = 0$ through $i = k-1$ and to stage k unless death occurs at some stage i ($i = 0, 1, 2, \ldots, k-1$). Thus, in this case the total rate of

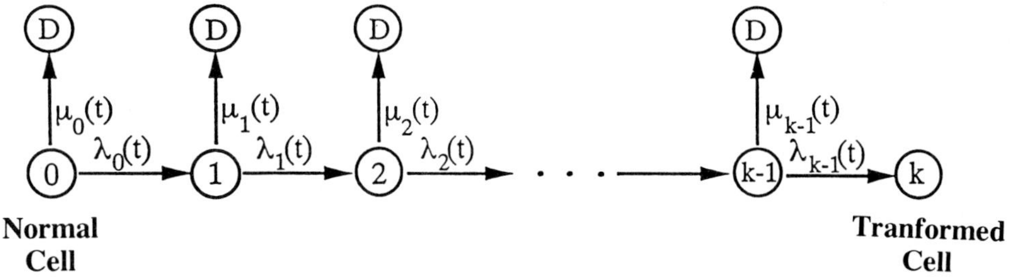

Figure 2.7 The Schematic Representation of the Multistage Theory of Cancer Formation.

disappearance of probability for some stage i ($i = 0, 1, 2, \ldots, k-1$), analogous to $r_0(t)$ in Equation (2.8), is given by the sum of the rates of transition $\lambda_i(t)p_i(t)$ and death $\mu_i(t)p_i(t)$; that is, $r_i(t) = [\lambda_i(t) + \mu_i(t)]p_i(t)$. Since the probabilities have the property

$$p_0(t) + p_1(t) + \ldots + p_k(t) + p_D(t) = 1 \tag{2.26}$$

they are conserved, and a conservation balance may be made on each stage in a manner analogous to that demonstrated for the one-stage model to give the following set of differential equations

$$\frac{dp_0(t)}{dt} = -\rho_0(t)p_0(t) \tag{2.27}$$

$$\frac{dp_i(t)}{dt} = -\rho_i(t)p_i(t) + \lambda_{i-1}(t)p_{i-1}(t) \qquad i = 1, 2, \ldots, k-1 \tag{2.28}$$

$$\frac{dp_k(t)}{dt} = \lambda_{k-1}(t)p_{k-1}(t) \tag{2.29}$$

$$\frac{dp_D(t)}{dt} = \sum_{i=0}^{k-1} \mu_i(t)p_i(t) \tag{2.30}$$

where

$$\rho_i(t) = \lambda_i(t) + \mu_i(t)$$

Since all cells are assumed to be alive and normal at time $t = 0$, the initial conditions are:

$$\begin{gathered} p_0(0) = 1 \\ p_i(0) = 0 \qquad i = 1, 2, \ldots, k \\ p_D(0) = 0 \end{gathered} \tag{2.31}$$

A comparison of Equations (2.16) and (2.27) and their initial conditions shows that their solutions are of the same form. Thus, the solution which satisfies Equation (2.27) and the initial condition $[p_0(t) = 1]$ is

$$p_0(t) = e^{-L_0(t)} \tag{2.32}$$

where

$$L_0(t) = \int_0^t \rho_0(\tau)d\tau$$

Now consider Equation (2.28) for $i = 1$; namely,

$$\frac{dp_1(t)}{dt} + \rho_1(t)p_1(t) = \lambda_0(t)p_0(t) \tag{2.33}$$

The solution of this linear differential equation with variable coefficients is well known,* and the solution that satisfies Equation (2.33) and the initial condition $p_1(0) = 0$, is given by

$$p_1(t) = e^{-L_1(t)} \int_0^t e^{L_1(\tau_0)}\lambda_0(\tau_0)p_0(\tau_0)d\tau_0 \tag{2.34}$$

where

$$L_1(t) = \int_0^t \rho_1(\tau)d\tau$$

Similarly, the solution that satisfies Equation (2.28) and the corresponding initial condition [see Equation (2.30)] for $i = 2$ is as follows:

$$p_2(t) = e^{-L_2(t)} \int_0^t e^{L_2(\tau_1)}\lambda_1(\tau_1)p_1(\tau_1)d\tau_1 \tag{2.35}$$

(The subscripts on the dummy variables are introduced because of the need for clarity in subsequent substitutions.) Thus, for the general case [$i = 1, 2, \ldots, k-1$], the solution

---

* The solution of the ordinary linear differential equation with variable coefficients,

$$dy/dx + P(x)y = Q(x)$$

is customarily stated in terms of indefinite integrals and an arbitrary constant K as follows:[9]

$$y = e^{-\int P(x)\,dx}\left[\int e^{\int P(x)\,dx} Q(x)\,dx + K\right]$$

When stated in terms of indefinite integrals of the form $\int_0^z f(\omega)d\omega$ and when the initial condition is of the form $y = y_0$ at $x = 0$, the solution is given by

$$y = e^{-\int_0^x P(\tau)d\tau}\left[\int_0^x e^{\int_0^\tau P(\omega)d\omega} Q(\tau)d\tau + y_0\right]$$

which satisfies Equation (2.28) and the initial condition given by Equation (2.31) are:

$$p_i(t) = e^{-L_i(t)} \int_0^t e^{L_i(\tau_{i-1})} \lambda_{i-1}(\tau_{i-1}) p_{i-1}(\tau_{i-1}) d\tau_{i-1} \qquad [i = 1, 2, \ldots, k-1] \tag{2.36}$$

For the case where $i = k$, the corresponding differential equation given by Equation (2.28) may be solved by separation of the variables to give

$$p_k(t) = \int_0^t \lambda_{k-1}(\tau_{k-1}) p_{k-1}(\tau_{k-1}) d\tau_{k-1} \tag{2.37}$$

Observe that the solution for each $p_i(t)$ [$i = 1, 2, \ldots, k$] contains the solution $p_{i-1}(t)$ [for $i = 1, 2, \ldots, k$] of the previous differential equation. Thus, the general solution of the complete set of differential equations and initial conditions may be obtained by successive substitution of the expression for $p_{i-1}(t)$ into the one for $p_i(t)$. This substitutional process is initiated by replacing $p_0(\tau_0)$ in Equation (2.34) by its solution given by Equation (2.32). The result so obtained is

$$p_1(t) = e^{-L_1(t)} \int_0^t \lambda_0(\tau_0) e^{L_1(\tau_0) - L_0(\tau_0)} d\tau_0 \tag{2.38}$$

Next when $p_1(\tau_1)$ in Equation (2.35) is replaced by the solution given by Equation (2.38), the following expression is obtained.

$$p_2(t) = e^{-L_2(t)} \int_0^t \left[\lambda_1(\tau_1) e^{L_2(\tau_1) - L_1(\tau_1)} \int_0^{\tau_1} \left[\lambda_0(\tau_0) e^{L_1(\tau_0) - L_0(\tau_0)} \right] d\tau_0 \right] d\tau_1 \tag{2.39}$$

Continuation of this process of substitution yields

$$\begin{aligned} p_{k-1}(t) = e^{-L_{k-1}(t)} & \int_0^t \left[\lambda_{k-2}(\tau_{k-2}) e^{L_{k-1}(\tau_{k-2}) - L_{k-2}(\tau_{k-2})} \right. \\ & \times \int_0^{\tau_{k-2}} \left[\lambda_{k-3}(\tau_{k-3}) e^{L_{k-2}(\tau_{k-3}) - L_{k-3}(\tau_{k-3})} \ldots \right. \\ & \times \left. \left. \int_0^{\tau_1} \left[\lambda_0(\tau_0) e^{L_1(\tau_0) - L_0(\tau_0)} \right] d\tau_0 \right] d\tau_1 \right] \cdots d\tau_{k-3} \right] d\tau_{k-2} \end{aligned} \tag{2.40}$$

When this result is substituted into Equation (2.37), the solution for the kth stage is obtained; namely,

$$\begin{aligned} p_k(t) = \int_0^t & \left[\lambda_{k-1}(\tau_{k-1}) e^{-L_{k-1}(\tau_{k-1})} \int_0^{\tau_{k-1}} \left[\lambda_{k-2}(\tau_{k-2}) e^{L_{k-1}(\tau_{k-2}) - L_{k-2}(\tau_{k-2})} \ldots \right. \right. \\ & \times \left. \left. \int_0^{\tau_1} \left[\lambda_0(\tau_0) e^{L_1(\tau_0) - L_0(\tau_0)} \right] d\tau_0 \right] d\tau_1 \right] \ldots d\tau_{k-2} \right] d\tau_{k-1} \end{aligned} \tag{2.41}$$

If it is assumed that $L_i(t) \ll 1, (i = 0, 1, 2, \ldots, k-1)$, then $e^{L_i(t)} \approx 1$, $e^{L_i(\tau_i) - L_{i-1}(\tau_i)} \approx 1$, and Equation (2.41) reduces to

$$p_k(t) = \int_0^t \lambda_{k-1}(\tau_{k-1}) \int_0^{\tau_{k-1}} \lambda_{k-2}(\tau_{k-2}) \ldots \int_0^{\tau_1} \lambda_0(\tau_0) d\tau_0 \ldots d\tau_{k-2} d\tau_{k-1} \tag{2.42}$$

The impact of the assumption that $L_i(t) \ll 1$ is discussed by Moolgavkar.[10] If it is assumed that each $\lambda_i(t)$ is independent of time, the integration implied by Equation (2.42) may be carried out to give

$$p_k(t) = \lambda_{k-1}\lambda_{k-2} \ldots \lambda_1 \lambda_0 \frac{t^k}{k!} \tag{2.43}$$

2.2.4 Effect of Dosage

Suppose that the transition probability λ_i is a function of both dosage and time, and let this dependency be denoted by $\lambda_i(t, d)$. In this case, Equation (2.42) implies immediately the following expression for $p_k(t, d)$,

$$p_k(t, d) = \int_0^t \lambda_{k-1}(\tau_{k-1}, d) \int_0^{\tau_{k-1}} \lambda_{k-2}(\tau_{k-2}, d) \ldots \int_0^{\tau_1} \lambda_0(\tau_0, d) d\tau_0 \ldots d\tau_{k-2} d\tau_{k-1} \tag{2.44}$$

Next consider the case where the transition function λ_i is independent of time and linearly dependent on dosage, and of the form:

$$\lambda_i(t, d) = \alpha_i + \beta_i d \tag{2.45}$$

where α_i and β_i are constants. Integration of Equation (2.44) under this condition yields,

$$p_k(t, d) = \left[(\alpha_{k-1} + \beta_{k-1} d)(\alpha_{k-2} + \beta_{k-2} d) \ldots (\alpha_0 + \beta_0 d) \frac{t^k}{k!} \right] \tag{2.46}$$

The importance of the assumption given by Equation (2.45) cannot be overemphasized because, as shown in subsequent developments, it leads to the implication that the probability $p(d)$ of cancer formation varies linearly with dose at very small doses (or as the dose d goes to zero). Although the linearity assumption is a common one in the analysis of physical systems, there is no mathematical requirement for making this assumption. A threshold dose could just as well have been postulated by assuming $\lambda_i(t, d)$ to be a step function instead of a linear function. For example, it could have been assumed that $\lambda_i(t, d)$ is of the following form:

$$\begin{aligned} \lambda_i(t,d) &= 0 \qquad 0 \le d \le d_p \\ \lambda_i(t,d) &= a_i + b_i d \qquad d > d_p \end{aligned} \tag{2.47}$$

where d_p is the threshold dose and a_i and b_i are constants.

2.2.5 Probability of the Formation of at Least One Tumor from N Independent Cell Lines

Equation (2.46) represents the probability of *one* cell in *one* animal progressing through the $0, 1, 2, \ldots, k-1$ stages to the kth stage and tumor formation. Assuming that an animal has N independent cell lines, and that the experimenter only observes the result (either at least *one* tumor or no tumor), it is desired to obtain an expression for the probability of the experimenter observing at least *one* tumor in time t for a given animal.

The probability $P(t)$ of observing at least *one* tumor at time t from the N independent cell lines is equal to one minus the probability $P_0(t)$ that all cells do not develop a tumor by time t; that is,

$$P(t) = 1 - P_0(t) \tag{2.48}$$

This expression is readily obtained by beginning with the fact that the sum of the probabilities of observing $X = 0,\ 1,\ 2, \ldots$ or N tumors in time t is equal to unity,

$$P(X = 0, t) + P(X = 1, t) + \ldots + P(X = N, t) = 1 \tag{2.49}$$

In order to simplify this expression the abbreviated notation is employed in which $P_R(t) = P(X = R, t)$, and $R = 0, 1, \ldots, N$. Thus Equation (2.49) becomes,

$$P_0(t) + P_1(t) + \ldots + P_N(t) = 1 \tag{2.50}$$

and since $P(t) = P(X \ge 1, t) = P_1(t) + \ldots + P_N(t)$, Equation (2.48) follows; that is,

$$P(t) = P_1(t) + P_2(t) + \ldots + P_N(t) = 1 - P_0(t) \tag{2.51}$$

As used here, $P_0(t) = P(X = 0; t)$, the probability that an animal having N cell lines will not have developed a tumor by time t. Also, observe that the variable X introduced above relates each outcome (tumors) of a random experiment with a number, and a variable of this type is called *random variable*. As used above, $P_R(t)$ $[P_R(t) = P(X = R, t)]$ is the probability of the specified outcome that exactly R tumors will be observed in a sequence of N independent Bernoulli trials [trials in which the outcome for each trial is either a success or a failure]. The probability $P_R(t)$ is given by the well-known binomial distribution formula (see Chapter 4),

$$P_R(t) = \left[\frac{N!}{R!(N-R)!}\right] p^R (1-p)^{N-R} \tag{2.52}$$

For convenience the dependency of the probability p on time has been dropped and

p = probability of success for any trial, or the probability that one particular cell line develops a tumor.

R = number of successes, or the number of tumors formed by all cell lines; $R = 0, 1, 2, 3, \ldots, N$.

N = the number of cell lines.

Thus, the probability that no tumors will develop by time t is obtained by setting $R = 0$ in Equation (2.52) and recalling that $0! = 1$, to give

$$P_0(t) = (1 - p)^N$$

This expression may be restated in the following form:

$$P_0(t) = e^{N \log_e (1-p)} \tag{2.53}$$

Since the probability p of a single cell line progressing to a tumor is exceedingly small, the term $\log_e (1 - p)$ in the above expression may be approximated with good accuracy by use of the first term of the series expansion of $\log_e (1 + x)$ [where $-1 < x \leq 1$] to give

$$\log_e (1 - p) \approx -p$$

Thus, Equation (2.53) reduces to

$$P_0(t) = e^{-Np} \tag{2.54}$$

Consequently, the probability of an experimenter observing at least *one* tumor by time t in an experiment involving *one* animal that has N cell lines is given by

$$P(t) = 1 - e^{-Np(t)} \tag{2.55}$$

The probability $p(t)$ is identically the same as the probability denoted by $p_k(t, d)$ in the multistage model [Equation (2.42)] for a single cell line exposed to a dose d. Therefore, the final result for the multistage model is that the probability of observing at least *one* tumor in *one* animal (or observing at least *one* tumor from all of the N cell lines of *one* animal) at dose d by time t is

$$P(X \geq 1, t; d) = P(t, d) = 1 - e^{-Np_k(t,d)} \tag{2.56}$$

2.2.6 Hazard Rate

Another quantity which is useful in the analysis of data is called the *incidence rate, specific hazard rate*, or simply the *hazard rate*. It is equal to the rate at which the tumor appears in previously tumor free tissue. More specifically the hazard rate $h(t)$ is defined as the rate of increase in the cumulative probability $P(t)$ of observing at least one tumor by time t divided by the probability that no tumor has been observed by time t. The probability of observing no tumors at time t is equal to $[1 - P(t)]$ where $P(t) = P(X \geq 1, t)$; see Equations (2.48) through (2.51). Since probabilities are conserved, it follows that the balance on $P(t)$ over the time period from t_n to $t_n + \Delta t$ is given by

$$\int_{t_n}^{t_n+\Delta t} [h(t)\,[1 - P(t)] - 0]\;dt = P(t)\Big|_{t_n+\Delta t} - P(t)\Big|_{t_n} \tag{2.57}$$

Application of the *mean value theorems* followed by the limiting process wherein Δt is allowed to go to zero and the recognition of the fact that t_n was arbitrarily selected yields the following differential equation upon rearrangement

$$\frac{dP(t)}{dt} - [1 - P(t)]\,h(t) = 0 \tag{2.58}$$

which is readily restated in the familiar form

$$h(t) = \frac{dP(t)}{dt}/[1 - P(t)]$$

Since $P(t)$ represents the cumulative probability $P(X \geq 1; t)$, it follows that at $t = 0, P(X \geq 0; 0) = 0$, since all cells are assumed to be in their normal state at time $t = 0$. Thus, the differential equation given by Equation (2.58) may be solved by separation of the variables followed by integration as follows:

$$\int_0^{P(t)} \frac{dP(\tau)}{1 - P(\tau)} = \int_0^t h(\tau)d\tau \tag{2.59}$$

Integration followed by rearrangement to the exponential form yields

$$P(t) = 1 - e^{-\int_0^t h(\tau)d\tau} = 1 - e^{-H(t)} \tag{2.60}$$

Comparison of the general result given by Equation (2.60), which is applicable for all models, with the result given by Equation (2.56) for the multistage model shows that the cumulative hazard rate for the multistage model is given by

$$H(t, d) = Np_k(t, d) \tag{2.61}$$

for the case where *one* animal having N cell lines is exposed to a daily dose d over time t.

When the transition rates are assumed to be linear functions of d as in Equation (2.45) and its corresponding form given by Equation (2.46), one obtains

$$H(t, d) = N\left[\prod_{i=0}^{k-1}(\alpha_i + \beta_i\,d)\right]\frac{t^k}{k!} \tag{2.62}$$

In many cases the time duration of the experiment is held fixed while the dosage is varied from one experiment to another. Since the product in Equation (2.62) can also be expressed as a power series, the multistage model is commonly stated in the following form and referred to as simply the multistage model or sometimes the Armitage-Doll[8] multistage model.

$$P(d) = 1 - e^{-H(d)} = 1 - \exp\left[-\sum_{i=0}^{k} q_i d^i\right] \tag{2.63}$$

where the number of cell lines N and the time period t have been included in the definitions of the $q_i' s$. For the single stage model, Equation (2.63) reduces to

$$P(d) = 1 - \exp\left[-(q_0 + q_1 d)\right] \tag{2.64}$$

Of all the proposed models for cancer formation, the multistage model is perhaps the most widely used.

2.2.7 The Armitage-Doll Multistage Model[8]

In evaluating the form of the multistage model given by Equation (2.63) from the general expression for $p_k(t,d)$ given by Equation (2.44), it was assumed that each of the transition rates $\lambda_i(t,d)$ is a function independent of time and linearly dependent on dosage. In some instances, one or both of these assumptions needs to be modified. For example, the dose level may be age-dependent and not constant over time. The starting point for these modifications is Equation (2.56) with $p_k(t,d)$ as given by Equation (2.44); namely,

$$P(t,d) = 1 - \exp\left[-N\int_0^t \lambda_{k-1}(\tau_{k-1},d)\int_0^{\tau_{k-1}} \lambda_{k-2}(\tau_{k-2},d)\right.$$

$$\left.\times \int_0^{\tau_1} \lambda_0(\tau_0,d)d\tau_0 \ldots d\tau_{k-2}d\tau_{k-1}\right] \tag{2.65}$$

This general form is often referred to as the Armitage–Doll multistage model.[8]

Any model which is explicitly represented as a function of time [e.g., $P(t,d)$] is referred to as a *time-to-response* or *time-to-tumor* model. For example, the Armitage-Doll model given by Equation (2.65) is a time-to-response model.

Since several different probabilities have been introduced in the above development, a summary of these probabilities and their interrelationship is presented at this point in the interest of avoiding confusion in subsequent developments. Thus, in summary, $p_k(t,d)$ [given by Equation (2.44)] denotes the probability that *one* cell [or *one* cell line] will pass through stages 0, 1, 2, ..., $k-1$ to stage k and to tumor formation as a consequence of having been exposed to a daily dose d over a fixed time period t. This probability [$p_k(t,d)$] becomes the *trial* or *test* probability in the determination of the probability $P(d)$ [Equations (2.56) and (2.63)] of *one* animal having N cell lines developing at least *one* tumor when exposed to the dose d over time period t. In Chapter 3 this probability [$P(d)$] becomes the trial or test probability $p(d)$ in the determination of the probability $P(X = r, d)$ of an experimenter observing exactly r tumors in an experiment in which n animals [each having

$p_k(d)$ = probability of *one* cell line developing *one* tumor in *one* animal. ⟶ $p_k(d)$ becomes the trial probability p in the calculation of the probability $P(d)$ of at least *one* tumor in N cell lines of *one* animal. ⟶ ⋯

⋯ ⟶ $P(d)$ becomes the trial probability p in the calculation of the probability $P(X = r)$ that an experimenter will observe exactly r animals that develop a tumor out of the n animals tested.

Figure 2.8 Flow Diagram of Probabilities Involved in Dose-Response Analysis of Animal Tests.

N cell lines] are exposed to a daily dose d over a fixed time period t. Further clarification of the progression of probabilities is provided by the flow diagram shown in Figure 2.8.

For a test involving n animals, one would expect to observe at least $nP(d)$ animals with at least one tumor [where $P(d)$ is given by Equation (2.63)] when the animals are exposed to a daily dose d over their lifetime. A continuation of this analysis leading to human risk assessment is presented in detail in Chapter 3.

2.2.8 The Multistage-Weibull Model

Let w denote the growth time required to form a tumor after the kth transformation has occurred. Assume that w is a constant and not a random variable. If t denotes the time required for the kth transition, then the total time to tumor T is given by

$$T = t + w$$

or

$$t = T - w \tag{2.66}$$

Then by use of Equations (2.60), (2.62), and (2.66), the following expression is obtained for the cumulative probability of the formation of a tumor in time T at dose d for an animal with N cell lines,

$$P(T, d) = 1 - \exp\left\{\left[-\prod_{i=1}^{k}(\alpha_{k-i} + \beta_{k-i}d)\right]\frac{(T-w)^k}{k!}\right\} \tag{2.67}$$

Note that the number of cell lines N has been absorbed in the definitions of the $\alpha's$ and $\beta's$. Also, $P(T, d)$ may be expressed as follows:

$$P(T, d) = 1 - \exp\left\{\left[-\sum_{i=0}^{k} q_i d^i\right]\frac{(T-w)^k}{k!}\right\} \tag{2.68}$$

2.2.9 The Hartley-Sielken Model

In a series of articles Hartley and co-workers [Hartley and Sielken,[11] and Hartley et al.[12]] proposed a model and demonstrated its application for the prediction of the *virtually safe dose levels* (or the more recent terminology *risk specific dose levels*) from animal tests. The form of this model is suggested by the form of the Armitage-Doll model given by Equations (2.60) through (2.63) and more generally in Equation (2.65) as well as the multistage-Weibull model given by Equation (2.68) in which the hazard function is seen to be a function of both dose d and time t. The Hartley-Sielken model in its simplest form consists of the assumption that the hazard function $h(t, d)$ may be expressed in product form; namely,

$$h(t, d) = g(d)f(t) \tag{2.69}$$

Thus, the cumulative hazard function $H(T, d)$ of the Hartley-Sielken model for the time T to tumor at dose d and for an animal having N cell lines is given by

$$H(T, d) = \int_0^T h(\tau, d)d\tau = \int_0^T g(d)f(\tau)d\tau = g(d)F(T) \tag{2.70}$$

where the dose d is independent of time. The function $g(d)$ is that part of the hazard function which depends on the dose d alone, while the function $F(T)$ is that part of the cumulative hazard function $H(T, d)$ which depends on the time to tumor T alone.

Equations (2.60) and (2.61) may be used to restate the Hartley-Sielken model in the form:

$$P(T, d) = 1 - \exp[-g(d)F(T)] \tag{2.71}$$

with the probability density function

$$p(T, d) = \frac{\partial P(T, d)}{\partial T} = g(d)f(T)\exp[-g(d)F(T)] \tag{2.72}$$

Furthermore, $P(T, d)$ is equal to the probability that *one* animal having N independent cell lines will develop at least *one* tumor when exposed to the daily dose d over the time period T. The most frequently used parameterization of the hazard function $H(T, d) = g(d)F(T)$ consists of

$$g(d) = \sum_{i=0}^{k} \alpha_i d^i \tag{2.73}$$

and

$$F(T) = \sum_{j=1}^{b} \beta_i T^i \tag{2.74}$$

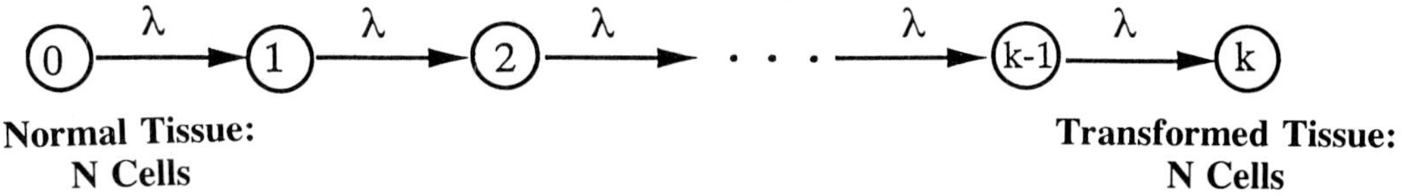

Figure 2.9 The Schematic Representation for the Multihit Model.

The product form assumes that hazard rates for different doses are proportional functions of time. If dose and time interact, then the more general non-product form of the cumulative hazard rate, $H(T, d)$, can be used. The usual parameterization of the non-product form of the cumulative hazard rate is

$$H(T, d) = \sum_{i=0}^{a} \sum_{j=1}^{b} K_{i,j} d^i T^j \tag{2.75}$$

2.2.10 The Multihit Models

Two developments of the multihit model are presented. Although these developments are based on entirely different suppositions, the final mathematical representations are identically the same.

The development of the multihit model consists of the development of an expression for the probability that *one* animal having N cells (or N cell lines) will develop at least *one* tumor caused by k hits in time t at dose d.

In the first development of the multihit model, it is supposed that at least k hits within the tissue containing the N cells are required for a response. That is, in this development, the multihit model consists of an expression for the probability that an entire collection of N cells will receive the k hits in time t at dose d.

$$P(tumor) = P(tissue\ containing\ N\ cells\ receives\ k\ hits) \tag{2.76}$$

Note that in the multihit model, each cell in the set N may experience a different number of hits; whereas, if in the multistage model the k transitions are attributed to k hits, one cell must receive k hits and these hits must occur in a specified order if the hits are physically different.

The number of hits occurring per unit time is a function of both the time t and the dose d. In the interest of simplicity, the development is carried out with the dose held fixed, and thus the number of hits becomes a function of the exposure time t at the fixed dose d.

The development of this model corresponds to the development of the *Poisson distribution process* for a *pure-birth process*. The initial state of the tissue is denoted by 0; after one hit the state is denoted by 1; ...; after k hits by k as shown in Figure 2.9.

The specific rate constant λ is assumed to be independent of time and dose. By use of the conservation balances demonstrated in the development of the multistage model, it is readily shown that the multihit model is represented by the following set of differential equations.

$$\frac{dP_0(t)}{dt} = -\lambda P_0(t) \tag{2.77}$$

$$\frac{dP_i(t)}{dt} = -\lambda P_i(t) + \lambda P_{i-1}(t) \qquad i = 1, 2, \ldots, k-1 \tag{2.78}$$

$$\frac{dP_k(t)}{dt} = \lambda P_{k-1}(t) \tag{2.79}$$

Note that in the multihit model the probability $P_i(t)$ refers to the whole tissue and not to a single cell line as $p_i(t)$ did in the multistage model. That is, $P_i(t)$ denotes the probability that the N cells have received i hits. Since the whole tissue of N cells must have received either 0 or $1, 2, \ldots, k$ hits, the probabilities $P_1, P_2, \ldots, P_k$ are conserved,

$$\sum_{i=1}^{k} P_i(t) = 1 \tag{2.80}$$

and the initial conditions are as follows:

$$P_0(0) = 1, \;\; P_i(0) = 0, \qquad i = 1, 2, \ldots, k \tag{2.81}$$

The above system of equations is readily solved in a consecutive manner by commencing with Equation (2.77). Separation of variables followed by integration yields

$$P_0(t) = e^{-\lambda t} \tag{2.82}$$

For $i = 1$, Equation (2.78) takes the following form on rearrangement

$$\frac{dP_1(t)}{dt} + \lambda P_1(t) = \lambda P_0(t) \tag{2.83}$$

The solution of this equation is given by the well–known relationship[9]

$$P_1(t) = e^{-\int \lambda dt} \left[\int e^{\int \lambda dt} \lambda P_0(t) dt + K \right] \tag{2.84}$$

where K is an arbitrary constant. After the expression given by Equation (2.82) for $P_0(t)$ has been substituted into Equation (2.84), the following results upon integration

$$P_1(t) = e^{-\lambda t} [\lambda t + K] \tag{2.85}$$

Since $P_1(0) = 0$, $K = 0$, and Equation (2.85) reduces to

$$P_1(t) = \lambda t e^{-\lambda t} \tag{2.86}$$

For $i = 2$, Equation (2.78) becomes

$$\frac{dP_2(t)}{dt} + \lambda P_2(t) = \lambda P_1(t). \tag{2.87}$$

As before,

$$P_2(t) = e^{-\int \lambda dt} \left[\int e^{\int \lambda dt} \lambda P_1(t) dt + K \right] \tag{2.88}$$

After the expression given by Equation (2.86) for $P_1(t)$ has been substituted into Equation (2.88), the following result is obtained by integration and evaluation of the arbitrary constant,

$$P_2(t) = \frac{(\lambda t)^2}{2} e^{-\lambda t} \tag{2.89}$$

Continuation of this procedure gives the Poisson probability distribution function for a pure birth process; namely,

$$P_{i-1}(t) = \frac{(\lambda t)^{i-1}}{(i-1)!} e^{-\lambda t} \qquad i = 1, 2, \ldots, k \tag{2.90}$$

The solution of Equation (2.79) is found by substituting Equation (2.90) for $i = k$ into Equation (2.79) followed by separation of the variables and integration to give

$$P_k(t) = \int_0^t \frac{\lambda(\lambda\tau)^{k-1} e^{-\lambda\tau}}{(k-1)!} d\tau = \int_{u=0}^{u=\lambda t} \frac{u^{k-1} e^{-u}}{(k-1)!} du \tag{2.91}$$

[Note the equivalence of the two integrals follows by making the change in variable $u = \lambda\tau$.] Since the development of Equation (2.91) was carried out at a fixed dose d, the parameter λ appearing in this equation can be a function of the dose d; that is, $\lambda = \lambda(d)$. Suppose, as is often the case, each experiment is carried out at a fixed dose d over a fixed length of time $t = T$. When the experiments are conducted in this manner, the upper limit λt in Equation (2.91) becomes

$$\lambda t = \lambda(d)T \tag{2.92}$$

Further suppose that $\lambda(d)$ is a linear function of d of the form: $\lambda(d) = ad$, where a is a constant. Let

$$\lambda(d)T = (aT)d = \lambda d \tag{2.93}$$

where in the interest of simplicity the symbol λ is used to represent the constant (aT). [Note this λ does not have the same meaning as the λ appearing on the left hand side of Equation (2.93).] Thus, Equation (2.91) becomes

$$P_k(T, d) = \int_{u=0}^{u=\lambda d} \frac{u^{k-1} e^{-u}}{(k-1)!} du \tag{2.94}$$

Since it is assumed that the probability of at least one tumor $P(T, d)$ is equal to the probability of a tissue of N cells receiving k hits, it follows that for the multihit model,

$$P(tumor) = P(T, d) = \int_{u=0}^{u=\lambda d} \frac{u^{k-1} e^{-u}}{(k-1)!} du \tag{2.95}$$

This function is called the *incomplete gamma function.*

An Alternate Development of the Multihit Model

An alternate derivation of the multihit model is based on the supposition that members of a population have different tolerances to a given dose d over a fixed time period $t = T$. Suppose that the response of the members of a population to a dose d is measured in terms of the tolerance τ. Further suppose that if

$$d \geq \tau, \quad \text{then } P(tumor) = 1 \tag{2.96}$$

and if

$$d < \tau, \quad \text{then } P(tumor) = 0 \tag{2.97}$$

The tolerance τ of each member of a population will vary. Suppose that the tolerance τ has a *gamma distribution*; that is, the probability density function is given by

$$f_\tau(\tau) = \begin{cases} \lambda^\alpha \tau^{\alpha-1} e^{-\lambda\tau}/\Gamma(\alpha) & \tau > 0 \\ 0 & \tau \leq 0 \end{cases} \tag{2.98}$$

where $\Gamma(\alpha)$ is the well-known *gamma function*, defined by

$$\Gamma(\alpha) = \int_0^\infty x^{\alpha-1} e^{-x}\, dx \qquad \alpha > 0 \tag{2.99}$$

For the case where α is equal to an integer k, the gamma function has the following property:

$$\Gamma(\alpha) = \Gamma(k) = (k-1)! \tag{2.100}$$

The probability that the tolerance lies between 0 and d is given by the cumulative distribution function evaluated at d, which is equal to the following integral of the probability density function [Equation (2.98)].

$$P(tumor) = P(\tau \leq d) = \int_0^d \frac{\lambda^k \tau^{k-1} e^{-\lambda\tau}}{(k-1)!} d\tau \tag{2.101}$$

This expression may be stated in the form given by Equation (2.95) by making a change of variable. Let

$$u = \lambda\tau \tag{2.102}$$

Then the incomplete gamma function is obtained.

$$P(tumor) = P(\tau \leq d) = \int_0^{\lambda d} \frac{u^{k-1} e^{-u}}{(k-1)!} du \tag{2.103}$$

Observe that Equations (2.95) and (2.103) are identical even though they were derived on the basis of different assumptions.

2.2.11 The One-Hit Model

If only one hit is required to produce a tumor in an animal having N cells (or N cell lines), the model is called the "one-hit model," and $k = 1$ in the multihit model. For this case, Equations (2.95) and (2.103) reduce to

$$P(tumor) = \int_0^{\lambda d} e^{-u}\, du$$

and thus, the cumulative probability given by Equation (2.103) becomes

$$P(tumor) = 1 - e^{-\lambda d} \tag{2.104}$$

The one-hit model is also a special case of the multistage model; see Equation (2.64).

2.2.12 The Probit Model

The probit model is based on the concept of tolerances introduced in Section 2.2.6 in the "Alternate Development of the Multihit Model." The formulation of the probit model makes use of the *cumulative normal distribution function* and the *standard normal distribution function*. Although these functions are treated in considerable detail in Chapter 4, the concepts needed in the development of the probit model are restated here.

Consider first the cumulative normal distribution function and its associated random variable X. In particular, the random variable X is said to be a *normal random variable* if the probability that it has a value lying between $-\infty$ and x is given by the cumulative normal distribution function,

$$P(X \leq x) = \int_{-\infty}^{x} \frac{\exp\left[-\frac{1}{2}\left(\frac{t-\mu}{\sigma}\right)^2\right]}{\sigma\sqrt{2\pi}}\, dt \tag{2.105}$$

where the parameters μ and σ^2 are the mean and the variance of the variable X (see Chapter 4).

When the change in variable $u = (t-\mu)/\sigma$ is made, Equation (2.105) can be expressed in terms of the *standard normal distribution function*; that is,

$$P(X \leq x) = P\left(\frac{X-\mu}{\sigma} \leq \frac{x-\mu}{\sigma}\right) = P(Z \leq z) = \int_{-\infty}^{z} \frac{e^{-u^2/2}}{\sqrt{2\pi}}\, du \tag{2.106}$$

The new random variable Z referred to as a *standard normal random variable* is defined by

$$Z = \frac{X-\mu}{\sigma} \tag{2.107}$$

and

$$z = \frac{x-\mu}{\sigma} \tag{2.108}$$

The above relationships are used in the development of the probit model which follows.

Suppose that an animal has a tolerance τ such that an individual in a population will develop a tumor if the logarithm of the dose d is equal to or greater than the logarithm of the tolerance τ, and will not develop a tumor if $\log \tau > \log d$. Further suppose that the common logarithm of the tolerance τ has a normal distribution with a mean μ and a variance σ^2. [This assumption is sometimes abbreviated by writing $\log_{10} \tau$ is $N(\mu, \sigma^2)$.] Thus, X and x in Equations (2.105) through (2.108) have been identified; namely,

$$X = \log_{10} \tau \;\; and \;\; x = \log_{10} d \tag{2.109}$$

Because $\log_{10} \tau$ is assumed to be normally distributed and an animal will develop a tumor if $\log_{10} \tau \leq \log_{10} d$, it follows from Equation (2.109) that the probability that a randomly selected member of the population will develop a tumor when the population is exposed to a dose d is given by

$$P(tumor) = P(\log_{10} \tau \leq \log_{10} d) = P\left(\frac{\log_{10} \tau - \mu}{\sigma} \leq \frac{\log_{10} d - \mu}{\sigma}\right) = P(Z \leq z) \tag{2.110}$$

Thus, in view of Equations (2.106) through (2.110), the probit model is given by

$$P(tumor) = P(Z \leq z) = \int_{-\infty}^{z} \frac{e^{-u^2/2}}{\sqrt{2\pi}}\, du \tag{2.111}$$

where as suggested by Equation (2.110)

$$Z = \frac{\log_{10} \tau - \mu}{\sigma}$$

$$z = \frac{\log_{10} d - \mu}{\sigma}$$

The upper limit z has been called the *probit* by Finney.[13] Thus, if the dose–response data can be represented by the probit model, a plot on normal probability paper of the proportion developing the specified response (tumor) versus the logarithm of the dose d will yield a straight line with slope $1/\sigma$ and intercept $-\mu/\sigma$.

2.2.13 The Logit Model

This model is applicable when the logarithm of the tolerance τ has a *logistic* distribution in which the probability density function is given by

$$f(\log_e \tau) = \frac{\beta e^{-[\alpha+\beta \log_e \tau]}}{[1 + e^{-[\alpha+\beta \log_e \tau]}]^2}; \quad \tau > 0 \tag{2.112}$$

where α and β are parameters. Thus, the probability that an individual having a tolerance τ and belonging to a population exposed to dose d will develop a tumor is given by

$$P(tumor) = P(\tau \leq d) = P\left(\log_e \tau \leq \log_e d\right)$$

The corresponding cumulative distribution function is given by

$$P(tumor) = P(\log_e \tau \leq \log_e d) = \int_{-\infty}^{\log_e d} \frac{\beta e^{-[\alpha+\beta \log_e \tau]}}{[1 + e^{-[\alpha+\beta \log_e \tau]}]^2} \, d \log_e \tau \tag{2.113}$$

After the indicated integration has been performed, one obtains

$$P(tumor) = P(\log_e \tau \leq \log_e d) = \frac{1}{1 + e^{-[\alpha+\beta \log_e d]}} \tag{2.114}$$

2.2.14 The Weibull Model

This model is applicable when the logarithm of the tolerance τ has an extreme value distribution in which the probability density function for τ is given by

$$f(\tau) = \alpha\beta\tau^{\beta-1} \exp[-\alpha\tau^{\beta}] \qquad \tau > 0 \tag{2.115}$$

where α and β are parameters. In the Weibull model, the probability that an individual having a tolerance τ and belonging to a population exposed to dose d will develop a tumor is given by the following cumulative distribution function,

$$P(tumor) = P(\tau \leq d) = \int_{0}^{d} \alpha\beta\tau^{\beta-1} \exp[-\alpha\tau^{\beta}] d\tau \tag{2.116}$$

so that

$$P(tumor) = 1 - \exp[-\alpha d^{\beta}] \tag{2.117}$$

The Weibull model can also be derived as a special case of the Armitage-Doll multistage model given by Equation (2.65). The cumulative distribution given by Equation (2.117) follows from Equation (2.65) if the transition rates $\lambda_i(t, d)$ are independent of time and dependent on the dose d alone,

$$\lambda_i(t, d) = \alpha_i d^{\beta_i} \tag{2.118}$$

where $\alpha_i > 0$, $\beta_i \geq 0$,

$$\alpha = N \prod_{i=0}^{k-1} \alpha_i \tag{2.119}$$

and

$$\beta = \sum_{i=0}^{k-1} \beta_i \tag{2.120}$$

2.2.15 The Generalized Multistage Model

This model consists of an expression for the probability that *one* cell (or *one* cell line) of *one* animal will develop a tumor from a daily dose d over a time period t.

Whittmore and Keller[5] proposed this model in response to some concerns that the multistage theory with $k > 2$ has some biological defects. The main one was the lack of any direct experimental evidence (at that time) that cancer occurs in more than two stages.

In the multistage theory only cells in the kth stage are assumed to multiply; whereas, in the generalized multistage theory, a cell in any stage i may produce an i-clone. In the generalized model, it is assumed that a cell in stage i produces an i-clone. Let x denote the age of an i-clone, which is just the time elapsed since its progenitor suffered its ith change. Note that x takes on the value zero each time a transition occurs. For example, at the instant an i-clone is formed from an $(i-1)$-clone, the newly formed i-clone has the age $x = 0$.

Let $p_i(x,t)$ denote the age distribution of i-clones at any time t, where $i = 0, 1, 2, \ldots, k$. That is, $p_i(x,t)$ denotes the relative likelihood that a cell is in stage i and has an i-clone of age x at time t, and it refers to any one of the N independent cell lines. Over a clone time Δx, the relative likelihood changes from $p_i(x,t)$ to $p_i(x+\Delta x, t)$. Also i-clones are lost by death at the rate $\mu_i(x,t)p_i(x,t)$ and by transition to $(i+1)$-clones at the rate $\lambda_i(x,t)p_i(x,t)$. Let the total rate at which i-clones are disappearing be denoted by $r_i(x,t)$. Then

$$r_i(x,t) = [\lambda_i(x,t) + \mu_i(x,t)]\, p_i(x,t) \tag{2.121}$$

Initially it is supposed that all cells are normal; that is,

$$p_0(0) = 1.$$

Furthermore, it follows from the assumption of no clones at time $t = 0$ that,

$$p_i(x,0) = 0, \quad i = 1, 2, \ldots, k \tag{2.122}$$

Since at any time t a cell either has no clones or has a clone of some age x (between 0 and t) in some stage i, it follows that

$$p_D(t) + \sum_{i=0}^{k} \int_0^t p_i(x,t)\, dx = 1 \tag{2.123}$$

or the $p_i(x,t)$'s and $p_D(t)$ [the probability of the death of a cell] are conserved over the clone age x and time t. Thus, a conservation balance on $p_i(x,t)$ over the time period from t_n to $t_n + \Delta t$ and the clone time from x_j to $x_j + \Delta x$ is given by

$$\int_{t_n}^{t_n+\Delta t} \left[\left[p_i|_{x_j,t} - p_i|_{x_j+\Delta x,t} \right] - \int_{x_j}^{x_j\Delta x} [r_i\, dx] \right] dt = \int_{x_j}^{x_j+\Delta x} \left[p_i|_{t_n+\Delta t,x} - p_i|_{t_n,x} \right] dx \tag{2.124}$$

where $r_i = (\lambda_i + \mu_i)p_i$. Beginning with the innermost terms and applying the *mean value theorems of integral and differential calculus* (see Appendix II) yields the following result

$$-\frac{\partial p_i(x,t)}{\partial x} - [\lambda_i(x,t)\mu_i(x,t)]\, p_i(x,t) = \frac{\partial p_i(x,t)}{\partial t} \tag{2.125}$$

To demonstrate the process by which this result was obtained, consider the first two terms in the integral on the left hand side of Equation (2.124). By the *mean value theorem of differential calculus* (see Appendix II),

$$p_i(x,t)\big|_{x_j,t} - p_i(x,t)\big|_{x_j\Delta x,t} = -\Delta x \frac{\partial p_i(x,t)}{\partial x}\bigg|_{x_j+\alpha_j(t)\Delta x,t} \tag{2.126}$$

where $\alpha_j(t)$ depends on t and is bounded, $0 \le \alpha_j(t) \le 1$. Next, by the *mean value theorem of integral calculus* (see Appendix II),

$$\Delta x \int_{t_n}^{t_n+\Delta t} \left[-\frac{\partial p_i(x,t)}{\partial x}\bigg|_{x_j+\alpha_j(\bar{t})\Delta x,\bar{t}} \right] dt = -\Delta x \Delta t \frac{\partial p_i}{\partial x}\bigg|_{x_j+\alpha_j(\bar{t})\Delta x,\bar{t}} \tag{2.127}$$

where $\bar{t} = t_n + \beta\Delta t$, $0 \le \beta \le 1$. For the third term,

$$-\int_{t_n}^{t_n+\Delta t} \int_{x_j}^{x_j+\Delta x} r_i \, dx\, dt = -\Delta x \int_{t_n}^{t_n+\Delta t} r_i\big|_{x_j+\gamma_1(t)\Delta x,t}\, dt \tag{2.128}$$

where $0 \le \gamma_1(t) \le 1$. Thus,

$$-\int_{t_n}^{t_n+\Delta t} \int_{x_j}^{x_j+\Delta x} r_i \, dx\, dt = -\Delta x \Delta t\, r_i\big|_{x_j+\gamma_1(\bar{t})\Delta x,\bar{t}} \tag{2.129}$$

where $0 \le \gamma_1(\bar{t}) \le 1$, and in this case $\bar{t} = t_n + \gamma_2\Delta t$, $0 \le \gamma_2 \le 1$. When the mean value theorems are applied to the right hand side of Equation (2.124), one obtains

$$\begin{aligned} \int_{x_j}^{x_j+\Delta x} \left[p_i\big|_{t_n+\Delta t,x} - p_i\big|_{t_n,x} \right] dx &= \Delta t \int_{x_j}^{x_j+\Delta t} \frac{\partial p_i}{\partial t}\bigg|_{t_n+\delta_1(x)\Delta t,x} dx \\ &= \Delta t \Delta x \, \frac{\partial p_i}{\partial t}\bigg|_{t_n+\delta_1(\bar{x})\Delta t,\bar{x}} \end{aligned} \tag{2.130}$$

where $0 < \delta_1(\bar{x}) < 1$, $\bar{x} = x_j + \delta_2\Delta x$, $0 \le \delta_2 \le 1$. Substitution of the results given above into Equation (2.124) followed by division by $\Delta x \Delta t$ and then passing to the limit as Δt and Δx go to zero gives the final expression, Equation (2.125), upon recognition that Δt and Δx were arbitrarily selected in the t and x domains of interest.

Numerical methods are now available for solving systems of partial differential equations such as Equation (2.125) by use of computers. However, a knowledge of the functional forms of the parameters $\lambda_i(x,t)$ and $\mu_i(x,t)$ would be required .

2.2.16 Summary

Expressions have been developed for the probability $p(t, d)$ that *one* cell (or *one* cell line) of *one* animal will develop a tumor from the exposure to a daily dose d over a time period t. Also, expressions have been developed for the probability $P(d)$ that one animal having N cell lines will develop a tumor as the result of the exposure to a daily dose d over a time period t. These probability functions $[P(d)]$ are used in the determination of the probability $[P(X = r)]$ that exactly r animals out of n test animals will develop tumors as a consequence of having been exposed to a daily dose d over time t. In the next chapter, these probabilities $[P(X = r)]$ are used in the estimation of virtually safe doses from dose-response data as well as the risk assessment for exposed populations.

PROBLEMS

1. Given the following ordinary linear differential equation with variable coefficients

$$\frac{dy}{dx} + P(x)y = Q(x)$$

The initial condition is

$$y = y_0 \quad \text{at} \quad x = 0$$

Show that the solution that satisfies the differential equation and the initial condition is given by

$$y = e^{-\int_0^x P(\tau)d\tau}\left[\int_0^x e^{\int_0^\tau P(\omega)d\omega} Q(\tau)d\tau + y_0\right]$$

Hint: Use the integrating factor $e^{\int_0^x P(\tau)d\tau}$.

2. Use the concept of the conservation of probabilities and the *mean value theorems* [see Appendix II] to show that the model in Figure 2.7 is described by the set of differential equations given by Equations (2.27) thorough (2.30).

3. Instead of the assumptions made in the integration of Equation (2.41); namely,
   (a) $L_i(t) << 1$ $(i = 0, 1, 2, \ldots, k-1)$, $e^{L_i(t)} \approx 1$ and $e^{L_i(\tau_i)-L_{i-1}(\tau_i)} \approx 1$
   (b) $\lambda(t) = \lambda_i$, a constant independent of time t,
   suppose that the following assumptions are made:
   (a) $L_i(t) << 1$ $(i = 0, 1, 2, \ldots, k-1)$, $e^{L_i(t)} \approx 1 + L_i(t)$, $e^{L_i(\tau_i)-L_i(\tau_i)} \approx 1 + (L_i(\tau_i) - L_{i-1}(\tau_i))$
   (b) $\lambda_i(t) = \lambda_i$ and $\rho_i(t) = \rho_i$, where both λ_i and ρ_i are indepedent of time t.
   Show that a power series of the third degree would have been obtained on integration of Equation (2.38) instead of the first degree. [This result suggests that Equation (2.43) represents only one term of the power series which would have been obtained under the second set of assumptions.]

4. Suppose that instead of assuming that $\lambda_i(t, d)$ varies linearly with the dose d over all doses as implied by Equation (2.45), it is supposed that $\lambda_i(t, d)$ has a threshold with respect to dose as given by Equation (2.47). Obtain the solution to Equation (2.44) corresponding to the threshold assumption.

5. To illustrate the use of the binomial distribution formula given by Equation (2.52), the following problem which may be solved by use of this formula is posed. Supposed 10 fair coins are tossed in a single throw. The probability that any one of them will show a head (success) is of course $p = 1/2$. What is the probability that (a) no coins will show heads (success), (b) 4 successes, (c) 5 successes, (d) 6 successes, and (e) 10 successes?

6. The purpose of this problem is to demonstrate that the development of the differential equation for the *hazard rate* on the basis of its definition and the fact that cumulative probabilities are conserved is analogous to the development of the differential equation for the net rate of reaction of a chemical compound on the basis of the definition of the rate and the law of conservation mass.

   (a) Let the net rate of appearance of a given compound B by a chemical reaction be defined as moles of compound B appearing per unit time per unit volume of the reacting mixture; that is,

$$r_B = \frac{(\textit{moles of B appearing})}{(\textit{time})(\textit{volume})}$$

   Furthermore, suppose that compound B is being produced in a perfectly mixed batch reactor. [In such a chemical reactor, it is supposed that B is produced at the same rate throughout the volume of the reacting mixture at any time t]. Let the moles of B in the reactor at any time t be noted by N_B and the volume of the reacing mixture by V. For definiteness, suppose that N_B is expressed in gram moles and that the molecular weight of B is denoted by M_B(g/g mol). Thus, the mass of B in the reactor at any time t is equal to $N_B M_B$. Make a mass balance over the time period from t_n to $t_n + \Delta t$ and show that in the limit as Δt approaches zero, one obtains,

$$r_B = \frac{1}{V}\frac{dN_B}{dt}$$

   (b) The hazard rate may be defined as the increase (or appearance) of the cumulative probability $P(t)$ of observing at least one tumor per unit time per unit of probability that no tumor has been observed at time t. The probability that no tumor has been observed by time t is equal to $1 - P(t)$, where

$$P(t) = P(X \geq 1, t) = P_1(t) + P_2(t) + \ldots + P_N(t)$$

   and

$$1 = \sum_{i=0}^{N} P_i(t)$$

   Thus if the hazard rate is defined by

$$h(t) = \frac{(\textit{increase in cumulative probability of observing at least one tumor})}{(\textit{time})(\textit{probability that no tumor has been observed})}$$

show that

$$h(t) = \frac{1}{1 - P(t)} \frac{dP(t)}{dt}$$

Also show that

$$h(t) = \frac{1}{P_0(t)} \frac{dP(t)}{dt}$$

(c) The definition of rates in terms of either appearance (increase) of disappearance (decrease) is arbitrary regardless of whether the entity (moles or probability) is appearing or disappearing. For example, suppose that instead of defining rates r_B and $h(t)$ in terms of appearance, they are defined in terms of disappearance as follows:

$$r_B = \frac{\textit{(moles of B disappearing)}}{\textit{(time)(volume)}}$$

$$h(t) = \frac{\textit{(decrease in cumulative probability of observing at least one tumor)}}{\textit{(time)(probability that no tumor has been observed)}}$$

Show that when r_B and $h(t)$ are defined as in terms of disappearance, the following differential equations are obtained

$$r_B = -\frac{1}{V} \frac{dN_B}{dt}$$

$$h(t) = -\frac{1}{1 - P(t)} \frac{dP(t)}{dt}$$

or

$$h(t) = -\frac{1}{P_0(t)} \frac{dP(t)}{dt}$$

7. Show that the multistage model given by Equation (2.46) may be stated in terms of the product form of the hazard rate [Equation (2.70)] proposed by Hartley and Sielken.[12]

8. If the movement of molecules A and B are independent and if it is supposed as in the kinetic theory of gases (see for example Reference 16), that a collision between A and B is a necessary condition for the chemical reaction

$$A + B \longrightarrow \textit{Products}$$

to occur between the two molecules A and B. Furthermore, it is postulated that the rate of reaction is proportional to the number of these collisions per unit time. Show that by the use of Theorem 4.2 of Chapter 4 that the rate of reaction may be expressed in terms of probabilities as follows:

$$r_p = K p_A p_B$$

where K is a proportionality constant and p_A is equal to the probability that A will collide with B and p_B is equal to the probability that B will collide with A. *Hint:* In the application of Theorem 4.2, observe that the movement of molecule A is independent of the movement of molecule B.

9. Consider the following variation of the multistage model for one animal with N cell lines. Supposed that when the number of cells in state 0 is very small, the rate at which cells are transformed from state 0 to state 1 is proportional to the square of the probability $p_0(t)$ that a cell is in state 0, that is,

$$r_{P_0} = \lambda_0 p_0^2(t) \tag{A}$$

and when the number of cells in state 0 is large, the rate of transformation of a cell from state 0 to state 1 is proportional to the first power of $p_0(t)$,

$$r_{P_0} = \tilde{\lambda}_0 p_0(t) \tag{B}$$

Show that this behavior can be explained by use of the following mechanism which was proposed for chemical reactions by Lindermann[14] and Hinshelwood.[15] Let A_0 denote the number (or moles) of normal cells in state 0 at any time t. Then suppose

$$A_0 + A_0 \underset{k_1'}{\overset{k_1}{\rightleftharpoons}} A_0^* + A_0 \tag{C}$$

where A_0^* is the number of activated normal cells at any time t. Next suppose that the activated normal cells A_0^* are transformed to cells in state 1 by the unidirectional reaction

$$A_0^* \xrightarrow{k_2} A_1 \tag{D}$$

Further suppose that the number of cells in the activated state at any time is very small and that a pseudo-steady-state[16] exists whereby the activated cells are transformed to state 1 at approximately the same rate at which they are formed; that is,

$$\frac{dA_0^*}{dt} \approx 0 \tag{E}$$

and that

$$k_1 \ll k_2$$

No restriction is placed on k_1' other than that it be finite and positive. Let the probability that a cell be in the activated state be denoted by $p_0^*(t)$. Suppose that the rates for the disappearance of probabilities can be treated in a manner analogous to that for the chemical reactions. That is, as a consequence of the pseudo-steady-state assumption given by Equation (E),

$$r_{A_0^*} = -\frac{dA_0^*}{dt} \approx 0 = k_1 A_0^2 - k_1' A_0^* A_0 - k_2 A_0^*$$

or

$$r_{p_0^*} = -\frac{dp_0^*(t)}{dt} \approx 0 = \alpha_1 p_0^2(t) - \alpha_1' p_0^*(t) p_0(t) - \alpha_2 p_0^*(t)$$

where it has been assumed that the probabilities $p_0(t)$ and $p_0^*(t)$ have the same role in the rate expresion $r_{p_0^*}$ that A_0 and A_0^* have in the rate expression $r_{A_0^*}$.

10. This problem is another variation of the multistage model for an animal having N cell lines. Suppose that cells in the normal state 0, denoted by A_0, react with an oxidant B to form an adduct C by the reaction

$$A_0 + B \longrightarrow C \tag{A}$$

The rate at which adduct cells C are formed, r_C, or the rate of disappearance of normal cells A_0, r_{A_0} is observed to be

$$r_C = r_{A_0} = kA_0 \tag{B}$$

The corresponding rate of disappearance (or decrease) in probability $p_0(t)$ is given by

$$r_{PC} = r_{P0} = \lambda_0 p_0(t) \tag{C}$$

To explain this result the following psuedo-steady-state mechanism is proposed

$$A_0 \xrightarrow{k_1} A_0^* \tag{D}$$

$$A_0^* + B \xrightarrow{k_2} C \tag{E}$$

where

$$k_1 \ll k_2$$

or the rate of change of the probability that a cell be in the activated normal state A_0^* is approximately equal to zero, $dp_0^*(t)/dt \approx 0$. Use this mechanism to verify the result given by Equation (C). Suppose that the amount of oxidant B remains nonzero with respect to time.

11. The concept of the rate-controlling step is frequently used as a mechanism in chemical kinetics in the analysis of a system of chemical reactions.[16] In this approach, one of the reactions is assumed to be the rate-controlling step ($r_2 \neq 0$) while the other reactions are assumed to be in dynamic equilibrium ($r_1 = 0$). Consider the following system of reactions

$$A_0 + A_0 \underset{k_1'}{\overset{k_1}{\rightleftharpoons}} A_0^* + A_0 \qquad r_1 = 0$$

$$A_0^* \underset{k_2'}{\overset{k_2}{\rightleftharpoons}} A_1 \qquad r_2 \neq 0$$

Suppose that the second reaction is the rate-controlling step and that the first is in dynamic equilibrium. Further assume that all of A_0 is either in the form of A_0 or A_1, which is assured by assuming $k_1/k_1' \ll 1$, $k_1 < k_2$, and $k_1' > k_2'$. That is by these assumptions

$$r_1 = k_1 A_0^2 - k_1' A_0^* A_0 = 0$$

and

$$r_2 = k_2 A_0^* - k_2' A_1$$

or

$$r_{p,1} = \alpha_1 p_0^2(t) - \alpha_1' p_0^*(t) p_0(t) = 0$$

and

$$r_{p,2} = \alpha_2 p_0^*(t) - \alpha_2' p_1(t)$$

Show that

$$r_{p0} = \lambda_0 p_0(t) - \lambda_0' p_1(t)$$

where

$$\lambda_0 = \frac{\alpha_1}{\alpha_1'}\alpha_2 \qquad \lambda_0' = \alpha_2'$$

12. Suppose that in problem 11, it is assumed that only a very small amount (a negligible amount) of A_0 is in the form of A_0^*, and thus $p_0(t) + p_1(t) \approx 1$, since $p_0^*(t) \approx 0$.

(a) Use this fact and the fact that a conservation balance on $p_1(t)$ gives the following expression for the net rate of appearance of $p_1(t)$,

$$r_{p,2} = \frac{dp_1(t)}{dt}$$

to show that

$$p_0(t) = \left[\frac{1}{\lambda_0 + \lambda_0'}\right]\left[\lambda_0' + \lambda_0 e^{-(\lambda_0+\lambda_0')t}\right].$$

(b) Show that at equilibrium ($t \to \infty$)

$$p_0(\infty) = \frac{\lambda_0'}{\lambda_0 + \lambda_0'}$$

NOTATION

A = mass of salt tracer introduced at $x = 0$ at $t = 0$; see Figure 2.1

cm = centimeter; 100 cm = *1 meter (m);* 1000 m = 1 *kilometer (km)*

d = daily dose in mass or volumetric units per animal or unit weight of the animal

$f(x)$ = function of x as indicated by the context; also used to denote the probability density function

$F(z)$ = cumulative distribution function which is equal to the area under the curve of $f(x)$ [the probability density function] from $x = -\infty$ to $x = z$; also $dF(z)/dz = f(z)$, defined by Equation (2.5)

g = symbol for *one gram mass;* 1000 *milligrams (mg)* = 1 *gram (g);* 1000 g = *1 kilogram (kg)*

$h(t)$ = hazard rate which is defined as the instantaneous rate at time t of the increase in the cumulative probability $P(t)$ of observing at least one tumor by time t divided by the probability that no tumor has been observed by time t

$H(t)$ = cumulative hazard rate: $H(t) = \int_0^t h(\tau)d\tau$

$K_{i,j}$ = parameter in the expression for the cumulative hazard rate given by Equation (2.75)

$L_i(t)$ = a function of t for stages $i = 0, 1, \ldots, k-1$; $L_i(t) = \int_0^t \rho_i(\tau)d\tau$

N = number of independent cell lines

p = probability of success for any trial, or the probability that one particular cell line develops a tumor

$p_i(t)$ = probability that a cell is in stage $i (i = 0, 1, \ldots, k-1)$ at time t

$p_D(t)$ = probability that the death of a cell occurs at time t at each of the stages $i = 0, 1, \ldots, k-1$

$P(t)$ = probability of observing at least one tumor at a time t from N independent cell lines

$P_R(t) = P(X = R, t)$ = probability of observing a tumor in each of R cell lines $R = 0, 1, \ldots, N$

q = volumetric flow rate of water past a plane at any location x of the system shown in Figure 2.1

q_i = parameters of the multistage model; see Equation (2.63)

$r_i(t)$ = rate of disappearance of probability

R = number of successes, or the number of cell lines in which tumors are found, $R = 0, 1, \ldots, N$

S = cross-sectional area; see Figure 2.1

Δt = increment of time

t = time

T = time to tumor

w = growth time required to form a tumor after transition to the kth stage has occurred

x = variable; used to denote distance in Figure 2.1 and clone age in Equation (2.121); also used to denote the number associated with an outcome from the sample space Ω of an experiment by the random number X

X = random variable which is a function that associates a number x with an outcome in the sample space Ω of an experiment

z = number associated with an outcome from the sample space Ω of an experiment by the standard normal random variable Z

Z = standard normal random variable defined in terms of the random variable X

GREEK LETTERS

α = constant

β = constant

$\Gamma(\alpha)$ = gamma function; defined by Equation (2.99)

$\lambda_i(t)$ = transition probability function of time for a cell in stage i $(i = 0, 1, \ldots, k-1)$

$\mu_i(t)$ = death rate probability function of time for a cell in stage i ($i = 0, 1, \ldots, k-1$); also, μ is used to denote the mean

$\rho_i(t) = \lambda_i(t) + \mu_i(t)$

σ = square root of the variance; see Equation (2.105)

τ = dummy variable

$\Psi(x)$ = concentration in mass per unit volume

REFERENCES

1. Welch, N.E., L.D. Durbin, and C.D. Holland "Mixing on Valve Trays and in Downcomers of a Distillation Column," *A.I.Ch.E. Journal*, **10**, 373 (1964).
2. Holland, C.D. *Unsteady State Processes with Application in Multicomponent Distillation*, Prentice Hall, Inc., Englewood Cliffs, N.J. (1966).
3. Iversen, S. and N. Arley "On the Mechanisms of Experimental Carcinogenesis,"*Acta Path. Microbiol. Scand.*, **27**, 773 (1950).
4. Arley, N. and S. Iversen "On the Mechanisms of Experimental Carcinogenesis, III. Further Development of the Hit Theory of Carcinogenesis," *Acta Path. Microbiol. Scand.*, **30**, 21 (1952).
5. Whittemore, Alice and J.B. Keller "Quantitative Theories of Carcinogenesis," *SIAM Review*, **20**, (No. 1), 1 (1978).
6. Muller, H.J. "Radiation Damage to Genetic Material," *Science Progress*, **7**, 93 (1951).
7. Nordling, C.O. "A New Theory on the Cancer Inducing Mechanisms," *British J. of Cancer*, **7**, 68 (1953).
8. Armitage, P. and R. Doll "The Age Distribution of Cancer and a Multistage Theory of Carcinogenesis," *British J. of Cancer*, **8**, 1 (1954).
9. Sokolnikoff, I.S. and E.S. Sokolnikoff, *Higher Mathematics for Engineers and Physicists*, Second Edition, McGraw-Hill Book Company, Inc., New York, N.Y. (1941).
10. Moolgavkar, S.H., "The Multistage Theory of Carcinogenesis and the Age Distribution of Cancer in Man," *J. Nat'l. Cancer Inst.*, **61**, (No. 1), 49 (1978).
11. Hartley, H.O. and R.L. Sielken, Jr. "Estimation of Safe Doses in Carcinogenic Experiments," *Biometrics*, **33**, 1 (1977).
12. Hartley, H.O., H.D. Tolley, and R.L. Sielken, Jr. "The Product Form of the Hazard Rate Model in Carcinogenic Testing," in *Statistics and Related Topics*, Editors: M. Csörgö, D.A. Dawson, J.N.K. Ras, and A.K. Md. E. Saleh, North-Holland Publishing Company (1981).
13. Finney, D.J. *Probit Analysis*, 3rd ed., Cambridge University Press, New York, N.Y. (1971).
14. Lindermann, F.A., *Trans. Faraday Soc.*, **17**, 298 (1922).
15. Hinshelwood, C.N., *Proc. Roy. Soc.*, **A113**, 230 (1927).

16. Holland, C.D. and R.G. Anthony, *Fundamentals of Chemical Reaction Engineering*, 2nd ed., Prentice-Hall, Englewood Cliffs, N.J. (1989).

3

Quantifying Virtually Safe Doses and Risk Assessment

A number of methods have been proposed for the use of animal data in the prediction of a *virtually safe dose* or more recently described as a *risk specific dose*. Of the methods that have been proposed only three are described herein in detail. The first method, proposed by Mantel and Bryan,[1] is presented because of its historical significance and because of the concepts introduced in this method. The second method presented is the one which is now used by the Environmental Protection Agency (EPA).[2] The third method appears to be the most general method which has been proposed. This method consists of an analysis of the experimental results, which does not rely on policy assumptions such as those utilized by Mantel and Bryan[1] and the EPA.[2] All of the methods for estimating virtually safe doses are based on the models developed in Chapter 2 for the probability $P(X \geq 1)$ that *one* animal having N cell lines will develop at least *one* tumor from an exposure to a daily dose d over a fixed time period.

In the interest of simplicity in the development and demonstration of these methods, it is supposed that the time period for all experiments is fixed and that the dose per day d is held fixed throughout the course of the experiment. Also, the transport process of the dose from the point of intake to the possible tumor site is neglected; that is, the dose at the tumor site is assumed to be proportional to the administered dose.

In the animal experiments commonly conducted for quantifying dose–response relationships, a fixed daily dose d is administered to a group of n animals over a fixed time period T, and the number of animals r that develop a tumor is noted. For example, suppose 3 animals develop tumors out of a total of 10 animals tested ($r = 3, n = 10$). This information is used to answer the question of primary interest to society, and that is: what is the probability that an animal will develop a tumor when exposed to the dose d? More importantly, what is the probability that a human from a given population will develop a tumor when exposed to a given dose? The answer to the latter question is deferred until the end of the chapter. The answer to the first question regarding the probability of an animal developing a tumor may be determined by use of expressions describing the probabilities of different outcomes of a binomial experiment, provided that the experiments satisfy the following conditions:

(a) The experiment consists of n trials (or n animals) with n fixed in advance.

(b) The trials are identical, and each trial can result in the same two outcomes, success or failure. [Each animal is identical and can experience the same two outcomes, it may develop a tumor (regarded as a success) or it may not develop a tumor (regarded as a failure).]

(c) The trials are independent; the outcome of one trial does not influence any other. [The development of a tumor by any one animal in no way influences the development of tumors in any of the other animals.]

(d) The probability of success p of each individual trial is constant from trial to trial.

If the experiments satisfy these conditions, they are said to be *binomial experiments*. The *binomial formula** for computing the probability of a given outcome in a binomial experiment follows. In particular, the probability of occurrence of exactly r successes and $(n - r)$ failures in n identical trials is given by

$$P(X = r) = \frac{n!}{r!(n-r)!} p^r (1-p)^{n-r} \tag{3.1}$$

where

n = total number of binomial trials, or the total number of animals used in a given experiment;

p = trial probability (probability of success), or the probability that an animal will develop a tumor;

---

* An intuitive development of the binomial formulas given by Equations (3.1) and (3.2) is presented in Chapter 4. Since the applications of these formulas are virtually independent of their development, the developments were deferred until Chapter 4 in order to avoid distracting from their application.

r = number of successes, or the number of animals that develop tumors among the n animals used in the given experiment;

X = binomial random variable relating an experimental outcome to the number of successes observed.

If it is desired to find the probability that as many as $r = 3$ animals will develop tumors (that is, the probability that 0, 1, 2, or 3 animals will develop tumors), the following *cumulative binomial distribution function** is applicable.

$$P(X \leq r) = \sum_{i=0}^{r} \binom{n}{i} p^i (1-p)^{n-i} \qquad (3.2)$$

where

$$\binom{n}{i} = \frac{n!}{i!(n-i)!}$$

This formula is used in the analysis of experimental results as discussed below.

3.1 BOUNDING A VIRTUALLY SAFE DOSE BY THE METHOD OF MANTEL AND BRYAN[1]

Mantel and Bryan[1] recognized that an absolutely safe dose (one which is noncarcinogenic) of any chemical could not be determined statistically. Instead of insisting on absolute safety, they recommended that some level of risk be specified regardless of how small. Furthermore, in the Mantel-Bryan method, an arbitrarily high statistical assurance level was specified, and finally a rule for extrapolation from observed data points to the virtually safe dose was given.

In the approach proposed by Mantel and Bryan,[1] the experimental data are utilized to determine the largest trial probability which can be reasonably expected. The development of the concepts for the selection of the largest trial probability which can be reasonably expected is initiated by use of the following example.

Example 3.1. Suppose that a binomial experiment is used to test a given substance for its carcinogenicity. Of the total of 10 animals used in the experiment, 3 developed tumors. Thus $n = 10$, and $r = 3$ in Equation (3.1), and the probability $P(X = 3)$ of observing exactly $r = 3$ tumors is seen to depend on the trial probability p that an animal will develop a tumor. To emphasize that the probability $P(X = 3)$ of the experimenter observing exactly 3 tumors depends on the individual probability p, the notation $L(p) = P(X = r)$ is used, and $L(p)$ is called the *likelihood function*; that is,

$$L(p) = P(X = 3) = \binom{n}{r} p^r (1 - p)^{n-r} \tag{3.3}$$

(a) Find the value of the individual probability p that maximizes the probability (or likelihood) of observing exactly 3 tumors. This value of p is the *most probable value* of p and is called the *maximum likelihood estimate* of p.

(b) Corresponding to the most probable value of p found in Part (a), find the probability that exactly 3 out of 10 animals will develop tumors.

Solution

(a) An analysis of the function $L(p)$ for $0 < r < n$ shows that as p is increased from $p = 0$ to $p = 1$, $L(p)$ increases from $L(0) = 0$ (at $p = 0$) to its maximum value, and then decreases to $L(1) = 0$ (at $p = 1$). Thus, the p found by setting $\partial L(p)/\partial p = 0$ and solving the resulting expression for p corresponds to the maximum value of $L(p)$. This value of p maximizes the probability of observing exactly 3 tumors. For convenience, let

$$l(p) = \log_e L(p)$$

Then

$$l(p) = \log_e \binom{n}{r} + r \log_e p + (n - r) \log_e(1 - p) \tag{3.4}$$

Thus, when $\partial l(p)/\partial p = 0$, it follows that

$$\frac{\partial l(p)}{\partial p} = \frac{\partial \log_e L(p)}{\partial p} = \frac{1}{L(p)} \frac{\partial L(p)}{\partial p} = 0 \tag{3.5}$$

Consequently, the p found by use of Equation (3.5) is the one that maximizes $L(p)$. This value of p may be found by any one of many search procedures which are available in the numerical literature. Because of the simplicity of this example, Equation (3.5) may be solved directly for p as follows. Differentiation of Equation (3.4) and setting the derivative equal to zero as implied by Equation (3.5) yields,

$$0 = 0 + \frac{r}{p} + \frac{n - r}{1 - p}(-1) \tag{3.6}$$

When this expression is solved for p, one obtains

$$p = \frac{r}{n} = \frac{3}{10} = 0.3 \tag{3.7}$$

which is the *Maximum Likelihood Estimate* of p; i.e., the most probable value of the trial probability p corresponding to the test result ($n = 10, r = 3$).

(b) The maximum value of the likelihood $L(p)$ is the one given when the most probable value $p = 0.3$ is substituted in Equation (3.3); namely,

$$L(p = 0.3) = \frac{10!}{3!7!}(0.3)^3(0.7)^7 = 0.2668 \tag{3.8}$$

The above procedure is commonly referred to as the *Maximum Likelihood Method.* Although only 3 animals out of the 10 animals in the above example developed tumors, other outcomes could be expected if additional experiments had been carried out. It is reasonable to expect that in some of the experiments, fewer than 3 animals would develop tumors and in others, more than 3 animals would develop tumors. From the standpoint of protecting the public, it is desired to find the largest trial probability that can be reasonably expected. The determination of this probability makes use of the following observations. First, for any trial probability p, the probabilities $P(X = r)$ of observing $r = 0, 1, 2, 3$ and $r = 4, 5, 6, 7, 8, 9, 10$ tumors have the sum of unity; that is,

$$\begin{aligned} P(X \le 10) = {} & \Big[P(X = 0) + P(X = 1) + P(X = 2) + P(X = 3)\Big] \\ & + \Big[P(X = 4) + \cdots + P(X = 10)\Big] = 1 \end{aligned} \tag{3.9}$$

Since the sums within the brackets are recognized as $P(X \le 3)$ and $P(X \ge 4)$, Equation (3.9) may be restated as follows:

$$P(X \le 10) = \Big[P(X \le 3)\Big] + \Big[P(X \ge 4)\Big] = 1 \tag{3.10}$$

For a trial probability of $p = 0.3$, the terms of Equation (3.9) may be evaluated by use of Appendix III to give

$$\begin{aligned} P(X \le 10) = {} & \Big[0.0282 + 0.1211 + 0.2335 + 0.2668\Big] \\ & + \Big[0.2001 + 0.1029 + 0.0368 + 0.0090 + 0.0014 + 0.0001 + 0.0000\Big] = 1 \end{aligned}$$

Thus,

$$P(X \le 10) = \Big[0.6496\Big] + \Big[0.3494\Big] = 1 \tag{3.11}$$

and the two terms $P(X \le 3)$ and $P(X \ge 4)$ in Equation (3.11) have the following corresponding values

$$\begin{aligned} P(X \le 3) &= 0.6496 \qquad (\text{for } p = 0.3) \\ P(X \ge 4) &= 0.3494 \qquad (\text{for } p = 0.3) \end{aligned} \tag{3.12}$$

Table 3.1 Variation of $P(X \leq 3)$ and $P(X \geq 4)$ for Example 3.1.

p	$P(X \leq 3)$	$P(X \geq 4)$
0.3	0.650	0.350
0.4	0.382	0.618
0.5	0.172	0.828
0.6	0.055	0.945
0.7	0.011	0.989
0.8	0.004	0.996
0.9	0.001	0.999

Thus, when $p = 0.3$, there is a 64.96 percent chance that 3 or fewer animals will develop tumors and a 34.94 percent chance that 4 or more will develop tumors. As the trial probability, p, is increased, $P(X \leq 3)$ decreases and $P(X \geq 4)$ increases as shown in Table 3.1.

To reflect the probability that additional tests could have resulted in 4 or more tumors, the value of the trial probability may be considered at any higher level. Observe, for example, that at $p = 0.7$, there is a 98.9 percent chance $[P(X \geq 4) = 0.989]$ that 4 or more tumors would be observed. This 98.9 percent chance is also called the *98.9 percent assurance or confidence level* that the trial probability is not greater than $p = 0.7$. Equivalently, $p = 0.7$ is the observed value of a *98.9 percent upper confidence limit* on the trial probability. In other words, the confidence level associated with the statement that the trial probability p is less than or equal to 0.7 is 98.9 percent. In practice it is customary to fix the confidence level and then find the corresponding value of the trial probability. For example, Mantel and Bryan[1] used a high confidence level of 99 percent in the analysis of their results.

In the next step of the Mantel-Bryan[1] extrapolation procedure, the *standard normal distribution function* is used to relate the trial probability found as described above to the dose. A review of some of the underlying assumptions involved in this step follows.

In experiments of the type described by Example 3.1, it is assumed that the members of a group of n animals used in the test may possess different tolerances to a given chemical. Those animals having tolerances below a given dose level respond by developing tumors and those having higher tolerances do not respond. Such responses are known as *all-or-nothing* or *quantal*.

Suppose that an animal has a tolerance τ such that an individual of a population will develop a tumor if the logarithm of the tolerance τ is equal to or less than the logarithm of the dose d, $(\log_{10} \tau \leq \log_{10} d)$. Further suppose that the common logarithm of the tolerance τ has a normal distribution with a mean μ and a variance σ^2. On the basis of this assumption, the probability P that a member of the population will develop a tumor when administered a dose d is given by the *standard normal distribution function* (see Chapter 2),

$$P(tumor) = P(Z \leq z) = \int_{-\infty}^{z} \frac{\exp(-u^2/2)}{\sqrt{2\pi}}\, du \tag{3.13}$$

where

$$Z = \frac{\log_{10} \tau - \mu}{\sigma}$$

and

$$z = \frac{\log_{10} d - \mu}{\sigma}$$

In the Mantel and Bryan[1] extrapolation method, the 99 percent upper confidence limit, say p_i^*, is determined for the fraction p_i of the members in the experiment i ($i = 1, 2, \ldots, m$) that have a tolerance equal to or less than the dose d_i in that experiment. The value of z_i is determined such that

$$p_i^* = \int_{-\infty}^{z_i} \frac{\exp(-u^2/2)\, du}{\sqrt{2\pi}} \tag{3.14}$$

where

$$z_i = \frac{\log_{10} d_i - \mu}{\sigma}$$

The next feature of the Mantel-Bryan method is the assumption of a very low risk of 1 tumor in a group of 100 million subjects. The corresponding tolerance z_0 is computed by use of Equation (3.13); namely,

$$10^{-8} = \int_{-\infty}^{z_0} \frac{\exp(-u^2/2)}{\sqrt{2\pi}}\, du \tag{3.15}$$

The final feature of the Mantel and Bryan[1] procedure is the technique used to extrapolate to the *virtually safe dose* (VSD). In particular, the extrapolation from each (z_i, d_i) to (z_0, d_0) is effected by use of the following linear function in $\log_{10} d_i$, assuming a slope of unity (i.e., assuming $1/\sigma = 1$).

$$z_i = \log_{10} d_i - \mu$$

Then, the candidate for the virtually safe dose d_0 is found as follows:

$$z_i - z_0 = (\log_{10} d_i - \mu) - (\log_{10} d_0 - \mu)$$

or

$$\log_{10} \frac{d_i}{d_0} = z_i - z_0 \tag{3.16}$$

which is readily solved for the dose d_0. In this case the dose d_0 would be the virtually safe dose for a 1 in 100 million risk; that is a risk of 10^{-8}.

Based on a number of observations of dose–response relationships, Mantel and Bryan[1] believed $1/\sigma = 1$ to be a lower bound on the slope $1/\sigma$, and hence the d_0 given by Equation (3.16) corresponds to a lower bound on the virtually safe dose.

To demonstrate the application of the Mantel and Bryan[1] method, the example presented by these authors in their original paper is used. This example, presented in Table 3.2, is based on the experimental results reported by Bryan and Shimkin.[3]

Example 3.2 Illustration of the Mantel-Bryan Method [Taken from N. Mantel and W.R. Bryan, by courtesy of *Journal of the National Cancer Institute*, 27 (No. 2), 455 (1961)].

Statement After a single injection of methylcholanthine into mice at the different dose levels shown below and after a fixed time period, the number of mice that developed tumors was noted. Find the virtually safe dose by the Mantel-Bryan method corresponding to a 99 percent upper confidence limit on the test probability and a risk of 1 in 100 million or 10^{-8}.

d Dose (*mg/mouse*)	r/n (*Number of tumor bearing animals/Number of mice*)
0.000244	0/158
0.000975	0/79
0.00195	0/38
0.0039	0/19
0.0078	3/17
0.0156	6/18
0.0312	13/20
0.0625	17/21
0.125	21/21

Solution The method of Mantel and Bryan consists of the following stepwise procedure.

Step 1 The 99 percent upper confidence limit p^* on the trial probability p for each experiment may be computed directly or looked up in a table for $P(X = r)$; see for example, Appendix III, Ref. 4. To illustrate the procedure, the 99 percent upper confidence p^* for a typical test [$d = 0.0312\,mg/mouse, r = 13$, and $n = 20$] is determined. For a 99 percent confidence level, p^* is the value of the trial probability p such that $P(X \geq 14) = 0.99$, or equivalently $P(X \leq 13) = 0.01$. Since $P(X \leq 13) + P(X \geq 14) = 1$, the same value of the trial probability p must satisfy both functions and may be computed by use of either one of them. Thus,

$$0.01 = P(X \leq 13) = \sum_{i=0}^{i=13} \binom{20}{i} p^i (1-p)^{20-i} \tag{3.17}$$

The value of p required to satisfy this function may be found in a set of tables for the *cumulative binomial distribution function* (see Appendix III or Reference 4). The value so obtained is

$$p = 0.872$$

Thus, the 99 percent upper confidence limit is $p^* = 0.872$.

Step 2 The value of the trial probability found in Step 1 is used to compute z, a measure of the tolerance of the animals to the dose d, by use of Equation (3.14).

$$0.872 = \int_{-\infty}^{z} \frac{\exp(-u^2/2)}{\sqrt{2\pi}} du \tag{3.18}$$

From the tables for the standard normal random distribution function (see Appendix IV),

$$z = 1.136$$

Step 3 The corresponding candidate for the virtually safe dose (VSD) is found use by use of Equation (3.16). In order to use this equation, the value of z_0 corresponding to some specified low risk is required. Mantel and Bryan[1] specified a risk of 1 tumor in a group of 100 million subjects. For this case Equation (3.15) is applicable,

$$10^{-8} = \int_{-\infty}^{z_0} \frac{\exp(-u^2/2)}{\sqrt{2\pi}} du$$

The corresponding value of z_0 is

$$z_0 = -5.612$$

Thus, Equation (3.16) becomes

$$\log_{10} \frac{0.0312}{d_0} = 1.136 - (-5.612) = 6.748$$

and

$$d_0 = \frac{0.0312}{5,597,576} = 5.5738 \times 10^{-9} mg/mouse \tag{3.19}$$

The values of p_i^*, z_i, and d_0 shown in Table 3.2 were determined as illustrated above.

Table 3.2 Calculated Values p_i^*, z_i, and d_0 for Example 3.2.

Dose (*mg/mouse*)	p_i^* (99 percent Upper Confidence Limit on Test Probability)	z_i (Tolerance Measure)	d_0 (VSD)
0.000244	0.0288	−1.899	4.73×10^{-8}
0.000975	0.0566	−1.584	9.14×10^{-8}
0.00195	0.1141	−1.205	7.64×10^{-8}
0.0039	0.2151	−0.789	5.86×10^{-8}
0.0078	0.480	−0.050	2.14×10^{-8}
0.0156	0.729	0.610	9.36×10^{-9}
0.0312	0.872	1.136	5.57×10^{-9}
0.0625	0.958	1.728	2.86×10^{-9}

Mantel and Bryan recommended that the virtually safe dose (VSD) be taken as the maximum value obtained for d_0. Examination of Table 3.2 shows that the VSD is given by

$$\text{VSD} = 9.14 \times 10^{-8} mg/mouse \tag{3.20}$$

3.2 BOUNDING A VIRTUALLY SAFE DOSE (VSD) BY THE EPA METHOD

The method presently used by the EPA to bound the virtually safe dose (VSD) from a given set of experiments such as those presented in Table 3.2 was described by Anderson et al.[2] in 1981. At present the multistage model is employed by the EPA to represent the trial probabilities; namely,

$$p(d) = 1 - \exp[-(q_0 + q_1 d + q_2 d^2 + \cdots + q_k d^k)] \tag{3.21}$$

Note that Equation (3.21) is obtained by replacing $P(d)$ of Equation (2.63) of Chapter 2 by the trial probability $p(d)$ for each of the n animals in an experiment. The basis for this substitution is as follows. $P(d)$ in Equation (2.63) of Chapter 2 denotes the probability of *one* animal having N cell lines developing at least *one* tumor as a result of having been exposed to a daily dose d over a fixed time period. The probability $P(d)$ becomes equal to the trial probability $p(d)$ (or simply p) in Equation (3.1) for the calculation of the probability $P(X = r)$ of an experimenter observing exactly r tumors in an experiment involving n animals exposed to a daily dose d over a fixed time period, where each animal has N independent cell lines.

For illustrative purposes, the linearized form of the multistage model is used in the following development,

$$p(d) = 1 - \exp[-(q_0 + q_1 d)] \tag{3.22}$$

Suppose that i experiments ($i = 1, 2, \ldots, m$) are carried out independently and that in each experiment i, a dose d_i [$i = 1, 2, \ldots, m$] is administered to a group of n_i ($i = 1, 2, \ldots, m$) animals, and after a fixed time period for all experiments, the number of animals X_i ($i = 1, 2, \ldots, m$) that have developed tumors is observed to be r_i ($i = 1, 2, \ldots, m$). For each experiment i, the probability $P(X_i = r_i)$ that an experimenter will observe exactly $X_i = r_i$ animals develop a tumor out of the n_i tested is given by Equation (3.1). The trial probability p_i in Equation (3.1) is equal to $p(d_i) = 1 - \exp[-(q_0 + q_1 d_i)]$. Thus, for m experiments, there are m equations ($i = 1, 2, \ldots, m$) of the form of Equation (3.1) namely, $P(X = r_1), P(X_2 = r_2), \ldots, P(X_m = r_m)$ involving the two unknown parameters q_0 and q_1. Thus, the problem to be solved is to find that set of parameters q_0 and q_1 such that the probability of the experimenter observing all outcomes $(X_1 = r_1, X_2 = r_2, \ldots, X_m = r_m)$ is maximized. Since the experiments are carried out independently, it follows from *Theorem 4.2* of Chapter 4 that

$$\begin{aligned} &P(\textit{observing m outcomes: } X_1 = r_1, X_2 = r_2, \ldots, X_m = r_m) \\ &\qquad = P(X_1 = r_1)P(X_2 = r_2) \cdots P(X_m = r_m) \end{aligned}$$

This function $P(\ldots)$ is called the *likelihood function* and denoted by $L(q_0, q_1)$. Thus when each $P(X_i = r_i)$ is replaced by its equivalent given by Equation (3.1), one obtains

$$L(q_0, q_1) = \prod_{i=1}^{m} \binom{n_i}{r_i} p_i^{r_i} (1 - p_i)^{n_i - r_i} \tag{3.23}$$

When each p_i in Equation (3.23) is replaced by its equivalent as given by Equation (3.22), the following result is obtained.

$$L(q_0, q_1) = \prod_{i=1}^{m} \binom{n_i}{r_i} \{1 - \exp[-(q_0 + q_1 d_i)]\}^{r_i} \{\exp[-(q_0 + q_1 d_i)]\}^{n_i - r_i} \tag{3.24}$$

Thus, the set $(\hat{q}_0, \hat{q}_1)$ that maximizes the probability that an experimenter will observe the outcomes $(X = r_1, X = r_2, \ldots, X = r_m)$ is that set that maximizes $L(q_0, q_1)$. [A further discussion of this method which is called the *Maximum Likelihood Method* is given in Chapter 4.] The values of q_0 and q_1 required to maximize $L(q_0, q_1)$ may be found by use of the technique shown in Chapter 4 or by one of the many optimization techniques which are described in the numerical literature.

After q_0 and q_1 have been estimated by use of the Maximum Likelihood Method, the estimated value of $p(d)$ at $d = 0$, called the *background probability*, may be found by setting $d = 0$ in Equation (3.22) to give

$$\hat{p}(0) = 1 - \exp(-\hat{q}_0) \tag{3.25}$$

Thus, Equation (3.22) may be rearranged to the following form:

$$\hat{p}(d) - \hat{p}(0) = [1 - \hat{p}(0)][1 - \exp(-\hat{q}_1 d)] \tag{3.26}$$

The virtually safe dose (VSD) is determined on the basis of a specified value of the *Added Risk** which depends on policy decisions, cost/benefits, etc. *Added Risk* is defined as follows:

$$p(\text{VSD}) - p(0) = \textit{Added Risk} \tag{3.27}$$

where

$$\textit{Added Risk} = \textit{specified number; say } 10^{-4}, 10^{-6}, \textit{ or } 10^{-8}$$

When this definition of Added Risk is combined with Equation (3.26) for d =VSD, one obtains

$$\textit{Added Risk} = [1 - \hat{p}(0)][1 - \exp(-\hat{q}_1 \hat{\text{VSD}})] \tag{3.28}$$

For a specified value of the Added Risk the corresponding Maximum Likelihood Estimate $\hat{\text{VSD}}$ of the VSD is found by use of Equation (3.28).

A digression at this point is made to point out that some investigators base the VSD on the specification of the *Extra Risk*, which is defined as follows:

$$\frac{p(\text{VSD}) - p(0)}{1 - p(0)} = \textit{Extra Risk} \tag{3.29}$$

When this definition is combined with Equation (3.22) for d =VSD one obtains

$$\frac{p(\text{VSD}) - p(0)}{1 - p(0)} = \textit{Extra Risk} = [1 - \exp(-q_1 \text{VSD})] \tag{3.30}$$

Thus, *Extra Risk* refers to the response rate among the portion of the population that would not have a spontaneous occurence of the response. *Added Risk* on the other hand, refers to the response rate in the whole population as opposed to a portion of the population. However, since the background $p(0)$ is usually much less than unity, there is little difference in the two definitions.

The formula for *Extra Risk* is based on Abbott's formula[4] for incorporating an independent *spontaneous* or *background* response rate into the total response rate at a given dose d. In Abbott's formula, the total probability of observing the specified carcinogenic response at dose d, $p(d)$, is the sum of the background response rate, $p(0)$, that is assumed to be independent of the effects of dose, plus $(1 - p(0))$ times the probability of developing the specified carcinogenic response given that a spontaneous response will not occur

$$p(d) = p(0) + [1 - p(0)]\textit{Extra Risk}$$

* The two quantities defined by Equations (3.27) and (3.29) as *Added Risk and Extra Risk* are very similar, but obviously different. Confusion exists in the literature because *Excess Risk* is frequently used to mean either of these. Note, however, as the background probability approaches zero, they all become identical.

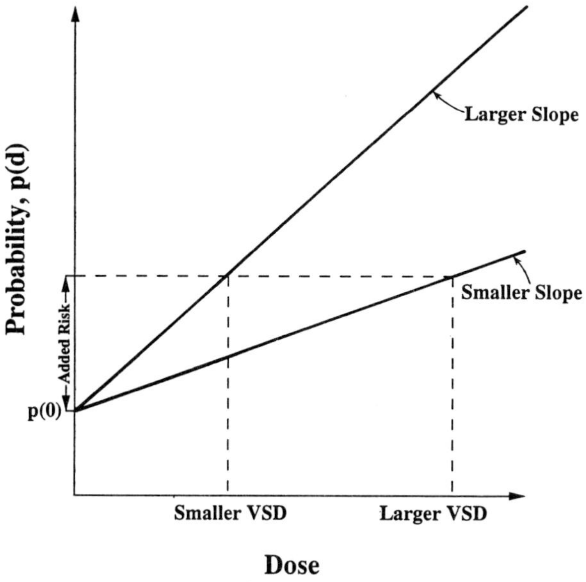

Figure 3.1 The Impact of the Slope of the Probability $p(d)$ on the VSD for a Specified Added Risk

where *Extra Risk* depends on the dose d rather than the specific dose $d = VSD$ as in Equation (3.29).

Instead of using the Maximum Likelihood Estimate of the VSD as given by Equation (3.28), a more conservative value is used by the EPA. In the EPA method, the VSD is found by use of a procedure that involves increasing the slope of $p(d)$. Observe that as the slope of $p(d)$ increases, the corresponding value of the VSD decreases as shown in Figure 3.1.

The procedure for increasing the slope of $p(d)$ as described by Anderson[2] follows. The value of q_1 is increased from its original value [the one found by maximizing $L(q_0, q_1)$] by successive increments. For each of the altered values of q_1, denoted by q_1^*, the corresponding q_0^* is found by the Maximum Likelihood Method with q_1 fixed at q_1^*. Observe that as q_1^* is increased, the slope of $p(d)$ increases (see Figure 3.1), and the corresponding value of VSD decreases.

For each set of the parameters $(\hat{q}_0, \hat{q}_1), (q_0^*, q_1^*)_1, \ldots, (q_0^*, q_1^*)_j$, the maximum likelihood function $L(q_0^*, q_1^*)$ is evaluated. The above procedure is continued until the largest q_1^* is found such that the set (q_0^*, q_1^*) satisfies the following condition that corresponds to a specified 95 percent upper confidence limit

$$-2\log_e\left[\frac{L(q_0^*, q_1^*)}{L(\hat{q}_0, \hat{q}_1)}\right] \le \chi^2_{1,\,0.90} = 2.71 \tag{3.31}$$

where $\chi^2_{1,\,0.90}$ = the 90th percentile value of the *chi-square distribution* for 1 degree of freedom. Thus, in this manner, the maximum slope q_1^* which satisfies the condition given by Equation (3.31) is found. This q_1^* is the largest slope not statistically detectable as being inconsistent with the experimental data using a particular statistical criterion. Then, this set (q_0^*, q_1^*) of parameters is used to evaluate the corresponding VSD_L^*, and this VSD_L^* is a lower bound on the true value of VSD.

The Added Risk curve corresponding to the set of parameters (q_0^*, q_1^*) is referred to as the 95 percent *upper confidence limit curve on risk.* The set of parameters (q_0^*, q_1^*) for the 95 percent *lower confidence limit curve on risk* is obtained in the same manner as that described for the 95 percent upper confidence limit curve on risk except that instead of increasing q_1 by successive increments, it is decreased by successive increments and the corresponding value of q_0 determined by the Maximum Likelihood Method. A 95 percent upper confidence limit VSD_U^* on the VSD can be obtained from the 95 percent lower confidence limit curve on risk.

To illustrate the application of the above equations in the determination of the VSD by the EPA method, the following numerical example is used.

Example 3.3 Illustration of the EPA Method. [This example is based on the experimental results reported in *National Toxicology Program Technical Report 398 on the Perinatal Toxicity and Carcinogenicity of Ethylene Thiourea (ETU) in F-344 Rats and B6C3F1 Mice*, Research Triangle, North Carolina.]

Statement In the following animal tests, the animals received the daily doses indicated over a fixed number of days, and the number of animals that developed tumors was noted.[5]

d Dose (ppm/day)	r/n (Number of tumor bearing animals/Number of mice)
0	9/99
100	4/28
333	136/150
1000	97/100

(a) Estimate the parameters (q_0, q_1) of the multistage model by use of the Maximum Likelihood Method.

(b) On the basis of an Added Risk= 10^{-6} compute the Maximum Likelihood Estimate of the VSD.

(c) Use the procedure described above Equation (3.31) to find the maximum and minimum values of q_1^* and the corresponding values of q_0^* that satisfy the 95 percent confidence limit condition, expressed by Equation (3.31).

(d) On the basis of the values of q_0^* and q_1^* found in Part (c) and an Added Risk$= 10^{-6}$, find VSD_L^* and VSD_U^* corresponding to the 95 percent lower and upper confidence limits.

Solution

(a) To fit the experimental results presented in Example 3.3, the linearized form of the multistage model [Equation (3.22)] was used. The estimated values of the parameters denoted by $\hat{q}_0$ and $\hat{q}_1$ as given by the Maximum Likelihood Method are as follows:

$$\hat{q}_0 = 0.087481$$
$$\hat{q}_1 = 0.005122$$

A graph of the data and the fitted model values [that is, the function $p(d)$ given by Equation (3.22) for the set of estimated parameters $(\hat{q}_0, \hat{q}_1)$] is presented in Figure 3.2.

(b) The estimates of the q's found in Part (a) are used to find the VSD corresponding to a specified value of the Added Risk $= 10^{-6}$ by use of Equation (3.28). The value of $(1 - \hat{p}(0))$ appearing in Equation (3.28) is evaluated by use of Equation (3.25) as follows:

$$1 - \hat{p}(0) = \exp(-\hat{q}_0) = 0.9162$$

By use of this result, Equation (3.28) may be solved for $\widehat{\text{VSD}}$ to give

$$\widehat{\text{VSD}} = 0.000213$$

[Because of the differences in small numbers involved in the intermediate calculations, several significant figures were carried.]

(c) By use of the procedure described above Equation (3.31), the maximum and minimum slopes q_1^* and the corresponding values of q_0^* which satisfied the condition given by Equation (3.31) for the 95 percent upper and lower confidence limits were found. The values so obtained for the 95 percent upper confidence limit on Added Risk were:

$$q_0^* = 0.056191$$
$$q_1^* = 0.005769$$

(d) On the basis of an Added Risk $= 10^{-6}$ and the parameters q_0^* and q_1^* found in Part (c) for the 95 percent upper confidence limit on Added Risk, Equation (3.28)

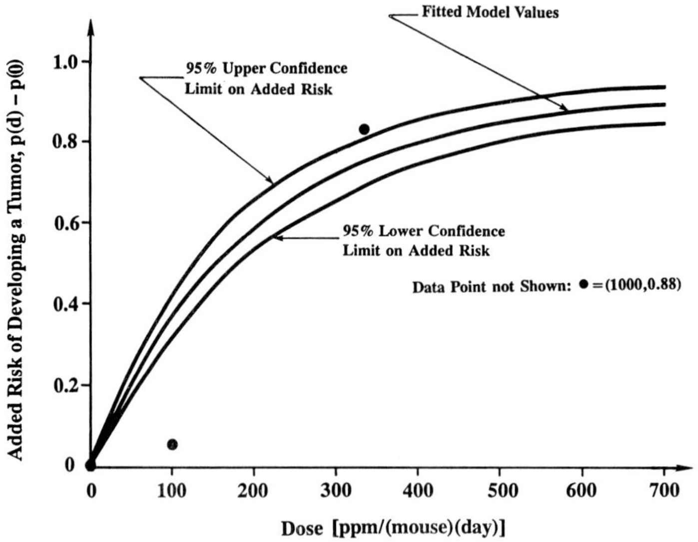

Figure 3.2 Graphs of the Curve Fits of the Experimental Data for Example 3.3. [Based on data taken from Reference 5. The parameters $q_0, q_1, \ldots, q_k$ for this and the other examples presented herein were estimated by use of the computer program, GEN.T, courtesy Sielken, Inc., Bryan, TX.]

may be solved for the corresponding VSD_L^* in the same manner as described in Part (b) to give

$$\text{VSD}_L^* = 0.00018$$

for the 95 percent lower confidence limit on the VSD.

The parameters q_0^*, and q_1^* for the 95 percent lower confidence limit on Added Risk were also determined,

$$q_0^* = 0.12396$$
$$q_1^* = 0.00446$$

and for an Added Risk $= 10^{-6}$, the virtually safe dose corresponding to the 95 percent upper confidence limit on the VSD was:

$$\text{VSD}_U^* = 0.000254$$

When the multistage model and the models corresponding to the 95 percent upper and lower confidence limits can be represented by a linearized form of the multistage model, their curves generally lie close together as shown in Figure 3.2.

Although the agreement between the $\hat{\text{VSD}}$ (the Maximum Likelihood Estimate) and VSD_L^* and VSD_U^* (the lower and upper bounds) is good for this particular example, these values may differ widely when the data are curve fit by use of the nonlinearized form of the multistage model as shown by some subsequent examples.

To illustrate the case where the nonlinear form of the multistage model given by Equation (3.21) is required to adequately describe the experimental results, the VSD was determined by the EPA method for Example 3.4 shown below.

Example 3.4 Illustration of the EPA Method for a Nonlinear Multistage Model. [Based on Battelle, Columbus Laboratories, "A Chronic Inhalation Toxicity Study in Rats and Mice Exposed to Formaldehyde." Battelle, Columbus Laboratories, Columbus, Ohio [*Chemical Industry Institute of Toxicology (CIIT) (1982).*]

Statement Different groups of rats were exposed to formaldehyde by inhalation for 6 hours per day, and 5 days per week for up to 24 months for the purpose of determining the probability of a rat developing a nasal cavity squamous cell carcinoma. The number in each group that developed tumors at each dose level was noted.[6] A summary of these results follows.

d Dose(ppm/day)	r/n (Number of tumors/Number of animals)
0.0	$0/199$
2.0	$0/200$
5.6	$2/200$
14.3	$103/199$

(a) Find the Maximum Likelihood Estimates of the parameters of the multistage model (linear, quadratic, or cubic) that gives the best fit of the data.

(b) Use the estimates of the parameters found in Part (a) for the multistage model to plot the probability function $p(d)$ versus the dose d.

(c) Find the Maximum Likelihood Estimate of the VSD corresponding to an Added Risk = 10^{-6}.

Solution

(a) In this case, the cubic form of the multistage model ($k = 3$) given by Equation (3.21) was needed to fit the curve to the experimental results. The estimated values of the parameters found by the Maximum Likelihood Method were as follows:

$$\hat{q}_0 = 0, \ \ \hat{q}_1 = 0, \ \ \hat{q}_2 = 0, \ \ \hat{q}_3 = 2.3286437 \times 10^{-4}$$

(b) A graph of the data and the curve based on the Maximum Likelihood Estimates of the parameters is presented in Figure 3.3. In this case, Equation (3.21)

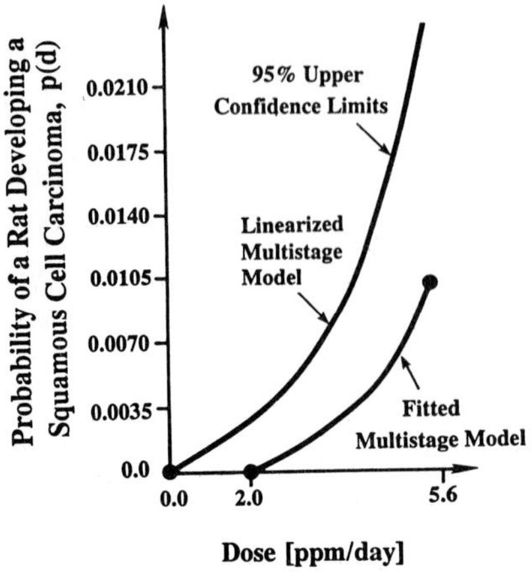

Dose (ppm)	Ratio: 95% Upper Confidence Limit / Fitted Model Value
5.6	2
2.0	41
1.0	368
0.5	3,140
0.1	417,000
0.01	423,000,000

Data Point not Shown: ● = (14.3,0.52)

Figure 3.3 Probability of a Rat Developing a Nasal Cavity Squamous Cell Carcinoma versus Dose, Example 3.4. [Based on data taken from Reference 6. Curve fit parameters by courtesy of Sielken, Inc.]

reduces to

$$\hat{p}(d) = 1 - e^{-\hat{q}_3 d^3} \approx \hat{q}_3 d^3$$

(c) Since $\hat{q}_0 = 0$, the background probability $\hat{p}(0) = 0$. Thus, for an Added Risk$= 10^{-6}$, the corresponding Maximum Likelihood Estimate of the VSD is given by

$$10^{-6} = [2.3286437 \times 10^{-4}][\hat{\text{VSD}}]^3$$

Thus,

$$\hat{\text{VSD}} = 0.163$$

3.3 DETERMINATION OF THE CONFIDENCE LIMITS ON RISK FOR EXAMPLE 3.4

For nonlinear multistage models, the problem of maximizing the slope q_1 subject to the 95 percent upper confidence limit constraint [Equation (3.31)] is different from that described above for the linear multistage models. In this case, the set of parameters $\mathbf{q}^*[\mathbf{q}^* = \{q_0^*, q_1^*, q_2^*, q_3^*\}]$ is found which maximize the Added Risk$= p(d) - p(0)$ at a small specified dose d' (in the region of regulatory interest) subject to the condition of constraint given by the multiparameter form of Equation (3.31) [see Equation (3.33)]. This approach for maximizing the slope q_1 may be stated as a maximization problem in which it is desired to find the $\mathbf{q}^*$ at a fixed $d = d'$ which gives the largest value of the Added Risk [Equation (3.32)] for which the general condition of constraint [Equation (3.33)] is satisfied;

that is,

$$\textit{maximize}: \quad f(d', \mathbf{q}^*) = p(d', \mathbf{q}^*) - p(q_0) \tag{3.32}$$

$$\textit{subject to}: \quad -2\log_e\left[\frac{L(\mathbf{q}^*)}{L(\hat{\mathbf{q}})}\right] \le \chi^2_{1,0.90} = 2.71 \tag{3.33}$$

where

$$\mathbf{q}^* = \{q_0^*, q_1^*, q_2^*, \ldots, q_k^*\}$$
$$\hat{\mathbf{q}} = \{\hat{q}_0, \hat{q}_1, \hat{q}_2, \ldots, \hat{q}_k\}$$

Many search techniques are available in standard texts on optimization for solving problems of this type. The general approach of these optimization techniques is to search over all possible values of $q_0, q_1, \ldots, q_k$ by some prescribed procedure for the set $\mathbf{q}^*$ that maximizes $f(d', \mathbf{q}^*)$ and satisfies the condition of constraint given by Equation (3.33) within a prescribed limit. Although a nonlinear form of $p(d)$ may be maximized in the above procedure, the final fit for function $p(d, \mathbf{q}^*)$ is commonly referred to as the "linearized model" because the linear term having the coefficient q_1^* usually dominates because of the small value of d' at which the maximization process is carried out.

For example, the parameters so obtained are as follows for the 95 percent upper confidence limit on Added Risk (and at $d' = 0.1$ ppm).

$$q_0^* = 0$$
$$q_1^* = 1.2091 \times 10^{-3}$$
$$q_2^* = 0$$
$$q_3^* = 2.2598 \times 10^{-4}$$

When this set of parameters is used in the multistage model for an Added Risk$= 10^{-6}$, one obtains

$$\begin{aligned} p(\mathrm{VSD}_L^*) - p(0) &= 10^{-6} \\ &= 1 - \exp\left[-\left(1.2091 \times 10^{-3}\mathrm{VSD}_L^* + 2.2598 \times 10^{-4}(\mathrm{VSD}_L^*)^3\right)\right] \end{aligned}$$

Solution of this equation for the VSD_L^* for the 95 percent lower confidence limit on VSD gives

$$\mathrm{VSD}_L^* = 0.000827$$

A graph of the function

$$p(d, \hat{q}) = 1 - \exp[-(\hat{q}_1 d + \hat{q}_3 d^3)]$$

based on the Maximum Likelihood parameters $\hat{\mathbf{q}}$ is presented in Figure 3.3 as well as the function

$$p(d, \mathbf{q}^*) = 1 - \exp[-(q_1^* d + q_3^* d^3)]$$

based on the 95 percent upper confidence limit on Added Risk parameters $\mathbf{q}^*$.

To find the corresponding parameters for the 95 percent lower confidence limit on risk, the same procedure as described above is followed except that the function given by Equation (3.32) is minimized rather than maximized. The parameters for the 95 percent lower confidence limit on risk are as follows:

$$q_0^* = 2.1293 \times 10^{-2}$$
$$q_1^* = -1.2069 \times 10^{-2}$$
$$q_2^* = 1.8235 \times 10^{-4}$$
$$q_3^* = 2.6025 \times 10^{-4}$$

For an Added Risk$= 10^{-6}$, the virtually safe dose corresponding to the 95 percent lower confidence limit on risk is a 95 percent upper confidence limit VSD_U^* on the VSD; namely,

$$\text{VSD}_U^* = 6.46$$

Since the Maximum Likelihood Estimate $\widehat{\text{VSD}} = 0.163$ is the most likely value based on the data and an Added Risk$= 10^{-6}$, one would expect values of VSD_L^* and VSD_U^* (the 95 percent confidence limits on the VSD) to lie in the same general neighborhood instead of being more than an order of magnitude away. A comparison of Examples 3.3 and 3.4 suggests that when the data can be adequately represented by the linearized form of the multistage model, the values of the $\widehat{\text{VSD}}$, VSD_L^* and VSD_U^* can be expected to be of the same order of magnitude as illustrated by Example 3.3. However, when the nonlinear form of the multistage model is used, $\widehat{\text{VSD}}$, VSD_L^* and VSD_U^* may differ by several orders of magnitude as illustrated by Example 3.4. The explanation for this difference in VSD values is suggested by graphs of the functions presented in Figures 3.2 and 3.3. In the case of the linearized form of the multistage model, the functions $p(d, \mathbf{q}^*)$ based on the $\mathbf{q}^*$ parameters follow closely the trace of the function $p(d, \hat{\mathbf{q}})$ based on the $\hat{\mathbf{q}}$ parameters as shown in Figure 3.3. Thus, one would expect the values of $\widehat{\text{VSD}}$, VSD_L^* and VSD_U^* to be of the same order of magnitude. However, when the nonlinear form of the multistage model is used, the functions $p(d, \mathbf{q}^*)$ are significantly different from the function $p(d, \hat{\mathbf{q}})$ for any given dose d, and consequently VSD_L^* and VSD_U^* are significantly different from $\widehat{\text{VSD}}$. These differences in the departures of the $p(d, \mathbf{q}^*)$ from $p(d, \hat{\mathbf{q}})$ (see Figure 3.3) result from the fact that the parameters $\mathbf{q}^*$ are found by maximizing or minimizing the Added Risk $= p(d', \mathbf{q}^*) - p(0, \mathbf{q}^*)$ [subject to the condition of constraint Equation (3.33)] at a small dose d' which is far to the left of the doses corresponding to that portion of $p(d, \hat{\mathbf{q}})$ which exhibits a steep slope.

3.4 DEVELOPMENT OF THE CONDITION GIVEN BY EQUATION (3.33)

Since the origin of the condition given by Equation (3.33) is far from obvious, a digression into the formulation of this condition is in order. First, consider a system with one degree of freedom, and suppose the random variable Z associated with the system is normally distributed; that is, it may be represented by Equation (2.106). The probability that Z lies in the confidence interval $100(1-2\alpha)$ percent is given by

$$P(-z_\alpha \le Z \le z_\alpha) = 1 - 2\alpha \tag{3.34}$$

where $P(Z \le -z_\alpha) = \alpha$, $P(z_\alpha \le Z < \infty) = \alpha$, $P(Z < \infty) = 1$, and $P(Z \le z_\alpha) = 1 - \alpha$. Then in terms of the *standard normal distribution function* $\Phi(z)$,

$$\Phi(z_\alpha) - \Phi(-z_\alpha) = 1 - 2\alpha \tag{3.35}$$

or

$$\int_{-\infty}^{z_\alpha} \phi(u)\,du - \int_{-\infty}^{-z_\alpha} \phi(u)\,du = \int_{-z_\alpha}^{z_\alpha} \phi(u)\,du = 1 - 2\alpha \tag{3.36}$$

where the probability density function $\phi(u)$ of the *standard normal distribution function* is given by

$$\phi(u) = \frac{e^{-u^2/2}}{\sqrt{2\pi}} \tag{3.37}$$

Thus, it follows that

$$\int_{-z_\alpha}^{z_\alpha} \phi(u)\,du = \int_{-z_\alpha}^{z_\alpha} \frac{e^{-u^2/2}}{\sqrt{2\pi}}\,du = 1 - 2\alpha \tag{3.38}$$

Furthermore, since the function $\phi(u)$ is an even function $[\phi(u) = \phi(-u)]$, it follows that

$$2\int_{0}^{z_\alpha} \frac{e^{-u^2/2}}{\sqrt{2\pi}}\,du = 1 - 2\alpha \tag{3.39}$$

Let the dummy variable u^2 be replaced by the dummy variable y; that is,

$$u^2 = y, \quad u = \sqrt{y}, \quad du = \frac{1}{2}\frac{dy}{\sqrt{y}}$$

When $u = 0, y = 0$, and when $u = z_\alpha, y = (z_\alpha)^2$. After this change of variable has been made, Equation (3.39) becomes

$$\int_{0}^{(z_\alpha)^2} \frac{e^{-y/2}\,dy}{\sqrt{2\pi}\sqrt{y}} = 1 - 2\alpha \tag{3.40}$$

The upper limit corresponds to the behavior of a standard normal random variable Z. That is, if Z is a standard normal random variable and $Y = Z^2$, then

$$P[Y \leq (z_\alpha)^2] = P[Z^2 \leq (z_\alpha)^2] = P[-z_\alpha \leq Z \leq z_\alpha] \tag{3.41}$$

and it follows from Equations (3.34), (3.40), and (3.41) that

$$P\left[Y \leq (z_\alpha)^2\right] = \int_0^{(z_\alpha)^2} \frac{e^{-y/2}}{\sqrt{2\pi}\sqrt{y}}\, dy = 1 - 2\alpha \tag{3.42}$$

For the case where there is one standard normal random variable involved (that is, one degree of freedom), the square of the standard normal random variable is denoted by χ_1^2 or

$$Z^2 = Y = \chi_1^2 \tag{3.43}$$

For one degree of freedom and a confidence level of $(1 - 2\alpha)$, $Z^2 = Y = \chi_1^2$, $\chi_{1,1-2\alpha}^2 = (z_\alpha)^2$, where $\chi_{1,1-2\alpha}^2$ is the $100\,(1-2\alpha)$th percentile of the *chi-square distribution function* which follows from Equations (3.42).

$$P\left(Y = \chi_1^2 \leq \chi_{1,1-2\alpha}^2\right) = \int_0^{\chi_{1,1-2\alpha}^2} \frac{e^{-y/2}}{\sqrt{2\pi}\sqrt{y}}\, dy = 1 - 2\alpha \tag{3.44}$$

To complete the development, a relationship given by Lehmann[7] is used without proof; namely, the particular chi-square random variable $Y = \chi_1^2$ is related to the ratio of the *likelihood functions* $L(\mathbf{q}^*)$ and $L(\hat{\mathbf{q}})$ as follows:

$$Y = -2\log_e \frac{L(\mathbf{q}^*)}{L(\hat{\mathbf{q}})} \tag{3.45}$$

where

$$\mathbf{q}^* = \{q_0^*, q_1^*, q_2^*, \ldots, q_k^*\}$$
$$\hat{\mathbf{q}} = \{\hat{q}_0, \hat{q}_1, \hat{q}_2, \ldots, \hat{q}_k\}$$

The development of Equations (3.34) through (3.44) implies that $Y = Z^2$ must be restricted to be equal to or less than its $100(1 - 2\alpha)$th percentile, in order to guarantee that Z is equal to or less than its $100(1 - \alpha)$th percentile. Similarly, in Equation (3.45) where

$$e^{-Y} = [L(\mathbf{q}^*)/L(\hat{\mathbf{q}})]^2$$

Y must be equal to or less than its 90th percentile, i.e.,

$$Y \leq \chi_{1,0.90}^2 = \chi_{1,1-2\alpha}^2 (\text{ for } \alpha = 0.05)$$

in order for $L(\mathbf{q}^*)/L(\hat{\mathbf{q}})$ not to exceed its 95th percentile, and thus Equation (3.33) follows.

To illustrate the relationship between the chi-square distribution function for one degree of freedom and the standard normal distribution function shown above, observe that according to Appendix V for the chi-square distribution function,

$$\chi_{1,1-2\alpha}^2 = \chi_{1,0.90}^2 = 2.70554$$

Then, as shown above,

$$Y = Z^2, \quad z_\alpha^2 = \chi^2_{1,1-2\alpha} = \chi^2_{1,0.90} = 2.70554$$

is equivalent to

$$Z = \sqrt{Z^2}, \quad z_\alpha = \sqrt{z_\alpha^2} = \sqrt{2.70554} = 1.6449$$

and by Appendix IV for the standard normal distribution function,

$$P(Z \leq z_\alpha \;= 1.6449) = 0.95$$

as expected since $P(Z \leq z_\alpha) = 1 - \alpha$ by Equation (3.34).

3.5 BOUNDING OF THE VIRTUALLY SAFE DOSE BY THE NONPARAMETRIC BOOTSTRAP PROCEDURE

This procedure, which was proposed by Sielken,[8] makes use of the original data and simulation techniques to generate any desired number of equally distributed replicates of the original data. The associated bounding procedure does not depend on policy assumptions such as those utilized by others.[1,2]

After the replicate experiments have been generated, a cancer model is selected such as the multistage stage model. Next the Maximum Likelihood Estimates of the parameters of this model are determined for the original set of data and each replicate set. After the parameters have been determined for each set of data, the corresponding function, $p(d)$ for each set is used to estimate the virtually safe dose (VSD). The observed distribution of these estimates of the VSD is then used to characterize the likelihood of the VSD being different numerical values and to bound the VSD.

The procedure for the generation of a set of replicate experiments is perhaps best described by use of a relatively simple example. In particular, suppose 4 test animals are exposed to a daily dose d over their lifetime, and that of these 4 test animals, 1 develops a tumor $[n = 4, r = 1]$. The corresponding value for the most probable trial probability p as determined by the Maximum Likelihood Method is given by Equation (3.7); namely,

$$p = \frac{r}{n} = 0.25 \tag{3.46}$$

The corresponding value of the probability of an experimenter observing this result $[n = 4, r = 1]$ is found by use of Equation (3.3) as follows:

$$L(p) = P(X = 1) = \frac{4!}{1!(4-1)!}(0.25)^1(0.75)^3 = 0.422$$

On the basis of the most probable value of the trial probability $p = 0.25$, the corresponding values of the cumulative probabilities $[P(X = 0), P(X \leq 1), P(X \leq 2), \ldots, P(X \leq 4)]$ that

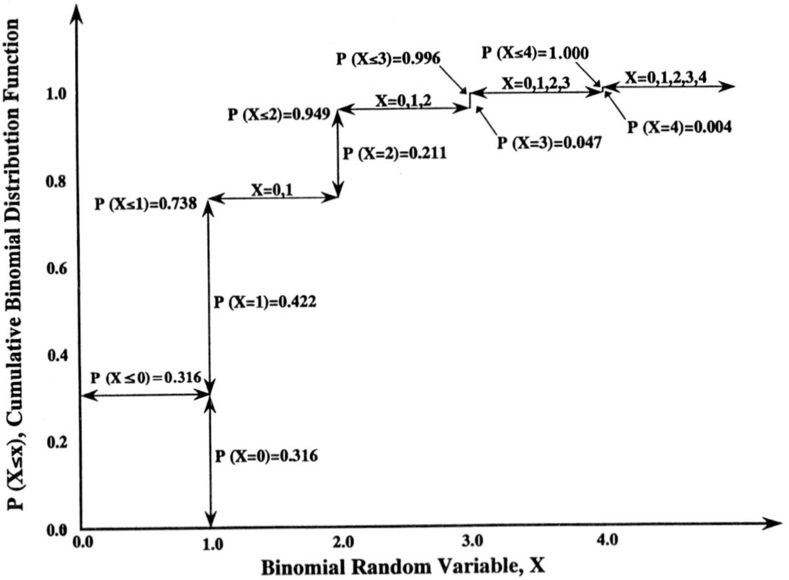

Figure 3.4 Graph of the Cumulative Binomial Distribution Function $P(X \leq x)$ for the Binomial Random Variable X. [Based on a binomial experiment with $n = 4$, $r = 1$, $p = r/n = 0.25$.]

an experimenter will observe either 0, 1 or less, 2 or less . . . , or 4 or less tumors is presented in Figure 3.4.

Also presented in this figure are the probabilities $[P(X = 0), P(X = 1), \ldots, P(X = 4)]$ that an experimenter will observe exactly 0, 1, 2, 3, or 4 tumors. Furthermore, observe that the sum of these probabilities is equal to unity, which is also equal to the length of the probability axis that ranges from 0 to 1. Thus, the lengths of the line segments that represent these probabilities $[P(X = 0), P(X = 1), \ldots, P(X = 4)]$ are also equal to the lengths of the corresponding line segments that make up the probability axis.

Next observe that each point $P(X = 0), P(X = 1), \ldots, P(X = 4)$ corresponds to one and only one experimental outcome $X = 0, X = 1, \ldots, X = 4$ (Note that for the general case of n outcomes, "4" is replaced by "n" in the previous statements and those that follow). Furthermore, the proportion of the probability axis corresponding to $X = i$ is equal to $P(X = i)$ for $i = 0, 1, 2, \ldots, 4$. Hence, if each number on the probability axis is equally likely to be generated, then the generated values are said to be uniformly distributed and the probability of generating a point corresponding to $X = i$ is equal to the proportion of the probability axis corresponding to $X = i$ which equals $P(X = i)$. Hence generating uniformly distributed values on the probability axis and assigning X the corresponding values $i = 0, 1, \ldots, 4$ (or n for the general case) is a procedure such that the probability of generating $X = i$ is $P(X = i)$. Figure 3.4 provides a graphical representation of the

Table 3.3 Replicate Experiments Corresponding to the Random Numbers and Outcomes.

Random Number	$X = r$	r/n
0.825	$X = 2$	$2/4$
0.848	$X = 2$	$2/4$
0.993	$X = 3$	$3/4$
0.676	$X = 1$	$1/4$
0.432	$X = 1$	$1/4$

one-to-one correspondence between the set of all numbers between 0 and 1 and the set of experimental outcomes, $X = 0, 1, \ldots, 4$ (or n for the general case).

The procedure described above is utilized in the following manner to generate replicate experiments. Suppose that it is desired to generate 5 replicate experiments. Corresponding to each replicate experiment desired, a uniformly distributed random number between 0 and 1 is required. Further suppose that the following set of random numbers has been selected from Reference 4 in an unbiased fashion:

$$0.825, 0.848, 0.993, 0.676, 0.432 \tag{3.47}$$

For this set of random numbers, the corresponding set of outcomes $X = r$ and replicate experiments (r/n) listed in Table 3.3 were found by use of Figure 3.4.

Two examples are presented that demonstrate the relationship between the Nonparametric Bootstrap method and the EPA method for characterizing the virtually safe doses (VSD). Example 3.5 shows that when the linearized form of the multistage model can be used to represent the dose-response relationship, the two methods give bounds on the VSD which are generally of approximately the same order of magnitude. However, when the nonlinear form of the multistage model is required to represent the dose-response data well, the bounds on the VSDs may differ significantly.

Example 3.5 Illustration of the Nonparametric Bootstrap Procedure When the Dose–Response is Linear.

In this example, the observed dose–response relationship can be well represented by a linearized form of the multistage model. The original data consists of two experiments at two different dose levels which is the first entry (see Group 1) of Table 3.4. This example was formulated by retaining only the high dose experiment and the control dose experiment of Example 3.4, which is based on the data reported in Reference 6 on the inhalation of formaldehyde by different groups of rats. The 19 replicates of each of these two original experiments (see Groups 2 through 20 of Table 3.4) were generated by the procedure described above.

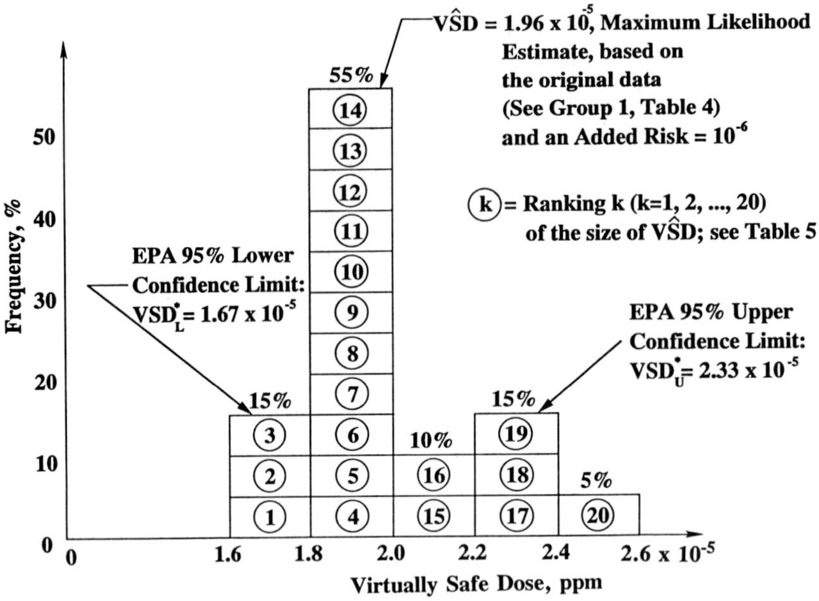

Figure 3.5 Histogram of the Virtually Safe Dose Estimates Obtained by the Nonparametric Bootstrap Method at an Added Risk = 10^{-6} for Example 3.5. [By courtesy of Sielken, Inc.]

To obtain the Maximum Likelihood Estimate of the VSD, the following procedure was used. First the parameters q_0 and q_1 were estimated using the Maximum Likelihood Method for each Group shown in Table 3.4. Then for an Added Risk = 10^{-6}, Equation (3.28) was solved for the $\hat{VSD}$, and the values so obtained are listed in Table 3.4. A ranking of the $\hat{VSD}$s shown in Table 3.4 is presented in Table 3.5.

A histogram of the 20 $\hat{VSD}$s is presented in Figure 3.5 in which the number of $\hat{VSD}$s falling within each given range of values is indicated. For example, 55 percent of the $\hat{VSD}$s fall within the range of 1.8×10^{-5} to 2.0×10^{-5}. The ordinate of 55 percent represents the frequency (in percent) with which the $\hat{VSD}$s fall within this range, and the circled numbers within each rectangle represents the ranking of the $\hat{VSD}$ according to size as given in Table 3.5. The most probable range is the one 1.8×10^{-5} to 2.0×10^{-5}, since it has by far the largest frequency of 55 percent. These results suggests that, if this experiment were repeated any number of times and the true proportion of responses at 14.3 *ppm* is near 103/199, then the most probable range for the $\hat{VSD}$s would be from 1.8×10^{-5} to 2.0×10^{-5}.

Next as should be expected, the Maximum Likelihood Estimate of the VSD of 1.96×10^{-5} for the original data (see Group 1 of Table 3.4) also falls in the most probable range, 1.8×10^{-5} to 2.0×10^{-5}. Also, VSD_L^* and VSD_U^* corresponding to the lower and upper 95 percent confidence limits of the EPA method are in approximate

Table 3.4 Original and Replicate Experiments for Example 3.5 and the Corresponding Maximum Likelihood Estimates of the VSD. [By courtesy of Sielken, Inc.]

Group No.	r/n at Dose 0 ppm	r/n at Dose 14.3 ppm	Maximum Likelihood Estimate at an Added Risk $= 10^{-6}$ $\hat{VSD} \times 10^5$
1*	0/199	103/199	1.96
2	0/199	107/199	1.85
3	0/199	106/199	1.88
4	0/199	107/199	1.85
5	0/199	96/199	2.17
6	0/199	94/199	2.24
7	0/199	93/199	2.27
8	0/199	107/199	1.85
9	0/199	93/199	2.27
10	0/199	116/199	1.64
11	0/199	104/199	1.93
12	0/199	105/199	1.91
13	0/199	111/199	1.75
14	0/199	106/199	1.88
15	0/199	106/199	1.88
16	0/199	103/199	1.96
17	0/199	103/199	1.96
18	0/199	101/199	2.02
19	0/199	88/199	2.45
20	0/199	110/199	1.78

* Group 1 denotes the experimental results based on data presented in Reference 6. Groups 2 through 20 are the replicates of the experimental results.

Table 3.5 Ranking of the $\hat{VSD}$s Found by the Nonparametric Bootstrap Method for Example 3.5. [By courtesy of Sielken, Inc.]

Ranking	Percentage Equal to or Greater than Ranked $\hat{VSD}$	$\hat{VSD} \times 10^5$ Added Risk $= 10^{-6}$	Ranking	Percentage Equal to or Smaller than Ranked $\hat{VSD}$	$\hat{VSD} \times 10^5$ Added Risk $= 10^{-6}$
1	100	1.64	11	55	1.93
2	95	1.75	12	60	1.96
3	90	1.78	13	65	1.96
4	85	1.85	14	70	1.96
5	80	1.85	15	75	2.02
6	75	1.85	16	80	2.17
7	70	1.88	17	85	2.24
8	65	1.88	18	90	2.27
9	60	1.88	19	95	2.27
10	55	1.91	20	100	2.45

agreement with the Nonparametric Bootstrap $\hat{VSD}$s. The VSD_L^* corresponding to the 95 percent lower confidence limit of 1.67×10^{-5} is of the same order of magnitude as the most probable range [1.8×10^{-5} to 2.0×10^{-5}] of the Nonparametric Bootstrap method while the upper confidence limit $VSD_U^* = 2.33 \times 10^{-5}$ of the EPA method is approximately equal to the 95th percentile value, 2.27×10^{-5}, in the Nonparametric Bootstrap distribution as shown in Table 3.5.

In general, relatively good agreement between the Nonparametric Bootstrap method and the EPA method can be expected when the dose–response data can be well represented by a linearized form of the multistage model as demonstrated by this example.

Example 3.6 Illustration of the Nonparametric Bootstrap Method when the Dose-Response is Nonlinear.

This example is based on all of the experimental results obtained by the exposure of different groups of rats to formaldehyde by inhalation as described in Reference 6. The experimental results as well as 19 replicate sets of these experiments are presented in Table 3.6. Also, the corresponding Maximum Likelihood Estimates of the VSD at an Added Risk $= 10^{-6}$ are shown in Table 3.6 for the original data and the 19 replicate sets. A ranking of the $\hat{VSD}$s so obtained is presented in Table 3.7, and the corresponding histogram is presented in Figure 3.6.

The histogram for Example 3.6 is similar to the one for Example 3.5 except that in this case the VSD_L^* and VSD_U^* corresponding to the EPA lower and upper 95 percent confidence limits on the VSD are outside the bounds of the $\hat{VSD}$s found by the Nonparametric Bootstrap method. The Maximum Likelihood Estimate of the VSD for the original experiments [line 1 of Table 3.6] lies within the most probable range [0.16 to 0.17]. Further observe that 65 percent of the $\hat{VSD}$s found by the Nonparametric Bootstrap method lie within this range [0.16 to 0.17] while the values of VSD_L^* and VSD_U^* (to the EPA lower and upper confidence limits) of 8.27×10^{-4} and 6.46, respectively, lie outside of the lower and upper bounds of all the $\hat{VSD}$s found by the Nonparametric Bootstrap method as shown in Figure 3.6.

The fit of the original data [see line 1 of Table 3.6] for Example 3.6 as well as the fit for the 95 percent upper confidence limits are the same as those shown in Figure 3.3 for Example 3.4.

3.6 LIMITATIONS OF THE EPA MODEL FOR RISK ASSESSMENT

The technique used by EPA to determine the upper bounds on risk from the linearized multistage model [see Equations (3.21) through (3.33)] generally leads to substantially higher values of the probability $p(d)$ than those given by estimates obtained from the multistage model whose parameters $(q_0, q_1, \ldots, q_k)$ have been estimated by the Maximum

Table 3.6 Original and Replicate Experiments for Example 3.6 and the Corresponding Maximum Likelihood Estimates of the VSD. [Based on data taken from CIIT Study.[6] The numerical results are by courtesy of Sielken, Inc.]

Group No.	r/n at Dose 0 *ppm*	r/n at Dose 2.0 *ppm*	r/n at Dose 5.6 *ppm*	r/n at Dose 14.3 *ppm*	Maximum Likelihood Estimate at an Added Risk $= 10^{-6}$ $\hat{VSD}$
1*	0/199	0/200	2/200	103/199	0.1625
2	0/199	0/200	2/200	106/199	0.1604
3	0/199	0/200	1/200	97/199	0.1677
4	0/199	0/200	2/200	95/199	0.1687
5	0/199	0/200	0/200	94/199	0.1707
6	0/199	0/200	3/200	104/199	0.1612
7	0/199	0/200	3/200	107/199	0.1591
8	0/199	0/200	3/200	107/199	0.1591
9	0/199	0/200	4/200	100/199	0.1636
10	0/199	0/200	2/200	95/199	0.1687
11	0/199	0/200	2/200	103/199	0.1625
12	0/199	0/200	2/200	102/199	0.1633
13	0/199	0/200	2/200	105/199	0.1610
14	0/199	0/200	3/200	97/199	0.1665
15	0/199	0/200	2/200	105/199	0.1610
16	0/199	0/200	2/200	118/199	0.1520
17	0/199	0/200	5/200	108/199	0.1574
18	0/199	0/200	2/200	103/199	0.1625
19	0/199	0/200	3/200	115/199	0.1536
20	0/199	0/200	2/200	90/199	0.1727

* Group 1 denotes the original data and results. Groups 2 through 20 are the replicates of the experimental results.

Table 3.7 Ranking of the $\hat{VSD}$s Found by the Nonparametric Bootstrap Method for Example 3.6.

Ranking	Percentage Equal to or Greater than Ranked $\hat{VSD}$	$\hat{VSD}$ at Added Risk $= 10^{-6}$	Ranking	Percentage Equal to or Smaller than Ranked $\hat{VSD}$	$\hat{VSD}$ at Added Risk $= 10^{-6}$
1	100	0.1521	11	55	0.1625
2	95	0.1536	12	60	0.1625
3	90	0.1574	13	65	0.1633
4	85	0.1591	14	70	0.1636
5	80	0.1591	15	75	0.1665
6	75	0.1604	16	80	0.1677
7	70	0.1610	17	85	0.1687
8	65	0.1610	18	90	0.1687
9	60	0.1612	19	95	0.1707
10	55	0.1625	20	100	0.1727

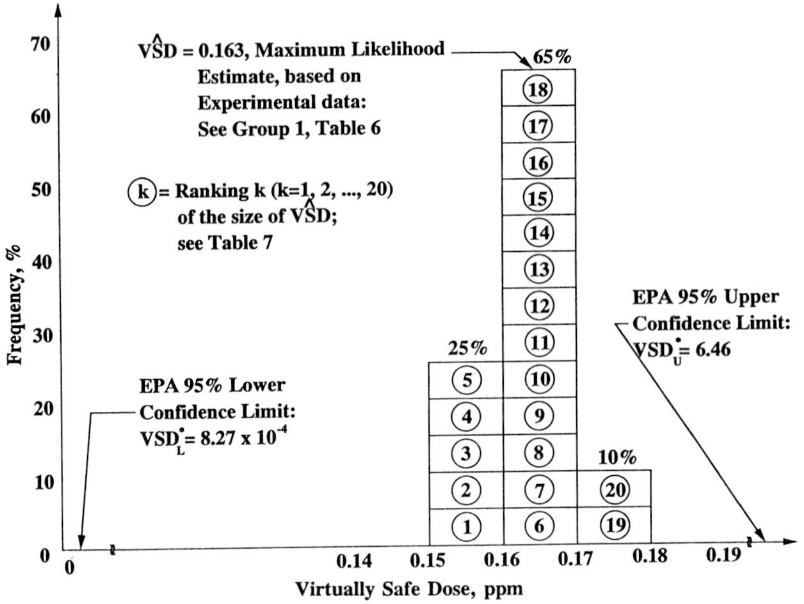

Figure 3.6 Histogram of the Virtually Safe Dose Estimates Obtained by the Nonparametric Bootstrap Method at an Added Risk = 10^{-6} for Example 3.6. [By courtesy of Sielken, Inc.]

Likelihood Method (see Chapter 4). The upper bound values are relatively near the fitted model values at high doses, but may be several thousand times as large as the fitted model values at low doses as shown in Figures 3.3 and 3.7. Observe that in the case of the CIIT study[6] shown in Figure 3.3, the ratio of the 95 percent upper confidence limit values to the corresponding fitted model values for $p(d)$ ranges from 2 at a dose of 5.6 *ppm* to 423,000,000 at a dose of 0.01 *ppm*. For the 1985 SRI chloroform-drinking water study,[9] the ratio of the 95 percent upper confidence limit values to the fitted model value range from 2.5 at a dose of 38 $mg/[(kg)(day)]$ to 9,300 at a dose of 0.01 $mg/[(kg)(day)]$; see Figure 3.7.

Although in many instances only the 95 percent upper bound or upper confidence limit is reported, both lower and upper bounds (or confidence limits) should be reported if bounds are reported. When only the 95 percent upper bounds are reported, there is the tendency by some to regard the fitted model values as the lower bounds instead of the most likely values of the actual risk. The fitted model is not the lower bound. The curves corresponding to the 95 percent lower and upper bounds on Added Risk were determined as described above [see Equations (3.31) through (3.33)] for the SRI data.[9] These curves as well as the one for the Maximum Likelihood Estimate are shown in Figure 3.8. The range of values between the lower and upper bounds gives an indication of the tightness or looseness of the bounding procedure. The values between the lower and upper bounds

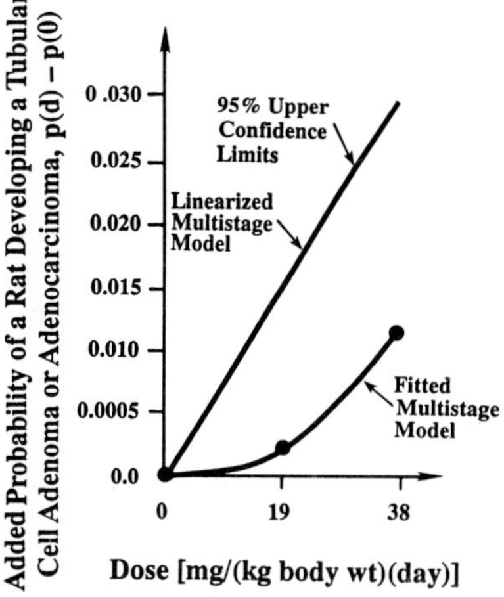

Dose (mg/kg/day)	Ratio: 95% Upper Confidence Limit / Fitted Model Value
38	2.5
19	4.9
10	9.3
1	93.0
0.1	930.0
0.01	9300.0

Data Points not Shown: ● = (81,0.05), ● = (160,0.13)

Figure 3.7 Added Probability of a Rat Developing a Tubular Cell Adenoma or Adenocarcinoma versus Dose. [Taken from R.L. Sielken, Jr., by courtesy *Toxic Substances Journal*, **9**, 353 (1989).]

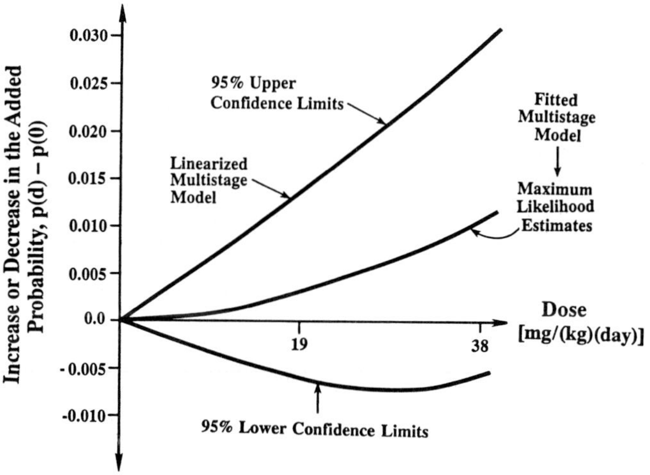

Figure 3.8 Comparison of the 95 percent Lower and Upper Confidence Limits and the Fitted Multistage Model for the 1985 SRI Chloroform–Drinking Water Study.[9] [Taken from R.L. Sielken, Jr., by courtesy *Toxic Substances Journal*, **9**, 353 (1989).]

are not all equally likely to represent the actual risk; the fitted model values (the Maximum Likelihood Estimates) are the most likely values of the actual risk under the assumed dose-response model (the multistage model here).

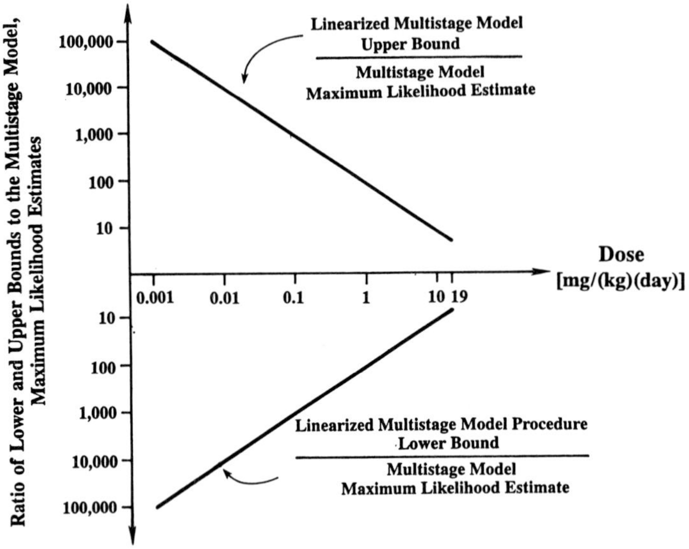

Figure 3.9 Divergence of the Responses of the 95 percent Lower and Upper Confidence Limits from the Fitted Multistage Model with Decreasing Dose for the 1985 SRI Chloroform-Drinking Water Study.[9] [Taken from R.L. Sielken, Jr., by courtesy *Toxic Substances Journal*, **9**, 353 (1989).]

Since the Added Risk is by definition zero when the dose is zero, the graph in Figure 3.8 might appear to suggest that the 95 percent lower and upper bounds are becoming more precise as the dose tends to zero. However, the contrary is true, the relative difference between lower and upper bounds and the fitted model values (the Maximum Likelihood Estimates) are diverging rapidly as the dose tends to zero as shown in Figure 3.9. This divergence of the bounds at low doses is most unfortunate because this is the region of primary interest in risk assessment.

The method used by EPA in risk assessment has another undesirable characteristic; namely, the slope q_1^* (which is used in risk assessment as shown in a subsequent section) of the 95 percent upper confidence limit on risk depends almost entirely on the value of the highest dose tested and is almost independent of the outcomes at the lower experimental dose levels. That is, the EPA method fails to adequately reflect the shape of the observed dose-response relationship and especially the outcomes in the low dose region, the region of primary interest in risk assessment. To illustrate this deficiency in the EPA model, Sielken[8] investigated the six experimental outcomes shown in Figure 3.10. Although the outcomes for each of the experiments are very different, the slopes q_1^* differ by less than one order of magnitude.

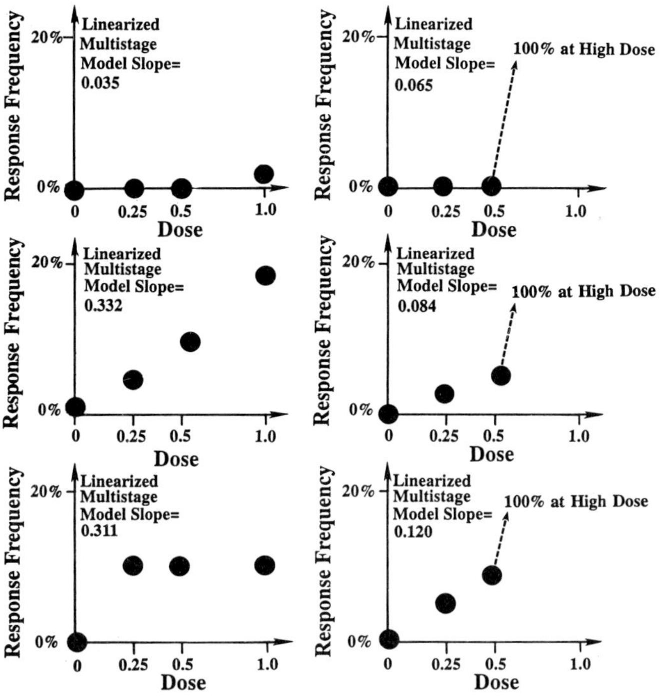

Figure 3.10 Nonresponsiveness of the 95 percent Upper Confidence Limit of the Linearized Multistage Model to Experimental Data.[8] [Taken from R.L. Sielken, Jr., by courtesy *Toxic Substances Journal*, **9**, 353 (1989).]

3.7 UPPER-BOUND UNIT RISK ESTIMATES AND THEIR USE IN RISK ASSESSMENT

The expression used by EPA for the *unit risk estimate* is obtained from the expression for the probability of a tumor on a *background free basis* or the probability of an *excess tumor* (a tumor in excess of those expected from the background exposure; that is, a tumor in the portion of the population which would not show background tumors). This probability expression is obtained in the following manner. First, the Maximum Likelihood Estimates of q_0 and q_1 in Equation (3.22) are replaced by the 95 percent upper confidence limit values q_0^* and q_1^* to give

$$p(d) = 1 - \exp\left[-(q_0^* + q_1^* d)\right] \tag{3.48}$$

The expression for the background at $d = 0$ becomes

$$p(0) = 1 - \exp(-q_0^*) \tag{3.49}$$

By use of these two expressions [Equations (3.48) and (3.49)], the following formula for the probability of a tumor on a background free basis (denoted by "$ER(d)$" for *Extra Risk* at dose d) is obtained

$$ER(d) = \frac{p(d) - p(0)}{1 - p(0)} = 1 - \exp[-q_1^* d] \tag{3.50}$$

For very small doses,

$$\exp(-q_1^* d) \approx 1 - q_1^* d \tag{3.51}$$

and thus Equation (3.50) reduces approximately to

$$ER(d) = q_1^* d \tag{3.52}$$

In Equation (3.52), the 95 percent upper confidence limit on the Extra Risk is a linear function of d with slope q_1^*. Hence, q_1^*, the 95 percent upper confidence limit on the slope in the linearized multistage model, is called the *slope factor* by the EPA. The relative potencies of different chemical substances are compared by the EPA on the basis of the slope factors. These slope factors are reported either on the basis of the weight of the chemical $[mg/(kg)(day)]$ (milligrams of chemical per kilogram body weight per day of exposure which is frequently stated as $[mg/kg/day]$) or the moles of the chemical $[mg\ moles/(kg)(day)]$.

The EPA makes use of a factor called the *Upper-Bound Risk Estimate*, or the *Unit Risk Factor*, which is defined as the excess lifetime risk associated with being exposed to a unit concentration of a given chemical over a 70 year life span for a 70 kg person. A unit concentration is either 1 $mg/(kg)(day)$ for food, 1 $\mu g/L$ (one microgram per liter) for drinking water (oral), or 1 $\mu g/m^3$ (one microgram per cubic meter) for air (inhalation). Thus, for a 95 percent confidence limit, the unit risk factor is evaluated by substituting $d = 1\ \mu g/m^3$ or 1 $mg/[(kg\ body\ weight)(day)]$ into Equation (3.52) to give

$$(Upper\ Bound\ on\ Risk) = ER(1) = q_1^* \tag{3.53}$$

It should be pointed out that q_1^* has the reciprocal units of d; that is, when d has the units of $\mu g/m^3$, the slope q_1^* has the units of $(\mu g/m^3)^{-1}$. Values of the unit risk factors for inhalation exposure of humans have been determined by EPA for the compounds shown in Table 3.8. Included in the unit risk factors are the assumptions for extrapolation from animal risk factors to human risk factors. One method is based on the assumption of the equivalence between species when q^* has the units of mg/(surface area)(day); see Problems 11 and 12.

Equations (3.48) through (3.53) are utilized fairly extensively by the EPA in making risk assessments of the number of people who can be expected to develop cancer as a

Table 3.8 Unit Risk Factors q_1^* for Inhalation Exposure. [Taken from U.S. Environmental Protection Agency: Integrated Risk Information System, EPA/600/8-86/ 032a, Washingon D.C.(1987).]

Compounds	Unit Risk Factors*	Compounds	Unit Risk Factors*
Acetaldehyde	2.2×10^{-6}	1,2-Diphenylhydrazine	4.5×10^{-1}
Acrylamide	1.3×10^{-3}	Epichlorohydrin	1.2×10^{-6}
Acrylonitrile	6.8×10^{-5}	Ethylene oxide	1.8×10^{-2}
Aldrin	4.9×10^{-3}	Formaldehyde	1.1×10^{-4}
Arsenic	4.3×10^{-3}	Heptachlor	1.3×10^{-3}
Asbestos	2.3×10^{-1}	Haptachlor epoxide	2.6×10^{-3}
Azobenzene	3.1×10^{-5}	Hexachlorobutadiene	2.2×10^{-5}
Benzene	8.3×10^{-6}	Hexachorocyclohexane	2.1×10^{-5}
Benzidine	6.7×10^{-2}	technical grade	2.0×10^{-1}
Beryllium	2.4×10^{-3}	alpha isomer	1.8×10^{-3}
1,3-Butadiene	2.8×10^{-4}	beta isomer	5.3×10^{-4}
Cadmium	1.8×10^{-3}	Hexacholordibenzodioxin	1.3×10^{-6}
Carbon tetrachloride	1.5×10^{-5}	Hydrazine/Hydrazine sulfate	4.9×10^{-3}
Chlordane	3.7×10^{-5}	Nickel refinery dust	2.4×10^{-4}
bis(2-chloroethyl)ether	3.3×10^{-4}	Nickel subsulfide	4.8×10^{-4}
Chloroform	2.3×10^{-5}	Nitroso-dimethylamine	1.4×10^{-2}
bis(chloromethyl)ether	6.2×10^{-2}	Di-butylamine	1.6×10^{-3}
Chromium VI	1.2×10^{-2}	Diethylnitrosamine	4.3×10^{-2}
DDT	9.7×10^{-5}	N-nitrosophyrrolidine	6.1×10^{-4}
1,2-Dibromoethane	2.2×10^{-4}	1,1,1,2-Tetrachloroethane	7.4×10^{-6}
Dibutylnitrosamine	1.6×10^{-3}	1,1,2,2-Tetrachloroethane	5.8×10^{-5}
1,2-Dichloroethane	2.6×10^{-6}	Toxaphene	3.2×10^{-4}
1,1-Dichloroethylene (Vinylidene chloride)	5.0×10^{-5}	1,1,2-Trichloroethane	1.6×10^{-5}
Dichloromethane	4.1×10^{-6}	Trichloroethylene	1.3×10^{-6}
Dieldrin	4.6×10^{-3}	2,4,6-Trichlorophenol	5.7×10^{-6}
Diethylnitrosamine	4.3×10^{-2}	Vinyl chloride	7.1×10^{-6}
Dimethylnitrosamine	1.4×10^{-2}		

* Estimated risk to humans from constant lifetime exposure in the units ($\mu g/m^3$)

consequence of having been exposed to a given dose d over a given time period. The equations needed to made these risk assessments are developed in the following manner.

Let n denote the total number of people in the group exposed to the dose d. Of this group, the number which would have developed cancer at the background level [without having been exposed to the dose d] is given by

$$\begin{pmatrix} \textit{Number of cancer cases} \\ \textit{expected from background} \end{pmatrix} = p(0)n \tag{3.54}$$

The number of cancer cases which could be expected as a consequence of having been exposed to the dose d is given by

$$\begin{pmatrix} \textit{Total number of cancer cases expected from} \\ \textit{dose d and from background} \end{pmatrix} = p(d)n \tag{3.55}$$

Thus, the excess number of cancer cases which could be expected over and above those resulting from the background is given by subtracting the members of Equation (3.54) from those of Equation (3.55) to give

$$\begin{pmatrix} \textit{Excess number of cancer cases} \\ \textit{expected from dose d} \end{pmatrix} = [p(d) - p(0)]n \tag{3.56}$$

From Equation (3.26), it follows that a 95 percent upper confidence limit on

$$\begin{pmatrix} \textit{Excess number of cancer cases} \\ \textit{expected from dose d} \end{pmatrix} = [1 - p(0)][1 - \exp(-q_1^* d)]n \tag{3.57}$$

which at small doses reduces approximately to:

$$\begin{pmatrix} \textit{Number of cancer cases} \\ \textit{expected from dose d} \end{pmatrix} \approx q_1^* d[1 - p(0)]n \tag{3.58}$$

It is of interest to note that the quantity $[1 - p(0)]n$ represents the number of people of group n who are at risk because of having been exposed to the dose d.

The utilization of the above relationships in making risk assessments is demonstrated by the following example. Consider the prediction of the expected number of cancer cases at the 95 percent upper-bound risk estimate for an exposure of 1 $\mu g/m^3$ for 24 hours per day over an average life span. The data on which this example is based were taken from Anderson et al.[2] and the EPA.[10]

Example 3.7 For copper smelters, the EPA[10] gives a value of $2.38 \times 10^{-3}\ (\mu g/m^3)^{-1}$ for the unit risk factor q_1^*, and Anderson et al.[2] estimated the number of exposed workers to be 43,800. At an assumed dose of 1 $\mu g/m^3$ per day of the chemical throughout the average life span of 70 years for a 70 kg person, compute the 95 percent upper confidence limit on the number of cancer cases expected per year.

Solution The 95 percent upper confidence limit on the number of cancer cases expected in excess of those resulting from the background may be found by use of Equation (3.58) and the assumption that the background cancer rate is negligible $[1 - p(0) \approx 1]$. On the basis of this assumption, a life span of 70 years, and a dose $d = 1\ \mu g/(m^3 day)$, Equation (3.58) becomes

$$\textit{Number of excess cancer cases expected per year} = \frac{q_1^* \cdot 1 \cdot n}{70}$$

Thus, a 95 percent upper confidence limit on the

$$
\begin{aligned}
&\textit{Number of excess cancer cases expected per year} \\
&= \frac{2.38 \times 10^{-3}\left(\mu g/(m^3)(day)\right)^{-1} \times 1\left(\mu g/(m^3)(day)\right) \times 43,800(workers)}{70(\textit{year life span})} \\
&= 1.5
\end{aligned}
$$

This result was given by Anderson et al.,[2] and the calculation used to obtain it assumes that the worker's average daily exposure was equivalent to having been exposed constantly to a dose of 1 $\mu g/m^3$ over their life span of 70 years instead of 8 working hours per day and 40 working years. Generally, workers are exposed only during working hours, and this fact is taken into account as shown below.

In addition to the compilation of unit risk factors by EPA, the American Conference of Government Industrial Hygienists (ACGIH) compiles TLV values (*Threshold Limit Values*) for the estimation of cancer risks resulting from occupational exposure. These TLVs were determined and compiled by the Chemical Substances Threshold Limit Values (CS–TLV) Committee of the American Conference of Governmental Industrial Hygienists (ACGIH).[11] The ACGIH list contains over 700 agents and those which have been classified by the Committee as confirmed human carcinogens and their respective TLV values are listed in Table 3.9. The TLVs shown in Table 3.9 are time weighted average concentrations (TWA) to which it is believed that nearly all workers may be repeatedly exposed day after day (8 hours per day, 40 hours per week) without adverse effect.[11]

The above defintion of the Threshold Limit Value (TLV) implies that a worker is at risk of developing cancer if his or her exposure level exceeds the TLV value, and not that the development of cancer is a certainty as is the case where the worker's exposure exceed the tolerance level in the Probit model; see the discussion relating to Equation (3.13).

Another set of exposure limits called the *Permissible Exposure Limits* (PELs) has been issued by OSHA. The PELs are similar to the TLVs, and the principle difference between them is that the PELs are legal requirements; whereas, the TLVs are not.

An analysis of the two measures of risk (unit risk factors and TLVs) was recently published by Alavanja et al.[12] In general they found substantial agreement in the relative potencies of the 16 chemicals considered, but substantial disparity in the actual levels proposed or recommended. In general, the EPA values were far more conservative.

As pointed out by Alavanja et al.,[12] industrial exposure is different from that of the public, and it is necessary to adjust the EPA unit risk factors accordingly. The EPA unit risk factor is based on an average exposure to a dose of 1 $\mu g/m^3$ over an average life span. Constant exposure is assumed for each week of 168 hours and each of the 52 weeks for each week of the average life span. Although Anderson et al.[2] took the average life span to be 70 years, Alavanja et al.[12] uses 74 years and the latter is used in the following calculations.*

* The average life span has been increasing over the years, and the different values used throughout the text generally reflect the year in which the referenced research was performed.

Table 3.9 Chemical Substances Classified as Carcinogens by ACGIH with Their Respective 1991–1992 Threshold Limit Values (TLVs). [By courtesy *American Conference of Government Industrial Hygienists (ACGIH)*, Cincinnati, OH (1990).]

Substance	TLV (mg/m^3)
Acrylamide–Skin	0.03, A2
Acrylonitrile–Skin	4.3, A2
4-Aminodiphenyl–Skin	A1
Anitomony trioxide production	A2
Arsenic trioxide production	A2
Asbestos	
Amosite	0.5 fiber/cc, A1
Chrysotile	2 fibers/cc, A1
Crocidolite	0.2 fiber/cc, A1
Other forms	2 fibers/cc, A1
Benzene	32, A2
Benzidine–Skin	A1
Benzo(a)pyrene	A2
Beryllium	0.002, A2
1,3-Butadiene	22, A2
Cadmium and compounds, as Cd (proposed)	0.01, A2, Total dust 0.002, A2, Respirable Fraction
Carbon tetrachloride–Skin	31, A2
Chloroform	49, A2
bis(Chloromethyl)ether	0.0047, A1
Chlormethyl methyl ether	A2
Chromium (VI), certain water insoluble compounds	0.05, A1
Chrysene	A2
Coal tar pitch volatiles as benzene solubles	0.2, A1

Since the working career of an employee is commonly taken to be 40 hours per week, 50 weeks per year, and 40 years, the EPA unit risk factor must be corrected accordingly. Also, the EPA assumes a normal respiration rate of 20 cubic meters in a 24 hour period while Alavanja et al.[9] assume a normal respiration rate of 10 cubic meters in an 8 hour period. Thus, the adjusted unit risk factor $\tilde{q}_1^*$ for workers is given by

$$\begin{aligned}\tilde{q}_1^* &= q_1^*\left(\frac{m^3 day}{\mu g}\right) \times \frac{8(hr/work\ day)}{24(hr/day)} \times \frac{5(work\ day/work\ wk)}{7(day/wk)}\\ &\times \frac{50(work\ wk/work\ yr)}{52(wk/yr)} \times \frac{40(work\ yr/life\ span)}{74(yr/life\ span)} \times \frac{(10\ m^3/8hr)}{(20\ m^3/24hr)}\\ &= 0.1856 q_1^*\left(\frac{m^3 day}{\mu g}\right)\end{aligned}$$

Table 3.9 (cont'd) Chemical Substances Classified as Carcinogens by ACGIH with Their Respective 1991–1992 Threshold Limit Values (TLVs). [By courtesy *American Conference of Government Industrial Hygienists (ACGIH)*, Cincinnati, OH (1990).]

3,3'-Dichlorobenzidine–Skin	A2
Dimethyl carbamoyl chloride	A2
1,1-Dimethylhydrazine–Skin	1.2, A2
Dimethyl sulfate–Skin	0.52, A2
Dinitroltoluene	1.5 (proposed A2)
Epichlorohydrin–Skin	7.6 (proposed A2)
Ethyl acrylate	20, A2
Ethylene dibromide–Skin	A2
Ethylene oxide	1.8, A2
Formaldehyde	1.2, A2
Heptachlor–Skin	0.5 (proposed A2)
Hexachlorobutadiene–Skin	0.21, A2
Hexamethyl phosphoramide– Skin	A2
Hyrazine–Skin	0.13, A2
Lead chromates as Cr, as Pb	0.05, A2
4,4'-Methylene bis(2-chloroaniline)–Skin	0.22, A2
Methylene chloride	174, A2
4,4'-Methylene dianiline–Skin	0.81, A2
Methyl hydrazine–Skin	0.38, A2
Methyl iodide–Skin	12, A2
β- Naphthylamine	A1
Nickel metal	1 (not a carcinogen at present; A1 proposed)
Nickle insoluble compounds, as Ni	1 (not a carcinogen at present; A1 proposed)
Nickle soluble compounds, as Ni	0.1 (not a carcinogen at present; A1 proposed)
Nickel sulfide roasting, fume & dust, as Ni	1, A1
4-Nitrodiphenyl–Skin	A1
2-Nitropropane	36, A2
N-Nitrosodimethylamine–Skin	A2
N-Phenyl-beta-naphthylamine	A2
Phenylhydrazine–Skin	0.44, A2
Propane sultone	A2
β-Propiolactone	1.5, A2
Propylene imine–Skin	4.7, A2
o-Tolidine–Skin	A2
o-Toluidine–Skin	8.8, A2
p-Toluidine–Skin	8.8, A2
Vinyl bromide	22, A2
Vinyl chloride	13, A1
Vinyl cyclohexene dioxide–Skin	57, A2
Zinc chromates, as Cr	0.01, A1

A1—Confirmed Human Carcinogen: The agent is carcinogenic to humans based on the findings of epidemiologic studies or, convincing clinical evidence in, exposed humans.

A2—The agent is carcinogenic in experimental animals at dose levels and by routes of administration that are considered relevant to worker exposure. Available epidemiologic studies are conflicting, controversial, or inadequate to confirm an increased risk of cancer in exposed humans.

where

$$\tilde{q}_1^* = \textit{adjusted value of the EPA unit risk factor } q_1^*$$

[Note the unit risk factors have the reciprocal units of the dose d.]

For a selected group of chemicals, the unit risk factors q_1^* for the public and the $\tilde{q}_1^*$ risk factors for workers (occupational exposure) are presented in Table 3.10. Also presented are the corresponding TLVs and the estimated lifetime cancer risk from the TLV exposure. For example, the adjusted unit risk factor $\tilde{q}_1^*$ shown in Table 3.10 for benzene is computed as follows:

$$\tilde{q}_1^* = q_1^*(0.1856) = 8.3 \times 10^{-6} \times 0.1856 = 1.5 \times 10^{-6} \left(\frac{\mu g}{m^3}\right)^{-1}$$

Then the estimated lifetime extra cancer risk from an exposure to a benzene dose d = TLV $= 30 \times 10^3$ $\mu g/m^3$ over the working career of an employee is computed as follows:

$$ER(d) = 1 - e^{-q_1^* d} \approx \tilde{q}_1^* d. \tag{3.59}$$

Thus,

$$ER(d) = (1.5 \times 10^{-6})(30 \times 10^3) = 45 \times 10^{-3}$$

which differs only slightly due to rounding from the 0.044 given in Table 3.10. Also observe that the values given for the TLV for benzene in Tables 3.9 and 3.10 are slightly different. (The TLVs are adjusted yearly by the ACGIH.[11]) The value shown in Table 3.10 was used in this calculation.

Also the unit risk factors may be used to compute the daily dose over a 40 year working career which would be required to reduce the excess risk to one cancer case in one million people.

$$d = \frac{ER(d)}{\tilde{q}_1^*} = \frac{1 \times 10^{-6}}{1.5 \times 10^{-6}} = 6.66 \times 10^{-1} \ \mu g/m^3$$

The daily doses corresponding to the extra risks of 10^{-6} and 10^{-3} for the chemicals shown in Table 3.11 were computed in this manner.

Instead of adjusting the unit risk factor corresponding to a constant exposure to a substance over a lifetime, the dose to which a worker is exposed over a working career may be adjusted. This approach was used by Tollefson et al.[13] in the analysis of the results of a mortality study reported by Hearne et al.[14] on Eastman Kodak employees at the plant in Rochester, New York. The study cohort consisted of 1013 men who were employed for at least 1 year between January 1, 1964 and December 31, 1970. The mean duration of exposure was 22 years and the exposure level by inhalation during each 8 *hr* working day (5 work days per week, 48 work weeks per year) was 26 *ppm* of methylene chloride. Both internal and external controls were used. The total number of deaths, from all causes,

Table 3.10 Risk Factors for the Public and for Workers; Threshold Limit Values (TLV), and Bounds on Lifetime Cancer Risks at TLV Exposures for Selected Chemicals. [Taken from M.C.R. Alavanja et al. by courtesy *Appl. Occup. Environ. Hyg.*, **5** (No. 8), 511–517 (1990).]

Compound	Unit Risk Factor, q_1^* $(\mu g/m^3)^{-1}$	Adjusted Unit Risk Factor, $\tilde{q}_1^*$ $(\mu g/m^3)^{-1}$	TLV $\mu g/m^3$	Estimated Lifetime Extra Cancer Risk from Exposure to TLV
Acrylonitrile	6.8×10^{-5}	1.3×10^{-5}	4,500	0.05700
Benzene	8.3×10^{-6}	1.5×10^{-6}	30,000	0.04400
1,3 Butadiene	2.8×10^{-4}	5.2×10^{-5}	22,000	0.68000
Carbon tetrachloride	1.5×10^{-5}	2.8×10^{-6}	30,000	0.08100
bis(chloromethyl)ether	3.3×10^{-4}	1.2×10^{-2}	5	0.05800
Chromium(VI)	1.2×10^{-2}	2.2×10^{-3}	50	0.10000
Ethylene oxide	1.8×10^{-2}	2.0×10^{-5}	2,000	0.03900
Hexachlorobutadiene	2.2×10^{-5}	4.1×10^{-6}	240	0.00098
Vinyl chloride	7.1×10^{-6}	1.3×10^{-6}	10,000	0.01300

Table 3.11 Daily Exposure Doses for Workers at Specified Extra Risks of $1/10^6$ and $1/10^3$. [Taken from M.C.R. Alavanja et al. by courtesy *Appl. Occup. Environ. Hyg.*, **5** (No. 8), 511–517 (1990).]

Compound	Adjusted Unit Risk Factor, $\tilde{q}_1^*$ $(\mu g/m^3)^{-1}$	Daily Exposure $(\mu g/m^3)$ of Workers Associated with an Extra Risk of $1/10^6$	$1/10^3$
Acrylonitrile	1.3×10^{-5}	7.7×10^{-2}	7.7×10^{1}
Benzene	1.5×10^{-6}	6.7×10^{-1}	6.7×10^{2}
1,3 Butadiene	5.2×10^{-5}	1.9×10^{-2}	1.9×10^{1}
Carbon tetrachloride	2.8×10^{-6}	3.6×10^{-1}	3.6×10^{2}
Bis(chloromethyl)ether	1.2×10^{-2}	8.3×10^{-5}	8.3×10^{-2}
Chromium(VI)	2.2×10^{-3}	4.5×10^{-4}	4.5×10^{-1}
Ethylene oxide	2.0×10^{-5}	5.0×10^{-2}	5.0×10^{1}
Hexachlorobutadiene	4.1×10^{-6}	2.4×10^{-1}	2.4×10^{2}
Vinyl chloride	1.3×10^{-6}	7.7×10^{-1}	7.7×10^{2}

among the cohort exposed to methylene chloride was 176 compared to the 206 expected deaths based on internal controls and 253 based on external controls. The total expected number of lung and liver cancer deaths was 17.1 based on internal controls (16.6 lung cancers and 0.5 liver cancers), which constitutes the background. Thus,

$$p(0)n = 17.1$$

and since $n = 1013$, it follows that

$$p(0) = \frac{17.1}{1013} = 0.01688$$

Risk factors for the excess cancers expected from methylene chloride exposures have been computed on the basis of the results of animal tests. The National Toxicology Program (NTP) sponsored carcinogenesis bioassays of the inhalation of methylene chloride by rats and mice, and the final results became available in 1986.

The Food and Drug Administration (FDA) calculated the carcinogenic potency, or unit risk, of methylene chloride to be

$$q_1^* = 4.4 \times 10^{-4} \left(\frac{mg}{(kg\ body\ wt)(day)} \right)^{-1} \tag{3.60}$$

for continuous lifetime exposure. By use of the same data on a linearized extrapolation model, the Environmental Protection Agency (EPA) estimated the upper 95 percent confidence limit on the potency of methylene chloride to be

$$q_1^* = 1.4 \times 10^{-2} (ppm)^{-1} \tag{3.61}$$

for continuous lifetime exposure. According to Tollefson et al.,[13] the disparity in the unit risk factors calculated by FDA and EPA is due to a difference in models (a factor of 2) and to body weight versus surface area interspecies scaling (a factor of 13). Since the risk factors are based on continuous exposures over a lifetime, the daily dose of methylene chloride exposure during working hours must be converted to the corresponding exposure over a lifetime. One method of computing the lifetime average daily dose corresponding to an average occupational exposure level of 26 *ppm* is as follows

$$d = 26\,(ppm) \times \frac{8(hr\ work/day)}{24(hr/day)} \times \frac{240(work\ day/yr)}{365(day/yr)} \times \frac{22(work\ yr/lifetime)}{74(yr/lifetime)} = 1.7\ ppm$$

(Instead of 74 years per lifetime, Tollefson et al.[13] used 50 years, based on 20 years of age at hire and an average latency of 30 years.)

Next, the 1.7 *ppm* is converted to $mg/[(kg\ body\ wt)(day)]$. To do so the following data are needed.

1. One gram mole of methylene chloride has a weight of 85×10^3 *mg* and a volume of 24.5 *L* at a room temperature of 25°C and 1 atmosphere pressure.
2. An average person has a weight of 70 *kg* according to the EPA.
3. The average breathing rate of a person is 12 *L/min*. Since the concentration of chemical is so small, it is assumed that 12*L* of the air mixture (air plus chemical) is equal to 12 liters of pure air.

Since

$$1.7ppm = \frac{1.7\ molecules\ of\ methylene\ chloride}{1,000,000\ molecules\ of\ air} = \frac{1.7\ L\ of\ methylene\ chloride}{1,000,000\ L\ of\ air}$$

it follows that

$$d = \frac{1.7\ L\ of\ methylene\ chloride}{1,000,000\ L\ air} \times \frac{85 \times 10^3\ mg}{24.5\ L} \times \frac{12\ L}{1\ min} \times \frac{1440\ min}{1\ day} \times \frac{1}{70\ kg} = 1.46 \frac{mg}{(kg\ body\ wt)(day\ over\ a\ lifetime)}$$

Then the FDA upper bound on the probability of an extra tumor $[ER(d) = q_1^* d]$ over and above the background is given by

$$ER(d) = 4.4 \times 10^{-4} \left[\frac{mg}{(kg\ body\ wt)(day)}\right]^{-1} \times 1.46 \left[\frac{mg}{(kg\ body\ wt)(day)}\right] = 6.42 \times 10^{-4}$$

Since

$$ER(d) = [1 - \exp(-q_1^* d)] \approx q_1^* d \tag{3.62}$$

it follows from Equation (3.56) that a 95 percent upper confidence limit on

$$\begin{pmatrix} Excess\ number\ of\ cancer\ cases\ expected \\ from\ exposure\ to\ dose\ d \end{pmatrix} = ER(d)[1 - p(0)]n \tag{3.63}$$

Thus, the number of excess lung and liver cancer cases expected from the cohort of 1013 is obtained by use of Equation (3.62) as follows

$$\begin{pmatrix} Number\ of\ excess\ cancer\ cases\ expected \\ from\ exposure\ to\ dose\ d \end{pmatrix} = [6.42 \times 10^{-4}][1 - 0.01688][1013] = 0.64$$

This would be a 95 percent upper confidence limit on the number of expected cancer cases among employees in the first 74 years of their lives. If the EPA upper bound is used, the corresponding results are:

$$ER(d) = 1.4 \times 10^{-2}\,(ppm)^{-1} \times 1.7\,(ppm)$$
$$= 2.38 \times 10^{-2}$$

and a 95 percent upper confidence limit on

$$\begin{pmatrix} \textit{Number of excess cancer cases expected} \\ \textit{from exposure to dose d} \end{pmatrix} = 2.38 \times 10^{-2}[1 - 0.01688][1013]$$
$$= 23.7.$$

PROBLEMS

1. This problem and the next one are based on the results presented in two papers by Kelly.[15,16] The objective of this problem is to compute the *Extra Risk (ER)* on the basis of the following information. For a known cadmium (Cd) concentration in the stack gas of an incinerator, the system was modeled to determine the maximum concentration of the metals at ground level.

For cadmium:
Maximum ground level exposure concentration = $3.5 \times 10^{-4} \mu g/m^3$

Other data given by Kelly and constants given by the Environmental Protection Agency in References 20–22 which are needed in the calculation of the Extra Risk follow:

Average human lifetime (US) = 75 *years*
Average body weight = 70 *kg*
Cd cancer potency factor = 6.1 $[\text{mg/(kg)(day)}]^{-1}$
Exposure duration (life of facility) = 20 *years*
Average human inhalation rate = 20 m^3*/(person)(day)*

(a) Some of the constants such as breathing rate differ from one author to another. Convert the average human inhalation rate of 12 [*liters/(min)(person)*] to the units of m^3*/(person)(day)* and compare with the above inhalation rate of 20 m^3*/(person)(day)* used by the Environmental Protection Agency (EPA).
Answer: Average breathing rate = 17.28 m^3*/(person)(day)*.

(b) The unit risk factor for cadmium as given by the EPA[20] is

$$q_1^* = 1.7 \times 10^{-3} (\mu g/m^3)^{-1}$$

When the risk factors are expressed in the units of *mg/(kg body weight)(day)*, they are called the *potency* (the term used by the FDA). In order to compare the value of the unit risk factor with the value given above for the potency factor, convert q_1^* of $1.7 \times 10^{-3} (\mu g/m^3)^{-1}$ to *[mg/(kg body weight)(day)]*$^{-1}$.

Answer: $q_1^* = 5.95\,[mg/(kg)(day)]^{-1}$ as compared to the value 6.1 given in the statement of the problem.

(c) The dose d that appears in Equation (3.52) is the daily dose over the lifetime of an individual. However, if a person is exposed for only 20 years, the daily dose is reduced by a factor of 20/75. Compute the corresponding effective maximum dose in *mg/(kg body weight)(day over a lifetime)* from the value given of $3.5 \times 10^{-4} (\mu g/m^3)$ for constant exposure over a lifetime of 75 years.

Answer: 2.66×10^{-8} [*mg/(kg)(day)*].

(d) On the basis of the value given for q_1^* of 6.1 $[mg/(kg)(day)]^{-1}$ in the statement of the problem and the dose found in part (c), calculate the Extra Risk for a person exposed to cadmium at the concentration stated over a 20 year period.

Answer: $ER(d) = 1.62 \times 10^{-7}$ or an Extra Risk of 1 chance in 6,172,840 of developing cancer.

2. Kelly[16] reported the results of an experimental study of emissions from an existing incinerator. On the basis of the concentration of metals in the stack gas presented below, the carcinogenic risk for the elements, arsenic (As), beryllium (Be), cadmium (Cd), chromium (Cr), and for the PCBs are to be computed.

Incineration Data

Item	As	Be	Cd	Cr*	PCB
Breathing Absorption Factor					
Conservative	1.0	1.0	1.0	1.0	1.0
Realistic	0.3	0.25	0.4	0.1	1.0
Potency $[mg/(kg)(day)]^{-1}$					
Offsite Exposure[22]	50.0	8.4	6.1	41.0 [Cr(VI)]	4.34
Concentration (ng/m^3)					
Maximum average exposed individual					
Conservative	< 0.007	< 0.005	0.01	0.04	$< 1 \times 10^{-5}$
Realistic	< 0.005	< 0.004	0.007	0.03	$< 1 \times 10^{-5}$
Exposure Duration					
Conservative (yr)	75	75	75	75	75
Realistic (yr)	20	20	20	20	20

* According to Kelly, chromium is believed to be emitted from waste incinerators primarily in the form of Cr_2O_3 or Cr(III), and not as Cr(VI) for which the unit risk factors have been developed. Trivalent chromium compounds are not believed to be carcinogenic. Calculating the chromium carcinogenic risk as Cr(VI) may therefore be a significant overestimate of the carcinogenic risk of the chromium in the emissions. In fact, on the basis of experimental results, Knoll[17] estimated that for the case where no Cr(VI) is in the feed, Cr(VI) in the emissions from a rotary kiln incinerator is less than 10%.

Constants given:
Average human lifetime = 75 *years*
Average body weight = 70 *kg*
Average human inhalation rate = 20 $m^3/(person)(day)$

(a) Calculate the conservative and realistic dose for each of the above elements and the PCBs. In the calculation of the conservative dose, the absorption factors are all taken equal to unity, and the length of exposure is taken to be the total lifetime of 75 years. In calculation of the realistic dose, the length of exposure is taken to be 20 years.

Answer:

Substance	Conservative Dose *d* [$mg/(kg)(day)$]	Realistic Dose *d* [$mg/(kg)(day)$]
As	2.0×10^{-9}	1.14×10^{-10}
Be	1.43×10^{-9}	7.62×10^{-11}
Cd	2.86×10^{-9}	2.13×10^{-10}
Cr(VI)	1.14×10^{-8}	2.29×10^{-10}
PCB	2.86×10^{-12}	7.62×10^{-13}

(b) Calculate both the conservative and the realistic values for the Extra Risk according to Equation (3.52).

Answer:

Substance	*ER*(*d*) Conservative	*ER*(*d*) Realistic
As	10.0×10^{-8}	5.70×10^{-9}
Be	12.0×10^{-9}	6.4×10^{-10}
Cd	1.74×10^{-8}	1.3×10^{-9}
Cr(VI)	4.67×10^{-7}	0.94×10^{-8}
PCB	1.24×10^{-11}	3.31×10^{-12}

(c) Calculate the total Extra Risk for the elements and the PCBs on the basis of no interaction. Since the risk for chromium may be highly overstated as Cr(VI), compute the total Extra Risk both with and without Cr(VI). Compare the Extra Risk of cancer from the PCBs with that of the elements.

Answer:

Total Extra Risk with Chromium (VI)
Conservative: $ER(d) = 5.96 \times 10^{-7}$ or 1 chance in 1,677,852
Realistic: $ER(d) = 1.70 \times 10^{-8}$ or 1 chance in 58,820,000
Total Extra Risk without Chromium
Conservative: $ER(d) = 12.94 \times 10^{-8}$ or 1 chance in 7,727,975
Relalistic: $ER(d) = 0.764 \times 10^{-8}$ or 1 chance in 130,890,052
Extra Risk from the PCB exposures
Conservative: $ER(d) = 1.24 \times 10^{-11}$ or 1 chance in 80,640,000,000
Realistic: $ER(d) = 3.31 \times 10^{-12}$ or 1 chance in 302,114,803,000

3. Kelly also gave the concentrations for the Maximum Exposed Individuals (MEI) in the same study on which Problem 2 was based. The concentration in ng/m^3 were as follows:

Item	As	Be	Cd	Cr	PCB
Conservative	< 0.15	< 0.1	0.3	0.7	< 0.0003
Realisitic	< 0.10	< 0.07	0.2	0.5	< 0.0002

(a) On the basis of the potency factors and absorption factors given in Problem 2, compute the corresponding Extra Risk for each element and for PCB.

Answer

Substance	Conservative	Realistic
As	2.15×10^{-6}	1.14×10^{-7}
Be	0.24×10^{-6}	0.112×10^{-8}
Cd	0.523×10^{-6}	0.372×10^{-7}
Cr(VI)	8.21×10^{-6}	1.56×10^{-6}
PCB	0.372×10^{-9}	0.662×10^{-10}

(b) Also compute the total Extra Risk with and without chromium.

Answer:

Total Extra Risk with chromium
Conservative: $ER(d) = 1.11 \times 10^{-5}$
Realistic: $ER(d) = 3.19 \times 10^{-7}$
Total Extra Risk without chromium
Conservative: $ER(d) = 2.89 \times 10^{-6}$
Realistic: $ER(d) = 1.62 \times 10^{-7}$

4. To illustrate the use of the Extra Risks calculated above, suppose that the maximum average exposed individuals consisted of a hypothetical population of 500,000. Further suppose that each member of this population was exposed to As, Be, Cd, Cr(VI), and PCBs. Use the Extra Risks found in Problem 2 to determine the upper bound on the number of expected excess cancer cases from exposure to each of the chemicals [Assume that the background probability $p(0)$ is equal to zero.] Also calculate the upper bound on the total number of estimated excess cancer cases with and without chromium.

Answer:

Upper Bound on the Expected Excess Cancer Cases

Substance	Conservative	Realistic
As	5.00×10^{-2}	2.85×10^{-3}
Be	0.60×10^{-3}	3.32×10^{-4}
Cd	0.87×10^{-2}	0.65×10^{-3}
Cr(VI)	2.34×10^{-1}	0.47×10^{-2}
PCB	0.62×10^{-5}	1.66×10^{-6}
Total excess cancer cases expected with chromium	0.299	0.00853
Total excess cancer cases expected without chromium	0.065	0.00383

5. According to Rogers et al.[17], the annual average concentration of benzene in U.S. cities ranged from 2 to 20 $\mu g/m^3$ in 1988. The corresponding TLV given in Table 3.9 is 32 mg/m^3.

(a) Calculate the range of the Extra Risks for an individual in a U.S. city. (*Hint:* use the Unit Risk Factor given in Table 3.8).

(b) The TLV given for benzene in Table 3.9 is 32 mg/m^3 and the OSHA limit for the workplace is 1 ppm. Both are averaged over an 8-hour day. Calculate the Extra Risk for a worker exposed over a working career of 22 years at the TLV and OSHA levels. (*Hint:* Use the Adjusted Unit Risk Factor given in Table 3.10 corrected to 22 work years. Use the constants given in Part (c) as needed.)

(c) The annual average maximum concentration of benzene recorded by the Houston Regional Monitoring Program[18] in the Houston Ship Channel area where a large chemical complex is located was 5.1 ppb for 1988[18]. Calculate the Extra Risk for an individual living at this location over a lifetime. Given:

1. 1 g mol of benzene has a molecular weight of 78 *g/g mol.*
2. Average human breathing rate = 12 L/min at 25° C and 1 *atm.*
3. 1 g mol of air has a volume of 24.5 L at 25° C and 1 *atm.*

Answer: (a) $ER(d) = 1.66 \times 10^{-5}$ and 1.66×10^{-4}, (b) For the TLV = 32 mg/m^3, $ER(d) = 0.0264$; For the OSHA limit of 1 *ppm*, $ER(d) = 0.00263$, (c) $ER(d) = 1.35 \times 10^{-4}$.

6. The Unit Risk Factor given in Table 3.8 for formaldehyde for an individual who is exposed to a dose over a lifetime is

$$q_1^* = 1.1 \times 10^{-4} (\mu g/m^3)^{-1}$$

(a) Compute the corresponding Adjusted Risk Factor $\tilde{q}_1^*$ for formaldehyde for an industrial worker who is exposed to the dose 8 hours per day, 5 days per week, 50 work weeks per year, and 40 work years per 74 year life span. Also following Alvanja et al.[12], assume a respiration rate of 10 $m^3/(24\ hour\ day)$ used by EPA. [Note: 10 $m^3/8\ hr\ day$ = 1.25 m^3/hr and 20 $m^3/24\ hr\ day$ = 0.833 m^3/hr.]

(b) For an industrial worker who is exposed at the TLV dose level of 1.2 mg/m^3 of formaldehyde over a working career of 40 years, compute the Extra Risk.

(c) Rogers[17] reported that the annual average of formaldehyde in the atmospehere of U.S. cities ranged from 4 to 6 $\mu g/m^3$. Calculate the Extra Risk for a person exposed to this level of formaldehyde over a lifetime.

Answer: (a) $\tilde{q}_1^* = 2.04 \times 10^{-5} (\mu g/m^3)^{-1}$; (b) $ER(d) = 0.0245$; (c) $ER(d) = 4.4 \times 10^{-4}$ and $ER(d) = 6.6 \times 10^{-4}$.

7. According to Kelly[16], residential wood burning (in say fireplaces) is one the major producers of the most toxic form of dioxin, namely, 2,3,7,8 TCDD (2,3,7,8 tetrachlorodibenzo-p-dioxin). Kelly reported that the analysis of the scrapings from locations of the wood burning showed that they contained from 26 to 600 *ppt* with a mean of 242 *ppt* on a weight basis of 2, 3, 7, 8, TCDD. Since this gives no information about the concentration of the dioxin in the air in a room with a fireplace, the following hypothetical situation is assumed in order to obtain an estimate of the possible exposure of an individual. In the pioneer days, food was frequently prepared over the hot coals in fireplaces. Suppose that one meal is prepared daily in this manner over a lifetime of an individual. Further suppose that one gram of the soot scrapings (assumed to be carbon plus dioxin) falls into each serving, and suppose that each gram of carbon and the associated dioxin is 100 per cent absorbed by the body with the ingestion of the food. The Unit Risk Factor given by Anderson[2] is

$$q_1^* = 1 (\mu g/m^3)^{-1}$$

or one cubic meter of air per microgram of dioxin. To make use of this factor, assume that one gram of carbon is contained in each 20 m^3 of air breathed per day. Further suppose that the carbon and the associated dioxin is perfectly (100 percent) absorbed.

(a) Express the dose of dioxin in $\mu g/m^3$.

(b) Calculate the Excess Risk per gram of carbon and the associated dioxin absorbed by the body of an individual per day at the mean value dioxin of 242 *ppt*.

Answer: (a) $d = 1.21 \times 10^{-5}$ $(\mu g/m^3)$; (b) $ER(d) = 1.21 \times 10^{-5}$.

8. Kelly[16] reported that the analysis of samples of the stack gases from seven municipal waste combustors in the U.S. showed that the concentration of 2, 3, 7, 8 TCDD ranged from 0.3 to 9.1 $ng/m.^3$ On the basis of the assumption that there is no dispersion of the stack gases and a Unit Risk Factor of 1.0 $(\mu g/m^3),^{-1}$ estimate the range of Extra Risks. [Note: the assumption of no dispersion is far too conservative because the purpose of a stack is to disperse the gases.]

Answer: $ER(d) = 3.0 \times 10^{-4}$ and $ER(d) = 9.1 \times 10^{-3}$.

9. A number of chemical complexes in Texas have contracted with an outside agency to monitor continuously the air quality in the vicinity of their plants. The oustide agency places air conditioned trailers containing analytical and sampling equipment at the fence lines of the plants, downwind of the plant, and between the plants and the community. At one of these locations air is continuously analyzed for the gases ozone (O^3), NO_2, NO_x, and NMHC (non methane hydrocarbons) and every twelfth day, a 24-hour cumulative sample is collected and subsequently analyzed on state of the art equipment for 50 chemical compounds. During the month of December, 1990, the outside agency reported that the highest concentrations of 1,3 butadiene observed in one large chemical complex were as follows:

Maximum concentration = 3.3 *ppb* (by volume)
Mean concentration for December 1990 = 1.4 *ppb* (by volume)

Consider the worst case where a person is exposed to the above concentrations of 1,3 butadiene over a lifetime. Compute the Extra Risks corresponding to

(a) the maximum concentration for December, 1990;

(b) the mean concentration for December, 1990.

Use the Unit Risk Factor given in Table 3.8 of:

$$q_1^* = 2.8 \times 10^{-4} (\mu g/m^3)^{-1}$$

Assume an average temperature of 25° C, and that the gas mixture behaves as a perfect gas. The molecular weight of 1,3 butadiene (C_4H_6) is 54 $g/g\ mol$.

Answers: (a) $ER(d) = 7.4 \times 10^{-4}$; (b) $ER(d) = 1.75 \times 10^{-3}$.

10. To illustrate the unique relationship between the standard normal distribution function $\Phi(x)$ and the chi-square distribution function for the case where the number of degrees of freedom $\nu = 1$, the following problem is posed.

(a) For the standard normal distribution, use the table for this function to find the negative z such that

$$\Phi(-z) = \alpha = 0.05$$

(b) From the same tables, find the positive value of z such that

$$\Phi(z) = 1 - \alpha = 0.95$$

[This corresponds to the 95th percentile = $100(1 - \alpha)$]

Also observe that

$$\Phi(z) - \Phi(-z) = (1 - \alpha) - \alpha = 1 - 2\alpha$$

(c) Show that

$$z^2 = (1.645)^2 = (-z)^2 = (-1.645)^2 = 2.706$$

(d) Use the table for the chi-square distribution function $\chi^2_{df,1-2\alpha}$ to show that for $df = 1$ and $1 - 2\alpha = 0.90$ that

$$\chi^2_{1,0.90} = 2.706$$

Observe that $(1 - 2\alpha)$ corresponds to the 90th percentile $[(1 - 2\alpha)100 = 90]$

11. According to Anderson[2], the Environmental Protection Agency (EPA) follows the suggestion of Mantel and Schneiderman[19] that the dose in *mg/(surface area)(day)* is an equivalent dose between species. On the basis of this assumption, it is desired to find the factor needed to convert the daily dose used in an animal test in *mg/(kg)(day)* to the corresponding human dose in *mg/(kg)(day)*. Show that these doses are related by the approximate relationship

$$d_h\left[\frac{mg}{(kg)(day)}\right] = \left[\frac{M_m}{M_h}\right]^{1/3} d_m\left[\frac{mg}{(kg)(day)}\right]$$

where d_h and d_m denote the doses for humans and mice, and M_h and M_m denote the corresponding masses.

1. Assume that the masses can be represented by spheres; that is,

$$M_h = \rho_h\frac{\pi D_h^3}{6} = 70\text{kg} \qquad M_m = \rho_m\frac{\pi D_m^3}{6} = 0.03\text{kg}$$

2. Also assume that the densities are equal

$$\rho_h = \rho_m$$

3. Assume the respective surface areas can be represented by that of a sphere

$$A_h = \pi D_h^2$$
$$A_m = \pi D_m^2$$

Show that

$$\left(\frac{M_m}{M_h}\right)^{2/3} = \frac{D_m^2}{D_h^2} = \frac{A_m}{A_h}$$

and then show that

$$d_m\left[\frac{M_m}{A_m}\right] = d_h\left[\frac{M_h}{A_h}\right]$$

and finally that

$$d_m = \left[\frac{M_h}{M_m}\right]^{1/3} d_h$$

For humans, mass (M_h) is 70 kg and for a mouse $M_m = 0.03\ kg$. Show that $d_m = 13.3 d_h$.

12. Show that the equivalency dose between species of

$$d[\textit{mass of dose/(surface area of species)(day)}]$$

may be expressed as

$$d\ [\textit{mass of dose/(body weight of species)}^{2/3}\textit{(day)}].$$

That is,

$$d\left[\frac{mass}{(area)(day)}\right] = k\,d\left[\frac{mass}{(body\ weight)^{2/3}\ (day)}\right]$$

where the proportionality constant k depends upon the precise units used for the dose.

(a) Estimate the value of k for the case where the dose is expressed in grams per square centimeter of surface area per day, and it is assumed that

$$\pi D^2 = \text{surface area of species}$$

$$\rho = \text{density of species} = 1(gm/gm^3)$$

$$\frac{\pi D^3}{6} = \text{volume of species}$$

(b) Repeat Part (a) for the case where d is expressed in $kg/(m^2)(day)$

Answer: (a) $k = 0.207$; (b) $k = 20.7$.

NOTATION

Added Risk = specified number for the risk as defined Equation (3.27), say 10^{-4}, 10^{-6}, or 10^{-8}

d = daily dose; d_i = daily dose for experiment i; d_0 = virtually safe dose in the Mantel-Bryan method

Extra Risk = specified number for the risk as defined by Equation (3.29) say 10^{-4}, 10^{-6}, or 10^{-8}

$ER(d)$ = Extra Risk at does d; see Equation (3.50)

$L(p) = P(X = r)$ = likelihood that exactly r animals out of n animals will develop tumors; $l(p) = \log_e L(p)$

$L(q)$ = likelihood of observing exactly m outcomes: $X_1 = r_1, X_2 = r_2, \ldots, X_m = r_m \cdot L(\mathbf{q}) = P(X_1 = r_1)P(X_2 = r_2)\ldots P(X_m = r_m)$; see Equation (3.23). $\mathbf{q} = (q_0, q_1, \ldots, q_k)$ = parameters of the cancer model

m = counting integer used to denote the number of experiments or outcomes

n = number of binomial trials, or the total number of animals used in a given experiment

p = trial probability (probability of success), or the probability that an animal will develop a tumor

p_i^* = trial probability corresponding to the 99 percent upper confidence limit. Used in the Mantel-Bryan method; see Equation (3.14)

$p(d)$ = trial probability for each of n animals exposed to a dose d; see Equation (3.21)

$p(0)$ = background probability = probability of an animal developing a tumor at dose $d = 0$

$P(X = r)$ = probability that exactly r animals out of n animals will develop tumors. The binomial formula for $P(X = r)$ is given by Equation (3.1)

$P(X \leq r) = P(X = 0) + P(X = 1) + \ldots + P(x = r)$: probability that as many as r animals out of n animals tested will develop tumors. The *cumulative binomial distribution function* as given by Equation (3.2)

$P(X \geq r) = P(X = r) + P(x = r + 1) + \ldots + P(x = n)$ = probability that r or more animals out of n animals tested will develop tumors

$P(Z \leq z)$ = probability that a member of a population will develop a tumor when administered a dose d as given by the *standard normal distribution function*; see Equation (3.13)

$\mathbf{q} = \{q_0, q_1, \ldots, q_k\}$ = parameters of the multistage model

$\hat{\mathbf{q}} = \{\hat{q}_0, \hat{q}_1, \ldots, \hat{q}_k\}$ = estimated values of the parameters of $\mathbf{q}$

$\mathbf{q}^* = \{q_0{}^*, q_1{}^*, \ldots, q_k{}^*\}$ = values of the parameter $\mathbf{q}$ corresponding to the EPA lower and upper bounds

r = number of successes; or the number of animals that develop tumors among the n animals used in a given experiment

VSD = virtually safe dose corresponding to a specified risk of say 10^{-4}, 10^{-6}, or 10^{-8}; see Equations (3.27) and (3.30)

$V\hat{S}D$ = value of the virtually safe dose based on values of the parameters $\hat{\mathbf{q}}$ obtained by the *Maximum Likelihood Method*

VSD_L^*, VSD_U^* = valued of the virtually safe dose on the parameters $\mathbf{q}^*$ corresponding to the EPA 95 percent lower and upper confidence limits

X = binomial random variable relating an experimental outcome to the number of successes x observed in n binomial trials

x = the number associated with an outcome in the sample space Ω of an experiment by the random number X: used herein to denote the number of outcomes that are successes

Y = random variable defined in terms of the standard normal random variable Z^2 ($Y = Z^2$)

y = the number associated with an outcome in the sample space Ω of an experiment by the random variable Y

Z = standard normal random variable defined in terms of the random variable X

z = number associated with an outcome in the sample space Ω of an experiment by the standard normal random variable Z

GREEK LETTERS

μ = mean value of a normal random variable

σ = square root of the variance of a normal random variable

τ = tolerance; see Equation (3.13)

$\phi(u)$ = probability density function of the *standard normal distribution function* defined by Equation (3.37)

$\Phi(z)$ = *standard normal random distribution function*; $\Phi(z) = P(Z \leq z)$, which is given by Equation (3.13)

$\chi^2_{1,p}$ = *chi-square distribution function* for one degree of freedom and the pth percentile

REFERENCES

1. Mantel, N. and W.R. Bryan, "Safety Testing of Carcinogenic Agents," *Journal of the National Cancer Institute*, **27** (No.2), 455 (1961).
2. Anderson, E.L. and the Carcinogen Assessment Group of the Environmental Protection Agency, "Quantitative Approaches in use to Assess Cancer Risk," *Society for Risk Analysis*, **3** (No. 4), 277 (1983).
3. Bryan, W.R. and M.B. Shimkin, "Quantitative Analysis of Dose—Response Data Obtained with Three Carcinogenic Hydrocarbons in Strain C3H Male Mice," *J. Nat. Cancer Inst.*, 503-531 (1943).
4. *CRC, Handbook of Tables for Mathematics*, Third Edition, R.C. Weast, Editor in Chief, The Chemical Rubber Co., Cleveland, OH.
5. National Toxicology Program (NTP) Technical Report 388 on the Perinatal Toxicity and Carcinogenicity of Ethylene Thiourea (ETU) in F-344 Rats and B6C3F1 Mice, Research Triangle, North Carolina.
6. Battelle Columbus Laboratories, "Final Report on A Chronic Inhalation Toxicity Study in Rats and Mice Exposed to Formaldehyde to Chemical Industry Institute of Toxicology, submitted September 18, 1981; revised December 31, 1981," Battelle Columbus Laboratories, Columbus, Ohio [*Chemical Industry Institute of Toxicology (CIIT)* Docket #10922, 1982].
7. Lehmann, E.L., *Testing Statistical Hypotheses*, pg. 306, John Wiley & Sons, Inc., New York, N.Y. (1959)

8. Sielken, R.L., Jr., "Useful Tools for Evaluating and Presenting More Science in Quantitative Cancer Risk Assessments," *Toxic Substances Journal*, **9**, 353 (1989).
9. Jorgenson, T.A., E.F. Meirhenry, C.J. Rushbrook, et al., [Stanford Research Institute (SRI)] "Carcinogenicity of Chloroform in Drinking Water to Male Osborne—Mendel Rats and B6C371 Mice," *Fundamental Application of Toxicology* (U.S.A.), **5** (No. 4), 760 (1985).
10. Carcinogen Assessment Group U.S. Environmental Protection Agency, "Final Risk Assessment on Arsenic," EPA–600/6–81–002 (May, 1981).
11. American Conference of Government Industrial Hygienists: Threshold Limit Values and Biological Exposure Indices for 1991–1992. ACGIH, Cincinnati, OH (1991).
12. Alavanja, M.C., R.C., Brown, R. Spirtas, and M. Gomez, "Risk Assessment for Carcinogens: A Comparison of Approaches of the ACGIH and the EPA," *Appl. Occup. Hyg.*, **5** (No. 18), 510 (1990).
13. Tollefson, L., R.J. Lorentzen, R.N. Brown, and J.A. Springer, "Comparison of the Cancer Risk of Methylene Chloride Predicted from Animal Bioassay Data with Epidemologic Evidence," *Risk Analysis*, **10** (No. 3), 429 (1990).
14. Hearne, F.T., F. Gross, J.W. Pifer, B.R. Friedlander, and R.L. Raleigh, "Methylene Chloride Mortality Study: Dose–Response Characterization and Animal Model Comparison," *Journal of Occupational Medicine*, **29**, 217 (1987).
15. Kelly, K.E., "Methodologies for Assessing Health Risks of Hazardous Waste Incinerator Stack Emissions to Surrounding Populations," *Hazardous Waste and Hazardous Materials*, **1** (No. 4) 507 (1984).
16. Kelly, K.E., "The Risks of Dioxins and Other Pollutants Emitted from Hazardous Waste Incinerator Facilities," Paper presented at the 3rd International Symposium on Operating European Hazardous Waste Incinerator Facilities, Odense, Denmark, September 16-19 (1986).
17. Rogers, B., J. Wiersema, S. Price, T. Porter, G. Dean, T. Driscoll, J. Gise, M. Jenks, K. Kilpatrick, J. Lindgren, C. McCauley, J. Panketh, V. Smith, D. Sullivan, and N. Zare, "Final Report: Gulf Coast Community Exposure Study," Texas Air Control Board, Austin, Texas, March (1988).
18. "An HRM Presentation to Joint Select Committee on Toxic Air Emissions and the Greenhouse Effect," Radian Corporation, Austin, Texas, January 11 (1990).
19. Mantel, N. and M.A. Schneiderman, "Estimating Safe Levels, a Hazardous Undertaking," *Cancer Research* **35**, 1379 (1975).
20. U.S. Environmental Protection Agency (USEPA): Exposure factors handbook, Office of Health and Environmental Assessment, U.S. EPA, EPA 600/8-89-043, Washington, D.C. (1989).
21. U.S. Environmental Protection Agency (USEPA): Human health evaluation manual, supplemental guidance: Standard default exposure factors, Office of Emergency and Remedial Response, OSWER Directive 9285.6-03, Washington, D.C. (1991).
22. U.S. Environmental Protection Agency (USEPA): Integrated Risk Information Systems (IRIS) database, records for arsenic, beryllium, cadmium, and chromium, Washington, D.C. (1992).

4

Concepts Used in the Statistical Analysis of Animal Tests

Analysis of the data from animal tests makes significant use of the concepts of probability and statistics. The purpose of this chapter is to present an abbreviated introductory development of most of those concepts utilized herein in the analysis of the experimental data. The first topic to be considered is probability. The introduction to probability is in the context of random trials where each possible outcome is equally likely to occur. More general developments of probability are possible.

4.1 PROBABILITY

Probability theory is applied herein to *random experiments*. Experiments whose outcomes are not known in advance but for which the set of all possible outcomes is known in advance are called *random experiments*. The set of all possible outcomes of a given experiment is called the *sample space* Ω. An *event* is any collection (subset) of outcomes contained in the sample space. To illustrate the meanings of these terms, the following example is used. Suppose each of three people toss a fair coin for which the outcome of any one toss is heads (H) or tails (T). For three people with one toss each, there are a total of eight outcomes, which comprise the sample space Ω; that is,

$$\Omega = \{TTT, HTT, THT, TTH, THH, HTH, HHT, HHH\} \tag{4.1}$$

The concept of event is illustrated by the selection of the following subsets. Let event A_1 denote the set of all outcomes involving one head or no heads,

$$A_1 = \{HTT, THT, TTH, TTT\} \tag{4.2}$$

An event could consist of a single outcome. Examples of such events are:

$$A_2 = [TTT] \tag{4.3}$$

$$A_3 = [HHH] \tag{4.4}$$

The role of probability in the analysis of the outcomes (or event) of a process is to assign to each event A a number $P(A)$, called the probability of event A, which will give a precise measure of the chance that A will occur.

Suppose that there are n equally likely outcomes for a random trial and that an event A corresponds to m of these outcomes. That is, the event A occurs if and only if one of these m outcomes occurs. Thus, there are m outcomes favorable to A or successes, and there are $n - m$ outcomes unfavorable to A or failures. Then the probability of the occurrence of the event A in a single trial is

$$P(A) = \frac{m}{n} = p \tag{4.5}$$

Let $Q(A)$ denote the probability of the failure of event A to occur in a single trial. Then

$$Q(A) = \frac{n-m}{n} = 1 - \frac{m}{n} = 1 - p \tag{4.6}$$

and it is evident that

$$P(A) + Q(A) = 1 \tag{4.7}$$

4.2 INDEPENDENT EVENTS

Definition 4.1 *A set of events is said to be independent if the occurrence of any one of them does not influence the probability of the occurrence of the others. If the occurrence of any one of the events affects the probability of the occurrence of the others, the events are said to be dependent.*

In the developments that follow, the concept called the *multiplication rule* is needed. This concept is contained in the following theorem.

Theorem 4.1 (Multiplication Principle) *If k tasks $A_1, A_2, \ldots, A_k$ are to be done in succession and the first task A_1 can be done in n_1 ways, and A_2 in n_2 ways after A_1 has been completed, A_3 in n_3 ways after A_1 and A_2 have been completed, ..., and A_k in n_k ways after $A_1, A_2, \ldots, A_{k-1}$ have been completed, then the total task $A_1, A_2, \ldots, A_k$ can be performed in $n_1 \times n_2 \times \cdots \times n_k$ ways.*

The proof for two tasks follows. With each of the n_1 different ways in which A_1 can be done, there are n_2 ways of doing task A_2. Thus with all of the n_1 different ways of doing task A_1, there are $n_1 n_2$ different ways of doing the tasks together in the order stated. The remainder of the proof for any number of events follows by mathematical induction.

Theorem 4.2 *If k processes or trials are independent and A_i is any set of outcomes for the ith trial ($i = 1, 2, \ldots, k$), then the probability that all outcomes will occur is*

$$P(A_1, A_2, \ldots, A_k) = P(A_1)P(A_2)\ldots P(A_k) \tag{4.8}$$

Proof. First the proof is given for two independent trials (or processes) with the respective outcomes A_1 and A_2. Let m_1 denote the number of outcomes of the first trial that are successes and let n_1 denote the total number of outcomes (successes plus failures) of the first trial. Similarly, let m_2 and n_2 denote the corresponding quantities for the second trial. Then the probabilities of success of the outcomes A_1 and A_2 for each of these respective trials is given by

$$P(A_1) = \frac{m_1}{n_1} = p_1 \quad \text{and} \quad P(A_2) = \frac{m_2}{n_2} = p_2 \tag{4.9}$$

From Theorem 4.1, the total number of ways in which both trials can succeed is $m_1 m_2$, and the total number of ways in which the two trials can succeed and fail is $n_1 n_2$. Hence, the probability of occurrence of success of the two trials

$$P(A_1 \textit{ and } A_2) = \frac{m_1 m_2}{n_1 n_2} = p_1 p_2 \tag{4.10}$$

The remainder of the proof is by mathematical induction.

Example 4.1 Suppose a coin is tossed 10 times. What is the probability that heads will appear on the 9th and 10th tosses?

Solution The probability of a head on any one toss is 1/2. Therefore, by Theorem 4.1, the probability of outcome A_1 (a head on the 9th toss) and outcome A_2 (a head on the 10 toss) is given by

$$P(A_1 \textit{ and } A_2) = \frac{1}{2} \times \frac{1}{2} = \frac{1}{4} \tag{4.11}$$

4.3 MUTUALLY EXCLUSIVE EVENTS

Definition 4.2 *If the occurrence of any one event prevents the occurrence of the other events, the events are said to be mutually exclusive.*

Theorem 4.3 *If the events A_1 and A_2 are mutually exclusive, then the probability of the occurrence of either A_1 or A_2 is equal to the sum of the probabilities of the respective outcomes.*

$$P(A_1 \text{ or } A_2) = P(A_1) + P(A_2) \tag{4.12}$$

Proof. Since the outcomes are mutually exclusive, A_1 and A_2 cannot occur simultaneously. Thus the possible cases are:

1. A_1 occurs and A_2 fails to occur,
2. A_2 occurs and A_1 fails to occur,
3. both A_1 and A_2 fail to occur.

Let the number of equally likely cases in which A_1 occurs and A_2 fails to occur be denoted by n_1, A_2 occurs and A_1 fails to occur by n_2, and both A_1 and A_2 fail to occur by n_3. Then the total number of equally likely cases n is given by

$$n = n_1 + n_2 + n_3 \tag{4.13}$$

The probability that A_1 occurs is given by

$$P(A_1) = \frac{n_1}{n} \tag{4.14}$$

and the probability that A_2 occurs is

$$P(A_2) = \frac{n_2}{n} \tag{4.15}$$

The probability that either A_1 or A_2 occurs is

$$P(A_1 \text{ or } A_2) = \frac{n_1 + n_2}{n} = P(A_1) + P(A_2) \tag{4.16}$$

Then for the case of k mutually exclusive events, $A_1, A_2, \ldots, A_k$, the probability that either A_1, or $A_2, \ldots$, or A_k occurs is given by the following extension of the above formula,

$$P(A_1, \text{ or } A_2, \ldots, \text{ or } A_k) = P(A_1) + P(A_2) + \cdots .P(A_k) \tag{4.17}$$

4.4 BINOMIAL EXPERIMENTS

The probability that, in a test involving n animals, r animals will develop tumors can be expressed in terms of the probability that an individual animal will develop a tumor. This expression is based on the concept of a *binomial experiment*. The definition of a binomial experiment according to Allen[1] follows.

Definition 4.3 *A binomial experiment is one that satisfies the following conditions.*

1. *The experiment consists of a sequence of n trials where n is fixed in advance.*
2. *The trials are identical, and each trial can result in one of two outcomes; namely, success or failure.*
3. *The trials are independent so that the outcome of any particular trial does not influence the outcome of any other trial.*
4. *The probability p of success is constant from trial to trial.*

4.5 DEVELOPMENT OF THE BINOMIAL PROBABILITY DENSITY FUNCTION

Here follows a development of the expression for calculating the probability that, in a binomial experiment of n trials, exactly x animals develop tumors (success) and the probability that the number of animals developing tumors is equal to or less than x, as well as the probability that the number of animals developing a tumor is equal to or greater than x. In the following development, which is based on the one presented by Devore[2], use is made of the *binomial random variable* X which relates the outcomes of an experiment to the number x that are successes.

Binomial Experiment: For an experiment of $n = 4$ trials (or $n = 4$ animals), the trial probability p that an animal develops a tumor is the same for each animal, because it is given that the experiment is binomial. An expression for the probability that exactly 3 animals will develop tumors as a result of having been administered the same dose of a toxic substance is found as follows.

Let S denote a success, an animal develops a tumor, and let F denote a failure, an animal fails to develop a tumor. The possible outcomes for 4 distinct animals in which 3 develop tumors follow.

$$SSSF, SSFS, SFSS, FSSS$$

The probability that the first three animals develop tumors and the fourth one does not (*SSSF*) is given by the product of the individual probabilities because the trials are independent (Theorem 4.2). That is,

$$P(SSSF) = P(S)P(S)P(S)P(F) = p^3(1-p) \tag{4.18}$$

because $P(S) = p$ and $P(F) = 1 - p$. Similarly, the probability of occurrence of each of the other possible results [*SSFS*, *SFSS*, *FSSS*] is also $p^3(1-p)$. Because these outcomes (*SSSF*, *SSFS*, *SFSS*, *FSSS*) are the only outcomes corresponding to exactly three animals developing tumors, the probability of observing exactly 3 animals with tumors (successes) is

$$
\begin{aligned}
P(X=3) &= P(SSSF) + P(SSFS) + P(SFSS) + P(FSSS) \\
P(X=3) &= ppp(1-p) + pp(1-p)p + p(1-p)pp + (1-p)ppp \\
P(X=3) &= 4p^3(1-p) \qquad (4.19)
\end{aligned}
$$

Observe that the above result can be written

$$
P(X=3) = \begin{pmatrix} \textit{number of outcomes} \\ \textit{with } X = 3 \end{pmatrix} \begin{pmatrix} \textit{probability of any particular} \\ \textit{outcome with } X = 3 \end{pmatrix} \qquad (4.20)
$$

The symbol $b(x : n, p)$ is often used in the literature to denote $P(X = x)$, and called the *probability density function (p.d.f.)*. Observe that the number of outcomes with $X = x$ is the number of ways of choosing x of the n trials to be successes.

Similarly, for the case where exactly 2 animals develop tumors, Equations (4.19) and (4.20) become

$$
\begin{aligned}
P(X=2) &= P(SSFF) + P(SFSF) + P(FSSF) + P(FSFS) + P(SFFS) + P(FFSS) \\
P(X=2) &= pp(1-p)(1-p) + \cdots + (1-p)(1-p)pp \\
P(X=2) &= 6p^2(1-p)^2
\end{aligned}
$$

and

$$
P(X=2) = \begin{pmatrix} \text{number of outcomes} \\ \text{with } X = 2 \end{pmatrix} \begin{pmatrix} \text{probability of any particular} \\ \text{outcome with } X = 2 \end{pmatrix}
$$

Thus the first factor is equal to the number of combinations of size x (number of successes) that can be constructed from n distinct trials (or animals). Further observe that in the expression for the probability of any particular outcome $X = x$ $(x = 0, 1, 2, 3, 4)$, the exponent of p is equal to x, and the exponent of $(1 - p)$ is equal to $(n - x)$. Thus the binomial probability density function (p.d.f.) is given by

$$
P(X = x) = b(x : n, p) = \binom{n}{x} p^x (1-p)^{n-x} \qquad (4.21)
$$

where

$$
\binom{n}{x} = \frac{n!}{x!(n-x)!}
$$

and in general, $m! = m(m-1)(m-2)\ldots 1$, and $0! = 1$.

4.6 DEVELOPMENT OF THE CUMULATIVE BINOMIAL DISTRIBUTION FUNCTION

Consider again the above binomial experiment involving $n = 4$ animals, and suppose it is desired to find the probability that $X \leq 3$. For $X \leq 3$, the possible outcomes are: no animal develops a tumor, $X = 0$; one animal develops a tumor, $X = 1$; two animals develop tumors, $X = 2$; and three animals develop tumors, $X = 3$. Because each of these events is mutually exclusive, it follows that $P(X \leq 3)$ is given by Theorem 4.3; that is,

$$P(X \leq 3) = P(X = 0) + P(X = 1) + P(X = 2) + P(X = 3) \tag{4.22}$$

where

$$P(X \leq 3) = P(X = 0, X = 1, X = 2, \text{ or } X = 3)$$

Thus

$$P(X \leq 3) = \sum_{i=0}^{i=3} \binom{n}{i} p^i (1-p)^{n-i} \tag{4.23}$$

Observe that $P(X \leq x)$ is the *cumulative binomial distribution function* which is often denoted by $B(x : n, p)$; see Reference 6. Thus the general result is given by

$$P(X \leq x) = B(x : n, p) = \sum_{i=0}^{i=x} \binom{n}{i} p^i (1-p)^{n-i} \tag{4.24}$$

The probability of observing at least $r + 1$ successes $[X = r+1, X = r+2, \ldots, X = n-1, X = n]$ is represented by $P(X \geq r+1)$, and may be computed by use of the following cumulative binomial distribution function:

$$P(X \geq r + 1) = \sum_{i=r+1}^{i=n} \binom{n}{i} p^i (1-p)^{n-i} \tag{4.25}$$

Thus,

$$\begin{aligned} P(X \leq n) = &\left[P(X = 0) + P(X = 1) + \cdots + P(X = r)\right] \\ &+ \left[P(X = r + 1) + P(X = r + 2) + \cdots + P(X = n)\right] = 1 \end{aligned}$$

or

$$P(X \leq n) = P(X \leq r) + P(X \geq r + 1) = 1 \tag{4.26}$$

Hence,

$$P(X \leq r) = 1 - P(X \geq r + 1) \tag{4.27}$$

4.7 APPLICATIONS OF THE BINOMIAL PROBABILITY DENSITY FUNCTION

Consider first the probability $P(X = x)$ that a success will happen exactly x times in n independent Bernoulli trials where the probability that a trial will result in success is p. (Trials with two possible outcomes are called *Bernoulli trials*.)

$$P(X = x) = \left[\frac{n!}{x!(n-x)!}\right] p^x (1-p)^{n-x} \tag{4.28}$$

An example of the usual application of this formula follows.

Example 4.2 Find the probability of observing exactly 9 heads in 10 tosses of a coin.

Solution Since getting a head or tail on any one toss of a fair coin is equally probable, the probability p of success for any trial is equal to 1/2. Thus, since $n = 10$, $x = 9$, and $p = 1/2$, the probability density function becomes

$$P(X = 9) = \left[\frac{10!}{9!(10-9)!}\right] (1/2)^9 (1/2)^{10-9}$$

$$P(X = 9) = \frac{10}{2^{10}} = \frac{10}{1024} = 0.00977$$

Observe that in this application, the *given* and *to find* are as follows:

Given: $n = 10,\ r = 9,\ p = 1/2$
To Find: $P(X = 9)$

(Note: In the application of the binomial functions to animal tests, r is frequently used instead of x to denote the number of animals that develop specified responses [tumors].)

In the application of the binomial density function $P(X = r)$ to animal experiments, the problem to be solved is the inverse of Example 4.2. That is, n and r are known, and it is desired to find the trial probability p corresponding to a specified value of $P(X = r)$. The problem then becomes

Given: $n,\ r,\ P(X = r)$
To Find: p

If instead of the probability of observing exactly r tumors, the probability of observing r or fewer tumors is specified, then the problem is of the type:

Given: $n,\ r,\ P(X \leq r)$
To Find: p

Alternatively, the probability of observing at least $r + 1$ tumors may be specified. Then the statement of the problem becomes

$$\begin{aligned} \textit{Given:} \quad & n,\ r,\ P(X \geq r + 1) \\ \textit{To Find:} \quad & p \end{aligned}$$

Example 4.3 If the probability $P(X = r)$ of observing 9 heads and 1 tail in 10 tosses of a fair coin is set at 1 percent, find the corresponding trial probability p required to satisfy the specified condition of 1 percent.

Solution In this case, $n = 10$, $r = 9$ (heads are counted as successes) and $P(X = 9) = 0.01$. Substitution of these values into Equation (4.21) yields

$$P(X = 9) = 0.01 = \frac{10!}{9!(10 - 9)!} p^9 (1 - p)^{10-9}$$

Although this equation may be solved by trial and error for the solution value of p, its solution may also be found directly by use of the tables for the binomial distribution functions such as those given in Appendix III or Reference 6. The result so obtained is

$$p = 0.5$$

or

$$p = 0.999$$

4.8 RANDOM VARIABLES AND FUNCTIONS OF RANDOM VARIABLES

A *random variable* X is any rule that associates a number with each outcome in the sample space Ω of an experiment. For example, suppose that the appearance of a head on the toss of a coin is regarded as a success S and a tail is regarded as a failure F. Then the sample space Ω consists of S and F, and denoted by

$$\Omega = \{S, F\} \tag{4.29}$$

A random variable X may be defined on the space Ω as follows

$$X(S) = 1, \qquad X(F) = 0 \tag{4.30}$$

More generally, if ω is an element of Ω, then

$$X = x \tag{4.31}$$

denotes the set of all ω such that

$$X(\omega) = x \tag{4.32}$$

Similarly,

$$X \leq x \tag{4.33}$$

denotes the set of all ω such that

$$X(\omega) \leq x \tag{4.34}$$

For each real $x, X \leq x$ represents an event or set. For each random variable X, its distribution function F evaluated at a real x is defined to be the probability that the random variable X will have a value equal or less than x; that is

$$F(x) = P(X \leq x) \tag{4.35}$$

This function is called the *cumulative distribution function (c.d.f.)*. Also associated with each random variable X, there is another function $f(x)$ called the *probability density function (p.d.f.)* of X. If X is discrete, the probability density function is defined by

$$f(x) = P(X = x) \tag{4.36}$$

for all real x. If X is a continuous random variable, the probability density function is defined by

$$f(x) = \frac{dF(x)}{dx} \tag{4.37}$$

for all real x. The definitions of discrete and continuous random variable are given in the next two sections.

4.9 DISCRETE RANDOM VARIABLES AND THEIR ASSOCIATED FUNCTIONS

In many instances the range of possible values for the random variable X is only discrete values $x_1, x_2, \ldots, x_n$. A random variable is said to be discrete if the set of all possible outcomes of X is finite or countably infinite. A countably infinite set is one whose elements can be placed in a one-to-one correspondence with the positive integers and thus enumerated $x_1, x_2, x_3, \ldots$. Suppose X is discrete, and let T denote the set of all possible outcomes of X. Then each outcome x_i is an element of T, which is denoted by $x_i \in T$. The notation $x_i \in T$ means that x_i is a member of the set of elements $T = [x_1, x_2, \ldots]$ for which $p(x_i) > 0$. The corresponding probability density function for discrete random variables is denoted by $p(x_i)$, and Equation (4.36) implies

$$p(x_i) = P(X = x_i) > 0 \tag{4.38}$$

and

$$\sum_{x_i \in T} p(x_i) = \sum_{x_i \in T} P(X = x_i) = 1 \tag{4.39}$$

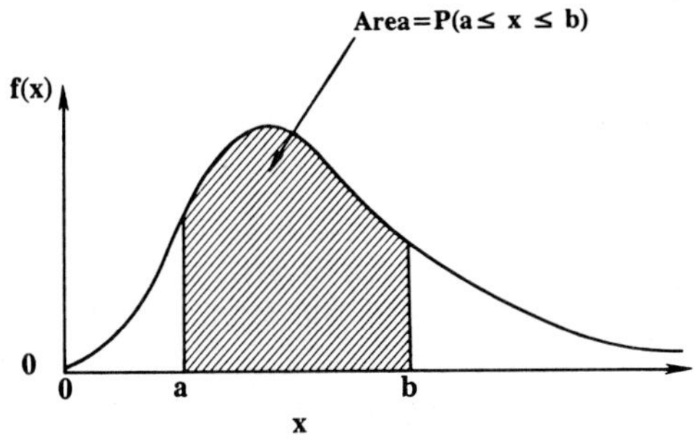

Figure 4.1 The Probability $P(a \leq X \leq b)$ that X Takes on a Value in the Interval $[a, b]$ Is Equal to the Area Under the Graph of the Density Function $f(x)$ for x in the Interval $[a, b]$.

4.10 CONTINUOUS RANDOM VARIABLES AND ASSOCIATED DISTRIBUTION FUNCTION

Continuous random variables can take on all values in one or more intervals. The probability that a continuous random variable X takes on a value in a set A is computed in terms of its probability density function (p.d.f.), $f(x)$, as follows:

$$P(A) = P(X \text{ } equals \text{ } a \text{ } value \text{ } in \text{ } A) = \int_A f(x)\,dx \tag{4.40}$$

and

$$P(a \leq x \leq b) = \int_a^b f(x)\,dx \tag{4.41}$$

for all real a, b with $a < b$. Thus the probability that X takes on a value in a closed interval [a,b] is equal to the area under the curve of $f(x)$ versus x between $x = a$ and $x = b$ as shown in Figure 4.1. The probability density function $f(x)$ is characterized by the additional properties:

$$f(x) \geq 0 \, for \text{ } all \text{ } real \text{ } x \tag{4.42}$$

$$\int_{-\infty}^{\infty} f(x)\,dx = 1 \tag{4.43}$$

The *cumulative distribution function F(x)* is the probability that $X \leq x$ and is given by

$$F(x) = \int_{-\infty}^{x} f(t)\,dt \tag{4.44}$$

4.11 NORMAL RANDOM VARIABLES AND THE NORMAL DISTRIBUTION FUNCTION

The *cumulative distribution function* and the *density function* associated with a given random variable are illustrated by consideration of the normal distribution functions. If a continuous variable X has the *probability density function*

$$f(x) = \frac{1}{\sigma\sqrt{2\pi}} \exp\left\{-\frac{1}{2}\left[(x-\mu)/\sigma\right]^2\right\} \tag{4.45}$$

for all real x, and for some parameters μ and $\sigma > 0$, then it is said to be a *normal random variable*. It is common to represent this fact by writing X *is* $N(\mu, \sigma^2)$.

The *cumulative normal distribution function* $F(x)$ is the probability that X lies between $-\infty$ and x and is given by

$$F(x) = P(X \leq x) = \int_{-\infty}^{x} \frac{\exp\left[-\frac{1}{2}\left(\frac{t-\mu}{\sigma}\right)^2\right]}{\sigma\sqrt{2\pi}}\,dt \tag{4.46}$$

A more convenient form of this function is called the *standard normal distribution function*, and it is obtained from Equation (4.46) by making the following change of variable. Let

$$u = \frac{t-\mu}{\sigma}, \qquad du = \frac{dt}{\sigma} \tag{4.47}$$

So when

$$\begin{aligned} t &= -\infty, \qquad u = -\infty \\ t &= x, \qquad u = \frac{x-\mu}{\sigma} \end{aligned} \tag{4.48}$$

After these substitutions have been made, the resulting form of the cumulative distribution function (the *standard normal distribution function*) is commonly denoted by $\Phi(z)$,

$$\Phi(z) = \int_{-\infty}^{z} \frac{\exp(-u^2/2)}{\sqrt{2\pi}}\,du \tag{4.49}$$

and the integrand by $\phi(u)$. Also, the upper limit $(x-\mu)/\sigma$ has been denoted by z; that is,

$$z = \frac{x-\mu}{\sigma} \tag{4.50}$$

and

$$Z = \frac{X-\mu}{\sigma} \tag{4.51}$$

where Z is called a *standard normal random variable*.

4.12 PARAMETERS OF RANDOM VARIABLES

The two most important parameters that are used to describe a random variable X are the *mean* μ or *expected value* $E(X)$ and the *variance* σ^2 or *Var*(X). The expected value $E(X)$ of the random variable X is commonly denoted by μ and defined as follows:

$$\mu = E(X) = \int_{-\infty}^{\infty} xf(x)\,dx \tag{4.52}$$

The variance $Var(X)$ of the random variable X is commonly denoted by σ^2 and defined as follows:

$$\sigma^2 = E\left\{[x - E(X)]^2\right\} \tag{4.53}$$

and

$$\sigma^2 = Var(X) = \int_{-\infty}^{\infty} [x - E(X)]^2 f(x)\,dx \tag{4.54}$$

The *standard deviation* of the random variable X is widely used, and it is defined as follows:

$$Standard\ Deviation = \sqrt{\sigma^2} = \sigma \tag{4.55}$$

For discrete variables, the mean and variance are defined as follows:

$$\mu = E(X) = \sum_{x_i \in T} x_i p(x_i) \tag{4.56}$$

$$\sigma^2 = Var(X) = \sum_{x_i \in T} [x_i - E(X)]^2 p(x_i) \tag{4.57}$$

where T is the set of all possible values of X. Examples of the parameters μ and σ^2 for a continuous random variable X are those associated with the normal distribution functions. For the cumulative normal distribution function given by Equation (4.46), the corresponding values for the expected value $E(X)$ and the variance $Var(X)$ are found by use of the definitions given by Equations (4.52) and (4.54) as follows:

$$E(X) = \int_{-\infty}^{\infty} \frac{[t] \exp\left[-\frac{1}{2}\left(\frac{t-\mu}{\sigma}\right)^2\right]}{\sigma\sqrt{2\pi}}\,dt = \mu \tag{4.58}$$

and

$$Var(X) = \int_{-\infty}^{\infty} \frac{[t-\mu]^2 \exp\left[-\frac{1}{2}\left(\frac{t-\mu}{\sigma}\right)^2\right]}{\sigma\sqrt{2\pi}}\,dt = \sigma^2 \tag{4.59}$$

These integrations may be carried out as described in most standard texts on statistics (see for example Allen[1]).

For the standard normal distribution function, the corresponding values of the expected value $E(X)$ and variance $Var(X)$ are found in a similar manner; namely,

$$E(X) = \int_{-\infty}^{\infty} \frac{ue^{-u^2/2}}{\sqrt{2\pi}}\,du = 0 \tag{4.60}$$

$$Var(X) = \int_{-\infty}^{\infty} \frac{(u-0)^2 e^{-u^2/2}}{\sqrt{2\pi}} du = 1 \tag{4.61}$$

or $\mu = 0$ and $\sigma^2 = 1$.

4.13 OTHER FUNCTIONS USED IN THE ANALYSIS OF ANIMAL TESTS

In the analysis of animal tests by the procedure employed by the Environmental Protection Agency (EPA), the *chi-square distribution function* is employed. This function is associated with the *chi-square random variable* Y. If

$$Y = X_1^2 + X_2^2 + \cdots + X_\nu^2 \tag{4.62}$$

where $X_1, X_2, \ldots, X_\nu$ are independent standard normal random variables, then the random variable Y is said to have a *chi-square distribution* with ν degrees of freedom. The corresponding probability density function is given by

$$f(x) = \begin{cases} x^{(\nu/2)-1} e^{-x/2} / 2^{\nu/2} \Gamma(\nu/2) & x > 0 \\ 0 & x \leq 0 \end{cases} \tag{4.63}$$

In this expression $\Gamma(\nu/2)$ denotes the *gamma function* of $\nu/2$. The gamma function is defined as follows:

$$\Gamma(t) = \int_0^{\infty} x^{t-1} e^{-x}\, dx \tag{4.64}$$

If n is an integer, it can be shown that

$$\Gamma(n+1) = n! \qquad n = 0, 1, 2, \ldots. \tag{4.65}$$

Tables are given in most standard statistic texts[1,2,3,4,6] that present the values of $\chi^2_{\nu,p}$, where ν represents the number of degrees of freedom and p represents the *percentile* of the chi-square distribution function. [In the tables for the chi-square distribution function presented in Appendix V, the degrees of freedom are denoted by *df* instead of *v*.] All of these quantities are related as follows:

$$p = \int_0^{\chi^2_{\nu,p}} f(x)\, dx \tag{4.66}$$

where the probability density function $f(x)$ is given by Equation (4.63).

4.14 CONFIDENCE INTERVALS

The idea of confidence intervals is similar to the concept of error in numerical analysis. In particular, suppose that the error of a calculated value $\tilde{x}$ of x does not exceed δ. Then the true value of x lies between $\tilde{x} - \delta$ and $\tilde{x} + \delta$; that is,

$$\tilde{x} - \delta \leq x \leq \tilde{x} + \delta \tag{4.67}$$

However, if a random variable X is an estimator of a parameter θ, then it is impossible to predict with certainty that θ is within a nontrivial interval on the basis of X. [For example, if θ is positive, a trivial interval would be 0 to ∞.] Instead, a *confidence interval* may be constructed such that the probability that the true value of θ lies within this interval is say 0.95 and the probability that it does not is 0.05. This probability is describing the method of constructing the confidence interval. In a $100(1 - \alpha)\%$ confidence interval, the $100(1 - \alpha)\%$ is the *confidence level*. The α is sometimes called the *level of significance* when confidence intervals are constructed in conjunction with hypothesis testing. Thus,

$$1 - \alpha = \textit{measure of confidence} \tag{4.68}$$

$$\alpha = \textit{measure of nonconfidence} \tag{4.69}$$

For example, if X is a normal random variable with a mean μ and variance σ^2, then the random interval

$$[X - \sigma z_{\alpha/2},\ X + \sigma z_{\alpha/2}]$$

is a $100(1 - \alpha)\%$ confidence interval on μ because

$$P\left(X - \sigma z_{\alpha/2} \leq \mu \leq X + \sigma z_{\alpha/2}\right) = 1 - \alpha^* \tag{4.70}$$

This follows because

$$P\left(-z_{\alpha/2} \leq Z \leq z_{\alpha/2}\right) = 1 - \alpha \tag{4.71}$$

Therefore, since the random variable Z is related to the random variable X by

$$Z = \frac{X - \mu}{\sigma} \tag{4.72}$$

it follows that

$$P\left(-z_{\alpha/2} \leq \frac{X - \mu}{\sigma} \leq z_{\alpha/2}\right) = 1 - \alpha \tag{4.73}$$

Rearrangement of the inequality yields the expression given by Equation (4.70).

Thus the interval of confidence is selected by the choice of $z_{\alpha/2}$, and the probability that the interval selected will contain μ is equal to $1 - \alpha$. The graphical representation of the portion of the distribution of Z used to construct the confidence interval is shown in Figure 4.2.

---

* A comparison of Equations (4.71) and (3.34) shows that they are equivalent statements of a confidence interval with Equation (4.71) being stated in terms of $-z_{\alpha/2}$, $z_{\alpha/2}$, and $(1 - \alpha)$, and Equation (3.34) in terms of $-z_{\alpha}$, z_{α}, and $(1 - 2\alpha)$.

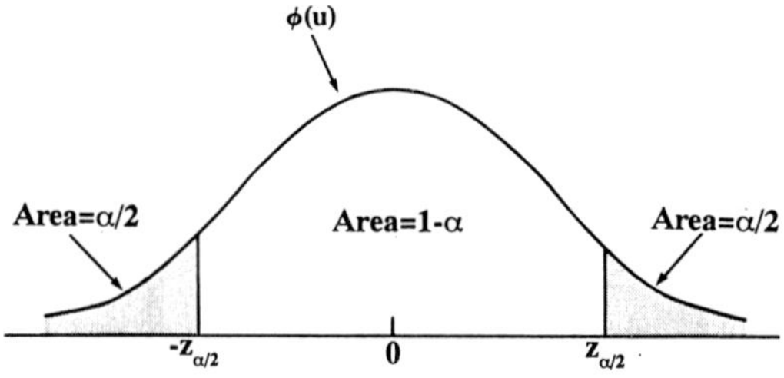

Figure 4.2 The Probability $P(-z_{\alpha/2} < Z < z_{\alpha/2})$ that the Random Variable Z Lies between $-z_{\alpha/2}$ and $z_{\alpha/2}$ Is Equal to Area $1 - \alpha$.

4.15 THE MAXIMUM LIKELIHOOD ESTIMATION METHOD FOR QUANTAL-RESPONSE MODELS

This procedure is often used to estimate the parameters pertaining to cancer formation that appear in the probability functions describing the outcomes of experiments. The procedure supposes that all of the experiments are carried out independently, and that each animal in each experiment is independent of the other animals in that experiment. Furthermore, in each experiment i, a dose d_i $[i = 1, 2, \ldots, m]$ is administered to a group of $n_i[i = 1, 2, \ldots, m]$ animals, and after a given time period T (for all experiments), the number of animals $X_i[i = 1, 2, \ldots, m]$ that have developed tumors is observed to be $r_i[i = 1, 2, \ldots, m]$.

The *Maximum Likelihood Estimation Method* makes use of the information or results $[d_i, n_i, r_i]$ in the determination of the most probable values of the parameters in the dose-response model for the test probabilities p_i. The expression for the *likelihood function* is developed in the following manner. From Equation (4.21), it follows that the probability of an experimenter observing exactly r_i tumors in any experiment i is given by

$$P(X_i = r_i) = \binom{n_i}{r_i} p_i^{r_i}(1 - p_i)^{n_i - r_i} \tag{4.74}$$

where

$$\binom{n_i}{r_i} = \frac{n_i!}{r_i!(n_i - r_i)!}$$

Since the m experiments are carried out independently, the probability of the experimenter observing all outcomes is given by the product of the probabilities of the outcomes of each of the experiments; that is,

$$P(observing\ m\ outcomes: \ X_1 = r_1, X_2 = r_2, \ldots, X_m = r_m)$$

$$= P(X_1 = r_1)P(X_2 = r_2) \cdots P(X_m = r_m) \tag{4.75}$$

The left hand side is called the *likelihood function* and denoted by L, and since the test probabilities p_i are unknown, the functional dependence can be represented by

$$L(p_1, p_2, \ldots, p_m)$$

The objective of the Maximum Likelihood Estimation Method is to pick the set $\{p_i\}$ that maximizes the likelihood $L(p_1, p_2, \ldots, p_m)$ that the experimenter will observe the experimental results $\{n_i, r_i\}$ for the m independent experiments.

The response probabilities p_i change as the respective doses d_i for each experiment i change. It is, of course, assumed that the same time period T is used for each experiment. Numerous models are presented in Chapter 2 for the test probability as a function of dose. To simplify the analysis of the behavior of the Maximum Likelihood Estimation Method, the following expression for the linearized form of the multistage model is used.

$$p_i(d_i) = 1 - \exp[-(q_0 + q_1 d_i)] \qquad i = 1, 2, \ldots, m \tag{4.76}$$

In the present situation, the dose d_i is known and the parameters q_0 and q_1 are unknown nonnegative numbers. The response probability p_i is regarded as a function of q_0 and q_1 and denoted by $p_i(q_0, q_1)$. Likewise the likelihood function becomes a function of q_0 and q_1 and is denoted by $L(q_0, q_1)$. Observe that with q_0 held fixed and q_1 allowed to vary, p_i increases from its smallest positive value at $q_1 = 0$ and approaches unity as q_1 is allowed to increase indefinitely. A similar trace of p_i for the case where q_1 is held fixed and q_0 allowed to vary is obtained. At $q_0 = q_1 = 0$, the likelihood function $L(0,0) = 0$ if $r_i > 0$ because of the term $p_i^{r_i}$. As q_0 and q_1 are increased indefinitely, the function $L(q_0, q_1)$ approaches zero because of the term $(1 - p_i)^{n_i - r_i}$ approaches zero, provided $r_i < n_i$. Since $0 \leq p_i \leq 1$, the function $L(q_0, q_1) \geq 0$ for all positive q_0 and q_1. Thus, the function must pass through at least one maximum as q_0 and q_1 are varied from zero to infinity. Numerous optimization techniques are available in the numerical literature for searching functions such as the likelihood function for their global maximum.

Of the possible methods for finding the set (q_0, q_1) that maximizes $L(q_0, q_1)$, only the Newton-Raphson[5] is presented. This method makes use of the fact that the necessary condition for a maximum to exist is that the partial derivatives be equal to zero; that is,

$$\frac{\partial L(q_0, q_1)}{\partial q_0} = 0 \quad \text{and} \quad \frac{\partial L(q_0, q_1)}{\partial q_1} = 0 \tag{4.77}$$

for unrestricted values of the parameters q_0 and q_1. A more convenient form of the likelihood function for computing the Maximum Likelihood Estimates $\hat{q}_0$ and $\hat{q}_1$ of the values q_0 and q_1 respectively is the logarithmic form. In particular, let

$$l = \log_e L(q_0, q_1) \tag{4.78}$$

Then

$$l = \sum_{i=1}^{m} \log_e \binom{n_i}{r_i} + \sum_{i=1}^{m} r_i \log_e p_i + \sum_{i=1}^{m} (n_i - r_i) \log_e (1 - p_i) \tag{4.79}$$

Thus,

$$\frac{\partial l}{\partial q_0} = 0 = 0 + \sum_{i=1}^{m} \frac{r_i}{p_i}\frac{\partial p_i}{\partial q_0} - \sum_{i=1}^{m} \frac{(n_i - r_i)}{(1 - p_i)}\frac{\partial p_i}{\partial q_0} \tag{4.80}$$

These terms may be combined to give the equation

$$0 = \sum_{i=1}^{m} \frac{(r_i - n_i p_i)}{p_i(1 - p_i)}\frac{\partial p_i}{\partial q_0} \tag{4.81}$$

Similarly,

$$0 = \sum_{i=1}^{m} \frac{(r_i - n_i p_i)}{p_i(1 - p_i)}\frac{\partial p_i}{\partial q_1} \tag{4.82}$$

For the linear form of the multistage model,

$$\frac{\partial p_i}{\partial q_0} = e^{-(q_0 + q_1 d_i)} \tag{4.83}$$

$$\frac{\partial p_i}{\partial q_1} = d_i e^{-(q_0 + q_1 d_i)} \tag{4.84}$$

Let the zeroes on the left hand sides of Equations (4.81) and (4.82) be replaced by $f_1(q_0, q_1)$ and $f_2(q_0, q_1)$, respectively. The set of values q_0 and q_1 that make $f_1(q_0, q_1) = f_2(q_0, q_1) = 0$ may be found by use of the Newton-Raphson method[5] which consists of the successive application of the equations

$$0 = f_1(q_{0,0}, q_{1,0}) + \Delta q_0 \frac{\partial f_1}{\partial q_0}\bigg|_{q_{0,0}, q_{1,0}} + \Delta q_1 \frac{\partial f_1}{\partial q_1}\bigg|_{q_{0,0}, q_{1,0}} \tag{4.85}$$

$$0 = f_2(q_{0,0}, q_{1,0}) + \Delta q_0 \frac{\partial f_2}{\partial q_0}\bigg|_{q_{0,0}, q_{1,0}} + \Delta q_1 \frac{\partial f_2}{\partial q_1}\bigg|_{q_{0,0}, q_{1,0}} \tag{4.86}$$

where

$$\Delta q_0 = q_{0,1} - q_{0,0}$$

$$\Delta q_1 = q_{1,1} - q_{1,0}$$

On the basis of the assumed values $(q_{0,0}, q_{1,0})$, the functions and derivatives appearing in Equations (4.85) and (4.86) are evaluated. Then Equations (4.85) and (4.86) are solved for Δq_0 and Δq_1. The values of q_0 and q_1 to be assumed for the next trial are then computed by use of the definitions of Δq_0 and Δq_1 as follows:

$$q_{0,1} = q_{0,0} + \Delta q_0 \tag{4.87}$$

$$q_{1,1} = q_{1,0} + \Delta q_1 \tag{4.88}$$

This process is continued until the Euclidean norm of the functions f_1 and f_2 has been reduced to some number equal to or less than a small preassigned number ϵ; that is,

$$[f_1^2 + f_2^2]^{1/2} \leq \epsilon \tag{4.89}$$

4.16 APPLICATION OF THE NEWTON-RAPHSON METHOD WHEN SOME OF THE PARAMETERS ARE CONSTRAINED

The Newton-Raphson technique described above implies that maximum likelihood estimates of the parameters q_j ($j = 0, 1, \ldots, c$) are unconstrained. If, however, some of the parameters are restricted to be nonnegative, then the Newton-Raphson method can be applied by solving each of several problems in which one or more of the parameters q_j ($j = 0, 1, \ldots, c$) are set equal to zero as described by Taha[7] or in similar texts on nonlinear programming. In particular, if the likelihood function is a concave function of the parameters q_j ($j = 0, 1, \ldots, c$), then the Kuhn-Tucker conditions[7] are necessary and sufficient conditions for identifying maximum likelihood estimates when some of the parameters are restricted to be nonnegative. The Kuhn-Tucker conditions imply that, in order for $\mathbf{q}^* = [q_0^*, q_1^*, \ldots, q_c^*]$ to be a maximum likelihood estimate of $\mathbf{q}$ either

$$\left.\frac{\partial L}{\partial q_j}\right|_{\mathbf{q}=\mathbf{q}^*} = 0 \qquad \text{if } q_j \text{ is unrestricted}$$

or

$$\left.\frac{\partial L}{\partial q_j}\right|_{\mathbf{q}=\mathbf{q}^*} = 0 \qquad \text{if } q_j \geq 0 \text{ and } q_j^* > 0$$

or

$$\left.\frac{\partial L}{\partial q_j}\right|_{\mathbf{q}=\mathbf{q}^*} \leq 0 \qquad \text{if } q_j \geq 0 \text{ and } q_j^* = 0$$

for $j = 0, 1, \ldots, c$.

For example, in order for

$$\mathbf{q}^* = [q_0^*, q_1^*, \ldots, q_c^*]$$

to be a maximum likelihood estimate of $\mathbf{q}$ when the components of $\mathbf{q}$ are restricted to be nonnegative, it is necessary and sufficient that either

$$\frac{\partial L}{\partial q_j} = 0\left.\vphantom{\frac{\partial L}{\partial q_j}}\right|_{\mathbf{q}=\mathbf{q}^*} = 0 \quad \text{and} \quad q_j^* \geq 0 \qquad \text{for } j = 0, 1, \ldots, c$$

or one or more of the q_j^* are zero and for those values of j

$$\left.\frac{\partial L}{\partial q_j}\right|_{\mathbf{q}=\mathbf{q}^*} \leq 0$$

while for the values of j with $q_j^* > 0$

$$\left.\frac{\partial L}{\partial q_j}\right|_{\mathbf{q}=\mathbf{q}^*} = 0$$

The use of the Newton-Raphson method in the solution of problems of this type is illustrated by use of the following example.

Example 4.4 Suppose that three quantal experiments are carried out and the following results are obtained:

Dose d_i	Number of Animals n_i	Number of Tumors r_i
0	100	2
5	100	10
10	100	50

These data are to be fit to

$$p_i = 1 - \exp[-(q_0 + q_1 d_i + q_2 d_i^2)]$$

where $q_0 \geq 0$, $q_1 \geq 0$, $q_2 \geq 0$.

Solution The nonnegative restrictions imply that, in order for q_0^*, q_1^*, q_2^* to be a maximum likelihood estimate for each q_j, then either

$$\left.\frac{\partial L}{\partial q_j}\right|_{\mathbf{q}=\mathbf{q}^*} = 0 \qquad \text{if } q_j^* > 0$$

or

$$\left.\frac{\partial L}{\partial q_j}\right|_{\mathbf{q}=\mathbf{q}^*} \leq 0 \qquad \text{if } q_j^* = 0$$

Thus, the Newton-Raphson technique is applied sequentially for solving up to 8 of the following problems that correspond to each of the 8 possible events in which some of the q_j^*'s may be zero.

1. Find q_0^*, q_1^*, q_2^* such that

$$\left.\frac{\partial L}{\partial q_0}\right|_{\mathbf{q}=\mathbf{q}^*} = 0 \qquad \left.\frac{\partial L}{\partial q_1}\right|_{\mathbf{q}=\mathbf{q}^*} = 0 \qquad \left.\frac{\partial L}{\partial q_2}\right|_{\mathbf{q}=\mathbf{q}^*} = 0$$

   If $q_0^* \geq 0$, $q_1^* \geq 0$, $q_2^* \geq 0$, this $\mathbf{q}^* = [q_0^*, q_1^*, q_2^*]$ is the maximum likelihood estimate, and stop.

2. Find $q_0^* = 0, q_1^*, q_2^*$ such that

$$\left.\frac{\partial L}{\partial q_1}\right|_{\mathbf{q}=\mathbf{q}^*} = 0, \qquad \left.\frac{\partial L}{\partial q_2}\right|_{\mathbf{q}=\mathbf{q}^*} = 0$$

   If $q_1^* \geq 0$, $q_2^* \geq 0$, and

$$\left.\frac{\partial L}{\partial q_0}\right|_{\mathbf{q}=\mathbf{q}^*} \leq 0$$

   then $\mathbf{q}^* = [q_0^* = 0, q_1^*, q_2^*]$ is the maximum likelihood estimate, and stop.

3. Find $q_0^*, q_1^* = 0, q_2^*$, such that

$$\left.\frac{\partial L}{\partial q_0}\right|_{\mathbf{q}=\mathbf{q}^*} = 0, \qquad \left.\frac{\partial L}{\partial q_2}\right|_{\mathbf{q}=\mathbf{q}^*} = 0$$

   If $q_0^* \geq 0$, $q_2^* \geq 0$, and

$$\left.\frac{\partial L}{\partial q_1}\right|_{\mathbf{q}=\mathbf{q}^*} \leq 0$$

   then $\mathbf{q}^* = [q_0^*, q_1^* = 0, q_2^*]$ is the maximum likelihood estimate, and stop.

4. Find $q_0^*, q_1^*, q_2^* = 0$, such that

$$\left.\frac{\partial L}{\partial q_0}\right|_{\mathbf{q}=\mathbf{q}^*} = 0 \qquad \left.\frac{\partial L}{\partial q_1}\right|_{\mathbf{q}=\mathbf{q}^*} = 0$$

   If $q_0^* \geq 0$, $q_1^* \geq 0$, and

$$\left.\frac{\partial L}{\partial q_2}\right|_{\mathbf{q}=\mathbf{q}^*} \leq 0$$

   then $\mathbf{q}^* = [q_0^*, q_1^*, q_2^* = 0]$ is the maximum likelihood estimate, and stop.

5. Find $q_0^* = 0, q_1^* = 0, q_2^*$ such that

$$\left.\frac{\partial L}{\partial q_2}\right|_{\mathbf{q}=\mathbf{q}^*} = 0$$

If $q_2^* \geq 0$ and

$$\left.\frac{\partial L}{\partial q_0}\right|_{\mathbf{q}=\mathbf{q}^*} \leq 0 \qquad \left.\frac{\partial L}{\partial q_1}\right|_{\mathbf{q}=\mathbf{q}^*} \leq 0$$

then $\mathbf{q}^* = [q_0^* = 0, q_1^* = 0, q_2^*]$ is the maximum likelihood estimate, and stop.

6. Find $q_0^* = 0$, q_1^*, $q_2^* = 0$ such that

$$\left.\frac{\partial L}{\partial q_1}\right|_{\mathbf{q}=\mathbf{q}^*} = 0$$

If $q_1^* \geq 0$ and

$$\left.\frac{\partial L}{\partial q_0}\right|_{\mathbf{q}=\mathbf{q}^*} \leq 0 \qquad \left.\frac{\partial L}{\partial q_2}\right|_{\mathbf{q}=\mathbf{q}^*} \leq 0$$

then $\mathbf{q}^* = [q_0^* = 0, q_1^*, q_2^* = 0]$ is the maximum likelihood estimate, and stop.

7. Find q_0^*, $q_1^* = 0$, $q_2^* = 0$ such that

$$\left.\frac{\partial L}{\partial q_0}\right|_{\mathbf{q}=\mathbf{q}^*} = 0$$

If $q_2^* \geq 0$ and

$$\left.\frac{\partial L}{\partial q_1}\right|_{\mathbf{q}=\mathbf{q}^*} \leq 0 \qquad \left.\frac{\partial L}{\partial q_2}\right|_{\mathbf{q}=\mathbf{q}^*} \leq 0$$

then $\mathbf{q}^* = [q_0^*, q_1^* = 0, q_2^* = 0]$ is the maximum likelihood estimate, and stop.

8. If $q_0^* = 0$, $q_1^* = 0$, $q_2^* = 0$ satisfies

$$\left.\frac{\partial L}{\partial q_0}\right|_{\mathbf{q}=\mathbf{q}^*} \leq 0 \qquad \left.\frac{\partial L}{\partial q_1}\right|_{\mathbf{q}=\mathbf{q}^*} \leq 0 \qquad \left.\frac{\partial L}{\partial q_2}\right|_{\mathbf{q}=\mathbf{q}^*} \leq 0$$

then $\mathbf{q}^* = [q_0^* = 0, q_1^* = 0, q_2^* = 0]$ is the maximum likelihood estimate, and stop.

4.17 THE MAXIMUM LIKELIHOOD ESTIMATION METHOD FOR TIME-TO-RESPONSE MODELS

The distinguishing feature of time-to-response models is the fact that they contain the time at which a response to a carcinogenic substance occurs; whereas, quantal response models include only the count of the individuals that have responded to the carcinogenic substance by the end of the experiment, and ignore the time at which the event occurs. For example, quantal response models do not differentiate between an event that occurs at age 5 and an event that occurs at age 60. In order to reflect this important health effect in the final risk assessment, the time at which events occur must be included in the model. The use of the Maximum Likelihood Estimation (MLE) Method for modeling two types of time-to-response data is demonstrated.

4.18 APPLICATION OF MAXIMUM LIKELIHOOD ESTIMATION METHOD TO INCIDENTAL RESPONSE EXPERIMENTS

These experiments are conducted in precisely the same manner as that described at the beginning of Section 4.15 for m quantal experiments except that the length of time T_i is varied for each experiment, $(i = 1, 2, \ldots, m)$. Thus, the procedure for fitting these data to a time-to-response model is analogous to that described for the quantal experiments except for the following differences.

In this case each p_i in Equation (4.74) is a function of both d_i and T_i; that is, $P_i = P_i(T_i; d_i)$. To illustrate the case where both T_i and d_i $(i = 1, 2, \ldots, m)$ differ for each experiment, the Multistage-Weibull model [Equation (2.68) of Chapter 2] is used. In the interest of simplicity, a one-stage model is used, and for this case Equation (2.68) reduces to

$$P(T; d) = 1 - \exp[-(q_0 + q_1 d)(T - w)^k] \tag{4.90}$$

where T is the time to response, and q_0, q_1, w, and k are parameters. Also, as a matter of convenience the "k!" appearing in the denominator of the exponential of Equation (2.68) has been absorbed in the parameters q_0 and q_1. The parameter w is interpreted as the time from the onset to the detectability of a tumor. Also in Equation (2.68), k is an integer that denotes the number of stages. If the constraint that k be an integer is removed and the parameters q_0 and q_1 containing k! are taken to be independent of k, then Equation (4.90) becomes an empirical expression having the same general form as the theoretical expression in which k is an integer and the absorption of k! in q_0 and q_1 is recognized. One method for fitting the experimental data to the empirical form of Equation (4.90) is the Newton-Raphson method, and a development of the equations needed in this method follows.

In each quantal response experiment i $(i = 1, 2, \ldots, m)$, $T = T_i$, the time of the observation or the end of experiment i at dose d_i. Thus, Equation (4.90) becomes

$$P_i(T_i; d_i) = 1 - \exp[-(q_0 + q_1 d_i)(T_i - w)^k] \tag{4.91}$$

Again, as in the quantal response experiments, the likelihood function is of the same form as Equation (3.23) of Chapter 3; namely,

$$L(q_0, q_1, k, w) = \prod_{i=1}^{m} \binom{n_i}{r_i} p_i^{r_i}(1 - p_i)^{n_i - r_i} \tag{4.92}$$

where $p_i = P_i(T_i; d_i)$. Let

$$l(q_0, q_1, k, w) = \log_e L(q_0, q_1, k, w) \tag{4.93}$$

Then the expressions given by Equation (4.79), (4.81), and (4.82) are obtained. In addition to Equations (4.81) and (4.82) for parameters q_0 and q_1, the following expressions are obtained for the parameters k and w,

$$0 = \prod_{i=1}^{m} \frac{(r_i - n_i p_i)}{p_i(1 - p_i)} \frac{\partial p_i}{\partial k} \tag{4.94}$$

$$0 = \prod_{i=1}^{m} \frac{(r_i - n_i p_i)}{p_i(1 - p_i)} \frac{\partial p_i}{\partial w} \tag{4.95}$$

Instead of Equations (4.83) and (4.84) the following expressions are obtained

$$\frac{\partial p_i}{\partial q_0} = (T_i - w)^k \exp[-(q_0 + q_1 d_i)(T_i - w)^k] \tag{4.96}$$

$$\frac{\partial p_i}{\partial q_1} = d_i(T_i - w)^k \exp[-(q_0 + q_1 d_i)(T_i - w)^k] \tag{4.97}$$

$$\frac{\partial p_i}{\partial k} = (q_0 + q_1 d_i)(T_i - w)^k \log_e(T_i - w) \exp[-(q_0 + q_1 d_i)(T_i - w)^k] \tag{4.98}$$

$$\frac{\partial p_i}{\partial w} = -k[q_0 + q_1 d_i][T_i - w](k - 1) \exp[-(q_0 + q_1 d_i)(T_i - w)^k] \tag{4.99}$$

When the zeroes on the left-hand sides of Equations (4.81), (4.82), (4.94), and (4.95) are replaced by $f_1(q_0, q_1, k, w), f_2(q_0, q_1, k, w), f_3(q_0, q_1, k, w)$, and $f_4(q_0, q_1, k, w)$, respectively, the functions to be solved for the solution set of the parameters (q_0, q_1, k, w) are obtained. In this case, the Newton-Raphson equations may be represented as follows:

$$\begin{bmatrix} \frac{\partial f_1}{\partial q_0} & \frac{\partial f_1}{\partial q_1} & \frac{\partial f_1}{\partial k} & \frac{\partial f_1}{\partial w} \\ \frac{\partial f_2}{\partial q_0} & \frac{\partial f_2}{\partial q_1} & \frac{\partial f_2}{\partial k} & \frac{\partial f_2}{\partial w} \\ \frac{\partial f_3}{\partial q_0} & \frac{\partial f_3}{\partial q_1} & \frac{\partial f_3}{\partial k} & \frac{\partial f_3}{\partial w} \\ \frac{\partial f_4}{\partial q_0} & \frac{\partial f_4}{\partial q_1} & \frac{\partial f_4}{\partial k} & \frac{\partial f_4}{\partial w} \end{bmatrix} \begin{bmatrix} \Delta q_0 \\ \Delta q_1 \\ \Delta k \\ \Delta w \end{bmatrix} = - \begin{bmatrix} f_1 \\ f_2 \\ f_3 \\ f_4 \end{bmatrix} \tag{4.100}$$

An iterative procedure similar to that described above for Equations (4.85) and (86) is repeated until the solutions set $[q_0, q_1, k, w]$ is found for which $f_1 = f_2 = f_3 = f_4 = 0$.

To fit the data to the theoretical form of Equation (4.90) [the one where k is an integer and the absorption of $k!$ in q_0 and q_1 is recognized], the following variation of the Newton-Raphson method shown above may be used. In particular, the three parameters

q_0, q_1, and w are determined for each choice of an integer value of k; namely, $k_1 = 1$, $k_2 = 2$, $k_3 = 3$, ... For example, for $k_1 = 1$, the set of parameters $\{q_0, q_1, w_1\}$ for which $f_1(q_{0,1}, q_{1,1}, w_1) = f_2(q_{0,1}, q_{1,1}, w_1) = f_4(q_{0,1}, q_{1,1}, w_1) = 0$ is found by use of the Newton-Raphson method in an analogous manner to that as shown above for four functions.

After each solution set of parameters $\{q_{0,j}, q_{1,j}, w_j\}$ for each choice $k = k_j$ has been found, the likelihood function $L(q_{0,j}, q_{1,j}, k_j, w_j)$ [Equation (4.92)] is evaluated. The set of the parameters that maximimzes the likelihood function is the desired solution set.

In addition to the two methods described above for maximizing the likelihood function $L(q_0, q_1, k, w)$, a number of other optimization methods are presented in standard texts on this topic. Like the two methods presented, these other optimization methods involve the searching of the parameter domain for the solution set for which the likelihood function $L(q_0, q_1, k, w)$ has its global maximum. In general the searches may be conducted either with or without k constrained to be an integer.

4.19 APPLICATION OF THE MAXIMUM LIKELIHOOD ESTIMATION METHOD TO DETECTABLE RESPONSE EXPERIMENTS

As an example of a set of detectable response experiments, suppose that the detectable response is death. In this case the experiments are carried out in the same general manner as described for quantal type experiments at the beginning of this section except for the following differences. Each animal in an experiment is followed with respect to time, and the time of the detectable response of death recorded. Death can result from cancer as a consequence of having been exposed to the carcinogenic substance or death can result from other causes including sacrifices. To illustrate, consider the following set of hypothetical experimental results.

Animal Number	Event	Time T(weeks)	Dose d
1	0*	$T_1 = 10$	d_1
2	0	$T_2 = 20$	d_2
3	1*	$T_3 = 30$	d_3
4	0	$T_4 = 50$	d_4
5	1	$T_5 = 75$	d_5
6	1	$T_6 = 100$	d_6*

* 0 = death by other cause, 1 = death due to cancer from exposure to carcinogenic substance.

Again suppose that the one-stage form of the multistage-Weibull given by Equation (4.90) is to be fitted to the data. The likelihood function for this experimental situation is formulated on the basis of the following considerations. First, observe that the function $P(T, d)$ at a fixed d_i and $T = T_k$ represents the probability that an animal will die of cancer at some time $T \leq T_k$, and is thus recognized as a cumulative probability. The probability that an animal will not die of cancer at some time $T \leq T_k$ is

$$P\begin{pmatrix} \textit{no response} \\ \textit{for } T \leq T_k \end{pmatrix} = 1 - P(T_k; d_i) \tag{4.101}$$

The probability that an animal will have a response at time $T = T_k$ (at a fixed dose d_i) is given by

$$P\begin{pmatrix} \textit{response} \\ \textit{at } T = T_k \end{pmatrix} = \frac{dP(T; d_i)}{dt}\bigg|_{T=T_k} = \frac{dP(T_k; d_i)}{dt} \tag{4.102}$$

Since the six events experienced by the six animals in the experiment are independent, it follows that the probability of observing all six events (which is the likelihood function) is equal to the product of their individual probabilities. Thus, in this case,

$$L(q_0, q_1, k, w) = \prod_{i=1,2,4} [1 - P_i(T_i; d_i)] \times \prod_{i=3,5,6} \frac{dP_i(T_i; d_i)}{dt} \tag{4.103}$$

Again when the function l is defined by Equation (4.93), one obtains

$$l = \sum_{i=1,2,4} \log_e[1 - P_i(T_i; d_i)] + \sum_{i=3,5,6} \log_e \left[\frac{dP_i(T_i; d_i)}{dt}\right] \tag{4.104}$$

The remainder of the procedure for finding the solution set of parameters $\{q_0, q_1, k, w\}$ which maximize the likelihood function l are found in a manner analogous to that outlined above for the quantal experiments.

4.20 DEFINITION AND EVALUATION OF THE EXPECTED VALUE OF THE TOTAL TUMOR RESPONSE FREE PERIOD

Before the ED_{01} study[8], almost all of the experimental toxicology data were quantal response data. Such response-rate data focus on the percentage of animals exhibiting a carcinogenic response to a specified exposure by a prescribed time—usually the end of the experiment; whereas, time-to-response data focus on the time required for a given specified response to occur.[8,9,10]

Actually, time has always been involved in toxicity experiments. Even in quantal response studies, the experimenter usually has to decide on a maximum length of exposure. Since time is a factor in toxicity, time should be meaningfully included in risk assessment. It makes a difference whether it takes 30 days or 30 years of exposure to a carcinogen to significantly increase the risk of developing a tumor. Yet the element of time is essentially missing from most current definitions of carcinogenic risks.

As a possible measure of the time required for a response to an exposure to a carcinogen, the expected time to response (see Equation (4.52)) or mean time to response is given by,

$$E(T;d) = \int_0^\infty t \left[\left. \frac{dP(T;d)}{dT} \right|_{T=t} \right] dt \tag{4.105}$$

where T is the random time to response. Although this mean might appear to be a good measure of the time to response, it would probably not be a good criterion for evaluating dose level d, because $E(T;d)$ is greatly influenced by the values of $P(T;d)$ at very large values of T and it is precisely these values of T for which $P(T;d)$ is hard to evaluate.

A more reasonable alternative criterion might be the *mean tumor response free period* from an exposure up until some time T^*. An expression for computing the expected value or mean of the tumor response free period is developed in the following manner. The development begins with a specific numerical example in which it is desired to find the number of tumor free years in the first $T^* = 70$ years of a person's potential lifetime. Suppose that at age $t = 50$ years the person develops a tumor. Then

$70 - 50 = 20$ years were not tumor free for this person that developed a tumor at age 50

and

$$70 - (70 - 50) = 50 \text{ years that were tumor free}$$

Thus, the amount of tumor free time in the period $[0, T^*]$ for the people who develop a tumor at time t is

$$T^* - (T^* - t) \qquad \text{if } t \leq T^*$$

and is

$$T^* \qquad \text{if } t > T^*$$

Thus, the expected amount of tumor free time in the period $[0, T^*]$ is

$$E\begin{bmatrix} \textit{tumor free time} \\ \textit{in } [0, T^*] \end{bmatrix} = \int_0^{T^*} [T^* - (T^* - t)] \left. \frac{dP(T;d)}{dT} \right|_{T=t} dt \int_{T^*}^\infty T^* \left. \frac{dP(T;d)}{dT} \right|_{T=t} dt \tag{4.106}$$

Since,

$$\int_0^{T^*} T^* \left. \frac{dP(T;d)}{dT} \right|_{T=t} dt = T^* P(T \leq T^*) \tag{4.107}$$

$$\int_{T^*}^\infty T^* \left. \frac{dP(T;d)}{dT} \right|_{T=t} dt = T^* P(T > T^*) \tag{4.108}$$

and

$$P(T \leq T^*) + P(T > T^*) = 1 \tag{4.109}$$

it follows that the expression for the expected or mean value of the tumor response free period given by Equation (4.106) reduces to

$$E\begin{bmatrix} \textit{tumor response} \\ \textit{free period} \end{bmatrix} = T^* - \int_0^{T^*} (T^* - t) \left. \frac{dP(T; d)}{dT} \right|_{T=t} dt \tag{4.110}$$

The contribution to the tumor response free period by those who do not develop a tumor before T^* and may not develop a tumor during their lifetime is often ignored thereby giving a misleading result. Suppose, as in the preceding example, that the average tumor free period among the proportion of the population developing a tumor by age 70 is 50 years. If this proportion is small, say 5 percent, and most of the population is tumor free for the first 70 years, then the mean tumor free period is

$$50 \times 0.05 + 70 \times 0.95 = 69 \ \textit{years}$$

Thus, for the whole population, the mean tumor free period is 69 years and not 50 years.

PROBLEMS

1. What is the probability that an odd number will appear in the single toss of a fair die?
   Answer: $p = 1/2$.
2. What is the probability that exactly one head will appear in three tosses of a fair coin?
   Answer: $P(X = 1) = 3/8$.
3. A single toss of a pair of fair dice is made.
   (a) What is the probability of observing a sum of 7?
   (b) Repeat Part (a) for each of the sums: 2, 3, 4, 5, 6, 8, 9, 10, 11, 12.

   Answer: (a) $p = 1/6$.
4. A ball is drawn at random from a box containing six red balls, four white balls, and five blue balls. What is the probability that it is
   (a) red
   (b) white
   (c) blue
   (d) not red
   (e) red or white?

   Answer: $p_{\text{red}} = 2/5, p_{\text{white}} = 4/15, p_{\text{blue}} = 1/3, p_{\text{notred}} = 3/5, p_{\text{redorwhite}} = 2/3$.
5. A fair die is tossed twice. Find the probability of getting a 4, 5 or 6 on the first toss and a 1, 2, 3, or 4 on the second toss.
   Answer: $P(A_1 \text{ and } A_2) = 1/3$.
6. A multiple choice test consists of 15 questions and for each question, five possible answers are listed. If for each question, an answer is selected in a completely random fashion,
   (a) what is the probability that at most eight of the questions are answered correctly (that is 8 or less)

(b) exactly 8
(c) at least 8 (that is 8 or more)
(d) between 4 and 7 (inclusive)?

Answer: (a) 0.9992, (b) 0.0035, (c) 0.0042, (d) 0.3476.

7. Two independent animal tests are carried out under the same conditions. In the first test, 8 of the 15 animals develop tumors ($r = 8$, $n = 15$). In the second test, 6 out of 13 animals develop tumors.
(a) Find the Maximum Likelihood Estimate of the trial probability.
(b) Find the values of the likelihood function $[L(p)]$ corresponding to the value of p found in part (a)

Answer: (a) $p = 1/2$, (b) $L(p) = 0.0411$.

8. Verify the results given by:
(a) Equation (4.58)
(b) Equation (4.59)
(c) Equation (4.60)
(d) Equation (4.61)

9. Beginning with Equations (4.81) and (4.82) of the text

$$\frac{\partial l(q_0, q_1)}{\partial q_0} = 0 = \sum_{i=1}^{m} \frac{(r_i - n_i p_i)}{p_i(1 - p_i)} \frac{\partial p_i}{\partial q_0}$$

$$\frac{\partial l(q_0, q_1)}{\partial q_1} = 0 = \sum_{i=1}^{m} \frac{(r_i - n_i p_i)}{p_i(1 - p_i)} \frac{\partial p_i}{\partial q_1}$$

show that

$$0 = \sum_{i=1}^{m} \frac{r_i}{1 - x_i} - \sum_{i=1}^{m} n_i$$

$$0 = \sum_{i=1}^{m} \frac{r_i d_i}{1 - x_i} - \sum_{i=1}^{m} n_i d_i$$

where

$$p_i = 1 - x_i$$
$$x_i = e^{-(q_0 + q_1 d_i)}$$

10. Let

$$f_1(q_0, q_1) = \sum_{i=1}^{m} \frac{r_i}{1 - x_i} - \sum_{i=1}^{m} n_i$$

$$f_2(q_0, q_1) = \sum_{i=1}^{m} \frac{r_i d_i}{1 - x_i} - \sum_{i=1}^{m} n_i d_i$$

Then the set of values (q_0, q_1) that make

$$f_1(q_0, q_1) = f_2(q_0, q_1) = 0$$

simultaneously is the set which maximizes the maximum likelihood function $l(q_0, q_1)$. One method for finding this solution set (q_0, q_1) is the Newton-Raphson method shown in the text. To apply this method, expressions for the following partial derivatives are needed:

$$\frac{\partial f_1}{\partial q_0}, \frac{\partial f_1}{\partial q_1}, \frac{\partial f_2}{\partial q_0}, \frac{\partial f_2}{\partial q_1}$$

Show that

$$\frac{\partial f_1}{\partial q_0} = -\sum_{i=1}^{m} \frac{r_i x_i}{(1-x_i)^2}$$

$$\frac{\partial f_1}{\partial q_1} = -\sum_{i=1}^{m} \frac{r_i d_i x_i}{(1-x_i)^2}$$

$$\frac{\partial f_2}{\partial q_0} = -\sum_{i=1}^{m} \frac{r_i d_i x_i}{(1-x_i)^2}$$

$$\frac{\partial f_2}{\partial q_1} = -\sum_{i=1}^{m} \frac{r_i (d_i)^2 x_i}{(1-x_i)^2}$$

where

$$x_i = e^{-(q_0 + q_1 d_i)}$$

11. **(a)** Verify for Example 4.8 that the unrestricted maximum likelihood estimate is approximately $q_0^* = 0.0202$, $q_1^* = -0.0332$, $q_2^* = 0.010$.

(b) Verify for Example 4.8 that $q_0^* = 0.016$, $q_1^* = 0$, and $q_2^* = 0.006$ satisfies the Kuhn-Tucker conditions (case 3 among the 8 cases), and hence is the maximum likelihood estimate of (q_0, q_1, q_2) under the restrictions: $q_j \geq 0, j = 1, 2, 3$.

12. Let "*lifetime*" denote the time interval between the start of observation (e.g., the beginning of an experiment) and the time the observation of an individual ends (e.g., the individual dies or the experiment ends). Note that *lifetime* is a well defined period of time, but that it may be a random variable because individuals may have different observed values for their lifetimes. In quantal response models $P(d)$ denotes the probability that a randomly chosen individual will develop the specified carcinogenic response during a lifetime (i.e., at some time during that individuals lifetime.)

(a) Does $P(d)$ predict the proportion of individuals in the given situation (e.g., the experiment) that would be expected to be observed developing the specified cacinogenic response? Explain your answer.

(b) Would $P(d)$ change if the length of the experiment were changed? Explain.

(c) Would $P(d)$ change if the length of the experiment remained unchanged, but the experiment was changed to lessen the possibility of non-cancer related diseases? Explain.

(d) Do particular quantitative values of $P(d)$ reflect a particular set of *competing risks*? Explain. Here *competing risks* are causes of death other than those related to the specified carcinogenic response.

(e) If $P(d)$ is estimated in one situation (e.g., an animal bioassay) and the results extrapolated to another situation (e.g., a human occupational or environmental exposure), will the difference in the competing risks between the two situations impact the accuracy of the extrapolation? Explain.

Answers: (a) Yes, (b) Yes, (c) Yes, (d) Yes, (e) Yes.

13. Let

T = time to tumor; i.e., the time to the occurrence of a specified carcinogenic response

S = survival time; i.e., the time to death from causes other than the specified carcinogenic response

Assume that T is observable; that is, the specifed carcinogenic response is detectable immediately when it occurs. Also, assume that T and S are independent. That is, assume that the carcinogenic response time (T) and the time (S) to death from other causes are independent.

(a) Let there be n individuals with the ith individual having dose d_i. Let

$$P_T(t; d) = P(T \leq t; d)$$

denote the probability that the time to tumor (T) does not exceed t when the dose is d. Let

$$P_S(s, d) = P(S \leq s; d)$$

denote the probability that the survival time (S) does not exceed s when the dose is d. Derive an expression for the likelihood function in this situation.

(b) Show that, in the situation described in Part (a), the maximum likelihood estimates of the parameters in $P_T(t; d)$ do not depend on the functional form of $P_S(s, d)$ or the parameters in $P_S(s, d)$.

(c) Explain why $P_T(t; d)$ can be described as the distribution function for the time to response *in the absence of competing risks*. Also, explain why the expected frequency of the specified carcinogenic response by a specific age, say age 65, in a population would not be less than $P_T(65, d)$.

14. The purpose of this problem is to introduce the concept of *competing risks* and the associated *cause-specific probability*. Specifically, in time-to-response models, $P(t; d)$ refers to the probability of a carcinogenic response in a fictitious world without competing risks. On the other hand, $P(T \leq t \text{ and } J = 1; d)$ is the probability of a carcinogenic response in the real world where there are competing risks and additional possible events other than cancer. These other possible causes of an observation are denoted by $J = 2, 3, \ldots,$ and the probabilities $P(T \leq t \text{ and } J = j; d)$ are called cause-specific probabilities. Consider the situation involving three possible events. Let

T_1	$=$	time to tumor; i.e., time to a specific carcinogenic response.
T_2	$=$	time to an observation other than the specific carcinogenic response or a scheduled end of observation.
T_3	$=$	scheduled end of observation; i.e., end of experiment, or an end of a specified time period.

Assume that T_1, T_2, and T_3 are observable when and if they occur. Do not assume that T_1, and T_2 are necessarily independent. Note that T_1 represents the time to tumor in the presence of the competing risks reflected in T_2. For an individual with a sacrifice time T_3 that exceeds t, the cause-specific probability for $j = 1, 2$ has the form

$$P(T \le t \text{ and } J = j; d) = \int_0^t \lambda_j(u; d) e^{-\int_0^u [\lambda_1(v;d)+\lambda_2(v;d)]dv} du \qquad (A)$$

The probability that the observation of an individual exposed to dose d will be terminated by some cause by time t is

$$P(T \le t; d) = \sum_{j=1}^{3} P(T \le t \text{ and } J = j; d) \qquad (B)$$

where, for example, $P(T \le t \text{ and } J = 1; d)$ is the probability that an individual exposed to dose d will escape unscheduled deaths ($J = 2$) and scheduled sacrifices ($J = 3$) long enough to develop a carcinogenic response by time t.

(a) For $T_3 > t$ and $j = 1, 2$, show that Equation (B) becomes

$$P(T \le t; d) = 1 - e^{-\int_0^t [\lambda_1(v;d)+\lambda_2(v;d)]dv} \qquad (C)$$

(b) In a manner analogous to the development of the hazard rate given by Equation (4.58) in Section 2.2.6 for the time-to-response model, the hazard rate for cause-specific model for event $J = j$ may be defined as follows:

$$h_j = \frac{\textit{Increase up to time t of the cause-specific probability of event j}}{\textit{Probability that no events have occurred by time } T \le t} \qquad (D)$$

Show that for $j = 1, 2$

$$h_j = \frac{1}{1 - P(T \le t; d)} \frac{dP(T \le t \text{ and } J = j; d)}{dt} \qquad (E)$$

(c) Use Equation (A) to show that for $j = 1, 2$ and $t < T_3$,

$$h_j = \lambda_j(t; d) \qquad j = 1, 2$$

(d) Because T_3 is a constant (the scheduled end of observation), for $J = 3$,

$$\lambda_3 = 1 \qquad \text{if } T_3 = t$$
$$\lambda_3 = 0 \qquad \text{if } T_3 \ne t$$

In this setting, what is the probability of observing a tumor ($J = 1$) by time t for an individual? Does this probability correspond to the real world where competing risks ($J = 2$) may occur before a tumor?

(e) How does $P(T \leq t \text{ and } J = 1; d)$ compare with $P_T(t; d)$ in Problem 13?

(f) Consider the general case where n independent individuals are being observed and each individual ($i = 1, 2, \ldots, n$) has a preassigned end of the experiment T_3 (i.e., a maximum observation time T_3). The *ith* individual's dose and observation time are d_i and t_i, respectively. Show that the likelihood L satisfies the equation

$$L = \prod_{i=1}^{n} \lambda_{J_i}(t_i, d_i) e^{-\int_0^{t_i} [\lambda_1(v; d_i) + \lambda_2(v; d_i)] dv}$$

where

$$\lambda_3(t_i; d_i) = 1$$

for an individual whose observation t_i is the end of the experiment T_3.

(g) If maximum likelihood estimation is used to estimate $P(T \leq t \text{ and } J = j; d)$, what additional parameters must be estimated compared to the parameters estimated for $P_T(t; d)$ in Problem 13?

NOTATION

A = an event which is a set of outcomes that have a common characteristic

A_1, A_2 = two different events or two sets of outcomes

$E(X)$ = expected value of the random variable X; defined by Equations (4.52) and (4.56)

$f(x)$ = probability density function. If X is a discrete random variable $f(x) = P(X = x)$. If X is a continuous random variable, $f(x) = dF(x)/dx$

$F(x)$ = cumulative distribution function, which is the probability that the random variable X will have a value equal to or less than x

l = logarithm of the likelihood function; defined by Equation (4.78)

L = likelihood function which is equal to the probability that an experimenter will observe the experimental outcomes $X_1 = r_1, X_2 = r_2, \ldots, X_m = r_m$ out of a total of $n_1, n_2, \ldots, n_m$ trials, respectively

n = a counting integer used to denote number of outcomes or number of trials

m = a counting integer used to denote the number of outcomes that are successes

p = trial probability or the number that represents the probability of success of a particular outcome. Also used to denote the percentile

$p(x_i)$ = probability density function for the outcome x_i, where x_i is a member of the set $x_1, x_2, \ldots,$ defined by Equation (4.38)

$P(A)$ = a number that represents the probability that event A will occur; see Equations (4.5) and (4.40)

$P(A_1, A_2, \ldots, A_k)$ = probability that all k events $(A_1, A_2, \ldots, A_k)$ of k independent trials will occur

$P(A_1 \text{ or } A_2)$ = probability of the occurrence of either one or the other or both of the events A_1 or A_2

$P(a \leq x \leq b)$ = the probability that the random variable X takes on a value in the closed interval $[a, b]$, and it is equal to the area under the curve of the probability density function $f(x)$ versus x between $x = a$ and $x = b$

$P(X = x)$ = binomial probability density function, and it is equal to the probability that exactly x successes out of n independent Bernoulli trials will occur

$P(X \leq x)$ = cumulative binomial distribution function, and it is equal to the probability that x or fewer successes will occur; defined by Equation (4.24)

x = the number associated with an outcome in the sample space Ω by the random variable X

X = a random variable is any rule that associates a number x with each outcome in the sample space Ω of an experiment

z = the number associated with an outcome in the sample space Ω by the random variable Z

Z = a standard normal random variable defined in terms of a random variable that associates a number z with each outcome in the sample space Ω of an experiment

GREEK LETTERS

$\alpha/2$ = an area under a curve; see Figure 4.2

$\Gamma(t)$ = gamma function; defined by Equation (4.64)

μ = mean value of a normal random variable

σ = square root of the variance of a normal random variable

$\chi^2_{\nu,p}$ = chi-square function for ν degrees of freedom and the pth percentile

$\phi(u)$ = probability density function of the standard normal distribution function; defined below Equation (4.49)

$\Phi(z)$ = standard random distribution function; defined by Equation (4.49)

REFERENCES

1. Allen, A.D., *Probability, Statistics and Queueing Theory*, Academic Press, Inc. Orlando, Florida (1978).
2. Devore, J.L., *Probability and Statistics for Engineering and the Sciences*, Brooks/Cole Publishing Company, Monterey, California (1987).
3. Kreyszig, E., *Introductory Mathematic Statistics*, John Wiley & Sons, Inc., New York, N.Y. (1970).
4. Kramer, H., *Mathematical Methods of Statistics*, Princeton University Press, Princeton, N.J. (1946).
5. Carnahan, B., H.A. Luther, and J.O. Wilkes, *Applied Numerical Methods*, John Wiley & Sons, Inc., New York, N.Y. (1969).
6. *CRC Handbook of Tables for Mathematics*, 3rd Edition, R.C. Weast, Editor, The Chemical Rubber Co., Cleveland, Ohio (1967).
7. Taha, H.A., *Operations Research: An Introduction*, The Macmillan Company, New York, N.Y. (1971).
8. Sielken, R.L., Jr., "Re-examination of the ED_{01} Study—Risk Assessments Using Time," *Fundamental and Appled Toxicology*, **1**, 88 (1981).
9. Sielken, R.L., Jr., "Use of the Hartley-Sielken Model in Low Dose Extrapolation," *Toxicological Risk Assessment*, Vol. 1, Editors: D.B. Clayson, D. Krewski, and I. Munro, CRC Press, Inc., Boca Raton, Florida (1985).
10. Sielken, R.L., Jr., "A Time-to-Response Perspective on Ethylene Oxide's Carcinogenicity," *The Risk Assessment of Environmental and Human Health Hazards*. Edited by D.J. Paustenback, John Wiley & Sons, Inc., New York, N.Y. (1989).

5

Incorporating Cell Proliferation and Physiologically Based Pharmacokinetics (PBPK) Into Dose-Response Models

The field of pharmacokinetics makes use of the concepts of chemical kinetics and catalysis. *Pharmacokinetics* is a combination of the Greek work *pharmakon* meaning drug or poison and kinetics which refers to the speed of a chemical reaction. When the rate of mass transfer of a chemical from its point of administration to its reaction site is included in the model, the combined model for mass transfer plus chemical reaction is called a *Physiologically Based Pharmacokinetic (PBPK) Model.* The development of the mathematical representation of these PBPK models parallels the corresponding development of the mathematical representation of systems of chemical reactions that occur in commercial reactors. The approach used in chemical kinetics and catalysis also can be used to formulate dose-response models. The use of the kinetic approach is exemplified first in terms of the development of the two-stage dose-response model,[1] called the *Moolgavkar-Venzon-Knudson* model. This

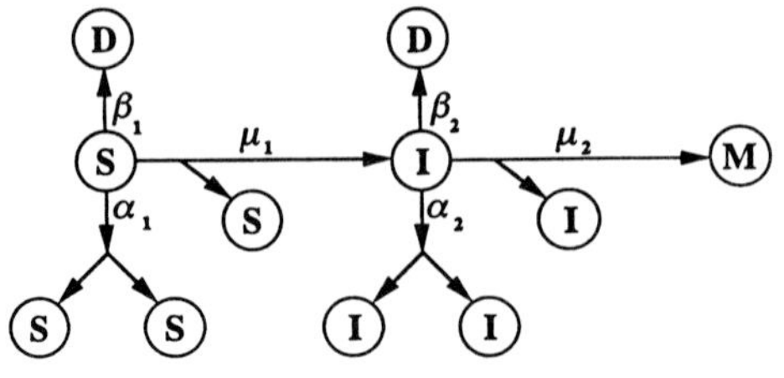

Figure 5.1 Schematic Diagram of the Two–Stage Model Proposed by Moolgavkar and Knudson.[1]

example is followed by the kinetic development and discussion of the *Michaelis-Menten rate equation* as well as physiologically based pharmacokinetic models.

5.1 A KINETIC DEVELOPMENT OF THE MVK TWO-STAGE DOSE-RESPONSE MODEL

Recently, Moolgavkar and Knudson[1] proposed a two-stage model to account for cancer formation. In this model, it is supposed that a normal cell S must undergo two mutations during the transition from a normal cell to a malignant cell. The first mutation state is represented by I in Figure 5.1 and the second one by M. Dead cells are denoted by D. On the basis of the proposed model represented by Figure 5.1, a combination of the concepts of chemical kinetics and the biological principles of cellular *mitosis* is utilized to develop an expression for the cumulative probability function for cancer formation.

In the following development, S, I, D, and M denote the concentrations of cells in their normal, one-hit, dead, and malignant states. These concentrations may be expressed as the number of cells, molecules, or moles per unit of tissue in volume or mass units. For definiteness the units of gram moles (g moles) and volume (say cubic centimeters) are used in the development that follows.

When a normal cell divides, the DNA divides and the left and right parts, denoted by E_L and E_R, are joined to the complementary right and left parts of the DNA. This process may be represented as follows. First, the normal cell divides

$$S \xrightarrow{\alpha_1} E_{L,0} + E_{R,0} \tag{5.1}$$

Then the original strands of the DNA unite with complementary stands formed from material in the near neighborhood, denoted by $E_{R,0}$ and $E_{L,0}$, as follows:

$$E_{L,0} + E_{R,0} \xrightarrow{k} S \tag{5.2}$$

$$E_{R,0} + E_{L,0} \xrightarrow{k} S \tag{5.3}$$

It will be supposed that the rate of reaction for the reaction given by Equation (5.1) is proportional to the first power of the concentration of S; that is,

$$r_1 \left(\frac{\textit{moles of S disappearing}}{\textit{time volume}} \right) = \alpha_1 S \tag{5.4}$$

where α_1 is the specific rate constant. In the interest of simplicity the rate controlling steps of the mechanisms shown in Figure 5.1 will be taken to be the cell division steps such as the one represented by Equation (5.1). More precisely it is assumed that the specific rate constants for the cell division steps are very much smaller than the rate constants for all other steps of the mechanism. In particular it is supposed that $\alpha_1 \ll k$. Thus, the individual strands $E_{L,0}$ and $E_{R,0}$ of the DNA formed by cell division [Equation (5.1)] are consumed by the reactions given by Equations (5.2) and (5.3) at approximately the same rate at which they are formed which further implies that the amount of S in the form of $E_{L,0}$ and $E_{R,0}$ is negligible. Let, $r_{L,0}$ and $r_{R,0}$ denote the rates of disappearance of $E_{L,0}$ and $E_{R,0}$ by Equations (5.2) and (5.3), respectively. Then it follows that

$$r_{L,0} = r_{R,0} \approx r_1 \tag{5.5}$$

Next, according to the mechanism shown in Figure 5.1, cell S dies at the rate r_2 by the reaction:

$$S \xrightarrow{\beta_1} D \qquad r_2 = \beta_1 S \tag{5.6}$$

The initial normal cell may also undergo its first hit in which a mutation occurs on the right strand of the DNA, which is represented by the reaction,

$$S \xrightarrow{\mu_1} E_{L,0} + E_{R,1} \qquad r_3 = \mu_1 S \tag{5.7}$$

The subscript 1 on $E_{R,1}$ is used to recognize that a mutation has occurred in the division process. Since a mutation of either the left or right strands of the DNA is equally likely, there is no loss of generality by assuming that the first mutation occurs on the right strand of the DNA. The cell division is followed by the formation of two new cells, I and S, by the reactions:

$$E_{R,1} + E_{L,1} \longrightarrow I$$
$$E_{L,0} + E_{R,0} \longrightarrow S$$

where $E_{L,1}$ is the mutated form produced in the surroundings that is required to mate with $E_{R,1}$ to give the new cell I which has undergone one mutation. The remainder of the mechanism is formulated in a similar manner. First, cell I may die

$$I \xrightarrow{\beta_2} D \qquad r_4 = \beta_2 I \tag{5.8}$$

Next, cell I may divide and recombine to form two new cells I as follows:

$$I \xrightarrow{\alpha_2} E_{L,1} E_{R,1} \qquad r_5 = \alpha_2 I \tag{5.9}$$

Then

$$E_{R,1} + E_{L,1} \longrightarrow I$$
$$E_{L,1} + E_{R,1} \longrightarrow I$$

Again, it is assumed that the division of I is the rate controlling step. That is, the specific rate constant α_2 for the cell division reaction [Equation (5.9)] is assumed to be very small relative to the rate constants for the above reactions by which new cells I are formed.

Finally, I may divide to form another I and a cell M which has undergone a second mutation.

These events are represented by the following reactions:

$$I \xrightarrow{\mu_2} E_{R,1} + E_{L,2} \qquad r_6 = \mu_2 I \tag{5.10}$$

and

$$E_{R,1} + E_{L,1} \longrightarrow I$$
$$E_{L,2} + E_{R,2} \longrightarrow M$$

The net rate of disappearance of S, denoted by r_S, is given by

$$r_S = r_1 + r_2 + r_3 - 2r_1 - r_3 = -r_1 + r_2 \tag{5.11}$$

By making a material balance on S in precisely the same manner as demonstrated for $p_0(t)$ [see Equations (2.9) through (2.15) of Chapter 2] the following differential equation is obtained in the limit as the time period Δt, over which the balance is made, is allowed to go to zero.*

$$r_S = -\frac{dS}{dt} \tag{5.12}$$

Similarly, the net rate of disappearance of I, denoted by r_I, is given by

$$r_I = -r_3 + r_4 + r_5 + r_6 - 2r_5 - r_6 = -r_3 + r_4 - r_5 \tag{5.13}$$

---

* Equation (5.12) is applicable when the volume V containing N_S moles of S is constant; that is, in general

$$r_S = -\frac{1}{V}\frac{dN_S}{dt}$$

and at constant volume V,

$$r_S = -\frac{1}{V}\frac{dN_S}{dt} = -\frac{d(N_S/V)}{dt} = -\frac{dS}{dt}$$

and

$$r_I = -\frac{dI}{dt} \tag{5.14}$$

The net rate of appearance of M, denoted by r_M, is given by

$$r_M = r_6 \tag{5.15}$$

and

$$r_M = \frac{dM}{dt} \tag{5.16}$$

It is desired to solve this set of linear differential equations with constant coefficients (α_1, α_2, β_1, β_2, μ_1, μ_2). Initially, the process begins with the normal cells. Thus, at $t = 0$,

$$S(0) = S^0,\ I(0) = 0,\ M(0) = 0 \tag{5.17}$$

Elimination of r_S from Equations (5.11) and (5.12) gives

$$\begin{aligned} -\frac{dS}{dt} &= -r_1 + r_2 \\ &= -\alpha_1 S + \beta_1 S \end{aligned} \tag{5.18}$$

Separation of the variables of Equation (5.18) followed by integration yields

$$\int_{S^0}^{S} \frac{dS}{(\beta_1 - \alpha_1)S} = -\int_0^t dt \tag{5.19}$$

Thus,

$$S = S^0 e^{-(\beta_1 - \alpha_1)t} \tag{5.20}$$

Next, elimination of r_I from Equations (5.13) and (5.14) gives

$$-\frac{dI}{dt} = -r_3 + r_4 - r_5 \tag{5.21}$$

Thus,

$$-\frac{dI}{dt} - \beta_2 I + \alpha_2 I = -\mu_1 S$$

or

$$\frac{dI}{dt} + (\beta_2 - \alpha_2)I = \mu_1 S \tag{5.22}$$

After the expression given by Equation (5.20) has been substituted into Equation (5.22), the following result is obtained

$$\frac{dI}{dt} + (\beta_2 - \alpha_2)I = \mu_1 S^0 e^{-(\beta_1 - \alpha_1)t} \tag{5.23}$$

The solution of this differential equation is well known*

$$I = e^{-\int(\beta_2-\alpha_2)\,dt}\left[\int e^{\int(\beta_2-\alpha_2)\,dt}\mu_1 S^0 e^{-(\beta_1-\alpha_1)t}\,dt + K\right] \tag{5.24}$$

Thus, integration followed by the use of the initial condition $I(0) = 0$ to evaluate the arbitrary constant K yields

$$I = \frac{\mu_1 S^0}{(\beta_2-\alpha_2)-(\beta_1-\alpha_1)}\left[e^{-(\beta_1-\alpha_1)t} - e^{-(\beta_2-\alpha_2)t}\right] \tag{5.25}$$

The next and final step in the solution of this set of differential equations consists of the elimination of r_M from Equations (5.15) and (5.16) to give

$$\frac{dM}{dt} = \mu_2 I \tag{5.26}$$

By substitution of the expression given by Equation (5.25) for I into Equation (26), followed by separation of the variables and integration, one obtains

$$\frac{M(t)}{S^0} = \frac{\mu_1\mu_2}{(\beta_2-\alpha_2)-(\beta_1-\alpha_1)}\left[\frac{1-e^{-(\beta_1-\alpha_1)t}}{(\beta_1-\alpha_1)} - \frac{1-e^{-(\beta_2-\alpha_2)t}}{(\beta_2-\alpha_2)}\right] \tag{5.27}$$

where $M(t)/S^0$ denotes the fraction of the original cells that forms tumors, or the probability of a tumor per cell line by time t. Thus, $M(t)/S^0$ has the same meaning as $p_k(t)$ in the expression for the cumulative hazard rate $H(t)$ as given by Equation (2.61) of Chapter 2. Also, S^0 corresponds to the number of cell lines N in this expression. Thus, in terms of the present notation, Equation (2.61) of Chapter 2 becomes

$$H(t) = Np_k(t) = S^0\left[\frac{M(t)}{S^0}\right] = M(t) \tag{5.28}$$

Thus, the probability of observing at least one tumor in S^0 cell lines is given by the following form of Equation (2.60) of Chapter 2; namely,

$$P(T) = 1 - e^{-H(T)} = 1 - e^{-M(T)} \tag{5.29}$$

where $M(T)$ is given by Equation (5.27).

* The solution of the linear, first-order, differential equation with variable coefficients of the form $dy/dx + P(x)y = Q(x)$ is shown by Sokolnikoff et al.[2] to be

$$y = e^{-\int P(x)\,dx}\left[\int e^{\int P(x)\,dx} Q(x)\,dx + K\right]$$

5.2 ANALYSIS OF THE MVK TWO-STAGE KINETIC MODEL

Since the kinetic model has six parameters, α_1, β_1, μ_1, α_2, β_2, and μ_2, it is possible to describe many possible behaviors.

First, suppose that the mutation rates are zero and that the metabolic process is at normal conditions; that is, the formation of new cells is exactly equal to cell deaths, or

1. $\alpha_1 = \beta_1,\ \alpha_2 = \beta_2,\ \mu_1 = 0, \mu_2 = 0$

   For this case Equation (5.18) reduces to

$$-\frac{dS}{dt} = 0$$

   and integration yields

$$S(t) = S^0$$

   Equation (5.23) gives

$$\frac{dI}{dt} = 0$$

   and since $I(0) = 0$, it follows that

$$I(t) = 0$$

   Also,

$$\frac{dM}{dt} = 0$$

   and since $M(0) = 0$

$$M(t) = 0$$

   Suppose that the birth and death rates are in balance, but that the mutation processes are possible, or

2. $\alpha_1 = \beta_1,\ \alpha_2 = \beta_2,\ \mu_1 \neq 0,\ \mu_2 \neq 0.$

   In this case, as before

$$S(t) = S^0$$

   and Equation (5.23) becomes

$$\frac{dI}{dt} = \mu_1 S^0$$

   Since $I(0) = 0$,

$$I(t) = \mu_1 S^0 t$$

   Then,

$$\frac{dM}{dt} = \mu_2 I = \mu_2 \mu_1 S^0 t$$

and integration subject to $M(0) = 0$, gives

$$M(t) = \frac{\mu_2 \mu_1 S^0 t^2}{2}$$

Observe that if the model shown in Figure 5.1 is expanded to include k stages, one obtains

$$M(t) = \mu_k \mu_{k-1} \ldots \mu_2 \mu_1 S^0 \frac{t^k}{k!}$$

which is the same result obtained by the multistage model [see Equations (2.43), (2.44), and (2.65) of Chapter 2].

Suppose that the birth and death rates are in balance for the first step ($\alpha_1 = \beta_1$) and the other rates are nonzero or

3. $\alpha_1 = \beta_1, \ \alpha_2 \neq \beta_2, \ \mu_1 \neq 0, \ \mu_2 \neq 0$

Again, as in the previous cases,

$$S(t) = S^0$$

Then Equation (5.23) becomes

$$\frac{dI}{dt} + (\beta_2 - \alpha_2) I = \mu_1 S^0$$

and

$$I(t) = \frac{\mu_1 S^0}{(\beta_2 - \alpha_2)} \left[1 - e^{-(\beta_2 - \alpha_2)t}\right]$$

Thus,

$$\frac{dM}{dt} = \frac{\mu_2 \mu_1 S^0}{(\beta_2 - \alpha_2)} \left[1 - e^{-(\beta_2 - \alpha_2)t}\right]$$

and

$$M(t) = \frac{\mu_2 \mu_1 S^0}{(\beta_2 - \alpha_2)} \left[t - \frac{\left[1 - e^{-(\beta_2 - \alpha_2)t}\right]}{\beta_2 - \alpha_2} \right]$$

If $\beta_2 > \alpha_2$, the concentration of intermediate cells I approaches a constant as $t \to \infty$,

$$I(\infty) = \frac{\mu_1 S^0}{\beta_2 - \alpha_2}$$

and as $t \to \infty$,

$$\frac{dM}{dt} = \frac{\mu_2 \mu_1 S^0}{(\beta_2 - \alpha_2)}$$

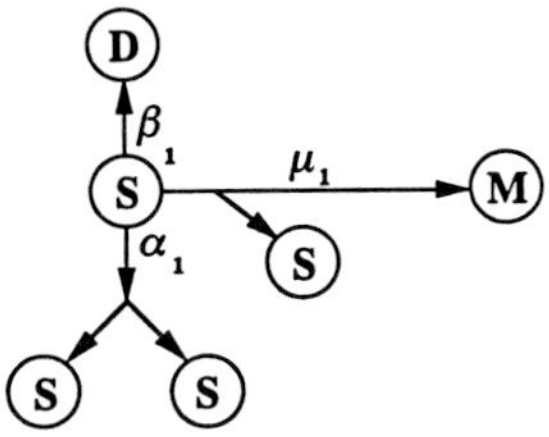

Figure 5.2 The MVK One–Stage Kinetic Model.

and

$$M(\infty) \to \infty$$

If $\beta_2 < \alpha_2$,

$$I(\infty) \to \infty$$
$$M(\infty) \to \infty$$

5.3 THE MVK ONE-STAGE KINETIC MODEL

In this case, the schematic representation shown in Figure 5.1 reduces to the one shown in Figure 5.2. The development down through Equation (5.7) is the same as shown above. Again, Equation (5.7) is given by

$$S \xrightarrow{\mu_1} E_{L,0} + E_{R,1} \qquad r_3 = \mu_1 S \tag{5.7}$$

In this case, however, the first mutation leads to a tumor; that is,

$$\begin{aligned} E_{R,1} + E_{L,1} &\longrightarrow M \\ E_{L,0} + E_{R,0} &\longrightarrow S \end{aligned} \tag{5.30}$$

The corresponding differential equations are as follows:

$$r_S = -\frac{dS}{dt} = (\beta_1 - \alpha_1)S \tag{5.31}$$

$$r_M = \frac{dM}{dt} = \mu_1 S \tag{5.32}$$

The solutions for S and M are readily shown to be

$$S(t) = S^0 e^{-(\beta_1 - \alpha_1)t} \tag{5.33}$$

and

$$M(t) = S^0 \mu_1 \left[\frac{1 - e^{-(\beta_1 - \alpha_1)t}}{(\beta_1 - \alpha_1)} \right] \tag{5.34}$$

so that the probability of observing at least one tumor in S^0 cell lines is given by Equation (5.29) where $M(t)$ is given by Equation (5.34).

5.4 DEVELOPMENT OF THE MICHAELIS-MENTEN RATE EXPRESSION

The Michaelis-Menten kinetics represents one of the first applications of pharmacokinetics. The development of the corresponding rate expression makes use of well-known concepts in the field of chemical kinetics and catalysis. [In the developments that follow, the concentration of a compound, say compound B, is denoted by C_B instead of simply B as was done in the above development.] To develop the *Michaelis-Menten equation* consider the case where the product B is formed from A by the reaction mechanism

$$A + S \underset{k_1'}{\overset{k_1}{\rightleftharpoons}} AS \overset{k_2}{\longrightarrow} B + S \tag{5.35}$$

S is a compound in the system which is consumed to produce AS, the active intermediate, and produced when B is formed from AS. Compound B is produced at the rate $r_2 = k_2 C_{AS}$, and thus,

$$\frac{dC_B}{dt} = k_2 C_{AS} \tag{5.36}$$

In the development which follows, expressions for C_{AS} and C_B in terms of C_A are needed. These expressions are obtained by use of the well-known *pseudo steady state assumption* from chemical kinetics. This assumption consists of the supposition that the active intermediate AS reacts to form B at approximately the same rate at which it is formed from A, which may be expressed as

$$\frac{dC_{AS}}{dt} \approx 0 \tag{5.37}$$

From the mechanism given by Equation (5.35), it follows that

$$\frac{dC_{AS}}{dt} \approx 0 = k_1 C_A C_S - k_1' C_{AS} - k_2 C_{AS}$$

which is readily solved for C_{AS} to give

$$C_{AS} = \frac{k_1 C_A C_S}{k_1' + k_2} \tag{5.38}$$

By material balance

$$C_S = C_S^0 - C_{AS} \tag{5.39}$$

where C_S^0 denotes the initial concentration of S, and initially $C_{AS}^0 = 0$. Elimination of C_S from Equations (5.38) and (5.39) yields

$$C_{AS} = \frac{C_S^0 C_A}{[(k_1' + k_2)/k_1] + C_A} \tag{5.40}$$

Substitution of this expression for C_{AS} into Equation (5.36) followed by rearrangement yields

$$\frac{dC_B}{dt} = \frac{k_2 C_S^0 C_A}{[(k_1' + k_2)/k_1]C_A} = \frac{VC_A}{K + C_A} \tag{5.41}$$

where V and K are the Michaelis-Menten parameters whose definitions follow immediately from Equation (5.41). [Note that in this case, V denotes a parameter and not the volume of the reacting mixture as it is commonly used in chemical kinetics.]

Next dC_B/dt is related to dC_A/dt by first observing that by material balance

$$C_A = C_A^0 - C_{AS} - C_B \tag{5.42}$$

where it has been assumed that $C_{AS}^0 = C_B^0 = 0$. Explicit differentiation of the members of Equation (5.42) yields

$$\frac{dC_A}{dt} = -\frac{dC_{AS}}{dt} - \frac{dC_B}{dt} \tag{5.43}$$

Then by use of the pseudo steady state assumption, Equation (5.37), it follows that

$$\frac{dC_A}{dt} \approx -\frac{dC_B}{dt} \tag{5.44}$$

and thus, the *Michaelis-Menten equation* is obtained by combining Equations (5.41) and (5.44) to give

$$-\frac{dC_A}{dt} = \frac{VC_A}{K + C_A} \tag{5.45}$$

Consequently, the rate expression for the rate of reaction of A is given by

$$r_A = \frac{VC_A}{K + C_A} \tag{5.46}$$

where r_A is defined in terms of disappearance.

5.4.1 Characteristics of the Michaelis-Menten Rate Expression

At small values of $C_A \ll K$, Equation (5.46) reduces to

$$r_A \approx \frac{V}{K} C_A \tag{5.47}$$

which is of the form known as a *first order* rate expression, a rate which varies with the first power of the concentration of the reactant A. As C_A^0 is increased, the value of C_A

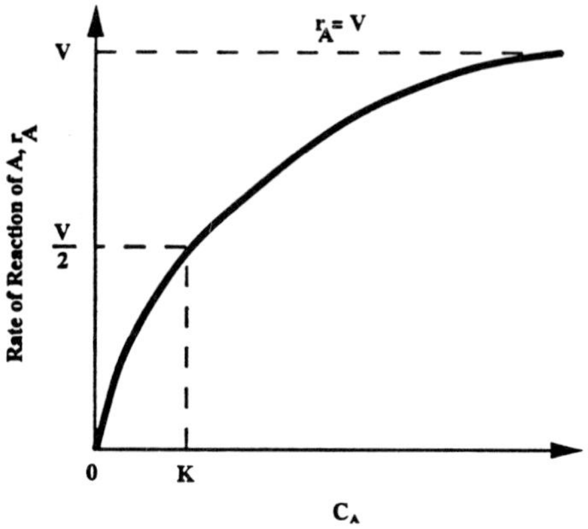

Figure 5.3 The Rate of Reaction of A Approaches its Maximum Value Asymptotically as C_A is Increased Indefinitely.

increases at any time t_k. The rate of reaction at any time t_k increases as C_A increases until it approaches its asymptotic maximum value. The validity of this statement is shown as follows:

$$\lim_{C_A \to \infty} r_A = \lim_{C_A \to \infty} \frac{VC_A}{KC_A} = \lim_{C_A \to \infty} \frac{V}{1 + K/C_A} = V \tag{5.48}$$

Also of interest is the fact that at $C_A = K$, r_A is equal to one-half its maximum value

$$r_A\big|_{C_A = K} = \frac{VK}{K + K} = \frac{V}{2} \tag{5.49}$$

A graph of r_A versus C_A is shown in Figure 5.3.

To obtain C_A as a function of time, Equation (5.45) is readily solved by separation of the variables followed by integration from $t = 0$ to $t = t$. At $t = 0$, the initial value (or dose concentration) is denoted by C_A^0. That is,

$$-\int_{C_A^0}^{C_A} \left[\frac{K + C_A}{VC_A}\right] dC_A = \int_0^t dt \tag{5.50}$$

Thus

$$\log_e \frac{C_A}{C_A^0} + \frac{1}{K}[C_A - C_A^0] = -\frac{V}{K}t \tag{5.51}$$

which is readily rearranged to the exponential form

$$C_A = C_A^0 e^{(C_A^0 - C_A)/K} e^{-Vt/K} \tag{5.52}$$

Of importance is the behavior of the concentration C_A as the initial concentration C_A^0 (or dose) is increased. In this analysis, let the time be fixed at $t = t_k$ for all choices of C_A^0. At values of $C_A^0 \ll K$, Equation (5.52) reduces to

$$C_A = C_A^0 e^{-Vt_k/K} \tag{5.53}$$

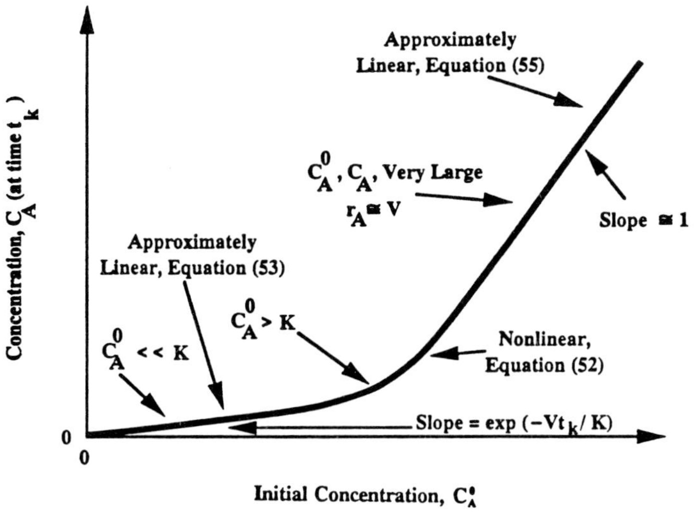

Figure 5.4 Variation of the Concentration C_A with the Initial Concentration C_A^0 as Given by the Michaelis–Menten Rate Expression.

Observe by Equation (5.42) C_A is always less than C_A^0 and if $C_A^0 \ll K$, then

$$e^{(C_A^0 - C_A)/K} \approx 1$$

A plot of C_A versus C_A^0 is shown in Figure 5.4. The approximately linear portion of the curve is given by Equation (5.53). As C_A^0 is increased, the relationship

$$e^{(C_A^0 - C_A)/K} > 1$$

holds for intermediate values of C_A^0 because C_A^0 is always greater than C_A and thus $C_A^0 - C_A > 0$. Consequently, for all choices of finite values C_A^0, the value of C_A given by Equation (5.52) will always be less than C_A^0 and the resulting curve is of the form shown in Figure 5.4. However, in the limit as C_A^0 approaches ∞, C_A likewise approaches infinity, and $C_A^0 - C_A$ is of the indeterminant form $\infty - \infty$. However, the variation of C_A versus C_A^0 in this region may be found by returning to Equations (5.45) and (5.48). At large values of C_A, $r_A \approx V$. Thus, as C_A becomes very large, it follows from Equations (5.45) and (5.48) that

$$-\frac{dC_A}{dt} = V \tag{5.54}$$

Separation of variables followed by integration yields

$$C_A = C_A^0 - Vt \tag{5.55}$$

Thus, at any $t = t_k$, the curve of C_A versus C_A^0 becomes linear at exceedingly high values of C_A^0 and its slope approaches unity. Also, it can be shown that the second derivative of

C_A with respect to C_A^0 is always positive, which does not permit a point of inflection, and thus the curve of C_A versus C_A^0 is of the form shown in Figure 5.4.

The parameters K and V of Equation (5.45) may be determined in a number of ways. One could use the relationships displayed in Figure 5.3 or one could simply rearrange Equation (5.45) to the linear form:

$$-\frac{1}{dC_A/dt} = \left(\frac{K}{V}\right)\frac{1}{C_A}\frac{1}{V} \tag{5.56}$$

The instantaneous rate dC_A/dt may be approximated from experimental data by noting that

$$\frac{dC_A}{dt} \approx \frac{C_A(t_2) - C_A(t_1)}{t_2 - t_1} = \frac{\Delta C_A}{\Delta t} \tag{5.57}$$

where $t_2 > t_1$ and $C_A(t_2)$, $C_A(t_1)$ denote the values of C_A at times t_2 and t_1. For small values of Δt, Equation (5.56) may be restated in the approximate form:

$$-\frac{1}{\Delta C_A/\Delta t} = \left(\frac{K}{V}\right)\frac{1}{C_A(t_{av})} + \frac{1}{V} \tag{5.58}$$

where $t_{av} = (t_2 + t_1)/2$. The straight line has the slope K/V and the intercept $1/V$, from which K and V may be obtained.

5.5 PHYSIOLOGICALLY BASED PHARMACOKINETIC (PBPK) MODELS

The dose scale used in the dose-response modeling can have a significant impact on the high-to-low-dose extrapolation of risks. The determination of that dose scale represents an important opportunity to incorporate available scientific information into the dose-response modeling process. *Delivered dose* scales refer to the amount of the active form of the chemical (parent compound or metabolite) that reaches the target site and reflects the route of dose administration as well as the biological processes associated with absorption, distribution, metabolism, and elimination. That is, the delivered dose reflects the transport of a chemical from its point of entry into the body to the reaction site within the body. The *biologically effective dose* reflects not only the amount of active compound delivered to the target site but also the net amount of relevant biological activity resulting from that delivery. For example, the biologically effective dose might be the amount of cell proliferation induced or the amount of DNA adducts formed, but not repaired. Pharmacokinetic modeling, especially physiologically based pharmacokinetic (PBPK) modeling, can be used to quantify the relationship between the administered dose and either the delivered dose, or preferably, the biologically effective dose. Typical of PBPK models of the biologically effective dose is the one shown in Figure 5.5. PBPK models were proposed and utilized in a series of papers by Gehring and Blau,[3] Reitz and Watanabe,[4] Andersen et al.,[5] and Clewell and Andersen.[6] These models consider both the reaction of mutagens with DNA to form DNA adducts, and the repair of DNA adducts. Mutagens are chemicals which react

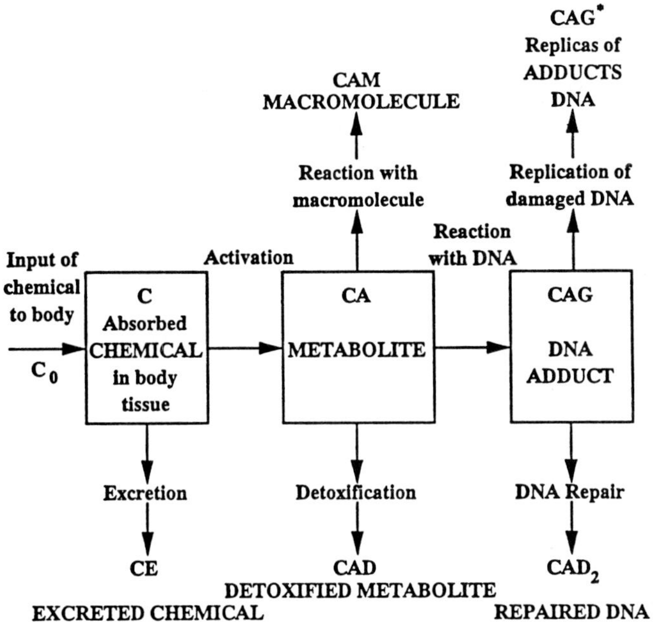

Figure 5.5 A Hypothetical Model of the Fate of a Carcinogen in the Body of a Mammal. [From Gehring, P.J., and G.E. Blau, *J. Environ. Pathol. Toxicol.*, **1**, 163 (1977).]

with the DNA thereby causing mutations. The initial findings by Miller and Miller were recently formalized and expanded in a recent article[7] in which they state that most chemical carcinogens, upon entering the body, are metabolized into a chemically active form called a metabolite. The metabolite is capable of reacting with many cellular macromolecules such as DNA, RNA, and proteins.[7] Some carcinogens such as alkylating agents are in their ultimate form as administered, but most require metabolism to the active metabolite form.[7]

Of particular importance is the reaction of the carcinogen or the metabolite with the DNA, since this macromolecule contains the genetic information for the cell. The given chemical's specific sites of reaction on the DNA are very important in determining the mutagenetic effect. Certain substitutions are more likely to result in miscoding than others. Furthermore, substitutions at some sites are much more readily excised from DNA than at other sites.

Experimental evidence that DNA repair is possible in metabolic systems was provided by Russel et al.[8,9] Ethylnitrosourea, the most potent mutagen for mice yet discovered, was administered to mice in two ways. In one test, one massive dose of 100 mg/kg (milligram of ethylnitrosourea per kilogram of mouse) was administered, and in the other test, doses of 10 mg/kg were administered weekly over a 10 week interval. Although it was anticipated that the 10 weekly doses would give the same number of mutations as the single large dose of 100 mg/kg, this was not the case; the weekly doses produced only 13 percent as many mutations as did the massive dose. Russel et al. interpreted the reduced mutagenic effect of the small weekly doses to the repair process for the damaged DNA. The repair process appeared to have been overwhelmed when the chemical was given as a single large dose of 100 mg/kg.

The hypothetical model shown in Figure 5.5 was used by Gehring and Blau and by Clewell and Andersen to represent the biochemical processes involved when a chemical carcinogen is introduced into the body of a mammal. After the chemical having concentration C_0 has entered the body, it is absorbed in the body tissue at the concentration C. Next, some of it may be excreted as CE and some of it bioactivated to the metabolite CA. The bioactivated molecule then reacts to form detoxified chemicals, noncritical macromolecules, or it may react with genetic material DNA to form CAG (damaged DNA or DNA adducts). The DNA adducts may be repaired by reaction to the form CAD_2 or a replication of the damaged DNA may occur to give CAG*. In this model, the formation of CAG* is the crucial event in the initiation of carcinogenesis because replication of the damaged DNA may produce new cells whose DNA no longer appears to be in need of repair by the repair system of the body. This model of the reaction system may be represented by a system of differential equations. The parameters and rate constants appearing in these equations can often be evaluated by use of *in vivo* and *in vitro* experiments as described by Clewell and Andersen.[6]

5.6 FORMULATION OF RATE EXPRESSIONS FOR THE CANCER MECHANISM SHOWN IN FIGURE 5.5

In the following mechanism proposed by Gehring and Blau,[3] the steps shown as equilibrium reactions are a *short hand* for the Michaelis-Menten mechanism. The absorbed chemical is denoted by C and its concentration is also denoted by C; the excreted chemical by CE and its concentration by C_E; the activated metabolites by CA and their concentration by C_A; the damaged DNA adducts by CAG and their concentration by C_{AG}; the detoxified metabolites by CAD and their concentration by C_{AD}; the macromolecules by CAM and their concentration by C_{AM}; the repaired DNA adducts by CAD_2 and their concentration by C_{AD_2}; and the replicates of the damaged DNA by CAG* and their concentration by C_{AG^*}. Also, k_M, k_g, and k_R are the rate constants shown, and the letters enclosed by parenthesis have the following meanings: (e) = excretion, (a) = activation, (d) = detoxification, and (r) = repair step.

$$
\begin{array}{ccccccc}
 & & & & CAM & & CAG^* \\
 & & & & \uparrow k_M & & \uparrow k_R \\
C_0 & \longrightarrow & C & \overset{(a)}{\rightleftarrows} & CA & \xrightarrow{k_G} & CAG \\
 & & \downarrow\uparrow (e) & & \downarrow\uparrow (d) & & \downarrow\uparrow (r) \\
 & & CE & & CAD & & CAD_2
\end{array}
\tag{5.59}
$$

To illustrate the Michaelis-Menten mechanism for the steps shown as equilibrium reactions, the complete mechanism for the reaction of C to CE and to CA is presented; namely,

$$
\begin{aligned}
C + S_e &\rightleftarrows CS_e \\
CS_e &\rightarrow CE + S_e \\
C + S_a &\rightleftarrows CS_a \\
CS_a &\rightarrow CA + S_a
\end{aligned}
\tag{5.60}
$$

where S_e and S_a denote the respective substrates involved in the respective reactions. In a manner analogous to that demonstrated in the development of the Michaelis-Menten relationship give by Equation (5.45), it is readily shown that

$$-\frac{dC}{dt} = \frac{V^e C}{K^e + C} + \frac{V^a C}{K^a + C} \tag{5.61}$$

Similarly,

$$-\frac{dC_A}{dt} = \frac{V^d C_A}{K^d + C_A} - \frac{V^a C}{K^a + C} + k_M C_A + k_G C_A \tag{5.62}$$

$$-\frac{dC_{AG}}{dt} = \frac{V^r C_{AG}}{V^r + C_{AG}} + k_R C_{AG} - k_G C_A \tag{5.63}$$

The rates of appearance of CE, CAD, CAM, CAD_2, and CAG* are given by

$$\frac{dC_E}{dt} = \frac{V^e C}{K^e + C} \tag{5.64}$$

$$\frac{dC_{AD}}{dt} = \frac{V^d C_A}{K^d + C_A} \tag{5.65}$$

$$\frac{dC_{AM}}{dt} = k_M C_A \tag{5.66}$$

$$\frac{dC_{AD_2}}{dt} = \frac{V^r C_{AG}}{K^r + C_{AG}} \tag{5.67}$$

$$\frac{dC_{AG^*}}{dt} = k_R C_{AG} \tag{5.68}$$

For an initial concentration of the chemical C and a set of values for all of the V and K parameters as well as the rate constants k_E, k_M, and k_R, the above set of ordinary differential equations may be solved simultaneously. From the results so obtained, graphs similar to those shown in Figure 5.6 may be prepared.

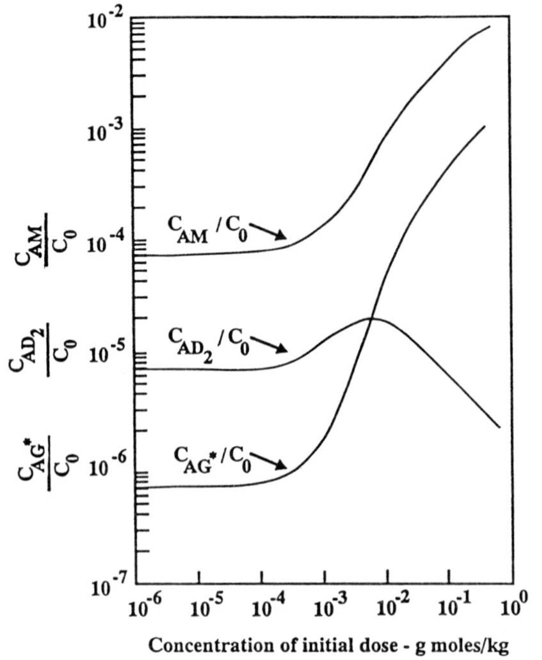

Figure 5.6 Variation of the Products CAM, CAD_2, and CAG* as a Function of the Initial Concentration. [CAM = concentration of macromolecules, CAD_2 = concentration of repaired DNA, and CAG* = concentration of replicated damaged DNA molecules; all concentrations are in g moles per kg of animal weight. (From Gehring, P.J., and Blau, *J. Environ. Pathol. Toxicol.*, **1**, 163 (1977)).]

5.7 OVERWHELMING REPAIR MECHANISMS OF DAMAGED DNA BY HIGH DOSES

To demonstrate that the model shown in Figure 5.5 describes well-known behavior, Gehring and Blau[3] selected a series of plausible values for the parameters and rate constants, and solved the above set of differential equations by use of a computer. Solutions were obtained for a wide variation of initial concentrations C_0 ranging from 10^{-6} to 1 (g moles/kg). The results are shown in Figure 5.6.

These graphs of the concentrations of the postulated compounds formed in the model are useful for the elucidation of the problem of high-to-low-dose extrapolations. First observe that for initial doses greater than 10^{-4}, the replicated–damaged DNA begins to form faster than the other products. Also the ability of the system to repair damaged DNA in proportion to the initial dose C_0 begins to decrease at 10^{-2}, which implies that the repair system is becoming overwhelmed; damaged DNA is being produced faster than it can be repaired. Production of macromolecules CAM also increases as C_0 is increased, but such molecules are not involved in the replication processes. For concentrations greater than $C_0 = 10^{-4}$, small increases in the initial concentration C_0 of the carcinogen give much larger increases in the concentration C_{AG^*} of the damaged adduct, which is illustrated by the following numerical example.

Example 5.1 Suppose that the concentration C_0 of the dose of the carcinogen is increased 100 fold from 10^{-4} to 10^{-2}. Use Figure 5.6 to find the concentration of the damaged DNA adduct at 10^{-2}.

Solution From Figure 5.6, it follows that at $C_0 = 10^{-4}$,

$$\frac{C_{AG^*}}{C_0} = 7 \times 10^{-7}$$

and

$$C_{AG^*} = 7 \times 10^{-7} \times 10^{-4} = 7 \times 10^{-11}$$

At $C_0 = 10^{-2}$

$$\frac{C_{AG^*}}{C_0} = 7 \times 10^{-5}$$

and

$$C_{AG^*} = 7 \times 10^{-5} \times 10^{-2} = 7 \times 10^{-7}$$

Thus, as C_0 is increased by a factor of 100, the concentration of damaged DNA adduct increases by a factor of 10,000; that is,

$$\frac{7 \times 10^{-7}}{7 \times 10^{-11}} = 10^4 = 10,000$$

This example demonstrates the effect of overwhelming the DNA repair mechanisms by use of high doses of the carcinogen. It also suggests the possibility of overestimation of the risk through the use of linear extrapolation methods when the slope of the linear extrapolation is assessed from the high dose experimental data. Note that the multiplication factor does not apply at low initial concentrations near the origin of the graph in Figure 5.6.

5.8 USE OF PHYSIOLOGICALLY BASED PHARMACOKINETICS (PBPK) MODELS IN RISK ASSESSMENT

Both *in vivo* and *in vitro* data are generally needed in order to evaluate the parameters of PBPK models. Reitz et al.[4] evaluated three types of model parameters [(1) physiological constants, (2) partition coefficients, and (3) metabolic rate constants] for methylene chloride by use of *in vivo* data from the literature and laboratory, and the *in vitro* laboratory studies. The model was validated by comparing computer simulations with experimental data gathered from mice, rats, and humans.

In order to reduce the uncertainties in the estimation of human hazards by extrapolation from animal studies, Clewell and Andersen[5] propose the use of PBPK models because they take into account actual physiological properties of the various species, the specific partitioning of different chemicals between tissues and blood, and the concentration dependent rates of metabolism. Because of the fundamentals on which the PBPK models are based, they are particularly useful for high-to-low-dose extrapolations as well as dose-route and interspecies extrapolations. As an example of the use of PBPK models to improve risk assessments, Clewell and Andersen[5] cite the estimations of Singh et al.[10] and Blancato et al.[11] By following the conventional default procedure for methylene chloride [without the use of PBPK modeling data], Singh et al.[10] estimated that the risk for continuous exposure to a concentration of 1 microgram per cubic meter of methylene chloride inhaled in air was 4.1×10^{-6}. Subsequently this estimated risk was lowered by Blancato et al.[11] through the use of PBPK modeling. Although a lower risk was obtained in this instance by PBPK modeling than classical methods, this is not always the case.

For those chemicals which form metabolites that react with DNA, Hoel et al.[12] has proposed the use of the concentration of the resulting DNA adducts to follow tumor formation. There is evidence that tumor response is linearly related to the appropriate DNA adducts in the target organ. PBPK models whose parameters have been accurately determined may be used to help predict the concentration of DNA adducts produced over a wide range of dose concentrations.

In summary, it is evident from the foregoing discussion that the development of the quantitative description of the cancer process is following the same familiar course as that followed in the developments of the fields of chemical kinetics, catalysis, and chemical reaction engineering. Although there are few reaction mechanisms that we understand on an atomic level well enough to compute the kinetic rate constants and mass transfer coefficients from theoretical considerations alone, we can nevertheless determine these parameters in the laboratory and pilot plants and use them in the design and control of chemical reactors. It should also be noted that the reaction engineering models, which are analogous to the cancer dose-response models, accurately predict the product response for a given change in the initial concentration of the chemical reactant.

PROBLEMS

1. Properties of the function I, which denotes the concentration of cells that have experienced one mutation in the MVK two-stage dose-response model, are investigated in this problem.

(a) By use of Equation (5.25) show that

$$\frac{dI}{dt} = \mu_1 S^0 \qquad \text{at } t = 0$$

$$\lim_{t\to\infty} \frac{dI}{dt} = 0$$

(b) Show that for all t

$$I \geq 0$$

(c) Show that I has a maximum at

$$t_{max} = \frac{\log_e(\beta_2 - \alpha_2)/(\beta_1 - \alpha_1)}{(\beta_2 - \alpha_2) - (\beta_1 - \alpha_1)}$$

(d) Show that I has an inflection point at

$$t_{inflection} = \frac{2\log_e(\beta_2 - \alpha_2)/(\beta_1 - \alpha_1)}{(\beta_2 - \alpha_2) - (\beta_1 - \alpha_1)}$$

2. For the function $M(t)$ which represents the concentration of cells that have experienced a second mutation in the MVK two-stage dose-response model given by Equation (5.27), show that

(a)

$$\frac{dM(t)}{dt} = 0 \qquad \text{at } t = 0$$

(b)

$$\frac{dM(t)}{dt} = 0 \qquad \text{as } t \to \infty$$

(c)

$$\frac{d^2M(t)}{dt^2} = \mu_1\mu_2 S^0 \qquad \text{at } t = 0$$

(d)

$$\frac{d^2M(t)}{dt^2} = 0 \qquad \text{as } t \to \infty$$

(e)

$$\lim_{t\to\infty} M(t) = \frac{\mu_1\mu_2 S^0}{(\beta_2 - \alpha_2)(\beta_1 - \alpha_1)}$$

(f) $M(t)$ has a point of inflection at

$$t_{inflection} = \frac{\log_e(\beta_2 - \alpha_2)/(\beta_1 - \alpha_1)}{(\beta_2 - \alpha_2) - (\beta_1 - \alpha_1)}$$

3. Show that for any set of finite values of V and K, the limit of the rate of reaction given by Equation (5.45) as C_A approaches ∞ is equal to V; that is, show that

$$\lim_{C_A\to\infty}\left[-\frac{dC_A}{dt}\right] = V$$

4. Show that C_A as a function of C_A^0 at a fixed $t = t_k$ does not have an inflection point by showing that the second derivative of C_A with respect to C_A^0 is always positive.

5. Instead of using the Michaelis-Menton mechansim for the reaction

$$A \to B$$

suppose that the rate-controlling step mechanism is used. In this approach it is assumed that all of the reactions are in equilibrium except for one which is the rate-controlling step. By this approach the net rate r_1 for the first reaction is assumed to be equal to zero, and that the rate–controlling step is assumed to be the second reaction; that is,

$$A + S \underset{k_1'}{\overset{k_1}{\rightleftharpoons}} AS \qquad r_1 = 0$$

$$AS \underset{k_2'}{\overset{k_2}{\rightleftharpoons}} B + S \qquad r_2 = k_2 C_{AS} - k_2' C_B C_S$$

which implies $k_1 \gg k_2, k_1' \gg k_2'$. Further, suppose that a very small amount of A is in the form AS, or $K_1 \ll K_2$, where $K_1 = k_1/k_1', K_2 = k_2/k_2'$.

(a) Show that

$$\frac{dC_B}{dt} = \frac{k[C_A - C_B/K]}{1 + K_1 C_A}$$

where

$$k = k_2 K_1 C_S^0 \qquad K = \frac{1}{K_1 K_2}$$

(b) Since $K_1 \ll K_2$, the amount of A is in the form of AS is very small; that is $C_A = C_A^0 - C_B$, where C_A^0 is the concentration of A at $t = 0$. Show that

$$-\frac{dC_A}{dt} = \bar{k}\left[\frac{C_A - C_A^0/\bar{K}}{1 + K_1 C_A}\right]$$

where

$$\bar{k} = k\left[1 + \frac{1}{K}\right] \qquad \bar{K} = 1 + K$$

(c) Obtain the expression for the time t as a function of C_A and C_A^0

6. Suppose that the rate-controlling step mechanism is assumed for steps (a), (e), (d), and (r) of the Gehring-Blau system of reactions instead of the Michaelis-Menten mechanism. That is, for step (e) of Equation (5.59) suppose that

$$C + S_e \underset{k_e'}{\overset{k_e}{\rightleftharpoons}} CS_e \qquad r_1 = 0$$

$$CS_e \underset{k_{CE}'}{\overset{k_{CE}}{\rightleftharpoons}} CE + S_e \qquad r_2 = r_{CE} = k_{CE} C_{CS_e} - k_{CE}' C_E C_{S_e}$$

and that $k_e \gg k_{CE}, k_e' \gg k_{CE}'$ and $K_e \ll K_{CE}$ where $K_e = k_e/k_e', K_{CE} = k_{CE}/k_{CE}'$. Suppose that S_e is available only for reaction (e), S_a is available only for reaction (a), S_d only for the reaction (d), and S_r only for reaction (r).
Show that

$$r_2 = \frac{k[C_C - C_E/K]}{1 + K_e C_C}$$

where

$$k = k_{CE} K_e C_{Se}^0 \qquad K = \frac{1}{K_e K_{CE}}$$

NOTATION

A = a chemical reactant; see Equation (5.35)
AS = chemical complex of A and S
C = absorbed chemical; see Equation (5.60)
C_0 = concentration of the dose
C_A = concentration of A in consistent units at any time t
C_A^0 = initial concentration of A at time $t = 0$
ΔC_A = change in concentration of A over the time interval Δt
CA = metabolite; see Figure 5.5
CAD = detoxified metabolite
CAD_2 = repaired DNA
CAG = DNA adduct
CAG^* = replicas of damaged DNA adducts
CAM = macromolecule
CE = excreted chemical
C_{AD} = concentration of detoxified metabolites
C_{AD_2} = concentration of repaired DNA
C_{AG} = concentration of DNA adduct
$C_{AG}{}^*$ = concentration of damaged DNA adducts
D = dead cells, and also denotes the concentration of these cells
$E_{L,0}, E_{R,0}$ = left and right strands of a normal DNA molecule; also denotes concentration of same
$E_{L,1}, E_{R,1}$ = left and right strands of DNA that have undergone mutation; also denotes concentration
$E_{L,2}, E_{R,2}$ = left and right strands of DNA that have undergone two mutations; also denotes concentration
I = cells that have experienced one mutation, and also used to denote the concentration of these cells
k = rate constant with subscripts used for identifiction of the particular reaction
K = constant in the Michaelis-Menten equation; see Equation (5.45)

M = cells that have experienced two mutations, and also used to denote the concentration for these cells

r_A = net rate of disappearance of A per unit time per unit volume

r_M = net rate of appearance of M per unit time per unit volume

r_I = net rate of disappearance of I per unit time per unit volume

r_S = net rate of disappearance of S per unit time per unit volume

S = normal cells, and also denotes the concentration of these cells

t = time

V = constant in the Michaelis-Menten equation; defined by Equation (5.41)

GREEK LETTERS

α_1, α_2 = rate constants; see Equations (5.4) and (5.9)

β_1, β_2 = rate constants; see Equations (5.6) and (5.8)

μ_1, μ_2 = rate constants; see Equations (5.7) and (5.10)

REFERENCES

1. Moolgavkar, S.H., and A.G. Knudson, Jr., "Mutation and Cancer: A Model for Human Carcinogenesis," *JNCI*, **66** (No. 6), 1037 (1981).
2. Sokolnikoff, I.S., and E.S. Sokolnikoff, *Higher Mathematics for Engineers and Physicists*, Second Edition, McGraw-Hill Book Company, Inc., New York, N.Y. (1941).
3. Gehring, P.J. and G.E. Blau, "Mechanisms of Carcinogenesis: Dose Response," *J. Environ. Pathol. Toxicol.*, **1**, 163 (1977).
4. Reitz, R.H., and P.G. Watanabe, *Mechanistic Considerations in the Formulation of Carcinogenic Risk Estimations*, Banbury Report 19, Risk Quantitation and Regulatory Policy, Cold Spring Harbor Laboratory, 241 (1985).
5. Andersen, M.E., H.J. Clewell III, M.L. Gargas, F.A. Smith, and R.H. Reitz, "Physiologically Based Pharmacokinetics and Risk Assessment Process for Methylene Chloride," *Toxicol and Appl. Pharmacology*, **86**, 341 (1987).
6. Clewell, H.J., III and M.E. Andersen, "Risk Assessment Extrapolations and Physiological Modeling," *Toxicology and Industrial Health*, **1** (No. 4), 111 (1985).
7. Miller, E.C., and J.A. Miller, "Searches for Ultimate Chemical Carcinogens and their Reactions with Cellular Macromolecules," *Cancer*, **47**, 2327 (1981).
8. Russell, W.L., E.M. Kelly, P.R. Hunsicken, J.W. Bangham, S.C. Maddux, and E.L. Phipps, "Specific-Locus Test Shows Ethylnitrosurea to be the Most Potent Mutagen in the Mouse," in *Proc. Nat. Acad. Sci. U.S.A.*, **76**, 5818 (1979).

9. Russell, W.L., P.R. Hunsicken, D.A. Carpenter, C.V. Cornett, and G.M. Guinn, "Effect of Dose Fractionation on the Ethynitorsourea Induction of Specific Locus Mutations in Mouse Spermatogonia," in *Proc. Nat. Acad. Sci. U.S.A.*, **79**, 3592 (1982).

10. Singh, D.V., H.L. Spitzer and P.D. White, Addendum to Health Assessment Document for Dichloromethane (Methylene Chloride). Updated carcinogenicity assessment of dichloromethane. EPA/600/8–82/004F (1985).

11. Blancato, J.N., J. Hopkins and L. Rhomberg, Update of the health assessment document and addendum for dichloromethane (Methylene Chloride): Pharmacokinetic mechanism of action, and epidemiology, External Review Draft, EPA/600/8–87/030A (1987).

12. Hoel, D.G., N.L. Kaplan, and M.W. Anderson, "Implication of Nonlinear Kinetics on Risk Estimation in Carcinogenesis," *Science*, **219**, 1032 (1983).

6

Biologically Based Dose Scales For Dose-Response Modeling

In previous chapters, a discussion of the mathematical development of *dose-response models* and their application in cancer risk assessment has been presented. Selecting an appropriate dose-response model that describes the carcinogenic mechanism is one of the most important tasks of cancer risk assessment. Another important task is the selection of the *dose scale* to be used in the dose-response model because the implications of the mathematical models depend heavily on the dose scale used. Furthermore, the theoretical development of the mathematical dose-response models is based on the assumption that the dose is expressed on a *biologically based dose scale* representing the actual dose level directly involved in the cancer processes. The dependency of dose-response models on the dose scale and the significant impact that the selection of a biologically based dose scale has in a risk assessment are the motivations for this chapter.

The dose scale can reflect the relationship between the external dose and the dose level actually directly involved in the physical processes associated with cancer mechanisms. Therefore, the dose scale also represents an excellent opportunity to incorporate available biological and toxicological information into the quantitative dose-response modeling.

The term *dose level* has been defined in the context of the dose-response model, but no discussion as to how to quantify the dose level has been presented so far. In this chapter, the alternative dose scales for dose-response modeling are discussed first. Next, the concepts of delivered dose and biologically effective dose are presented. The roles of administered dose, background dose and susceptibility in dose-response modeling are then discussed. The last four sections of this chapter are devoted to the practical implementation of the biologically based dose scales in cancer risk assessment, the incorporation of interindividual variation into dose-response modeling, the extrapolation from the experimental situation to the inference situation, and the differences between individual and population inferences.

6.1 ALTERNATIVE DOSE SCALES FOR DOSE-RESPONSE MODELING

The dose level in all of the dose-response models used to estimate cancer risk may be expressed as either

1. an *administered dose, d* (exposure level, applied dose, external dose, environmental level, etc.),
2. an *intermediate dose* (amount of the carcinogenic agent reaching the target individual),
3. a *delivered dose,* d_{DD} (the amount of the carcinogenic agent reaching the target cells of a particular tissue), or
4. a *biologically effective dose,* d_{BED} (the amount of the carcinogenic agent or metabolite that interacts with DNA, the net amount of cell damage, etc.).

The biologically effective dose reflects not only the amount of the carcinogenic agent or metabolite delivered to the target organ, but also the net generation of cancer related activity, including cell turnover or regeneration, DNA repair, and immune system responses. Figure 6.1 shows an example of the different dose scales in an inhalation exposure situation.

There are several advantages to using biologically based dose scales as opposed to administered dose scales. One advantage is that the theoretical development of the mathematical dose-response models in Chapter 2 is based on the assumption that the dose is expressed on the biologically effective dose scale. A second advantage is that, by incorporating the available biological, physiological, and pharmacokinetic knowledge, the uncertainty and the number of unknowns in the dose-response model may be reduced. The more biologically based the dose scale is, the better the model's capability to extrapolate from high to low doses, from species to species, from one target organ to another, from one exposure route to another, and from one exposure pattern to another. The closer the dose-response model's dose scale is to the biologically effective dose, the simpler the remainder that must be explained by the rest of the model and the smaller the differences between alternative models. As the following example illustrates, a third advantage is that the shape of the curve for the dose-response model becomes simpler as the dose scale becomes more biologically based. Such simplifications are important because they make the simple

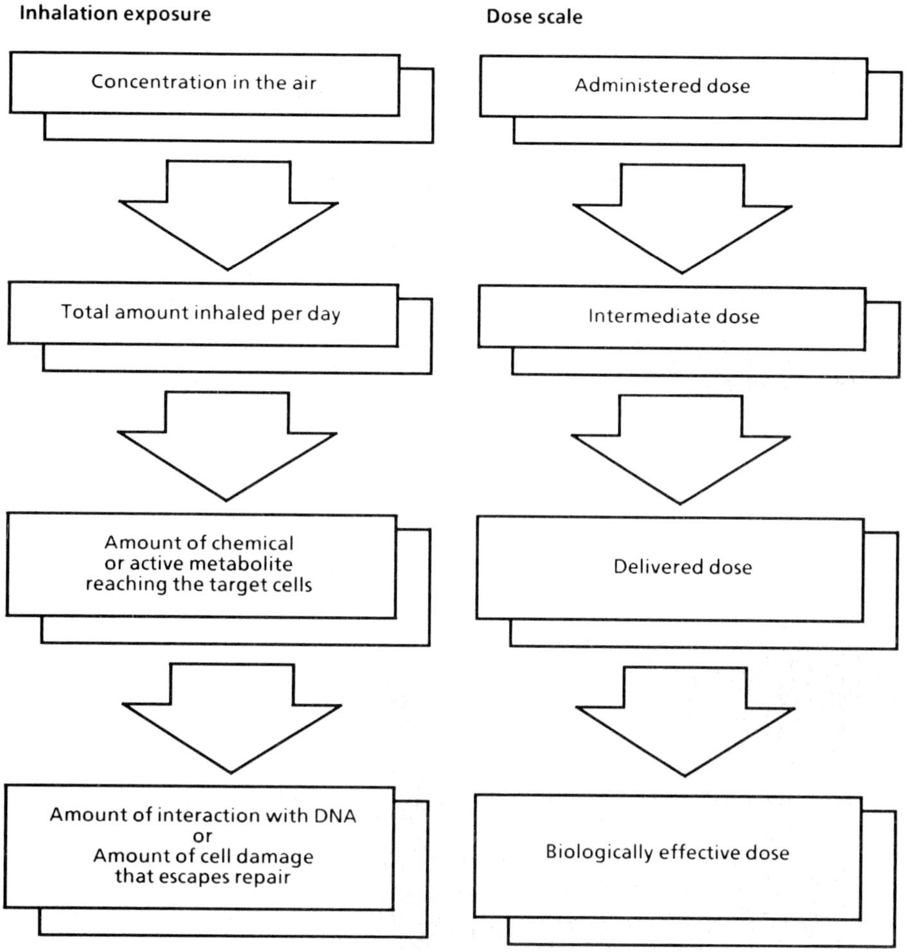

Figure 6.1 Using More Biologically Relevant Dose Scales in an Inhalation Exposure Situation.

default linear extrapolations often used in the decision making of risk management more meaningful.

Example 6.1 Suppose that a dose-response model is to be fit to the cancer dose-response data in an inhalation situation similar to that in Figure 6.1. If the dose-response model is fit using the amount of cell damage that escapes repair in the lung as the dose scale (the biologically effective dose, d_{BED}), then there is a linear relationship between the probability of cancer and low levels of d_{BED} (Figure 6.2a). In particular,

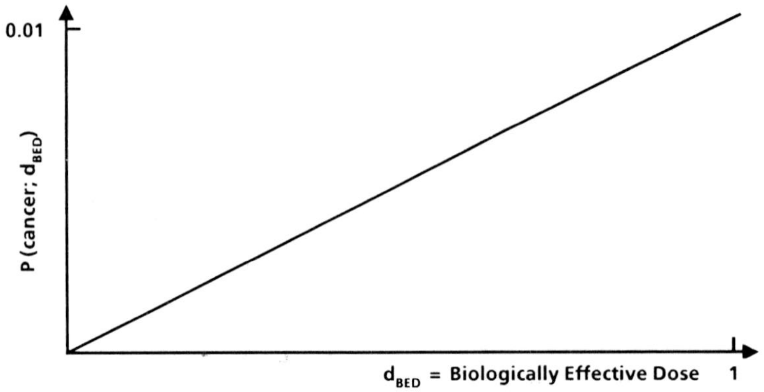

a) P (cancer; d_{BED}) = $1 - e^{-0.01 d_{BED}}$

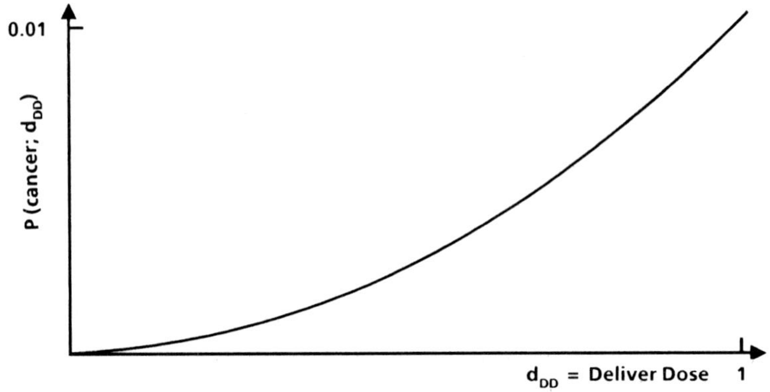

b) P (cancer; d_{DD}) = $1 - e^{-0.01 (d_{DD})^2}$

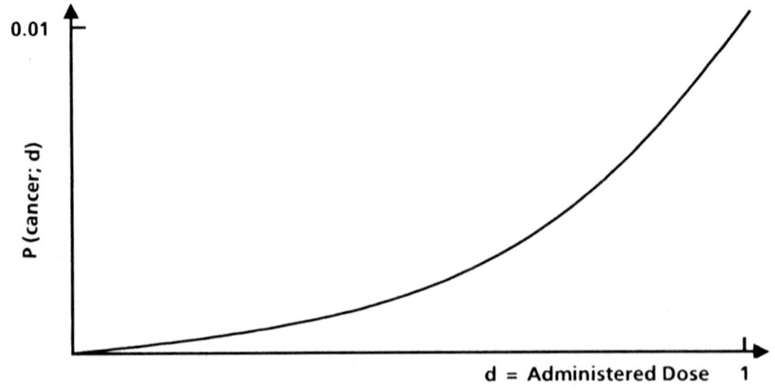

c) P (cancer; d) = $1 - e^{-0.01 d^3}$

Figure 6.2 Low-Dose Model Fit to the same Cancer Dose-Response Data using the Dose Scales of d_{BED}, d_{DD}, d.

$$P(\text{cancer}; d_{BED}) = 1 - e^{-0.01 d_{BED}}$$
$$\approx 0.01 d_{BED} \qquad \text{for small values of } d_{BED} \tag{6.1}$$

Suppose, further, that research has shown that the relationship between the amount of cell damage that escapes repair in the lung (d_{BED}) and the amount of the chemical under consideration that reaches the lung cells (delivered dose, d_{DD}) is given by

$$d_{BED} = d_{DD}^2 \tag{6.2}$$

as illustrated in Figure 6.3a. If the model to predict cancer risk uses the delivered dose instead of the biologically effective dose, then the resulting relationship between the probability of cancer and d_{DD} is quadratic in d_{DD} (Figure 6.2b)

There is also the possibility of using the concentration in the air (administered dose, d) to predict the risk of cancer. Suppose that, in this hypothetical example, the relationship between d_{DD} and d is given by

$$d_{DD} = d^{1.5}$$

as illustrated in Figure 6.3b, and thus

$$d_{BED} = d_{DD}^2 = (d^{1.5})^2 = d^3$$

as illustrated in Figure 6.3c. If the model to predict cancer risk uses the administered dose instead of the delivered dose, the relationship between the probability of cancer and d is cubic in d (Figure 6.2c). These dose-response models, namely,

$$P(\text{cancer}; d_{BED}) = 1 - e^{-0.01 d_{BED}}$$
$$P(\text{cancer}; d_{DD}) = 1 - e^{-0.01 d_{DD}^2} \tag{6.3}$$
$$P(\text{cancer}; d) = 1 - e^{-0.01 d^3}$$

are mathematically equivalent in the sense that they all three imply the same probability of cancer at a given administered dose d. For example, at $d = 0.001$,

$$\begin{aligned} d_{DD} &= d^{1.5} &= 0.001^{1.5} &= 3.16228 \times 10^{-5} \\ d_{BED} = d_{DD}^2 &= d^3 &= 0.001^3 &= 1 \times 10^{-9} \end{aligned} \tag{6.4}$$

and the probabilities of cancer are

$$\begin{aligned} P(\text{cancer}; d_{BED} = 1 \times 10^{-9}) &= 1 - e^{-0.01(1\times 10^{-9})} &= 1 \times 10^{-11} \\ P(\text{cancer}; d_{DD} = 3.1623 \times 10^{-5}) &= 1 - e^{-0.01(3.1623\times 10^{-5})^2} &= 1 \times 10^{-11} \\ P(\text{cancer}; d = 1 \times 10^{-3}) &= 1 - e^{-0.01(1\times 10^{-3})^3} &= 1 \times 10^{-11} \end{aligned} \tag{6.5}$$

However, it is obvious that the shape (linear, quadratic, cubic) of the dose-response probability curve changes with the dose scale. The differences in the shapes have significant impacts on *low-dose linear extrapolations*. For example, the low-dose linear extrapolation of probabilities using the administered dose scale results in an

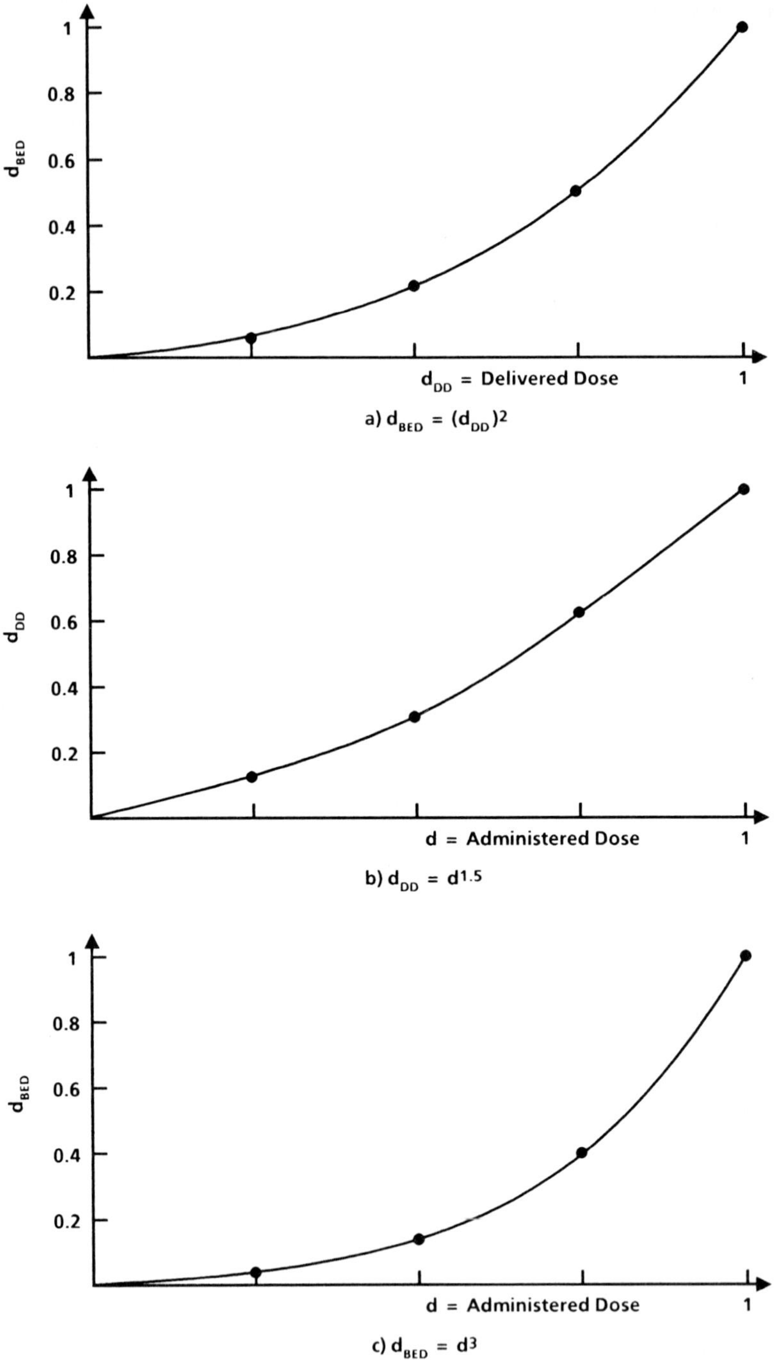

Figure 6.3 Relationship Among the Different Dose Scales Used to Fit the Hypothetical Situation Given in Example 6.1

overestimation of risk by several orders of magnitude; whereas, low-dose linear extrapolation using d_{BED} generates estimates that are closer to the dose-response model values. Specifically, suppose the risk at an administered dose of 0.001 is to be computed using low-dose linear extrapolation starting at an administered dose level of 0.1. The extrapolated risks obtained by use of d_{BED}, d_{DD} and d dose scales are considerably different; namely,

Dose Scale	Target Dose Corresponding to $d = 0.001$	Starting Dose for Linear Extrapolation	Risk at Starting Dose	Extrapolated Risk	Actual Risk	Ratio = Extrapolated/ Actual
d_{BED}	1×10^{-9}	1×10^{-3}	1×10^{-5}	1×10^{-11}	1×10^{-11}	1
d_{DD}	3.1623×10^{-5}	3.1623×10^{-2}	1×10^{-5}	1×10^{-8}	1×10^{-11}	1000
d	1×10^{-3}	1×10^{-1}	1×10^{-5}	1×10^{-7}	1×10^{-11}	10000

The above extrapolated risks are computed by use of the equation for the straight line from the starting dose x_1 ($x_1 = d_1 = 0.1$, or $x_1 = d_{DD_1} = (0.1)^{1.5}$, or $x_1 = d_{BED_1} = (0.1)^3$) to any dose x which is obtained as follows. Because $P(\text{cancer}; 0) = 0$ in the dose-response models given in Equation (3), it follows that the linearly extrapolated risk for any dose x ($x = d$, $x = d_{DD}$, $x = d_{BED}$) is given by

$$P(\text{cancer}; x)_{\text{extrapolated}} = \left[\frac{P(\text{cancer}; x_1) - 0}{x_1 - 0}\right] x \tag{6.6}$$

The starting doses x_1 and corresponding risks $P(\text{cancer}; x_1)$ are computed in a manner analogous to that shown by Equation (6.3) through (6.5). The actual risks corresponding to $d = 0.001$ are also computed by use of the dose-response models given by Equations (6.3) through (6.5).

The dose scale used in cancer risk assessment should be expressed in terms of the most biologically relevant scale that is available. If there is insufficient scientific information available to establish the complete transformation from the administered dose to the biologically effective dose, then using a partial transformation or the best approximation on the basis of what is known should result in a better risk assessment than using the administered dose.

6.2 BIOLOGICALLY BASED DOSE SCALES

Biologically based dose scales refer to measures that reflect the biological and physiological processes involved in the absorption of external dose levels and the formation of cancer, as opposed to only simple measures of the level of exposure to a substance. The *delivered dose* (d_{DD}) is a biologically based dose scale that represents the amount of substance that

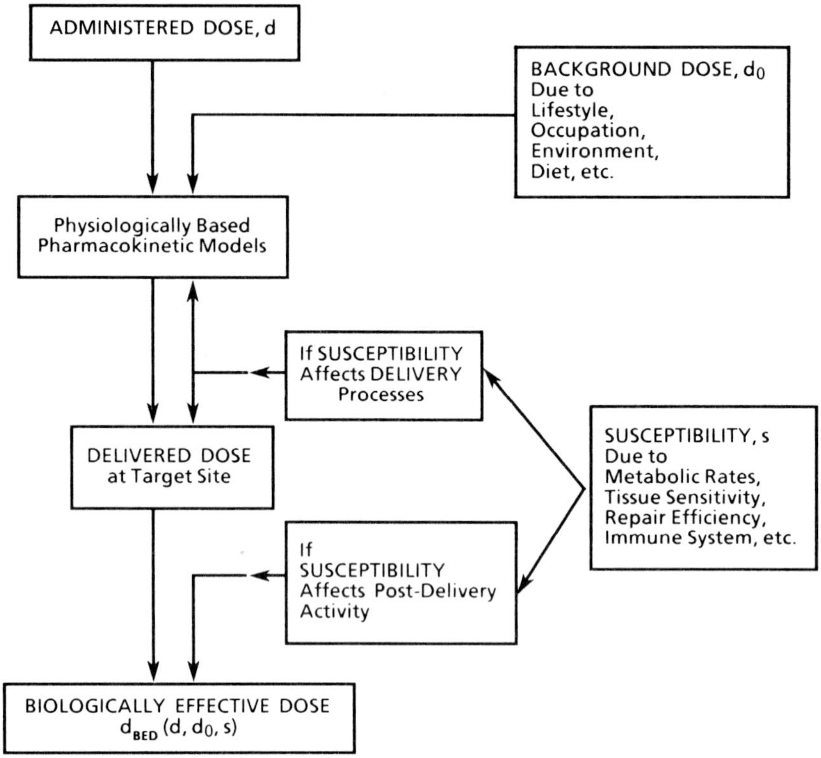

Figure 6.4 Graphical Representation of the Interaction of Administered Dose, Background Dose and Susceptibility in the Determination of more Biologically Based Dose Scales (Delivered Dose and Biologically Effective Dose).

reaches the target tissue. Delivered dose scales refer to the amount of the active form of the substance (parent compound or metabolite) that reaches the target site and reflects the route of administration as well as the biological processes associated with absorption, distribution, metabolism, and elimination. The d_{DD} for a given species is dependent upon the level of exposure as well as the substance itself. The delivered dose can be obtained through direct experimentation or, as illustrated schematically in Figure 6.4, through physiologically based pharmacokinetic modeling. Physiologically based pharmacokinetic (PBPK) modeling was discussed in Chapter 5.

The dose scale incorporating the greatest extent of biological information is the *biologically effective dose* (d_{BED}). The d_{BED} can reflect not only the amount of the carcinogenic agent or metabolite delivered to the target tissue, but also the net generation of cancer related activity, including cell turnover (or cell regeneration), repair processes, cellular defense mechanisms, and immune system responses. The biologically effective dose can represent the net amount of the intracellular receptor binding, the amount of

DNA adducts not repaired, the amount of cell proliferation in a tissue, and the changes in intercellular communication. The d_{BED} may be influenced by several factors in addition to the administered dose.

Delivered doses and biologically effective doses have been studied in different animal experiments (e.g., Andersen et al.[1], Anderson et al.[2], Chen and Blancato[3], Cohen and Ellwein[4,5], Reitz et al.[6], and Starr and Buck[7]). The results show that the relations between delivered doses, biologically effective doses and administered doses are nonlinear in several cases. The nonlinear relation is caused by factors such as saturation of transport pathways, saturation of clearance pathways, saturation of metabolization pathways, organ sizes, and immune system responses.

The delivered dose and biologically effective dose, in addition to being functions of the administered dose, can depend on some other factors that may introduce more nonlinear effects. Figure 6.4 illustrates the potential dependency of delivered dose and biologically effective dose on the administered dose, the background dose, and the susceptibility in the delivery process and the postdelivery activity. Detailed discussion of the delivered dose and the biologically effective dose is deferred to Sections 6.5.1 and 6.5.2, after the administered dose, background dose and susceptibility have been presented.

6.3 ADMINISTERED DOSE

The amount of the substance in the exposure medium is often referred to in the literature as the *administered dose*. The administered dose may be introduced to the individual by inhalation, ingestion, dermal absorption or injection. The units of the administered dose are often in terms of concentration (e.g., parts per million (*ppm*) or parts per billion (*ppb*)) or in terms of normalized intake (e.g., milligrams of substance per kilogram of body weight per day or milligrams of substance per unit body surface area per day).

6.4 BACKGROUND DOSE

The *background dose* is usually defined as the total amount of the substance being evaluated that the individuals receive from all sources other than the source of the administered dose. The background dose may also include substances, other than the substance being tested, which contribute in any way to the total delivered dose or biologically effective dose. For example, suppose that the biologically effective dose is the number of adducts that are formed of a particular type. Then the background dose refers to all substances, excluding the portion of these substances corresponding to the administered dose, that are associated with the formation of that particular adduct.

In animal experiments, the environment is normally controlled such that the only substance affecting the animals on test comes from an established administered dose. That is, the habitat and diet are usually controlled in animal experiments to avoid confounding factors in the resulting carcinogenic responses. However, when animals are exposed to the same substance in some way other than via the administered dose or exposed to different substances that may affect the occurrence of the response, the risk assessment should incorporate this background dose.

6.5 SUSCEPTIBILITY

Susceptibility is another relevant component of biologically based dose scales. Species, and individuals from the same species, vary in their ability to suppress carcinogenic mechanisms from a particular exposure to a potentially hazardous substance due to genetic traits, pre-existing diseases, etc. The ability to suppress cancer formation as well as the ability to enhance or diminish delivered doses is called susceptibility.

Susceptibility can play two roles and may have a significant impact on the determination of biologically based dose scales (see Figure 6.4).

1. *Delivery susceptibility.* Susceptibility may reflect the factors which amplify or diminish the normal delivery process in some individuals. For example, people with different metabolic rates may have different delivered doses even though they were exposed to the same administered dose. In such circumstances, susceptibility becomes a multiplier of the normal delivered dose with the value of the multiplier being a function of the individual's metabolic rates.
2. *Postdelivery susceptibility.* Susceptibility may also affect the biologically effective dose by reflecting the postdelivery activity. In such circumstances, the net amount of cancer related activity within the cells (the d_{BED}) may be expressed as a function of the individual's susceptibility which has a value determined by the capabilities of the cell defense mechanisms, repair processes, immune system responses, etc. to suppress a carcinogenic response within that individual. As a consequence of susceptibility, the biologically effective dose may take the form of a *hockey stick* shaped function of the delivered dose.

In general, the role that susceptibility plays in the delivery process and postdelivery activity is not the same for different carcinogenic substances.

Oftentimes the postdelivery susceptibility in the carcinogenic process takes the form of a *susceptibility frontier*. The susceptibility frontier is defined as the delivered dose level corresponding to the transition from substantially lower carcinogenic potency to the dose region of higher potency where the predominant defensive mechanisms resisting or suppressing carcinogenesis have become overwhelmed (Sielken[8]). An example of the susceptibility frontier is provided by the physiologically based pharmacokinetic (PBPK) model proposed by Gehring and Blau[9] and described in Chapter 5; see Figures 5.5 and 5.6, and Equations (5.59) through (5.68), and Example 5.1. In this example, when the administered doses are low, the repair processes for the damaged DNA offset the mutagenic effect of the carcinogen. However, the repair processes for the damaged DNA become overwhelmed by the carcinogenic effect of the chemical as the administered dose increases. An examination of Figure 5.6 shows that the susceptibility frontier for the example given occurs at an administered dose of approximately 10^{-3} g mol per kg of animal body weight.

A susceptibility frontier implies a different functional relationship between the biologically effective dose and the delivered dose than does either a threshold or a tolerance level. *Susceptibility frontiers*, *thresholds*, and *tolerance levels* are different and should not be confused. All three are particular delivered doses at which a transition occurs in the d_{BED} as a function of the delivered dose. However, the nature of the transition may be very different for susceptibility frontiers, tolerance levels, and thresholds.

Thus, the susceptibility frontier may be interpreted as the delivered dose level at which the normal functioning of the body's defensive mechanisms are overwhelmed and the amount of carcinogenic activity above this delivered dose level is much greater than below it. In more mathematical terms, the d_{BED} as a function of the delivered dose increases more slowly below the susceptibility frontier and increases much faster above it. A threshold is an extreme case of a susceptibility frontier transition in that below a threshold the d_{BED} is assumed to be zero and not merely slowly increasing. A tolerance level is even more extreme than a threshold; a tolerance level is a delivered dose such that the d_{BED} is zero below the tolerance level, and the d_{BED} is essentially infinite above the tolerance level (so that, the probability of the specified carcinogenic response in an individual is 1.0 whenever the delivered dose exceeds that individual's tolerance level). In general, a susceptibility frontier neither forces the d_{BED} to be zero below it nor infinite above it.

More specifically, let $d_{DD,tol}$ be a tolerance level, $d_{DD,th}$ a threshold level, and s a susceptibility frontier.

In the case of tolerances:

$$d_{BED}(d_{DD}, s) = \begin{cases} 0 & \text{if } d_{DD} \leq d_{DD,tol} \\ \infty & \text{if } d_{DD} > d_{DD,tol} \end{cases} \tag{6.7}$$

$$P(\text{tumor; dose} = d_{BED}) = \begin{cases} 0 & \text{if } d_{DD} \leq d_{DD,tol} \\ 1 & \text{if } d_{DD} > d_{DD,tol} \end{cases} \tag{6.8}$$

In the case of thresholds:

$$d_{BED}(d_{DD}, s) = \begin{cases} 0 & \text{if } d_{DD} \leq d_{DD,th} \\ g(d_{DD}) & \text{if } d_{DD} > d_{DD,th} \end{cases} \tag{6.9}$$

$$P(\text{tumor; dose} = d_{BED}) = \begin{cases} 0 & \text{if } d_{DD} \leq d_{DD,th} \\ f(d_{DD}) & \text{if } d_{DD} > d_{DD,th} \end{cases} \tag{6.10}$$

where $g(d_{DD})$ and $f(d_{DD})$ are nondecreasing functions.

In the case of susceptibility frontiers:

$$d_{BED}(d_{DD}, s) = g(d_{DD}, s) \tag{6.11}$$

$$P(\text{tumor; dose} = d_{BED}) = f(d_{DD}) \qquad \text{for all } d_{DD} \geq 0 \tag{6.12}$$

where $g(d_{DD}, s)$ and $f(d_{DD})$ are nondecreasing functions and the rate of change of the functions immediately above s is greater than the rate of change immediately below s. More precisely,

$$g'(s^+, s) > g'(s^-, s) \tag{6.13}$$

and

$$f'(s^+) > f'(s^-) \tag{6.14}$$

That is, as d_{DD} approaches s from the right, the slopes of $g(d_{DD}, s)$ and $f(d_{DD})$ are greater than when d_{DD} approaches s from the left. Figure 6.5 illustrates the effects that a tolerance, threshold and susceptibility frontier in terms of the delivered dose have on the probability of cancer.

The concept of a threshold was introduced in conjunction with the transition probabilities for the multistage model (Equation (2.47), Chapter 2). Tolerance levels were introduced in Chapter 2 in the development of the multihit, probit, logit, and Weibull models. The concept of susceptibility frontier may be further clarified by the following example adapted from Sielken[8]:

Example 6.2 Suppose that for a particular individual the exposure to a substance causes a particular number of specific molecules to reach and invade a target cell. Also, suppose that the target cells have, for simplicity, a single cancer defense mechanism relative to these invaders—say a detoxification process—and that the cell begins with n opportunities to carry out the detoxification of an invading molecule. However, at each opportunity the probability of detoxifying an invader is, for example, only 0.9 (not 1.0), and a successful detoxification reduces the number of detoxification opportunities the next invader must face by one. In such circumstances the expected number of invaders that avoid random detoxification can be shown to be approximately $10^{-((n+1)-X)}$ if there are X invaders and $X \leq n$. If the number of invaders X exceeds the number of detoxification opportunities n (that is, $X > n$), then the expected number of invaders that avoid detoxification is given by $X - n$.

Suppose that both the probability of a carcinogenic response and the dose d_{BED} are proportional to the number of invaders that avoid detoxification. Then the d_{BED} and the probability of carcinogenic response undergo a slow increase (nearly linear at very low doses) as the delivered dose of the substance increases until it generates approximately n invaders. At this point further increases in the delivered dose correspond to more rapid linear increases in the d_{BED} and the probability of a carcinogenic response.

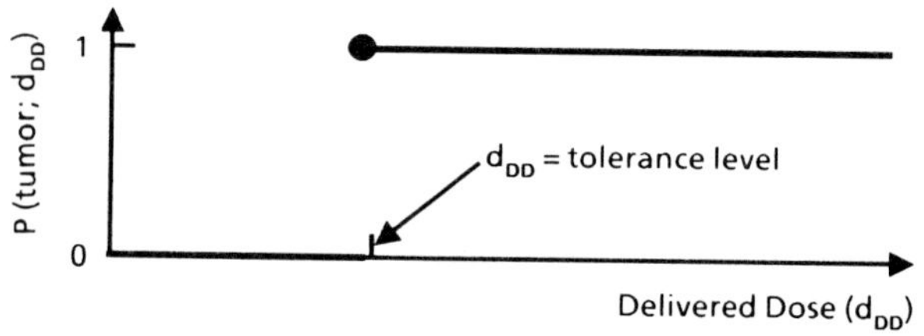

(a) Effect of Tolerance Level on Probability of Tumor Formation

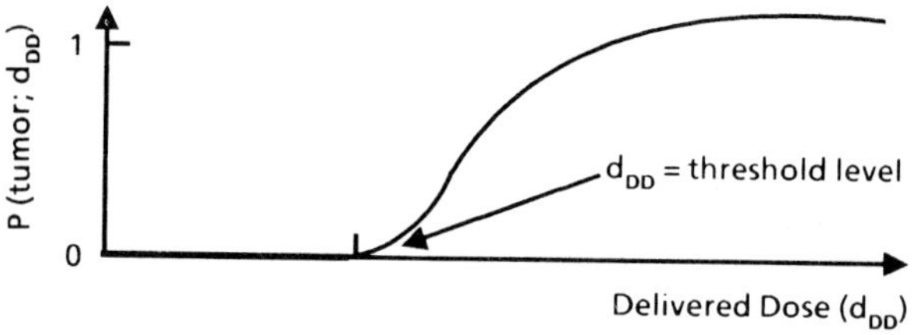

(b) Effect of Threshold Level on Probability of Tumor Formation

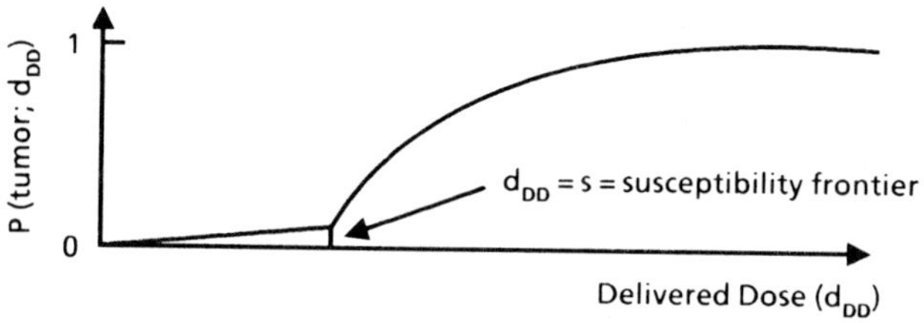

(c) Effect of Susceptibility Level on Probability of Tumor Formation

Figure 6.5 Graphical Representation of the Effects of Tolerance, Threshold, and Susceptibility Frontier on the Probability of Tumor Formation.

In general, if the susceptibility frontier for an individual is greater than zero, then the susceptibility frontier is the delivered dose level at which any increase in the delivered dose will change the relation between the biologically effective dose and the delivered dose from a slowly increasing function to a more rapidly increasing function. In the previous example, the delivered dose level, say $d_{DD}(n)$, expected to generate n invaders would be called the individual's susceptibility frontier; that is, $s = d_{DD}(n)$.

The previous example can be used to further clarify the differences illustrated in Figure 6.5 between a susceptibility frontier, a threshold, and a tolerance. In Figure 6.5c, for values of d_{DD} less than the susceptibility frontier $s = d_{DD}(n)$, the probability of a tumor increases slowly as d_{DD} increases because the expected number of invaders avoiding detoxification increases from near 0 to 0.1. However, for delivered doses exceeding $d_{DD}(n)$, the expected number of invaders avoiding detoxification increases rapidly and so does the probability of a tumor. In this example, it is more reasonable to consider $d_{DD}(n)$ to be a susceptibility frontier (Figure 6.5c) rather than a threshold (Figure 6.5b). This follows because the expected number of invaders avoiding detoxification is not zero below $d_{DD}(n)$ but rather positive and slowly increasing. Hence, the probability of a tumor should not be zero below $d_{DD}(n)$ as it would have to be if $d_{DD}(n)$ represented a threshold instead of a susceptibility frontier. Also, it is more reasonable to consider $d_{DD}(n)$ to be a susceptibility frontier (Figure 6.5c) rather than a tolerance (Figure 6.5a). This follows because the expected number of invaders is not zero below $d_{DD}(n)$ and does not become infinite and a tumor become a certainty for all delivered doses exceeding $d_{DD}(n)$ which would be the case if $d_{DD}(n)$ were a tolerance.

6.5.1 Delivered Dose

The *delivered dose* is the amount of administered dose and background dose that reaches the target tissue. The delivered dose is also influenced by the susceptibility effects on the delivery process and the substance and species being analyzed. In general, the delivered dose is affected by parameters such as:

1. level of the administered dose,
2. level of the background dose,
3. susceptibility level,
4. route of exposure (inhalation, oral ingestion, intravenous, dermal, gavage implantation, etc.),
5. metabolic rates (in the liver, kidney, lungs, etc.),
6. saturable pathways,
7. size of the different organs,
8. clearance rates of substances (through feces from the intestinal lumen, through urine from the kidneys, through exhalation from the lungs, through sweat from the muscles, etc.),
9. partition coefficients relating tissue concentrations to the blood concentration,
10. blood flow rates through the different organs and the total cardiac output.

Most of the items listed above differ between species and often differ between strains within the same species. Because of these differences, the delivered dose to the organs is uniquely defined for each substance, species and strain. Other factors affecting the delivered dose in PBPK modeling are the tissue-dependent parameters; that is, the parameters that are specific to the target organs. The delivered dose is clearly different for different organs due to metabolic rates, clearance rates, organ size, blood flow rate through the tissue, etc. Figure 6.6 illustrates a physiologically based compartmental model that has been used to simulate delivered doses to several organs. The model presented in this figure includes

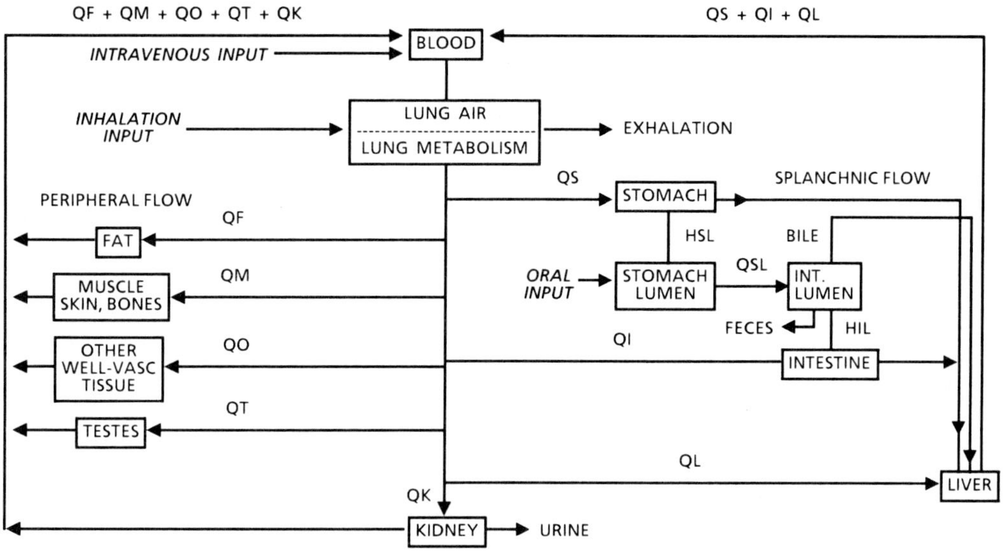

Figure 6.6 A Compartmentalized PBPK Model Showing the Interrelationship of Body Organs in the Determination of the Delivered Dose to Different Target Tissue. (The arrow labels represent flow rates of blood QE, QM, QO, . . . or other fluids).

three routes of exposure; namely, intravenous, inhalation and oral input. The body is divided into twelve body regions or compartments and the delivered dose can be simulated for any body region. Substances can be eliminated via three pathways; namely, feces, exhalation, and urine. The arrows represent the flow of the substance through the different body regions and the labels on the arrows represent transport rates of blood or other fluids.

In view of the complexity of the model shown in Figure 6.6 and the other factors affecting the delivered dose, a nonlinear relation between the exposure levels (administered and background dose levels) and the delivered dose should be expected. For example, even if the clearance and the intake rates are linearly related, the metabolization rates of saturable pathways are not linearly related to the intake rates of a substance. Risk assessment extrapolations from high to low doses may introduce large errors in the resulting inference situations if the assessment is performed using an administered dose scale and there is a significant nonlinear relationship between delivered dose and administered dose. Examples of the nonlinear relation between administered dose and delivered dose are given in Hoel et al.[10] and Starr and Buck[7]. Figure 6.7 shows the typical form of the delivered dose as a function of the administered dose. For very small administered dose levels, the delivered dose increases very slowly. At high levels, the delivered dose increases more rapidly because the elimination and detoxification pathways have become saturated.

Modeling delivered doses to organs of animals exposed to administered doses that vary with time has been described by Andersen et al.[1], Clewell and Andersen[12], Gehring

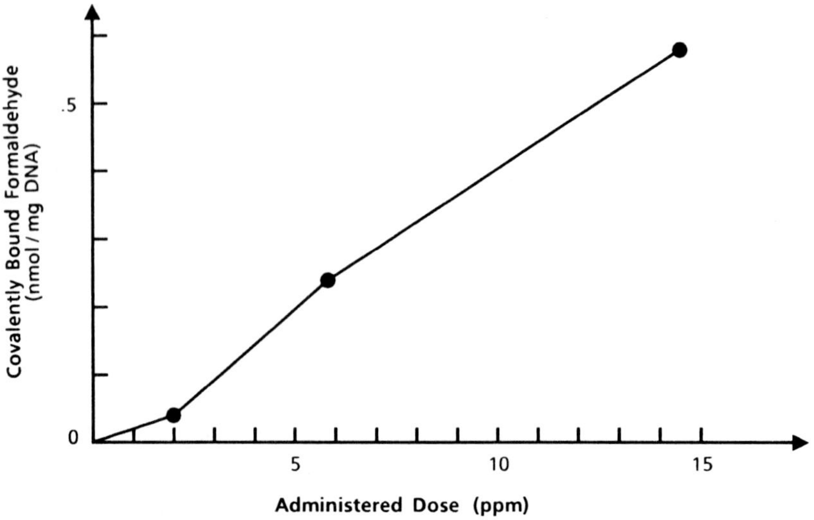

a) Covalently Bound Formaldehyde in Respiratory Muscosal DNA in Fischer-344 Rats[11]

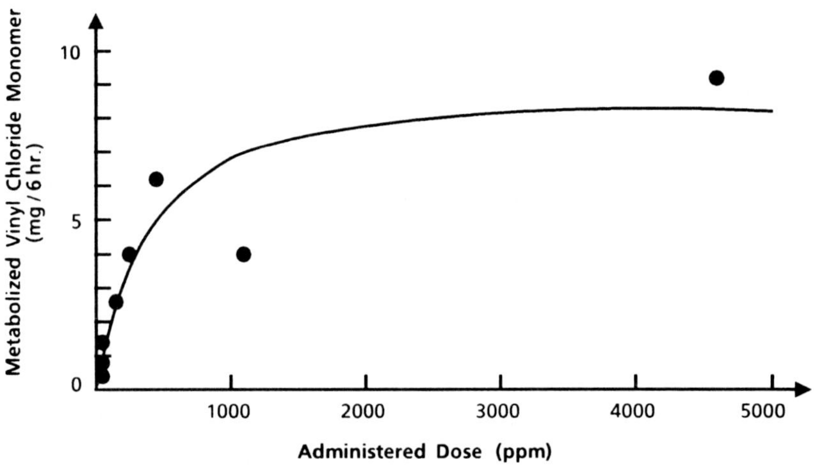

b) Metabolized Vinyl Chloride Monomer in Sprague-Dawley rats[11]

Figure 6.7 Examples of Delivered Dose as a Function of Administered Dose in Rats Exposed to Chemicals via Inhalation.

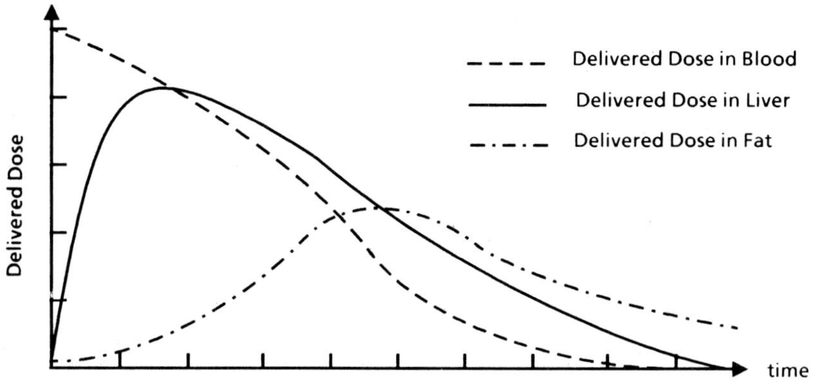

a) Intravenous administered dose given only at time zero

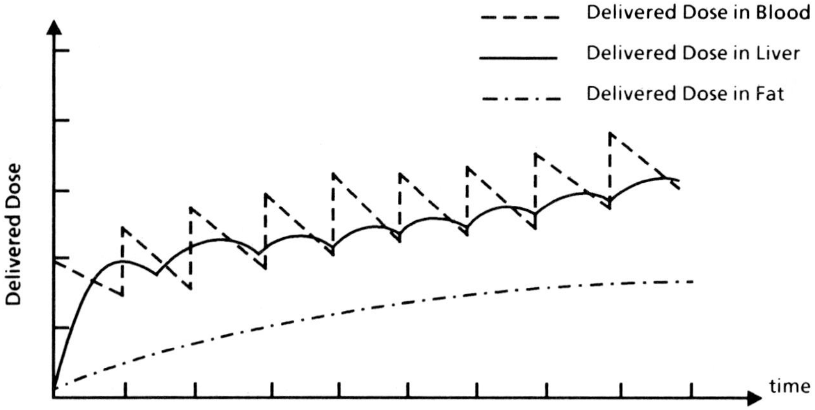

b) Intravenous administered dose given at regular intervals

Figure 6.8 Examples of Possible Behavior of Delivered Dose as a Function of Time for Different Administered Dosing Patterns.

and Blau[9], and others. Figure 6.8 shows how the delivered dose can change over time for different dosing patterns and different organs. Figure 6.8a demonstrates how the delivered dose to the blood, liver and fat may change over time after a single intravenous dose at time zero. The delivered dose to the blood is essentially equal to the administered dose immediately after injection, while the delivered dose to the liver builds up rapidly through the interchange of chemicals with the blood. The fatty tissue normally has a very low blood flow rate and the exchange of the dose with the blood is slow, and thus the build up of delivered dose in the fat is slow. Likewise, the delivered dose in the fatty tissue is depleted slowly due to the slow blood flow rate through this tissue. The concentration in the different organs show similar effects with varying degrees of build-up and depletion of the delivered dose. The concentration in the blood decreases rapidly because of the constant clearance of the chemical and the interchange between blood and other organs is fast.

Figure 6.8b illustrates the effect of intermittent intravenous dosing on the delivered dose. Here, blood concentration decreases rapidly between dose injections, and there is a steady build up in the blood concentration. The concentration in the liver increases rapidly first, and then the concentration build-up slows down. There is some lag between the peaks of concentrations in the blood and liver. This lag is caused by the differences in the time it takes for a substance to reach the different tissues. The concentration in the fatty tissue builds up gradually and tends to stabilize sooner than the concentrations in the blood and liver. Notice that there is no decrease in the concentration in the fatty tissue due to the lack of effective elimination pathways and slow blood flow rate through this body region.

6.5.2 Biologically Effective Dose

The *biologically effective dose* (d_{BED}) reflects the net effect of the delivered dose and postdelivery susceptibility on the carcinogenic mechanisms. This net effect includes both the adverse effects of the delivered dose as well as any repair or remediation. The adverse effects of the delivered dose are a function of both the delivered dose itself and the postdelivery susceptibility level. The delivered dose is a function of the administered dose, background dose, and delivery susceptibility. The terms *delivery susceptibility* and *postdelivery susceptibility* are used herein to differentiate between the two possible roles of susceptibility.

If all of the individuals in a population were identical with respect to the biological processes that respond to the delivered dose, then d_{BED} would be simply a function of just the delivered dose and postdelivery susceptibility would only be a useful parameter in describing that functional relationship. However, if all of these individuals are not identical, then the functional relationship between d_{BED} and the delivered dose is not necessarily the same for every individual. When the functional relationship for d_{BED} differs among individuals, postdelivery susceptibility is a biologically based component of the d_{BED} that allows the differences in individuals' functional relationships for d_{BED} to be incorporated into the dose-response modeling. By explicitly introducing a postdelivery susceptibility s into the functional relationship for d_{BED}, individual differences in the functional relationship between d_{BED} and the delivered dose can be reflected.

The susceptibility frontier is one representation of a postdelivery susceptibility that reflects the individual differences in the functional relationship between d_{BED} and the delivered dose. The differences between a susceptibility frontier and thresholds and tolerance levels have already been discussed in this section. The range of effects that postdelivery susceptibility may have on the d_{BED} are illustrated in Figure 6.9. In Figure 6.9a the susceptibility has no effect; that is, the d_{BED} is a function of the delivered dose only, or

$$d_{BED}(d_{DD}, s) = f(d_{DD}) \tag{6.15}$$

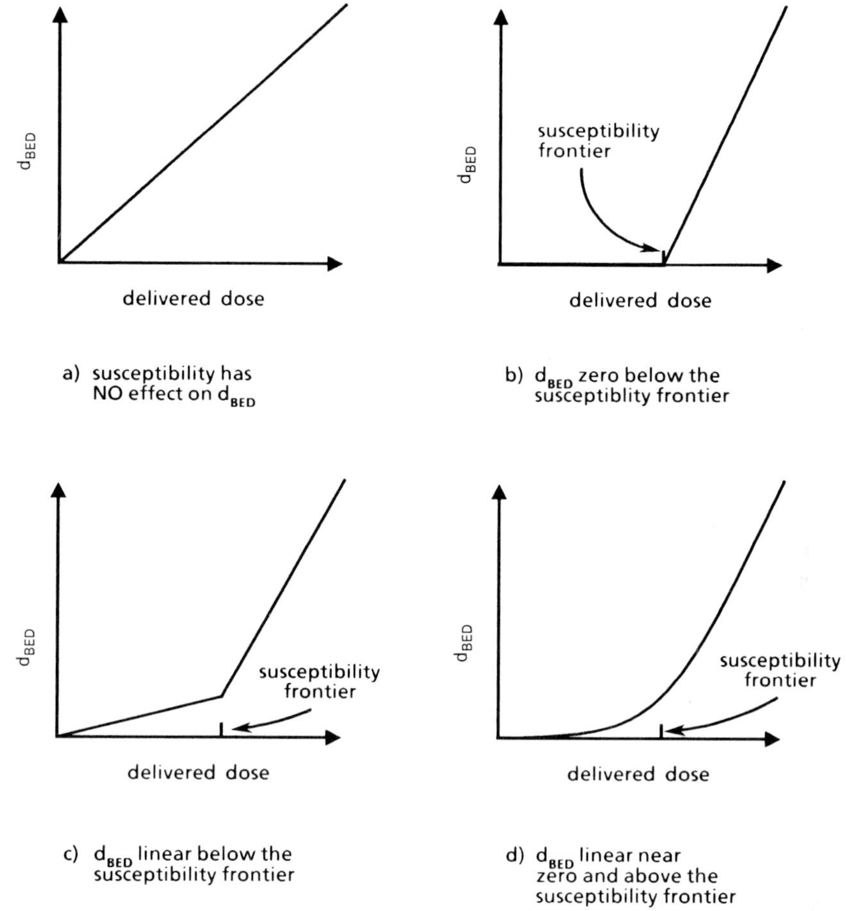

Figure 6.9 Some Possible Relationships Between Susceptibility Affecting the Postdelivery Process, and Delivered Dose, and the Biologically Effective Dose.

Figure 6.9b presents the case in which the delivered dose has no net effect and, hence, results in a zero biologically effective dose when the amount of the chemical reaching the target tissue is below the susceptibility frontier,

$$d_{BED}(d_{DD}, s) = \begin{cases} 0 & \text{if } d_{DD} \leq s \\ f(d_{DD} - s) & \text{if } d_{DD} > s \end{cases} \tag{6.16}$$

In this case the susceptibility frontier acts like a threshold on the d_{BED}. Figures 6.9c and 6.9d show examples in which the d_{BED} increases slowly for delivered doses below the susceptibility frontier and more rapidly for delivered doses above the susceptibility frontier, or

$$d_{BED}(d_{DD}, s) = f(d_{DD}, s) \qquad \text{for all } s \text{ and } d_{DD} \geq 0 \tag{6.17}$$

where $f(d_{DD}, s)$ is a nondecreasing function of the delivered dose and the rate of change of the function immediately above the susceptibility frontier is greater than the rate of change immediately below it. Notice that the concept of susceptibility frontier means that the higher the susceptibility of an individual to a given substance, the smaller the susceptibility frontier, and conversely the lower the susceptibility of an individual, the higher the amount of substance necessary to overwhelm the normal functioning of the defense mechanisms of the body.

Because the development of biologically based dose-response models for cancer risk assessment assumes d_{BED} scales, the use of any other dose scale in model fitting and risk estimation implicitly assumes that the d_{BED} scale is proportional to the dose scale used. As discussed previously, the use of d_{BED} scales in risk assessment reduces the amount of uncertainty and bias associated with the utilization of less relevant biologically based dose scales. The importance of using more biologically based dose scales (delivered dose and biologically effective dose) in risk assessment and the bias introduced by less relevant dose scales (administered dose) in low-dose extrapolations have been the subject of numerous papers (e.g., Sielken[13], Starr and Buck[7]).

6.6 AGE DEPENDENCY AND INTERINDIVIDUAL VARIABILITY IN DOSE SCALES

In animal experiments, the administered dose is controlled by the experimenter and often held constant throughout the duration of the experiment. However, there are some experiments in which the administered dose levels are time dependent as shown in Figures 6.10, 6.11, and 6.12. In controlled experiments, the administered dose is usually assumed to be known with certainty and is, therefore, usually not treated as a random variable. All the members of the experimental population who are subject to a given administered dose level are assumed to be exposed to the same dose level. However, human exposures to a substance from a given source, as opposed to animal exposures in controlled experiments, may vary randomly from individual to individual and the exposures may also be different at different times.

A human's background exposure depends upon such factors as environment, diet, lifestyle, occupation, and hygiene. Because the factors affecting background exposures may not be the same for each individual in a population, the background dose levels may be different for different members of a population. For example, the background dose may depend on the length of time an individual holds different types of jobs and lives in different locations. Hence, the background dose levels could differ among individuals who do not hold the same jobs and live in the same locations for the same durations.

An individual's susceptibility level depends upon such factors as genetic traits, age, and previous diseases. Because these factors are not the same for each individual in a

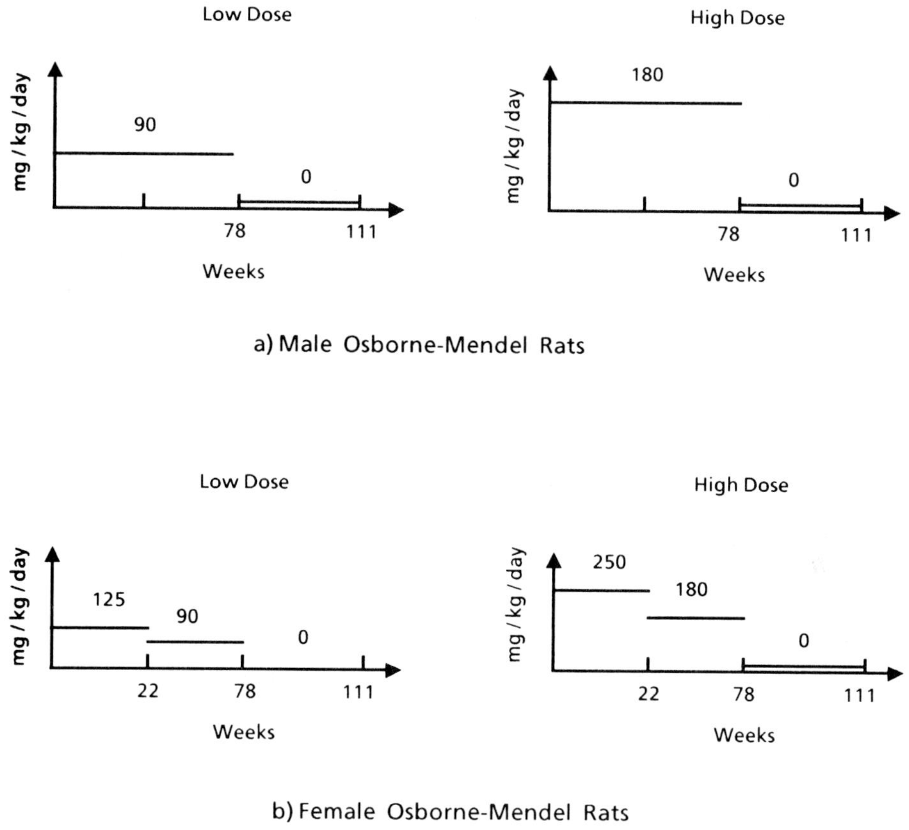

Figure 6.10 Time-Dependent Administered Doses: 1976 NCI Chloroform Rat Gavage Study.[14]

population, the susceptibility dose level may vary among individuals as well as being age dependent.

Because the administered dose, background dose and susceptibility may vary from individual to individual, the dose scale components d, d_0, and s can be considered more generally as the random variables D, D_0, and S rather than constants. Use of the random variables permits the randomness in the population due to interindividual variability to be incorporated into the dose scales d, d_{DD}, and d_{BED}. In addition, the age or time dependence in the dose scales and their components can be reflected by the notation $D(t)$, $D_0(t)$, $S(t)$, $d_{DD}(t)$, and $d_{BED}(t)$. Both interindividual variability and age dependency in dose can be reflected in some current dose-response modeling computer software (e.g., GEN.T[16]). The state of the art is for these computer tools to incorporate deterministic changes in dose over time rather than a more general treatment of the dose as a stochastic process with random pathways through time. The incorporation of variation in d, d_0 and s should be particularly

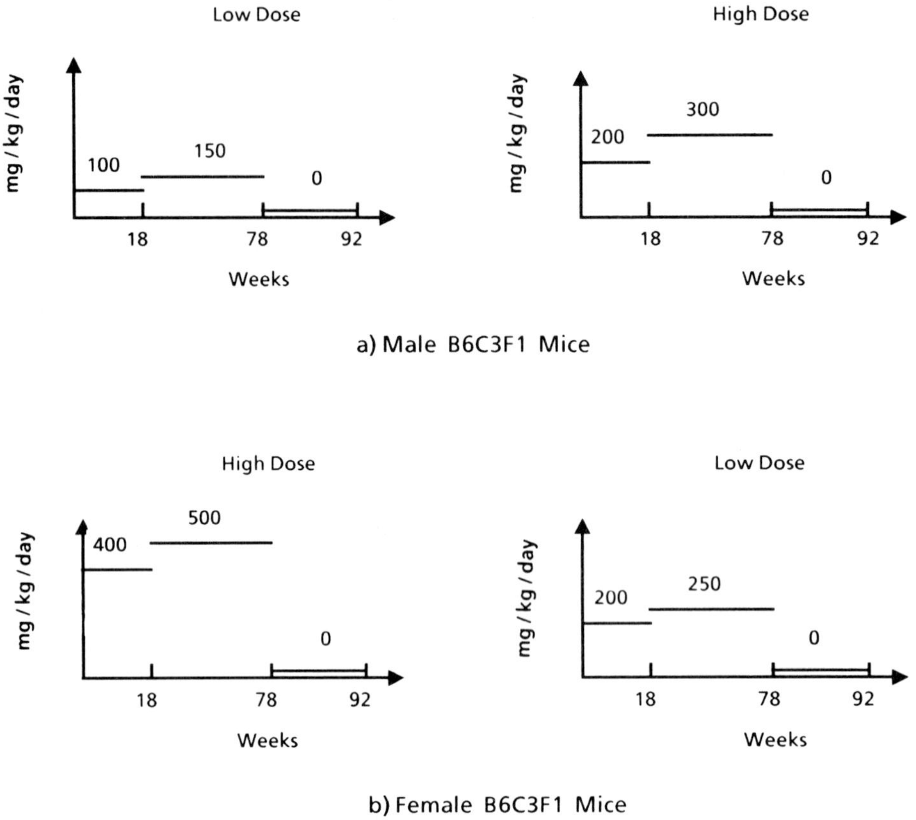

Figure 6.11 Time-Dependent Administered Doses: 1976 NCI Chloroform Mouse Gavage Study.[14]

useful when risk assessments are performed on heterogeneous populations with different behaviors, sociological strata, etc.

6.7 DOSE SCALES IN A NUTRITION EXAMPLE

The concept of the different dose scales can be further illustrated by the nutrition example shown in Figure 6.13. In this figure, some of the biological processes involved in human protein metabolism are illustrated. Here the dietary protein intake is the administered dose. The total amount of daily protein that enters the gastrointestinal tract is made up of the proteins ingested and the digestive enzymes and cells sloughed off from the lining of intestinal tract that are digested and reabsorbed as amino acids (intermediate dose). Most of the free amino acids are then transported to the liver. The amino acids reaching the

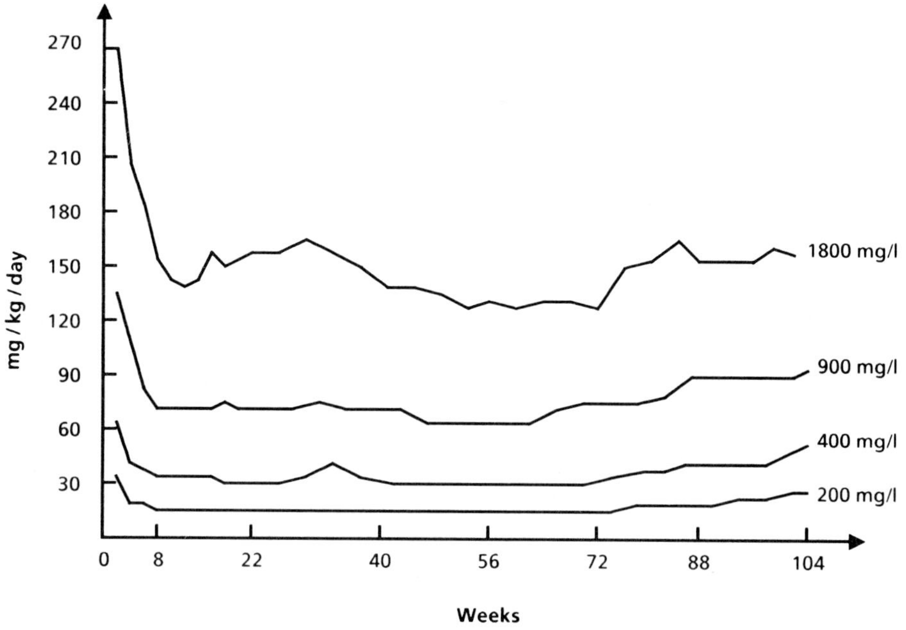

Figure 6.12 Time-Dependent Administered Dose: The Jorgenson Drinking Water Study (Jorgenson, T.A., E.F. Meierhenry, C.J. Rushbrook, R.J. Bull, and M. Robinson, "Carcinogenicity of Chloroform in Drinking Water to Male Osborne-Mendel Rats and Female B6C3F1 Mice," *Fundamental and Applied Toxicology*, **5**, 760 (1985)).

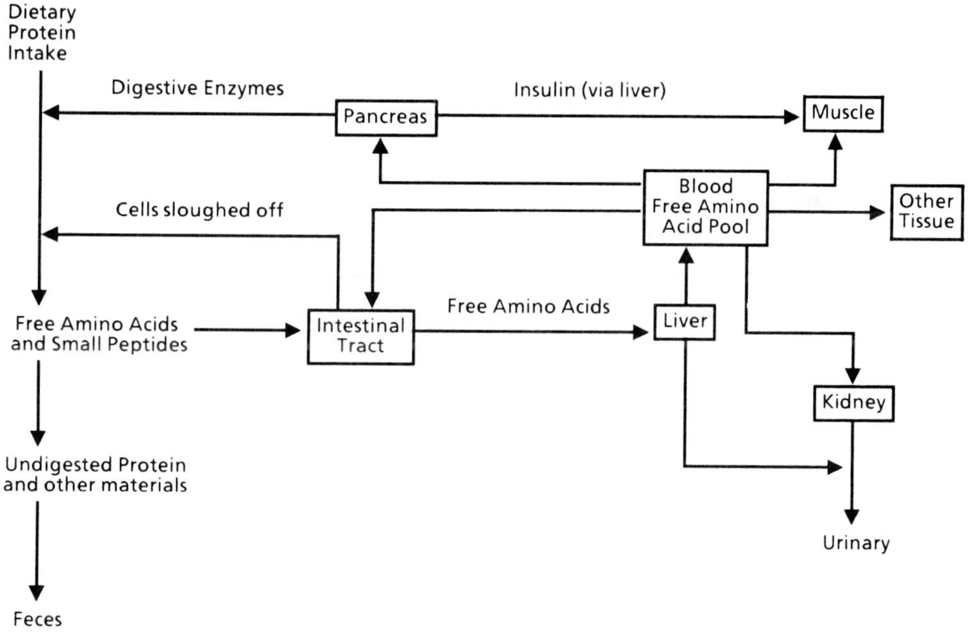

Figure 6.13 Simplified Block Diagram of Protein Intake, Elimination and Metabolism in Humans.

liver may be regarded as the intermediate dose or delivered dose to the liver. Other amino acids are absorbed by cells on the wall of the intestinal tract. Undigested protein and other materials not used by the body are eliminated in the feces. Upon entering the liver, the free amino acids are processed and the excess amino acids are degraded. The synthesis of proteins in the liver and muscle is sensitive to amino acid influx from the diet. Muscle protein synthesis and part of the effect on liver protein synthesis is mediated by insulin. The amount of insulin secreted (biologically effective dose) is a function of the influx of amino acids and/or glucose according to Marreiro Rocha et al.[17].

In this illustration the amount of amino acids reaching a particular organ could be regarded as the delivered dose. Every organ uses the amino acids for different purposes and metabolizes them differently. The effect of the amino acids in an organ such as the effect on insulin secretion or the amount of certain metabolites could be taken as the biologically effective dose (d_{BED}).

The amount of metabolites generated from the protein reaching the target organ or the net amount of "effect" on organ functions could also be considered as the d_{BED} in the nutrition example. Clearly, these d_{BED}s are not necessarily linearly related to the administered dose (the amount of dietary protein intake).

Linder[18] uses another measure for the biologically effective dose, called the *biological value*, which is the change in nitrogen excretion, relative to the nitrogen intake, when an individual subjected to a diet with no protein is switched to a diet with protein. This biological value is defined by Linder as follows:

$$\text{Biological value} = \frac{\text{Dietary } N - (\text{Urinary } N - \text{Urinary } N_0) \times (\text{Fecal } N_0)}{\text{Dietary } N} \tag{6.18}$$

where

N_0 = nitrogen content in the protein diet or in the urine

N = nitrogen content in the protein-free diet or in the urine or in the feces.

The metabolization of ingested protein seems to be affected by the presence of vitamin B_6 according to Linder. Thus, an individual consuming greater amounts of proteins has greater requirements for vitamin B_6 than those ingesting less proteins. Other factors affecting protein metabolization include diseases such as homocystinuria, phenylketonuria, food allergies, and protein malnutrition. All these diseases and the insufficiency of vitamin B_6 may be regarded as the susceptibility of an individual to protein ingestion. In other words, the "biological value" of protein defined by Linder is affected by this individual susceptibility.

The fate and metabolism of different substances are not necessarily similar. How the body absorbs, eliminates and metabolizes substances depends on the substance, the susceptibility, and the route of exposure. Thus, the biologically effective dose in a target tissue varies for different substances, different individuals, and different routes of exposure. In the nutrition example, the total protein reaching the blood would be different if the protein were injected into the blood stream as opposed to being ingested. It is also known that the metabolites formed and the compounds eliminated are different for different nutrients (Linder[18]).

Because there is a saturation level in the liver where excess amino acids are metabolized or eliminated, the nutrition example illustrates the case where the amount of protein reaching the organs is not linearly related to the dietary protein intake. Just as in the case of proteins, the intake levels of other substances (administered dose levels) are not necessarily linearly related to either the amount of substances reaching the organs (delivered doses) or the biological activity produced in that organ (biologically effective doses). The potential nonlinearity in the relationships between administered doses, delivered doses, and biologically effective doses makes the selection of a biologically based dose scale for dose-response modeling an important consideration in cancer risk assessment.

6.8 INCORPORATING d_{BED} AND INTERINDIVIDUAL VARIATION INTO DOSE-RESPONSE MODEL FITTING

The carcinogenic mechanism of a suspected substance is the principal factor in the selection of a particular dose-response model. After the model has been selected, the next concern is how to fit it to the cancer dose-response data from a particular experiment. Because the theoretical development of a cancer dose-response model assumes that the dose scale in the model is either equal to the biologically effective dose (d_{BED}) or proportional to the d_{BED}, the first step is the identification and characterization of the d_{BED}. The d_{BED} can depend on the administered dose, background dose, susceptibility, and the delivery process. It has already been noted that at least two of these components of d_{BED}, namely, the background dose and susceptibility, can vary among the individual members of the experimental population. Hence, the dose-response model fitting should incorporate the available information on the d_{BED} as well as the possible variability in the d_{BED} among the experimental population.

In experimental settings, the administered dose levels are fixed for the different groups of animals and for each animal within each group. In other words, the administered dose does not vary among animals of the same group. In experimental situations, the variability of the background dose and susceptibility is minimized by controlling the environment and by selecting animals of the same species, sex, and strain. Thus, the analysis of animal bioassay data does not require the use of distributions to describe the administered doses, but distributions are sometimes necessary to model the random nature of background doses and susceptibilities. Figure 6.14 shows how the interindividual variation in background dose and susceptibility combine to produce a distribution of biologically effective doses, and consequently, a distribution of probabilities of cancer is obtained for a given administered dose. Figure 6.15 sketches the procedure for estimating the probability of a carcinogenic response by time t for a given administered dose d. To illustrate, consider the case of a fixed administered dose level d, and suppose that the distributions of D_0 and S consist of

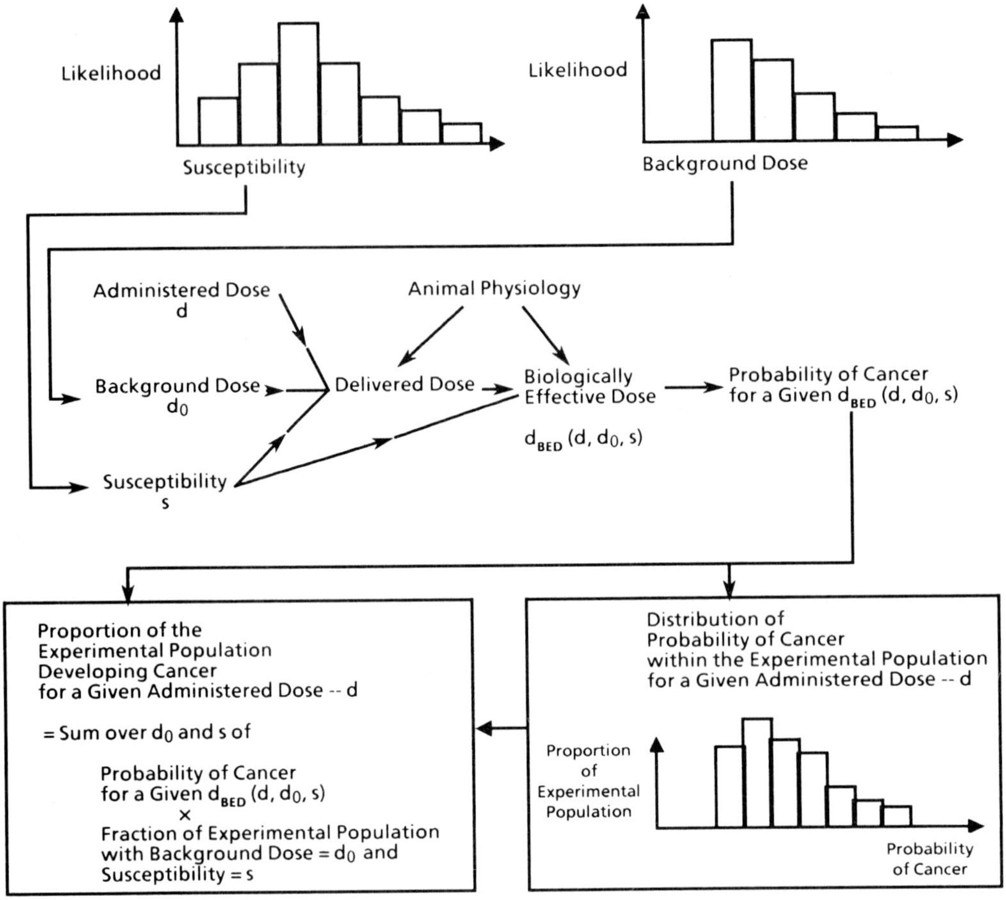

Figure 6.14 Incorporating d_{BED} and Interindividual Variation of Background Dose and Susceptibility in the Experimental Situation.

only two values each; namely,

$$D_0 = \begin{cases} d_{0,1} \\ d_{0,2} \end{cases} \quad \text{and} \quad S = \begin{cases} s_1 \\ s_2 \end{cases} \tag{6.19}$$

Corresponding to each of these four different values of D_0 and S, there are four distinguishable possibilities,

$$(d_{0,1}, s_1), (d_{0,1}, s_2), (d_{0,2}, s_1), (d_{0,2}, s_2).$$

Thus, corresponding to this situation, there are four probabilities of cancer; namely,

$$P[T \le t; d_{BED}(d, d_{0,i}, s_j)] \qquad i = 1, 2 \text{ and } j = 1, 2$$

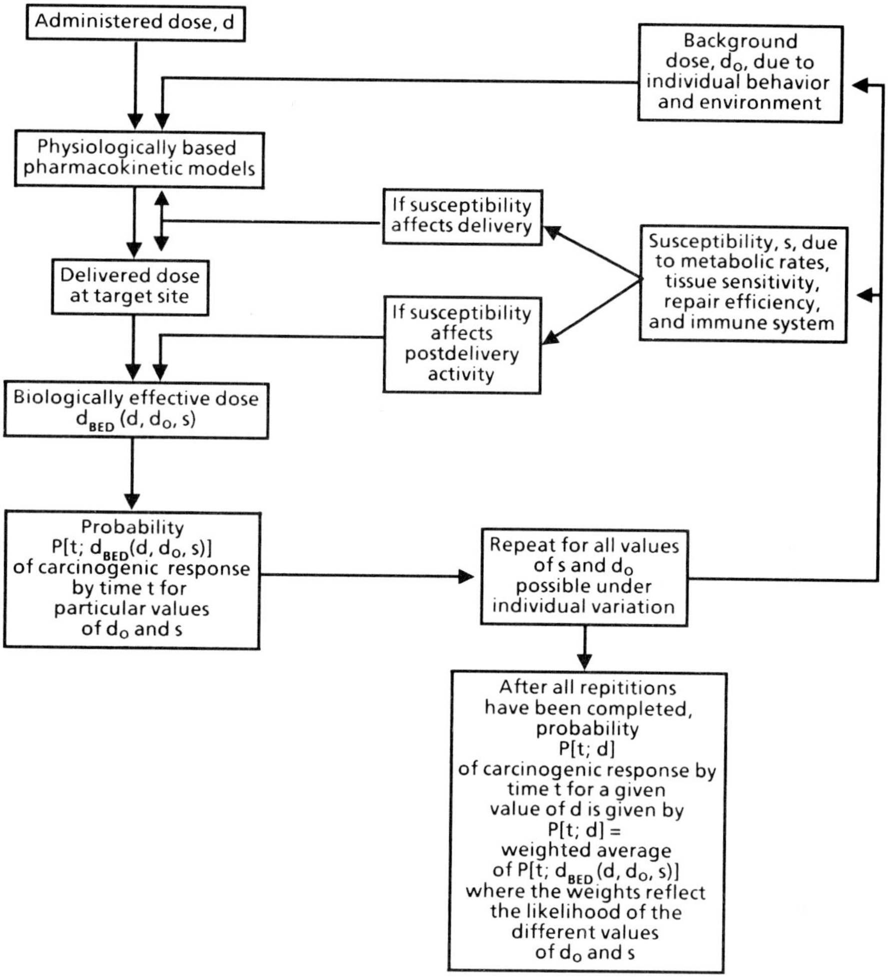

Figure 6.15 A Dose-Response Model Fitting Procedure Incorporating Pharmacokinetics, Delivered Dose, Biologically Effective Dose, Background Dose Variability and Interindividual Variation in Susceptibility into the Estimation of the Cancer Probability for a Given Administered Dose in a Chronic Bioassay.

where T is the time to response. That is, for each of the above four distinguishable pairs of background doses and susceptibility values ($D_0 = d_{0,i}, S = s_j$), there exists a corresponding probability of cancer. That is, $P[T \leq t; d_{BED}(d, d_{0,i}, s_j)]$ denotes the probability that an individual of a population will develop cancer by time t, when the administered dose is d, the background dose is $d_{0,i}$ and the susceptibility is s_j. Let $P(D_0 = d_{0,i})$ denote the probability that an individual of a given population has a background dose $d_{0,i}$ (or the fraction of the population having this background dose). Also, let $P(S = s_j)$ denote the probability of an individual of a given population having a susceptibility s_j (or the fraction of the population having susceptibility s_j). Thus, the probability of observing members of a population having a background dose $d_{0,i}$ and susceptibility s_j (or the fraction of the population having a background dose $d_{0,i}$ and susceptibility s_j) is given by

$$P(D_0 = d_{0,i} \text{ and } S = s_j) = P(D_0 = d_{0,i})\, P(S = s_j) \qquad i = 1, 2 \text{ and } j = 1, 2 \tag{6.20}$$

The equality in Equation (6.20) is a consequence of the assumed independence of the background dose and susceptibility. (A more general treatment without the assumption of independence is also possible). Thus, the contribution of the fraction of the population with background dose $d_{0,i}$ and susceptibility s_j to the probability that any individual from the given population, subject to administered dose d, develops cancer by time t is given by

$$\begin{aligned} &P(T \le t \text{ and } D_0 = d_{0,i} \text{ and } S = s_j; d) \\ &\qquad = P[T \le t; d_{BED}(d, d_{0,i}, s_j)]\, P(D_0 = d_{0,i})\, P(S = s_j) \end{aligned} \tag{6.21}$$

Thus, the probability of cancer for a given administered dose is computed by estimating the probability of a carcinogenic response by time t for a given $d_{BED}(d, d_0, s)$ and every possible value of D_0 and S, and by taking the weighted average of these probabilities, where the weights $P(D_0 = d_{0,i})$ and $P(S = s_j)$ reflect the likelihood distributions of D_0 and S. That is, for the given example,

$$P(T \le t; d) = \sum_{j=1}^{2} \sum_{i=1}^{2} P[T \le t; d_{BED}(d, d_{0,i}, s_j)]\, P(D_0 = d_{0,i})\, P(S = s_j) \tag{6.22}$$

In general, for discrete distributions of D_0 and S,

$$P(T \le t; d) = \sum_{s} \sum_{d_0} P[T \le t; d_{BED}(d, d_0, s)]\, P(D_0 = d_0)\, P(S = s) \tag{6.23}$$

and for continuous distributions of D_0 and S,

$$P(T \le t; d) = \int_s \int_{d_0} P[T \le t; d_{BED}(d, d_0, s)]\, f(d_0) f(s)\, dd_0\, ds \tag{6.24}$$

where $f(d_0)$ and $f(s)$ are the probability density functions of the background dose and the susceptibility, respectively. The resulting probability of $P(T \le t; d)$ is the probability used to determine how good the dose-response model fits the chronic bioassay cancer frequency.

In the development of the expression for $P(T \le t; d)$, there are several considerations which merit additional discussion. Figure 6.16 provides a flowchart of the interaction of the multiple factors that determine the probability of cancer for a given d_{BED} in the experimental situation for animals. The figure shows that the probability for a given d_{BED} depends directly on the mathematical dose-response model utilized, the chronic bioassay cancer dose-response data, and the d_{BED}. Given the chronic bioassay cancer dose-response data, the only decisions a risk assessor can make refer to the selection of a plausible dose-response model and to the determination of a relevant dose scale. The dose-response model should

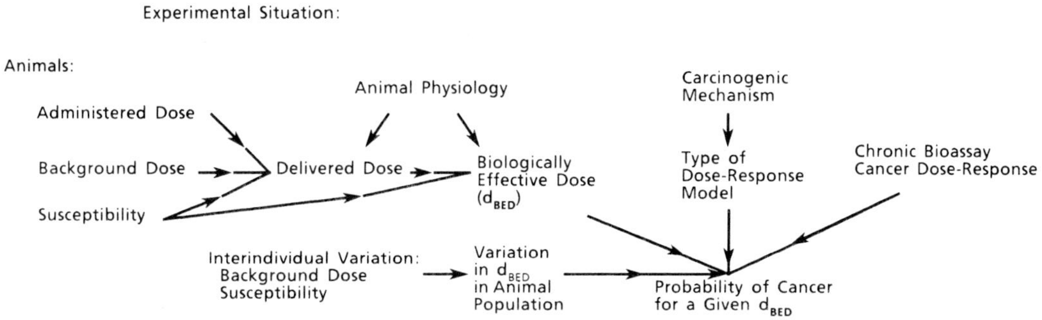

Figure 6.16 Schematic Representation of the Interaction of Administered Dose, Background Dose, Susceptibility, Carcinogenic Mechanism and Chronic Bioassay Data in the Determination of the Probability of Tumor Formation within the Bioassay Situation.

be selected on the basis of the carcinogenic mechanism induced by the substance under investigation. In other words, the mathematical dose-response models have been developed to emulate the carcinogenic mechanisms of the substances studied. Therefore, it is important for the risk assessor to be aware of the biological assumptions of the model selected and to fix or estimate the parameters that correspond to the carcinogenic mechanism to be modeled. The biological assumptions and carcinogenic mechanisms represented by the dose-response models were discussed extensively in Chapter 2. For example, in the theory of the two-stage model (see Chapter 2), normal stem cells go through a two-stage process to become malignant cells. The first stage transforms normal stem cells into premalignant cells; the second stage affects premalignant cells and produces malignant cells (cancerous cells). There are substances that affect the first stage of the carcinogenic process by either increasing the number of stem cell divisions or the rate of transformation per division or both and, thereby, increasing the rate of formation of premalignant cells. There are also substances that affect the second stage of the carcinogenic process. Analogously, these substances increase the rate of formation of malignant cells from premalignant cells by either increasing the number of premalignant cell divisions or the rate of transformation per division or both. Thus, for the two-stage model the parameters to be estimated or fixed should depend on how the substance under study impacts the carcinogenic process.

Figure 6.16 also shows that the biologically effective dose has a direct impact on the estimation of the probability of cancer. The d_{BED} defined for an experimental situation should reflect the physiology and carcinogenic mechanisms of the animal species under experimentation. The previous sections have discussed how the administered dose, background dose, and susceptibility combine to define a d_{BED}. Methods for incorporating the variability in the animal background dose and the animal susceptibility into the determination of the biological effective dose have also been discussed. The physiological mechanisms by which administered dose, background dose and susceptibility combine to determine a d_{BED} should be those pertaining to the experimental situation (animal species and strain, route of exposure, etc.) whenever possible. In some instances where there is less information and greater uncertainty about the d_{BED}, extrapolating physiological information from one species to another or one situation to another, rather than using a less biologically relevant dose, may result in a better risk assessment.

The experimental situation normally involves chronic bioassay cancer dose-response data reported for animals exposed to different fixed levels of administered doses. The dose-response model should be the model that best describes the carcinogenic mechanism induced by the substance under study. The parameters of the dose-response model selected should be those that best predict the chronic bioassay cancer dose-response data at the administered dose levels under consideration.

If the experimental animals have either constant or variable background doses and susceptibilities, then these factors should be combined with the administered dose as in Figure 6.15 to reflect the biologically effective dose and give a predicted value for $P(T \leq t; d)$ to be used in the determination of the best prediction.

6.9 EXTRAPOLATING FROM THE EXPERIMENTAL SITUATION TO THE INFERENCE SITUATION

Cancer risk assessment usually starts with the estimation of carcinogenic responses of animals subject to the application of an administered substance in a controlled environment. The mathematical dose-response model used to predict the number of responses should be the model that best emulates the carcinogenic mechanism of the substance being applied to the animals under experimentation. By use of the dose-response model, the best available biologically based dose scale, and the experimental dose-response data, the model parameters that provide the best fit to the results of the experiment are estimated. The resulting estimated model can be applied to predict the probability of cancer for a given biologically effective dose in the species, strain, route of exposure, etc. utilized in the study. This is called the experimental situation and is illustrated in Figure 6.16.

In order to use the dose-response model fit for the experimental situation to estimate the probability of cancer for a different species, strain, route of exposure, etc., the fitted parameters should be adjusted to reflect interspecies differences in life span (time scale factor) and responsiveness to biologically effective doses (dose scale factor). Figure 6.17 illustrates how the parameters from the fitted dose-response model for the experimental situation are adjusted when the dose-response model is used in the inference situation.

For example, if the parameters of a model were estimated using mice in the experimental situation, time and dose scale factors should be used to adjust the estimated parameters when the model is being used in the assessment of cancer risk for humans (the inference situation). A mouse's average lifetime is approximately 2 years; whereas, a human's average lifetime is approximately 70 years. That is, humans live 35 times longer than mice, and the time-dependent parameters of the dose-response model should be adjusted to reflect this fact. This implies that a time of t_h for humans is assumed to be equivalent (with respect to the probability of a carcinogenic response) to a time $t_m = (2/70)t_h$ for

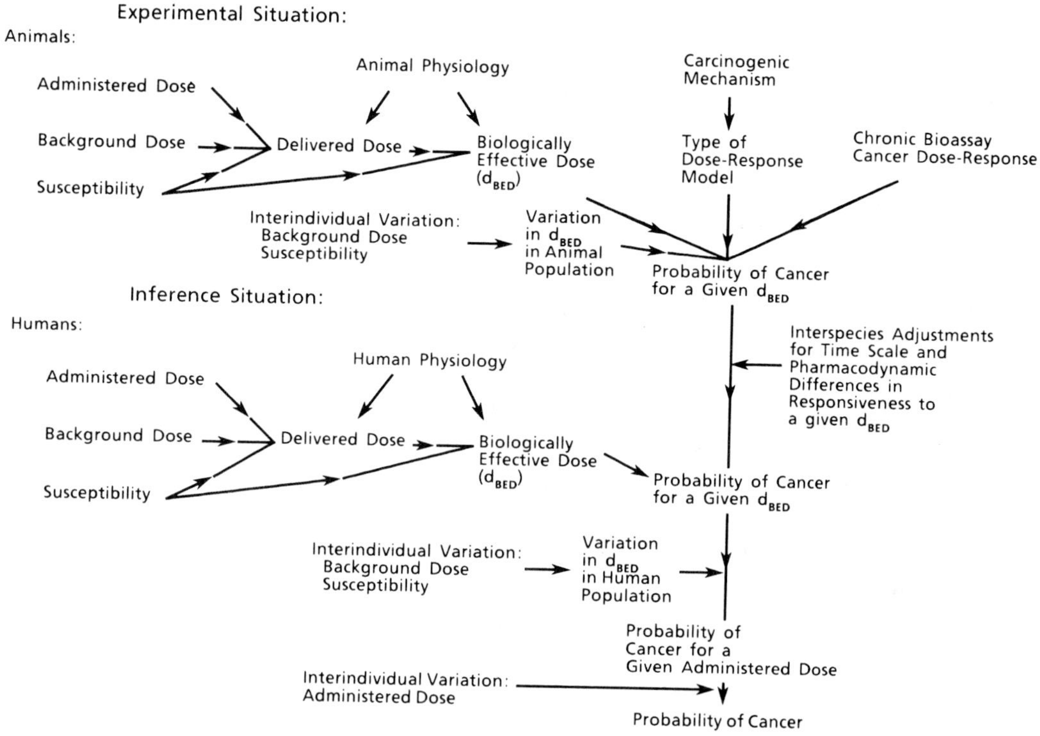

Figure 6.17 A Generalized Framework and Flowchart for Incorporating Physiological Processes, Carcinogenic Mechanisms, Individual Variation, and Species Adjustments for Differences in Life Span and Pharmacodynamic Sensitivity in Cancer Dose-Response Modeling and Extrapolation.

mice (assuming that the time units used in fitting the model were years and the time units used in the inference situation were also years). The ratio (2/70) is often called the *time scale factor*. Mathematically, the time scale factor is the value such that $P(T \leq t; d_{BED})$ in humans is equal to $P(T \leq t \times \text{time scale factor}; d_{BED})$ in mice, where the dose d_{BED} is regarded to be the same for both species.

Using the same example as before, the dose scale factor is the value such that humans respond to a biologically effective dose in the same way as the mice respond to a biologically effective dose of $d_{BED} \times$ *dose scale factor*. Thus, $P(T \leq t; d_{BED})$ in humans is equal to $P(T \leq t; d_{BED} \times \text{dose scale factor})$ in mice, where the life span and time units are assumed to be the same for both species. In rough terminology, humans are *dose scale factor* times "more" sensitive (or "more" responsive) to a given biologically effective dose than mice. The dose scale factor often reflects the pharmacodynamic differences in species and situations. In general, both time and dose scale factors are required to go from the experimental situation to the inference situation, and in this case $P(T \leq t; d_{BED})$ in humans is equal to $P(T \leq t \times \text{time scale factor}; d_{BED} \times \text{dose scale factor})$ in mice.

Both time and dose scale factors can be greater than, equal to, or less than one. A dose scale factor greater than one indicates that humans are more sensitive than mice to a given d_{BED}; whereas, a dose scale less than one indicates that humans are less sensitive than mice to a given d_{BED}. The time scale factor has a slightly more complicated interpretation in that it reflects not only species differences but also possibly different units (weeks, months, years, etc.). A time scale factor smaller than one in the previous example implies that the average lifetime of humans, measured in the time units of the inference situation, is greater than the average lifetime of mice, measured in the time units used to fit the dose-response model. In the previous example, the mice data were fit using years as time units. The inference situation used years also, and the time scale factor was

$$\frac{\text{life span of mice in years}}{\text{life span of humans in years}} = \frac{2}{70} \tag{6.25}$$

However, if the mice data were fit using weeks as time units and the inference situation used years, then the time scale factor would have been

$$\frac{\text{life span of mice in weeks}}{\text{life span of humans in years}} = \frac{104}{70} \tag{6.26}$$

Caution should be exercised when extrapolating from the experimental situation to the inference situation. If the parameters of the dose-response model are not adjusted to reflect time differences and differences in dose responsiveness, then it implies that the species in the experimental situation and the inference situation are being assumed to be physiologically and biologically identical.

6.10 THE INFERENCE SITUATION

The inference situation should reflect the exposure levels, background doses, susceptibilities, and biological and physiological processes for the target population, and not for the species in the experimental situation. For example, individuals in the experimental situation will be subject to different administered dose levels than those individuals in the inference situation.

The flowchart in Figure 6.17 indicates that the dose-response model estimated for the experimental situation is adjusted for time and dose responsiveness factors in order to extrapolate to an inference situation. The inference situation also includes its own administered dose, background doses, susceptibilities, and physiological characteristics which determine the delivered dose and the biologically effective dose.

The population in the inference situation has its own distributions of background doses and susceptibilities, and these distributions are not necessarily equal to the distributions that described the background doses and susceptibilities in the experimental situation. The way in which administered dose, background dose and susceptibility combine to produce a delivered dose and a biologically effective dose can be completely different for the experimental and inference situations.

The biologically effective dose in the inference situation should measure the same phenomenon or characteristic as in the experimental situation, even though the functional relationships may be completely different. For example, if in the experimental situation the d_{BED} is the number of a particular adduct formed and not repaired, then in the inference situation the d_{BED} should be the number of that same adduct that are formed and not repaired.

When facing the problem of specifying the dose scales for use in the experimental situation and the inference situation, the risk assessor may contemplate several alternative courses of action. A discussion of four such alternatives follows.

1. Use the d_{BED} for both situations. If the biologically effective dose is known for both the experimental and inference situations, then the dose scale for dose-response modeling should be the d_{BED}. In this ideal case, the risk assessor has no difficult decision to make because all of the uncertainty regarding physiological and biological extrapolation from one species to another is eliminated if the model is fit using the d_{BED} for the experimental situation and extrapolations are made using the d_{BED} for the inference situation. There may be instances, however, where the transformation from the administered dose to the biologically effective dose scale is unknown or too uncertain in either the experimental situation or the inference situation or both. In such instances, alternatives (2), (3), and (4) below may be considered.
2. Use the most biologically based dose (MBBD) scale known for *both* situations. For example, if the administered dose, d, the delivered dose, d_{DD}, and the biologically effective dose, d_{BED}, are known in the experimental situation but only d and d_{DD} are known in the inference situation, then the MBBD known for *both* situations is d_{DD}. Using d_{DD} as the dose scale for both the experimental and inference situations is workable; however, the additional information on the d_{BED} in the experimental situation is not used.
3. Use the most biologically based dose (MBBD) scale known for *either* situation. For example, if the administered dose, d, the delivered dose, d_{DD}, and the biologically effective dose, d_{BED}, are known in the experimental situation but only d and d_{DD} are known in the inference situation, then the MBBD known for *either* situation is d_{BED} in the experimental situation and the dose scale used for dose-response modeling and inference would be the d_{BED}. However, the MBBD is not known for the other situation and must be estimated. In this example, the d_{BED} in the inference situation would have to be estimated. A reasonable candidate for that estimate is to use the d_{DD} in the inference situation and assume that the functional relationship between d_{DD} and d_{BED} in the inference situations is the same functional relationship as held in the experimental situation. The appropriateness of this alternative compared to the second alternative above depends on the substance and the available information.

4. Use a different dose scale in the inference situation than in the experimental situation. This alternative is *not* workable. For example, if the administered dose, d, the delivered dose, d_{DD}, and the biologically effective dose, d_{BED}, are known in the experimental situation but only d and d_{DD} are known in the inference situation, then the dose-response model fit on the d_{BED} scale could not be used to make inferences on the d_{DD} scale. This approach is clearly incorrect in that it violates the requirement that the dose scale in the inference situation must measure the same phenomenon or characteristic that is being measured in the dose scale used for model fitting.

It is apparent that the first alternative is the best, and that either the second or third approach is the most desirable otherwise. If a decision has to be made as to whether the second or third approach should be used, then a decision analysis might be preferable to using either single approach. Decision analysis for cancer risk assessment is discussed in Chapter 7.

6.11 INDIVIDUAL AND POPULATION INFERENCES

After fitting a dose-response model to chronic animal bioassay data and adjusting the parameters by the dose scale and time scale factors, population and individual estimations for the inference situation can be made. The resulting probability of cancer in the inference situation can be described in terms of a probability distribution if the background dose or the susceptibility, or both, are described by a probability distribution.

Figure 6.17 shows how the variability in background dose and susceptibility combine to generate a probability distribution of cancer in the inference situation. If the probability of cancer for a specific individual is desired, then that individual's administered dose (exposure level), background dose, and susceptibility should be used. On the other hand, if the probability of cancer of any individual of the population exposed to an administered dose d in the inference situation is desired, the weighted sum of the probability of cancer for a given d_{BED} should be computed. The weights used in computing this sum should reflect the likelihood of the particular values of background dose and susceptibility. This weighted sum of probabilities would also be equal to the fraction of the population that would be expected to develop cancer from an administered dose d.

Suppose that a dose-response model has been estimated for the experimental situation and the probability of cancer by time t for a given individual with administered dose d, background dose d_0 and susceptibility s is desired. The probability of cancer under these conditions is found by evaluating the fitted dose-response model to obtain

$$P[T \leq t; d_{BED}(d, d_0, s)]$$

If the probability of cancer for any individual of the inference population exposed to an administered dose d is desired, the model fit to the experimental situation should be evaluated (after adjustment for time and dose responsiveness differences have been made) for all the possible combinations of background dose d_0 and susceptibility s in the inference situation. Thus, the probability of cancer for an individual exposed to an administered dose d in the inference population is given by

$$P(T \leq t; d) = \sum_{s} \sum_{d_0} P[T \leq t; d_{BED}(d, d_0, s)] \; P(D_0 = d_0) \; P(S = s) \qquad (6.27)$$

where appropriate adjustments have been made for time and dose scale factors as discussed in Section 6.9. A distribution on the probability of cancer gives the risk assessment manager complete information to determine such quantities as the proportion of individuals in a given population that are at risks greater than a specified level. This capability should prove useful in establishing regulatory standards with respect to suspected carcinogenic substances.

The concept of distributions of background dose and susceptibility may be extended to accommodate population variation in exposure to an administered dose. For example, there may be an interest in determining the probability of cancer for a population exposed to a substance disseminated over some area in different concentrations, and the exposure level of the individuals is dependent upon residence location. In such a case, $P(T \leq t; d)$ should be computed for every possible value of d as in Equation (6.27) and the distributions of D_0 and S that correspond to the inference population. The probability of cancer for any individual in the inference population should then be computed as the weighted average of $P(T \leq t; d)$, where the weights reflect the likelihood of the particular values of d (or the proportion of the inference population exposed to an administered dose level of d). Thus, for any individual in the inference situation, the probability of cancer by time t is given by

$$P(T \leq t) = \sum_{d} P(T \leq t; d) \; P(D = d) \qquad (6.28)$$

or, combining with the previous expression, (Equation (6.27))

$$P(T \leq t) = \sum_{d} \sum_{s} \sum_{d_0} P[T \leq t; d_{BED}(d, d_0, s)] \; P(D_0 = d_0) \; P(S = s) \; P(D = d) \qquad (6.29)$$

where T is the time to cancer and D is the random variable denoting the exposure level of the inference population. Figure 6.17 and 6.18 illustrates how the interindividual variation in exposure levels (administered dose) combines with the probability of cancer for a given administered dose to produce the probability of cancer for an individual randomly selected from the population of interest. Thus, Figure 6.18 shows the extension to the consideration of the administered dose (exposure level) as a random variable.

PROBLEMS

1. A model has been fit to an experimental situation using a species whose average life span is two years. Inferences are needed for humans with an average life span of 70 years and 13.5 times

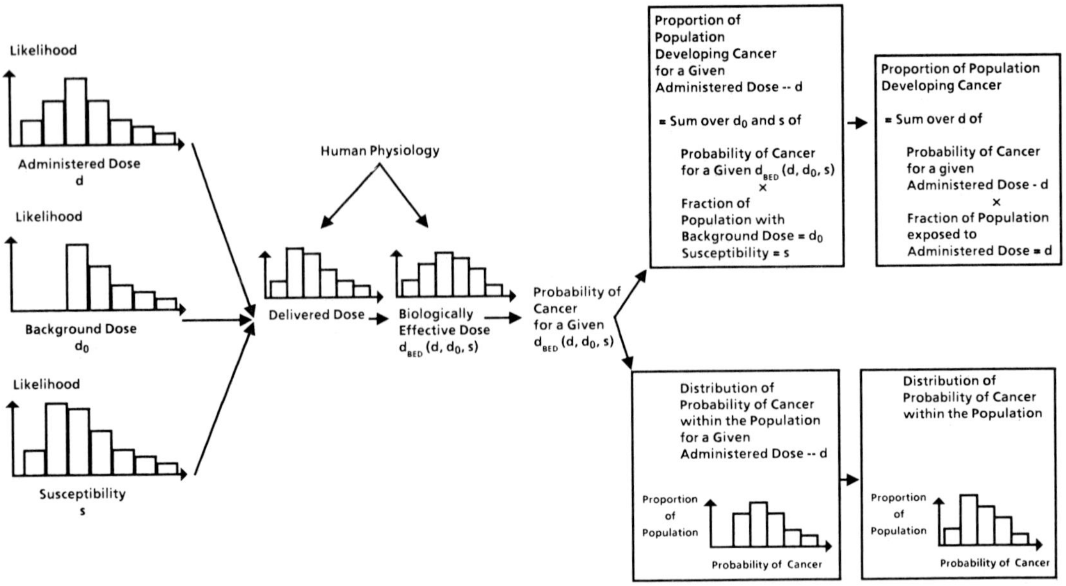

Figure 6.18 Incorporating Biologically Effective Dose and Interindividual Variation in the Inference Situation to Generate Useful Information for Decision Making.

greater sensitivity to the carcinogen under study than that of the species in the experimental situation. Based on this information, make the necessary adjustments to the parameters of the following fitted models. Let q_i represent the values of the fitted model, and define the $q_i(h)$s for the human inference situation in terms of the dose scale, time scale and q_is. In the equations, d and t represent dose and time for the experimental situation, respectively. Find the corresponding values of the parameters $q_i(h)$s in terms of the q_is for the case where d_h and t_h refer to the human inference situation.

(a) The multistage model,

$$P(d) = 1 - \exp[-(q_0 + q_1 d + q_2 d^2 + q_3 d^3)]$$

Answer: $q_i(h) = (13.5)^i q_i$, and $P(d_h) = 1 - \exp\left[-(q_0(h) + q_1(h)d_h + q_2(h)d_h^2 + q_3(h)d_h^3)\right]$

(b) The logit model,

$$P(d) = \frac{1}{1 + \exp[-(q_0 + q_1 \log_e d)]}.$$

Answer: $q_0(h) = q_0 + q_1 \log_e 13.5$; $q_1(h) = q_1$

(c) If the time units used for the inference situation are years and the time units used in fitting the experimental data were months (assume 12 months per year), find the values of the $q_i(h)$s in terms of the q_is for the Weibull-Weibull model (a time-to-response model generalization of the Weibull model),

$$P(t; d) = 1 - \exp[-(q_0 + q_1 d^{q_2})(t - q_4)^{q_3}]$$

Answer: $q_0(h) = q_0 \left(\frac{24}{70}\right)^{q_3}$; $q_1(h) = q_1 \left(\frac{24}{70}\right)^{q_3} (13.5)^{q_2}$; $q_2(h) = q_2$; $q_3(h) = q_3$; $q_4(h) = \left(\frac{70}{24}\right) q_4$

(d) Repeat Part (c) for the case where the time units used in fitting the data were weeks (assume 52 weeks per year) instead of months.
Answer: $q_0(h) = q_0 \left(\frac{104}{70}\right)^{q_3}$; $q_1(h) = q_1 \left(\frac{104}{70}\right)^{q_3} (13.5)^{q_2}$; $q_2(h) = q_2$; $q_3(h) = q_3$; $q_4(h) = \left(\frac{70}{104}\right) q_4$

2. Suppose that, in a given situation, the d_{BED} is proportional to the administered dose; i.e.,

$$d_{BED} = \beta_1 d,$$

although the specific value of $\beta_1 > 0$ may be unknown. In such a situation, the fitted dose-response model using the d_{BED} scale provides exactly the same fit to the experimental data as the fitted dose-response model using the administered dose scale. Furthermore, low-dose linear extrapolations using either the d_{BED} scale or the administered dose scale will yield equivalent results. However, the low-dose linear extrapolations using the d_{BED} scale will not necessarily be equivalent to low-dose linear extrapolations using the administered dose scale if the d_{BED} is a nonlinear function of the administered dose.
In the problems that follow, assume that the dose-response model family is

$$P(\text{cancer}; d_{BED}, \mathbf{q}) = 1 - \exp[-(q_0 + q_1 d_{BED} + q_2 d_{BED}^2)]$$

Also, assume that, when the d_{BED} is equal to the administered dose d and the qs are restricted to be nonnegative, the maximum likelihood estimates of (q_0, q_1, q_2) are $(\hat{q}_0, \hat{q}_1, \hat{q}_2)$.
Note that analogous results would hold if the d_{BED} were linearly related to d

$$d_{BED} = \beta_0 + \beta_1 d \text{ and } \beta_0 \geq 0,\ \beta_1 \geq 0$$

provided that the dose-response model did not restrict q_0 to be zero (that is, the dose-response model did not exclude q_0) and the nonnegativity restrictions were not prohibitive.

(a) Let $\hat{\mathbf{q}} = \{\hat{q}_0, \hat{q}_1, \hat{q}_2\}$ denote the nonnegative maximum likelihood estimates corresponding to the experimental administered dose d. Show that, if $d_{BED} = \beta_1 d$ with $\beta_1 > 0$, then there exist nonnegative maximum likelihood estimates $\mathbf{q}^* = \{q_0^*, q_1^*, q_2^*\}$ which satisfy

$$P(\text{cancer}; d, \hat{\mathbf{q}}) = P(\text{cancer}; d_{BED}, \mathbf{q}^*)$$

for every experimental dose d and corresponding biologically effective dose $d_{BED} = \beta_1 d$. This last characteristic implies $P(\text{cancer}; d, \hat{\mathbf{q}})$ and $P(\text{cancer}; d_{BED}, \mathbf{q}^*)$ are equivalent "fits" to the experimental data.
Answer: $q_i^* = \hat{q}_i / \beta_1^i$

(b) Repeat Part (a) for the case where $d_{BED} = \beta_0 + \beta_1 d$.
Answer: $q_0^* = \hat{q}_0 - \beta_0[(\hat{q}_1/\beta_1) - 2\beta_0\hat{q}_2/\beta_1^2] - \beta_0^2(\hat{q}_2/\beta_1^2)$; $q_1^* = (\hat{q}_1/\beta_1) - 2\beta_0\hat{q}_2/\beta_1^2$; $q_2^* = \hat{q}_2/\beta_1^2$

(c) Consider again the case in Part (a) where $P(\text{cancer}; d_{BED}, \mathbf{q}^*) = P(\text{cancer}; d, \hat{\mathbf{q}})$, and $d_{BED} = \beta_1 d$. Show that the low-dose linear extrapolation from $d_{BED} = \beta_1$ using $P(\text{cancer}; d_{BED}, \mathbf{q}^*)$ and from $d = 1$ using $P(\text{cancer}; d, \hat{\mathbf{q}})$ to $P(\text{cancer}; 0, \mathbf{q}^*)$ and $P(\text{cancer}; 0, \hat{\mathbf{q}})$, respectively, give the same result; that is, show that

$$P(\text{cancer}; \beta_1, \mathbf{q}^*) - P(\text{cancer}; 0, \mathbf{q}^*)w$$
$$= P(\text{cancer}; 1, \hat{\mathbf{q}}) - P(\text{cancer}; 0, \hat{\mathbf{q}})$$

Also, show that for $d_{BED} = 1$ and $d = 1$, the same results are not necessarily obtained by a linear extrapolation; that is, show that

$$P(\text{cancer}; 1, \mathbf{q}^*) - P(\text{cancer}; 0, \mathbf{q}^*)$$
$$\neq P(\text{cancer}; 1, \hat{\mathbf{q}}) - P(\text{cancer}; 0, \hat{\mathbf{q}})$$

where β_1 is positive and unequal to unity.

3. A population is at risk from a substance at environmental levels of 10 ppm. An animal experiment with the same substance had been previously analyzed using a time-to-response model. The experimental data have been fit using the d_{BED} for the species under study. The delivery process of the chemical to the target organs in humans has been widely accepted. The relationship between the biologically effective dose and delivered dose is also known to be affected by a susceptibility frontier. The population also has a very diverse ethnic origin and the susceptibility to the substances in question is believed to vary among ethnic groups. Due to different lifestyles, the exposure to a background substance that contributes to the carcinogenic effects of the primary substance is considered a random variable. The following model has already been adjusted for life span (70 years for the individuals in the inference situation) and dose responsiveness differences between the experimental and inference situations.

$$P[T \leq t; d_{BED}(d, d_0, s)] = 1 - \exp[-(0.00001 + 0.01 d_{BED})t^2]$$

where

$$d_{BED} = \begin{cases} 0.3 d_{DD} \exp[-(7/3)(s - d_{DD})/s] & \text{if } d_{DD} \leq s \\ 0.3s + (d_{DD} - s) & \text{if } d_{DD} > s \end{cases}$$

$$d_{DD} = 0.025 \exp[-200(d + d_0)^{-1.5}]$$

$$P(D_0 = 1 \text{ ppm}) = 0.10 \qquad P(S = 0.0001) = 0.50$$
$$P(D_0 = 2 \text{ ppm}) = 0.30 \qquad P(S = 0.0003) = 0.35$$
$$P(D_0 = 3 \text{ ppm}) = 0.60 \qquad P(S = 0.0005) = 0.15$$

Using the information given above:

(a) Compute the lifetime probability of cancer for an individual whose background exposure is 2 ppm and susceptibility level is 0.0003. *Answer:* $P[T \leq 70;\ d_{BED}(d = 10 \text{ ppm}, D_0 = = 2 \text{ ppm}, S = 0.0003)] = 0.049162$.

(b) By observation, determine the combinations of constant values for D_0 and S that will make the lifetime probability of cancer for individuals in the population inference a maximum and a minimum.
Answer: $P[T \leq 70;\ d_{BED}(d = 10\text{ ppm}, D_0 = 3\text{ ppm}, S = 0.0001)] = 0.060822$; $P[T \leq 70;\ d_{BED}(d = 10\text{ ppm}, D_0 = 1\text{ ppm}, S = 0.0005)] = 0.048048$.

(c) Compute the lifetime probability of cancer for an individual whose background exposure is 2 *ppm*. (*Hint*: First, for each of the three possible values of susceptibility, compute the conditional probability of cancer for an individual whose background exposure is 2 *ppm* and whose susceptibility is that given value. Then compute the weighted sum of these probabilities. The weight for a particular probability corresponding to a particular susceptibility is the proportion of the population with that susceptibility. The lifetime probability for a randomly selected individual whose background exposure is 2 *ppm* and whose environmental exposure level is 10 ppm is equal to this weighted sum of probabilities.)
Answer: $P[T \leq 70; d = 10ppm, D_0 = 2ppm] = 0.05150$.

(d) Compute the lifetime probability of cancer for an individual whose susceptibility level is 0.0003. (*Hint*: First, for each of the three possible background dose values, compute the conditional probability of cancer for an individual whose susceptibility level is 0.0003 and at an administered dose $d = 10\ ppm$. Then compute the weighted sum of these probabilities. The weight for a particular probability corresponding to a particular background dose is the proportion of the population exposed to that background dose.)
Answer: $P[T \leq 70; d = 10\text{ ppm}, S = 0.0003] = 0.052176$.

(e) Compute the lifetime probability of cancer for a randomly selected individual of the population. (*Hint*: Compute the probability of cancer for each combination of susceptibility levels and background doses. Then compute the weighted sum of these probabilities. The weight for a particular probability is the product of the proportion of the population exposed to the corresponding background dose times the proportion of the population with the corresponding susceptibility.)
Answer: $P[T \leq 70; d = 10\text{ppm}] = 0.05451$.

4. For each of the following situational descriptions, write in the space provided the dose-response modeling component (administered dose, background dose, susceptibility, delivered dose, or biologically effective dose) that best matches the description given.

(a) ______________________ Experimental animals are exposed to a substance whose presence was the result of an uncontrolled release. The substance may affect the carcinogenic responses of the animals in the experiment.

(b) ______________________ The amount of a given substance that reaches a particular organ.

(c) ______________________ The net amount of carcinogenic activity caused by all substances reaching a given organ.

(d) ______________________ The amount of dose required to overwhelm the defensive mechanisms suppressing cancer formation.

(e) ______________________ The amount of a substance under study to which individuals are directly exposed.

5. An animal experiment was analyzed using the two-stage growth model. The data were fit on the basis of the d_{BED}s corresponding to three different assumptions. The closer the dose scale was to the true biologically effective dose, the better the fit. The assumptions about the potential d_{BED} scales were as follows:

d_{BED} = administered dose plus background dose, $(d + d_0)$,

d_{BED} = delivered dose, d_{DD}, a function of the sum of the administered dose plus the background dose, and

d_{BED} = actual biologically effective dose.

The parameterization of the two-stage model used was as follows:

$$P[T \le t; d_{BED}(d, d_0, s)] = 1 - \exp\{-\int_0^{t-\tau} \lambda_2(u, d_{BED}) \int_0^u \lambda_1(v, d_{BED}) N_0(v, d_{BED}) \times \exp[\int_v^u (\beta(w, d_{BED}) - \delta(w, d_{BED}))\, dw]\, dv\, du\},$$

where:

τ =	latency period	$= 0$
$\lambda_2(t, d_{BED})$ =	rate per intermediate cell per unit time that intermediate cells are transformed at time t into malignant cells	$= 1$
$\lambda_1(t, d_{BED})$ =	rate per normal cell per unit time that normal cells are transformed at time t into intermediate cells	$= \alpha_0 + \alpha_1 d_{BED}$
$N_0(t, d_{BED})$ =	number of normal stem cells at time t	$= 1$
$\beta(t, d_{BED})$ =	birth rate or replication rate of intermediate cells at time t	$= 0.00005$
$\delta(t, d_{BED})$ =	death rate (including terminal differentiation rate) of intermediate cells at time t	$= 0$

When the d_{BED} was assumed to be proportional to the administered dose plus the background dose,

$$\alpha_0 = 5.44682 \times 10^{-10}, \alpha_1 = 4.33005 \times 10^{-4}$$

When the d_{BED} was assumed to be proportional to the delivered dose,

$$\alpha_0 = 1.20698 \times 10^{-4}, \alpha_1 = 1.941637$$

When the d_{BED} was assumed to be the actual biologically effective dose,

$$\alpha_0 = 1.32542 \times 10^{-4}, \alpha_1 = 2.07346$$

The delivered dose is given by

$$d_{DD} = 0.025 \exp[-200(d + d_0)^{-1.5}]$$

The biologically effective dose is given by

$$d_{BED} = \begin{cases} 0.3 d_{DD} \exp[-(7/3)(s - d_{DD})/s] & \text{if } d_{DD} \le s \\ 0.3s + (d_{DD} - s) & \text{if } d_{DD} > s \end{cases}$$

The background dose $d_0 = 0$, and the susceptibility frontier $s = 0.001$ for all members of the inference situation population, and $d_0 = 0$ and $s = 0.001$ in the problems below. The parameters have been adjusted for life span and dose responsiveness differences between the population in the inference situation and the population in the experimental situation. However, a further adjustment has to be made to account for the limits of integration.

(a) Show that, when all the parameters are constant over time, the two-stage model given above simplifies to

$$P[T \leq t; d_{BED}(d, d_0, s)] = 1 - e^{-\left[\frac{\lambda_1 \lambda_2 N_0}{(\beta-\delta)^2}\right]\left[e^{(\beta-\delta)(t-\tau)} - (t-\tau)(\beta-\delta) - 1\right]}$$

where λ_1, λ_2, N_0, β and δ can be a function of the d_{BED}, but not a function of time.

(b) Assume that all the parameters have been adjusted for differences in dose-responsiveness in the inference situation and the experimental situation. Show that the simplified two-stage model obtained in Part (a) has to be adjusted to account for life span differences in the limits of the integration as follows,

$$P[T \leq t; d_{BED}(d, d_0, s)] = 1 - e^{-\left[\frac{\lambda_1 \lambda_2 N_0}{(\beta-\delta)^2}\left[e^{(\beta-\delta)(t\mathcal{T}-\tau)} - (t\mathcal{T}-\tau)(\beta-\delta) - 1\right]\right]}$$

where $\mathcal{T}$ is the time scale factor.

(c) Compute the lifetime risk of cancer using the simplified model of Part (b), for $\mathcal{T} = 24/70$, administered dose of 10 *ppm*, the three dose scales considered for d_{BED}, background dose $d_0 = 0$, and the susceptibility frontier $s = 0.001$. Compute the ratios of the probability obtained using the administered dose to the probability obtained using the delivered dose as well as the probability obtained using the actual biologically effective dose. Explain the differences encountered in the probabilities computed. (*Hint*: Plot the d_{DD} versus the administered dose, the d_{BED} versus the administered dose, and d_{BED} versus d_{DD}.)
Answer: $P[T \leq 70; d_{BED} = d] = 0.7128$; $P[T \leq 70; d_{BED} = d_{DD}] = 0.0581$; $P[T \leq 70; d_{BED}] = 0.0383$.

(d) Compute the lifetime risk of cancer using the simplified model of Part (b), for $\mathcal{T} = 24/70$, administered dose of 8 *ppm*, the three dose scales considered for d_{BED}, background dose $d_0 = 0$, and the susceptibility frontier $s = 0.001$. Compute the ratios of probabilities obtained using the delivered dose to the probabilities computed using the biologically effective dose. Compare the results with those found in Part (c), and explain the differences that occurred when the d_{DD} and d_{BED} scales were used for an administered dose of 8 as opposed to 10.
Answer: $P[T \leq 70; d_{BED} = d] = 0.6314$; $P[T \leq 70; d_{BED} = d_{DD}] = 0.0361$; $P[T \leq 70; d_{BED}] = 0.0375$.

(e) Compute the administered dose for which the delivered dose overwhelms the defensive mechanisms suppressing cancer formation. That is, find the administered dose such that the delivered dose equals the susceptibility frontier (background dose $d_0 = 0$ and the susceptibility frontier $s = 0.001$).
Answer: $d = 15.6874$.

REFERENCES

1. Andersen, M.E., H.J. Clewell III, M.L. Gargas, F.A. Smith, and R.H. Reitz, "Physiologically Based Pharmacokinetics and Risk Assessment Process for Methylene Chloride," *Toxicology and Applied Pharmacology*, **87**, 185 (1987).
2. Anderson, M.W., D.G. Hoel, and N.L. Kaplan, "A General Scheme for the Incorporation of Pharmacokinetics in Low-Dose Risk Estimation for Chemical Carcinogenesis: Example—Vinyl Chloride," *Toxicology and Applied Pharmacology*, **55**, 154 (1980).
3. Chen, C.W., and J.N. Blancato, " Role of Pharmacokinetic Modeling in Risk Assessment: Perchloroethylene as an Example," in *Pharmacokinetics in Risk Assessment: Drinking Water and Health*, volume 8, edited by National Research Council, National Academy Press, Washington, D.C. (1987).
4. Cohen, S.M., and L.B. Ellwein, "Cell Proliferation in Carcinogenesis," *Science*, **249**, 1007 (1990).
5. Cohen, S.M., and L.B. Ellwein, "Proliferative and Genotoxic Effects in 2-Acetylaminofluorene Bladder and Liver Carcinogenesis: Biological Modeling of the ED01 Study," *Toxicology and Applied Pharmacology*, **104**, 79 (1990).
6. Reitz, R.H., J.N. McDougal, M.W. Himmelstein, R.J. Nolan, and A. M. Schumann, "Physiologically Based Pharmacokinetic Modeling with Methyl Chloroform: Implications for Interspecies, High Dose/Low Dose, and Dose Route Extrapolations," *Toxicology and Applied Pharmacology*, **95**, 185 (1988).
7. Starr, T.B., and R.D. Buck, "The Importance of Delivered Dose in Estimating Low-Dose Cancer Risk from Inhalation Exposure to Formaldehyde," *Fundamental and Applied Toxicology*, **4**, 740 (1984).
8. Sielken, R.L., Jr., "Cancer Dose-Response Extrapolations," *Environmental Science & Technology*, **21**, 1033 (1987).
9. Gehring, P.J. and G.E. Blau, "Mechanisms of Carcinogenesis: Dose Response," *J. Environ. Pathol. Toxicol.*, **1**, 163 (1977).
10. Hoel, D.G., N.L. Kaplan, and M.W. Anderson, "Implication of Nonlinear Kinetics on Risk Estimation in Carcinogenesis," *Science Magazine*, **219**, 1032 (1983).
11. Krewski, D., D.J. Murdoch, and J.R. Withey, "The Application of Pharmacokinetic Data in Carcinogenic Risk Assessment," in *Pharmacokinetics in Risk Assessment: Drinking Water and Health*, volume 8, edited by National Research Council, National Academy Press, Washington, D.C. (1987).
12. Clewell, H.J. III, and M.E. Andersen, "Risk Assessment Extrapolations and Physiological Modeling," *Toxicology and Industrial Health*, **1**, 111 (1985).
13. Sielken, R.L., Jr., "The Capabilities, Sensitivity, Pitfalls, and Future of Quantitative Risk Assessment," in *Environmental Health Risks: Assessment and Management*, edited by S.R. McColl, University of Waterloo Press, Ontario (1987).
14. NCI (National Cancer Institute), *Report on Carcinogenesis Bioassay of Chloroform*, NTIS PB-264018 (1976).
15. Jorgenson, T.A., E.F. Meierhenry, C.J. Rushbrook, R.J. Bull, and M. Robinson, "Carcinogenicity of Chloroform in Drinking Water to Male Osborne-Mendel Rats and Female B6C3F1 Mice," *Fundamental and Applied Toxicology*, **5**, 760 (1985).
16. GEN.T: *A General Tool for Quantitative Risk Analysis*, version 4.0, Sielken, Inc., Bryan,

Texas (1991).

17. Marreiro Rocha, D., G.R. Faloona, and R.H. Unger, "Glucagon-Stimulating Activity of 20 Amino Acids in Dogs,"*Journal of Clinical Investigation*, **51**, 2346 (1972).

18. Linder, M.C., "Nutrition and Metabolism of Proteins," in *Nutritional Biochemestry and Metabolism with Clinical Applications*, edited by M.C. Linder, Elsevier Science Publishing Company, Inc., New York, N.Y. (1985).

7

A Weight-of-Evidence Approach to Quantitative Cancer Risk Assessment

In the preceding chapters, it has become increasingly apparent that quantitative cancer risk assessment involves a large number of possible components. Furthermore, there are several competing alternatives for many of these components, and the current state of knowledge is not sufficient to prove that one of these alternatives is *right* and the other alternatives are *wrong*.

There are basically two approaches to the reality of multiple alternative risk analyses. The simplest and most widely followed approach today is to generally choose the alternative which portrays the risk to be the largest. This approach is usually described as the "conservative" approach in the sense that a risk assessor who continually overstates the perceived risk believes that he is being protective of public health. There is considerable controversy surrounding this approach.[1,2]

There are several issues which make the conservative approach controversial. For example, the conservative approach may confuse risk assessment with risk management. It may also distort science in order to influence policy. The conservative approach may be motivated by a desire to emphasize safety over other considerations, such as cost; however, the conservative bias may lead to an inefficient allocation of health protection and risk reduction resources because the degree of conservatism varies widely across different risk assessments. Failure to accurately portray the relative magnitudes of the risks increases the difficulty in differentiating between hazards. Misallocation of resources can actually lead to less safety rather than more safety (e.g., Nichols and Zeckhauser[3]).

The second approach to quantitative cancer risk assessment is an emerging approach which is referred to herein as *information analysis.* The information-analysis approach is based on the concept that all of the available relevant information on the cancer risk should be incorporated into the quantitative cancer risk assessment.[4,5] Because the different sources of information have differing levels of scientific support and relevance, these sources are weighted, and not all given equal emphasis. Information analysis utilizes many of the techniques of decision analysis to construct a weight-of-evidence analysis which reflects all of the available, relevant information.[6–12]

Information analysis has also been described as *weight-of-evidence analysis, decision analysis, the distributional method of risk characterization, and comprehensive methodology.*[13]

Information analysis describes risk in terms of a probability distribution indicating the relative likelihood of the different magnitudes of risk. By indicating a probability distribution on risk instead of just an upper bound, information analysis allows the public and the other risk managers to evaluate the magnitude of risk reduction and actual benefits to the public of actions.[14–16]

7.1 AN EXAMPLE: THE QUANTITATIVE CANCER RISK ASSESSMENT OF FORMALDEHYDE

There are often a large number of possible quantitative evaluations in a cancer risk assessment[17–19]. Figure 7.1 displays several of the dose-response calculations made concerning the possible cancer risk associated with the inhalation of formaldehyde.[20,21] The objective of a weight-of-evidence approach to quantitative cancer risk assessment is to incorporate all of these calculations and other relevant calculations in the dose-response characterization.[4,13]

In Figure 7.1, the data on the incidence of nasal cavity squamous cell carcinoma in three species (rat, mouse, and hamster) are considered. There was no observed increased experimental risk to hamsters[22,23], and only two mice developed the specified response.[24,25] In the four-dose rat study[24,25], there were no nasal cavity squamous cell carcinomas in the controls and in the 2 *ppm* treatment group. Approximately, a 1 percent response rate was observed in the 5.6 *ppm* treatment group, and just over 50 percent of the rats at 14.3 ppm developed nasal cavity squamous cell carcinoma. Two quantal response models are explicitly considered in Figure 7.1, namely, the Weibull and multistage models. Two forms of the multistage model are considered—the three-stage and five-stage models. For each specific form of the quantal response model, three descriptions of the added risk at 1 *ppm* are indicated. The maximum likelihood estimate or *fitted model value* is given, and also one pair of upper and lower bounds on the risk. The impact of the dose scale used for

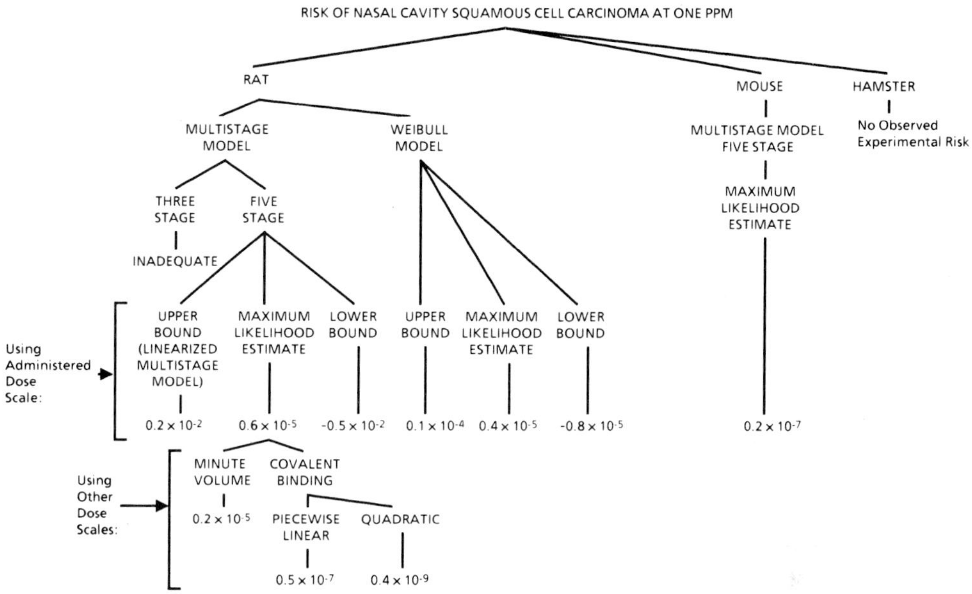

Figure 7.1 Added Risk [$P(1) - P(0)$] of Nasal Cavity Squamous Cell Carcinoma at 1 *ppm*.

dose-response modeling on the five-stage multistage model's maximum likelihood estimate of the added risk is also shown. In addition to the administered dose, a delivered dose based on minute volumes and two forms of the dose scale based on covalent binding to DNA are considered. The two dose scales reflecting the covalent binding information differ in their fit to the observed binding data below 6 *ppm*; one form assumes linearity below 2 *ppm*, and the other form utilizes a fit of a quadratic polynomial to the binding data below 6 *ppm*.

There are ten risk calculations shown in Figure 7.1. All of these ten numbers refer to the risk of nasal cavity squamous cell carcinoma at one ppm. The number of calculations, even at a single dose level, increases dramatically when other elements of the dose-response characterization are considered. For example, in addition to the risk of nasal squamous cell carcinoma at one *ppm*, the definition of the response could be expanded to include nasal cavity nonsquamous polypoid adenomas. Additional elements could also be the different methods of extrapolating the dose-response relationship from an experimental species to humans, and the use of human epidemiological data. There are, of course, other quantal dose-response models and time-to-response models that could have been indicated as well as additional risk attributes such as the nonparametric bootstrap distribution of maximum likelihood estimates. Furthermore, the fitted model values shown only reflect one set of assumptions or restrictions on the mathematical form of those models and one set of restrictions on the model parameters.

This example has not gone into any specific details about the data, modeling, or the underlying biological considerations, and hence is not intended to represent a complete quantitative risk assessment of formaldehyde. Instead, the purpose of this example is to simply illustrate that there are a large number of calculations that can be made in a quantitative risk assessment. Each of these calculations contributes some information. However, no one number conveys all the available information.

The two approaches to quantitative cancer risk assessment characterize the risk associated with formaldehyde inhalation quite differently in this example. The conservative approach essentially identifies the largest number calculated (0.2×10^{-2}) and describes the available quantitative information in terms of a *plausible upper bound* on the cancer potency of 0.002, a single number. On the other hand, the information-analysis approach tries instead to combine the information in all of the calculated numbers into a more reflective characterization. Information analysis identifies the range of risk numbers (here, −0.005 to 0.002) as well as the relative likelihood of the different numbers in that range. A more complete development and presentation of an information analysis for formaldehyde is given in Section 7.4.

7.2 OVERVIEW OF FACTORS AFFECTING QUANTITATIVE DOSE-RESPONSE CHARACTERIZATION

Dose-response characterization involves multiple alternatives. Some of these alternatives are suggested in the formaldehyde example in the preceding section. Figure 7.2 provides an overview of the factors affecting the quantitative dose-response characterization.

The high-to-low-dose extrapolation modeling involves three principal components. One of these components is the experimental data which may include several studies, two sexes, multiple strains, multiple species, different definitions of a carcinogenic response reflecting different response sites and severities, different routes of exposure, and different temporal dosing patterns as well as decisions concerning which experimental dose levels and subjects are to be analyzed (e.g., all doses versus only doses at or below the maximum tolerated dose, and all animals at a dose versus only those animals that survived until the time the first animal developed a tumor).

A second high-to-low-dose extrapolation modeling component is the dose scale used for dose-response modeling. As discussed in the Chapter 6, the dose scale used in the actual dose-response modeling can be either an administered dose, a delivered dose reflecting not only the external dose but also the delivery process, or a biologically effective dose reflecting the delivery process and the net amount of resulting cancer related effects of that delivery.

The third component of the high-to-low-dose extrapolation is the mathematical form of the dose-response model. That is, whether the model is a quantal or time-to-response model, the type of cancer mechanism reflected in the model, the components of the model allowed to be dose and/or time dependent, and any restrictions on the parameter values in the model. Many of these aspects have been discussed in Chapters 2 and 4.

In addition to the several alternatives associated with the high-to-low-dose extrapolation components, there are also several alternatives associated with the extrapolation of

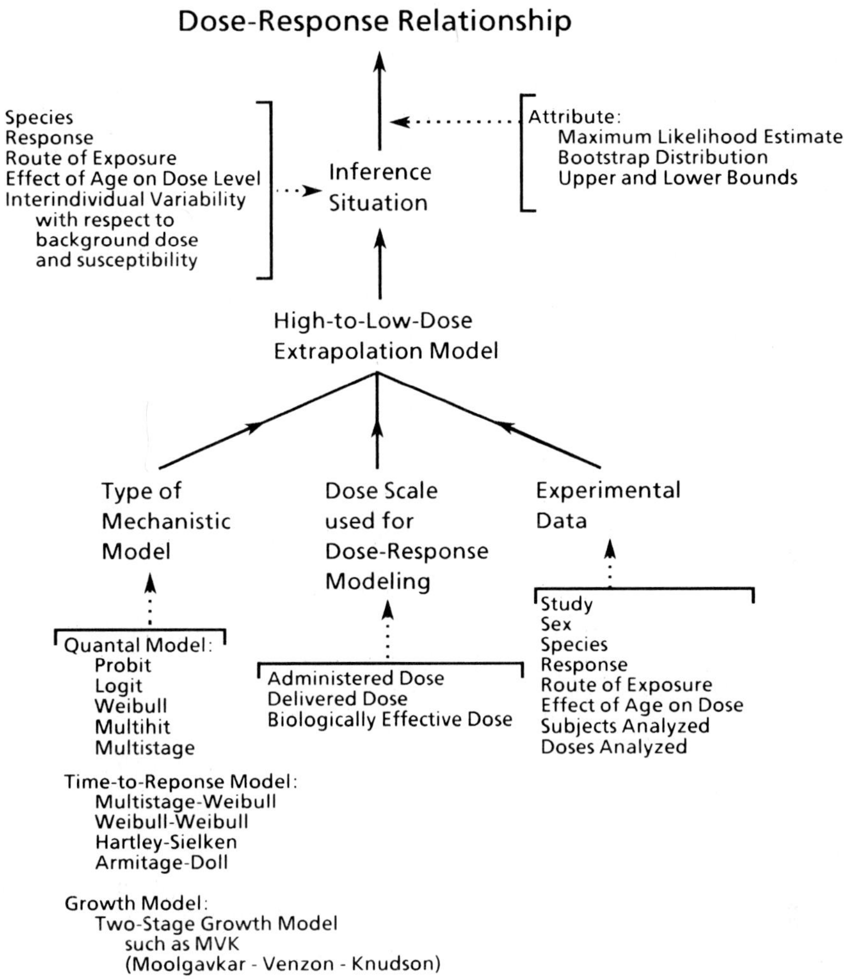

Figure 7.2 An Overview of the Factors Affecting a Quantitative Dose-Response Characterization.

the high-to-low-dose extrapolation models from an experimental situation to the inference situation of interest. For example, the experimental situation might refer to rats, and the inference situation refer to humans. The experimental situation might refer to continuous lifetime oral exposures while the inference situation might refer to intermittent inhalation exposures. There are several alternative methods of implementing these situation extrapolations (that is, interspecies, route-to-route, and temporal extrapolations).

There are also alternatives with respect to the attribute used to describe a particular dose-response relationship. Alternative attributes include maximum likelihood estimates, upper bounds, lower bounds, ranges, and bootstrap distributions indicating the impact of experimental variability on the maximum likelihood estimates.

7.3 INFORMATION-ANALYSIS BASED DOSE-RESPONSE CHARACTERIZATIONS

Information analysis characterizes the dose-response relationship in terms of a probability distribution that reflects a weight-of-evidence assessment of all of the available relevant information.[4,13]

A major improvement in the current practice of quantitative dose-response modeling would be the use of information-analysis based dose-response characterizations reflecting weight-of-evidence evaluations of all of the available dose-response information instead of focusing on only one experimental data set, one dose scale, one dose-response model, one assumption about interspecies differences, and one method for describing the implications of the dose-response model.[16,26–30] An information analysis of the dose-response relationship utilizes the techniques of decision analysis to reflect the current state of knowledge, emphasize weight-of-evidence characterization, and identify the factors having the greater quantitative impacts.[4,20,31–34] Information analysis also provides a means of realistically reflecting the quantitative impacts of uncertainty.[27,35–37]

Information analysis identifies the factors (e.g., relevant human target tissue, the chemical's mode of action, dose scale, dose-response model, data set, interspecies extrapolation method, and risk attribute) entering into the extrapolation of risks. Then it identifies each relevant alternative for each factor. (For example, administered dose, delivered dose, and biologically effective dose are alternatives for the dose scale factor.) Each combination of alternatives for the factors is explicitly evaluated, and the specified attribute (e.g., maximum likelihood estimate) of a particular dose-response feature (e.g., potency or added risk at a specified dose level) computed. These quantitative attributes are reported individually and then summarized (not averaged).[38,39] Summaries can be frequency distributions indicating how often a particular attribute value occurs or, preferably, weighted frequency distributions indicating the proportion of scientific support for each combination of factor alternatives. Weights can reflect sample sizes, statistical analyses, or expert judgments of the appropriateness of particular alternatives.[31,35,40–43] Weighting allows a relevant alternative to be evaluated without requiring unattainable proof that another alternative is *wrong*.[44] In this manner information analyses also encourage additional data collection and stimulate research. Sensitivity analyses using alternative weights help identify the critical factors in the quantitative assessment and, thereby, help prioritize and direct research as well as focusing discussions.[4,31]

Information analyses characterize dose-response attributes in terms of a probability distribution that describes the current state of knowledge concerning the relative likelihood of each possible value of that attribute.[41] Probability distribution characterizations of the dose-response attributes can be legitimately combined with probability distribution characterizations of exposure to yield the most accurate risk characterizations available.[20,34]

Such characterizations reflect the current state of knowledge without censoring the available information. These characterizations provide more than *bright lines* and avoid the *false* impression of mathematical precision associated with single number characterizations of risk.[27,35] Furthermore, by indicating the differing levels of evidence supporting different risk values, such characterizations allow the risk manager to more fully utilize the tools of risk management in evaluating alternative actions.[14,20]

7.4 AN EXAMPLE OF INFORMATION ANALYSIS

An illustrative example of an information-analysis based dose-response characterization is developed and discussed in this section. This example focuses on the formaldehyde inhalation study in rats conducted by the Chemical Industry Institute of Toxicology.[24,25] This study has been the primary focus of efforts to quantify the carcinogenic dose-response relationship for formaldehyde.[45–48]

CIIT also conducted a similar four-dose inhalation study in mice in which only two nasal cavity squamous cell carcinomas were observed, and these responses were at the highest dose tested.[24] There was a formaldehyde inhalation study in hamsters in which no increased cancer risk was observed. In addition, there is some important human epidemiological evidence.[49] These additional sources of information have been used primarily in the qualitative evaluation of the carcinogenic potential of formaldehyde. Efforts to utilize human epidemiological data in quantitative dose-response characterizations are expanding. New epidemiological data and modeling techniques are expected to be increasingly helpful in the future.

This example is intended to be illustrative of the information-analysis approach and is not intended as a definitive dose-response characterization of formaldehyde.

7.4.1 Decision Tree

In the CIIT formaldehyde inhalation study of rats, the only increased carcinogenic responses were in the nasal cavity.[24,25] The six major Factors in the quantitative dose-response characterization based on this study and the alternatives within each Factor are explicitly identified in Table 7.1 and their interrelationship shown figuratively in the *decision tree* in Figure 7.3.

A key feature of decision analysis as a tool is its focus on defining the problem, its major components, and the alternatives within these components. Decision trees are helpful tools for visualizing this structure.[50] Each relevant combination of possibilities or analytical methodologies in the decision tree is explicitly evaluated, and the quantitative outcome presented. This feature encourages the explicit consideration and evaluation of non-default approaches as well as default approaches. (A *default* approach is an approach dictated by agency policies or legislative guidelines as opposed to an approach that has been demonstrated to be scientifically applicable to the case at hand.[51])

Table 7.1 The Decision Tree: The Alternatives for the Six Major Dose-Response Factors in the Decision Tree for the Example Information-Analysis based Dose-Response Characterization of Formaldehyde

Factor 1: Human Carcinogenicity: Relevant Human Target Tissue
1. A Human Carcinogen
2. Not a Human Carcinogen

Factor 2: Mode of Action: Carcinogenic Mechanism
1. Cell Proliferation Involved But Not Genotoxicity
2. Genotoxicity Involved But Not Cell Proliferation
3. Cell Proliferation and Genotoxicity Both Involved

Factor 3: Dose Scale
1. Formaldehyde Concentration in the Air Inhaled (ppm)
2. Daily Intake of Formaldehyde
3. Amount of Formaldehyde Induced DNA protein cross-links (DPX)

Factor 4: Dose-Response Model
1. Threshold: Probit
2. Sublinear: Multistage (5 Stage)
3. Sublinear and Low-Dose Linear: Multistage (5 Stage) and Linear below 1.0 ppm [Abbreviation = Sublinear (LDL)]
4. Linear: One-Hit

Factor 5: Experimental Data Set
1. Malignant Squamous Cell Carcinoma in the Rat Nasal Cavity (Abbreviation = M)
2. Malignant Squamous Cell Carcinoma and/or Benign Polypoid Adenoma in the Rat Nasal Cavity (Abbreviation = M&B)

Factor 6: Interspecies Extrapolation
1. Human and Rat Response Probabilities are Equal when the Dose in Humans Equals the Dose in Rats (Abbreviation = Same)
2. Human and Rat Response Probabilities are Equal when the Dose in Humans is $\{[\text{Rat Body Weight}]/[\text{Human Body Weight}]\}^{1/4}$ Times the Dose in Rats
3. Human and Rat Response Probabilities are Equal when the Dose in Humans is $\{[\text{Rat Body Weight}]/[\text{Human Body Weight}]\}^{1/3}$ Times the Dose in Rats

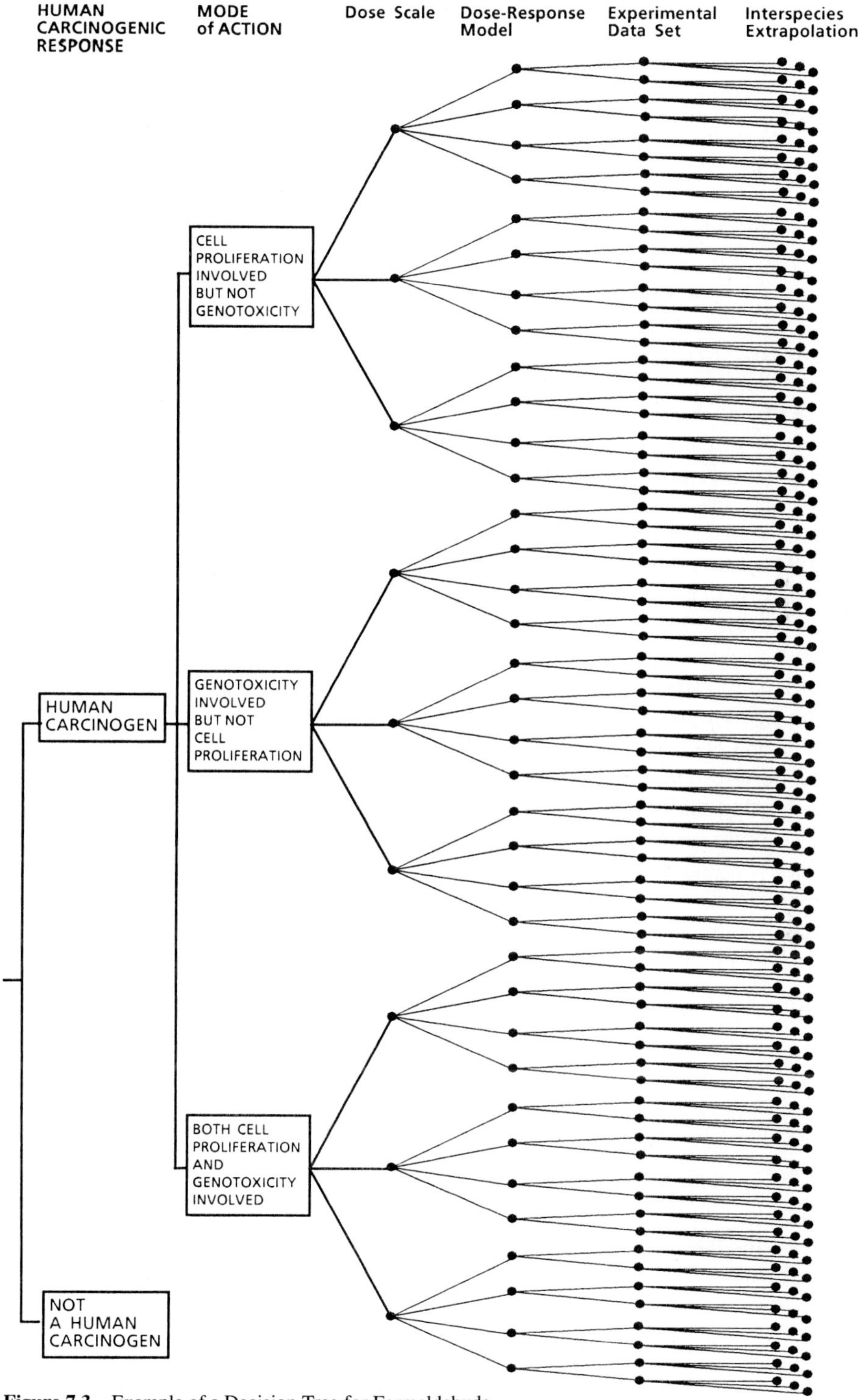

Figure 7.3 Example of a Decision Tree for Formaldehyde.

The decision tree shown in Figure 7.3 for the formaldehyde cancer dose-response characterization is growing from left to right and hence is sideways relative to nature's trees. The *branches* in the *tree* are the alternatives. For example, the first two branches in the tree are *Human Carcinogen* and *Not a Human Carcinogen* which represent the two alternatives for the first Factor *Human Carcinogenic Response*. A *path* through the decision tree is a sequence of individually connected branches starting at the left and continuing to its end at the right. A path corresponds to an analysis of what the dose-response relationship for formaldehyde would be if each branch in the path occurred.

As discussed in the remainder of Section 7.4, at the end of each path in the decision tree there is a weight and one or more *dose-response attributes*. The *weight* indicates the relative likelihood or subjective probability that the combination of alternatives along the path is the true *state of nature*. *Dose-response attributes* or *risk attributes* refer to a user-specified feature of the dose-response relationship and include the maximum likelihood estimate, upper and lower bounds, confidence limits, and bootstrap distributions for that feature. The *decision* or *action* at the end of a path is the dose-response attribute (description of the dose-response relationship) which corresponds to each alternative along the path being the true *state of nature*.

The weights and dose-response attributes are not explicitly shown in Figure 7.3 but are shown in Figures 7.4 through 7.9. In Figures 7.4 through 7.9 the particular feature of the dose-response relationship being described is the added cancer risk (defined in Chapter 3) of inhaling air containing 1 ppb (0.001 *ppm*) of formaldehyde for a lifetime. Figures 7.4 through 7.6 indicate the maximum likelihood estimate of this added risk as well as the 95th and 5th percentiles of the nonparametric bootstrap distribution of these estimates for all dose-response models plus the 95th upper and lower confidence limits on the added risk using the linearized multistage model procedure. Figures 7.7 through 7.9 indicate the nonparametric bootstrap distribution characterization of the impact of experimental variability on the maximum likelihood estimate of the added risk.

As discussed in more detail in Section 7.4.4, the weights in Figures 7.4 through 7.9 indicate the relative emphasis or weight of evidence associated with each alternative and each combination of alternatives; that is, the weight associated with each branch and path (and its dose-response attribute value).

Different chemicals and different data may have different decision trees with different alternatives and other factors.

Factor 1. Human Carcinogenic Response: Relevant Human Target Tissue

Is formaldehyde a human carcinogen by the routes and at the dose levels to which people are likely to be exposed? Does the human epidemiological evidence, the experimental data, the mechanistic information, and the rest of the biological information indicate that formaldehyde is a human carcinogen in the envisioned human exposure scenarios? Does the quantitative characterization of the cancer dose-response relationship need to be subdivided on the basis of different human target tissues? In the decision tree for formaldehyde shown in Figure 7.3, the alternatives for the human carcinogenicity are simply that in the envisioned human exposure situations either formaldehyde is a human carcinogen or it is not. In this decision tree, the human carcinogenic response of concern is defined to be any cancer regardless of site or severity.

Factor 2. Mode of Action: Carcinogenic Mechanism

Formaldehyde appears to have three possible modes of action with respect to cancer.[52–54] One potential carcinogenic mechanism is that formaldehyde affects cell proliferation but does not affect genotoxicity. A second possibility is that formaldehyde affects genotoxicity but not cell proliferation. The third possible mode of action is that formaldehyde affects *both* cell proliferation and genotoxicity. No other possible modes of action are considered to be suggested by the current available information.

Factor 3. Dose Scale

The dose scale used for formaldehyde's cancer dose-response modeling is a Factor that has received considerable attention.[45,55–57] The three primary dose scales are the concentration of formaldehyde in the air being inhaled, the total daily intake of formaldehyde based on minute volumes of inhaled air[58,59], and the amount of formaldehyde induced *DNA protein cross-links* (DPX).[60–62] Herein, the assumption has been made that humans have the same relationship between the concentration (*ppm*) of formaldehyde in the air and the total daily intake (per unit of nasal cavity surface area) as the rats. However, the relationship between the concentration of formaldehyde in the air and the amount of DPX in humans has been assumed to equal that observed in monkeys. Each of these three alternative dose scales is considered in conjunction with each of the three modes of action.

Factor 4. Dose-Response Model

The time-to-response information has not usually been considered. The quantal response data in Example 3.4, Chapter 3, have been the usual focus of attention. The shape of the dose-response relationship implied by these data depends on the dose scale being used as well as formaldehyde's carcinogenic mechanism. As discussed in Chapter 6, the shape of the relationship between the administered dose (here, the concentration of formaldehyde in the air) and the dose scale used in dose-response modeling is incorporated in the dose scale itself. Thus, the dose-response model need only reflect the shape of the portion of the carcinogenic process linking the dose scale and the cancer incidence. The shape of the dose-response relationship in this remaining portion of the carcinogenic process depends upon the carcinogenic mechanism. Herein, the probit model is used to describe very nonlinear,

HUMAN CARCINOGENIC HAZARD	MODE OF ACTION	DOSE SCALE	DOSE-RESPONSE MODEL	EXPERIMENTAL DATA SET	INTERSPECIES EXTRAPOLATION	WEIGHT ON PATH	MAXIMUM LIKELIHOOD ESTIMATE	95TH PERC. OF THE BOOTSTRAP DISTRIBUTION	5TH PERC. OF THE BOOTSTRAP DISTRIBUTION	95TH UPPER CONFIDENCE LIMIT	95TH LOWER CONFIDENCE LIMIT
HUMAN CARCINOGEN 0.8	CELL PROLIFERATION INVOLVED BUT NOT GENOTOXICITY 0.800	PPM 0.1	THRESHOLD 0.50	M 0.8	Same 0.20	0.005120	0.0D + 00	0.0D + 00	0.0D + 00	N/A	N/A
					$BW^{3/4}$ 0.40	0.010240	0.0D + 00	0.0D + 00	0.0D + 00	N/A	N/A
					$BW^{2/3}$ 0.40	0.010240	0.0D + 00	0.0D + 00	0.0D + 00	N/A	N/A
				M&B 0.2	Same 0.20	0.001280	0.0D + 00	0.0D + 00	0.0D + 00	N/A	N/A
					$BW^{3/4}$ 0.40	0.002560	0.0D + 00	0.0D + 00	0.0D + 00	N/A	N/A
					$BW^{2/3}$ 0.40	0.002560	0.0D + 00	0.0D + 00	0.0D + 00	N/A	N/A
			SUBLINEAR 0.45	M 0.8	Same 0.20	0.004608	5.5D - 18	6.3D - 14	0.0D + 00	2.2D - 06	-2.6D - 05
					$BW^{3/4}$ 0.40	0.009216	1.1D - 15	2.7D - 12	7.6D - 19	8.3D - 06	-8.3D - 05
					$BW^{2/3}$ 0.40	0.009216	3.6D - 14	1.1D - 11	7.7D - 18	1.3D - 05	-6.2D - 05
				M&B 0.2	Same 0.20	0.001152	5.5D - 06	1.2D - 05	0.0D + 00	1.2D - 05	-2.2D - 06
					$BW^{3/4}$ 0.40	0.002304	2.3D - 05	4.4D - 05	3.5D - 18	4.6D - 05	-6.2D - 06
					$BW^{2/3}$ 0.40	0.002304	4.2D - 05	7.1D - 05	4.7D - 15	7.3D - 05	-1.3D - 05
			SUBLINEAR (LDL) 0.05	M 0.8	Same 0.20	0.000512	6.4D - 09	6.5D - 08	1.0D - 09	2.2D - 06	-1.8D - 05
					$BW^{3/4}$ 0.40	0.001024	1.7D - 06	5.7D - 06	7.7D - 07	8.8D - 06	-2.4D - 05
					$BW^{2/3}$ 0.40	0.001024	1.2D - 05	2.8D - 05	7.0D - 06	2.9D - 05	-2.4D - 05
				M&B 0.2	Same 0.20	0.000128	5.5D - 06	1.2D - 05	1.5D - 09	1.2D - 05	-1.6D - 06
					$BW^{3/4}$ 0.40	0.000256	2.4D - 05	4.4D - 05	1.0D - 06	4.6D - 05	-3.8D - 08
					$BW^{2/3}$ 0.40	0.000256	4.8D - 05	7.6D - 05	1.0D - 05	7.7D - 05	6.0D - 06
			LINEAR 0.00	M 0.8	Same 0.20	0.0	2.9D - 05	3.4D - 05	2.5D - 05	3.4D - 05	2.5D - 05
					$BW^{3/4}$ 0.40	0.0	1.1D - 04	1.3D - 04	9.4D - 05	1.3D - 04	9.4D - 05
					$BW^{2/3}$ 0.40	0.0	1.7D - 04	2.0D - 04	1.5D - 04	2.0D - 04	1.5D - 04
				M&B 0.2	Same 0.20	0.0	3.4D - 05	3.8D - 05	2.9D - 05	3.9D - 05	2.9D - 05
					$BW^{3/4}$ 0.40	0.0	1.3D - 04	1.4D - 04	1.1D - 04	1.5D - 04	1.1D - 04
					$BW^{2/3}$ 0.40	0.0	2.0D - 04	2.2D - 04	1.7D - 04	2.3D - 04	1.7D - 04
			THRESHOLD 0.50	M 0.8	Same 0.50	0.038400	0.0D + 00	0.0D + 00	0.0D + 00	N/A	N/A
					$BW^{3/4}$ 0.25	0.019200	0.0D + 00	0.0D + 00	0.0D + 00	N/A	N/A
					$BW^{2/3}$ 0.25	0.019200	0.0D + 00	0.0D + 00	0.0D + 00	N/A	N/A
				M&B 0.2	Same 0.50	0.009600	0.0D + 00	0.0D + 00	0.0D + 00	N/A	N/A
					$BW^{3/4}$ 0.25	0.004800	0.0D + 00	0.0D + 00	0.0D + 00	N/A	N/A
					$BW^{2/3}$ 0.25	0.004800	0.0D + 00	0.0D + 00	0.0D + 00	N/A	N/A
			SUBLINEAR 0.40	M 0.8	Same 0.50	0.030720	1.9D - 21	3.8D - 14	0.0D + 00	1.2D - 06	-1.5D - 05
					$BW^{3/4}$ 0.25	0.015360	1.4D - 18	1.5D - 13	1.2D - 18	4.5D - 06	-7.2D - 05
					$BW^{2/3}$ 0.25	0.015360	1.3D - 17	2.1D - 13	1.1D - 17	7.0D - 06	-9.5D - 05
				M&B 0.2	Same 0.50	0.007680	2.4D - 06	8.5D - 06	0.0D + 00	9.1D - 06	-3.8D - 06
					$BW^{3/4}$ 0.25	0.003840	9.1D - 06	3.2D - 05	0.0D + 00	3.4D - 05	-2.7D - 04
					$BW^{2/3}$ 0.25	0.003840	1.4D - 05	4.9D - 05	1.0D - 17	5.3D - 05	-1.8D - 04

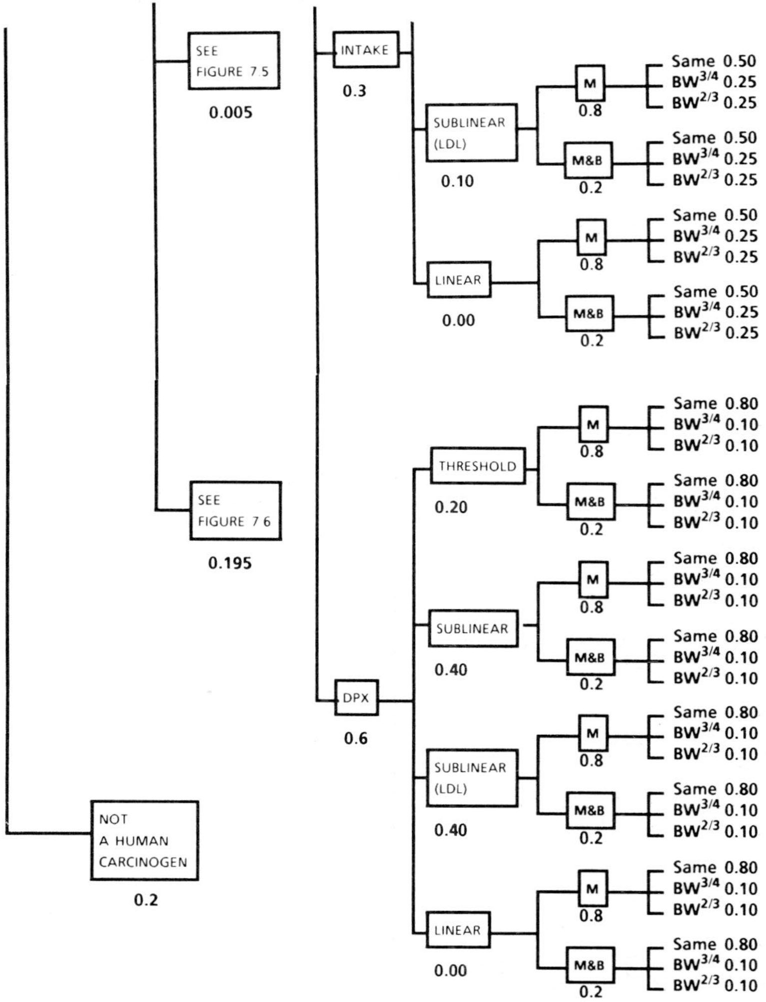

INTAKE 0.3	SUBLINEAR (LDL) 0.10	M 0.8	Same 0.50	0.007680	1.9D - 09	2.6D - 09	1.6D - 09	1.2D - 06	-1.4D - 05
			$BW^{3/4}$ 0.25	0.003840	1.4D - 06	1.7D - 06	1.2D - 06	5.9D - 06	-3.8D - 05
			$BW^{2/3}$ 0.25	0.003840	1.3D - 05	1.6D - 05	1.1D - 05	2.1D - 05	-3.8D - 05
		M&B 0.2	Same 0.50	0.001920	2.4D - 06	8.4D - 06	1.7D - 09	9.0D - 06	-4.2D - 06
			$BW^{3/4}$ 0.25	0.000960	1.0D - 05	3.3D - 05	1.2D - 06	3.5D - 05	-1.1D - 05
			$BW^{2/3}$ 0.25	0.000960	2.6D - 05	6.1D - 05	1.1D - 05	6.2D - 05	-8.0D - 06
	LINEAR 0.00	M 0.8	Same 0.50	0.0	2.9D - 05	3.4D - 05	2.5D - 05	3.4D - 05	2.5D - 05
			$BW^{3/4}$ 0.25	0.0	1.1D - 04	1.3D - 04	9.5D - 05	1.3D - 04	9.4D - 05
			$BW^{2/3}$ 0.25	0.0	1.7D - 04	2.0D - 04	1.5D - 04	2.0D - 04	1.5D - 04
		M&B 0.2	Same 0.50	0.0	3.4D - 05	3.8D - 05	2.9D - 05	3.9D - 05	2.9D - 05
			$BW^{3/4}$ 0.25	0.0	1.3D - 04	1.4D - 04	1.1D - 04	1.5D - 04	1.1D - 04
			$BW^{2/3}$ 0.25	0.0	2.0D - 04	2.2D - 04	1.7D - 04	2.3D - 04	1.7D - 04
DPX 0.6	THRESHOLD 0.20	M 0.8	Same 0.80	0.049152	0.0D + 00	0.0D + 00	0.0D + 00	N/A	N/A
			$BW^{3/4}$ 0.10	0.006144	0.0D + 00	0.0D + 00	0.0D + 00	N/A	N/A
			$BW^{2/3}$ 0.10	0.006144	0.0D + 00	0.0D + 00	0.0D + 00	N/A	N/A
		M&B 0.2	Same 0.80	0.012288	0.0D + 00	0.0D + 00	0.0D + 00	N/A	N/A
			$BW^{3/4}$ 0.10	0.001536	0.0D + 00	0.0D + 00	0.0D + 00	N/A	N/A
			$BW^{2/3}$ 0.10	0.001536	0.0D + 00	0.0D + 00	0.0D + 00	N/A	N/A
	SUBLINEAR 0.40	M 0.8	Same 0.80	0.098304	5.8D - 14	2.7D - 13	0.0D + 00	6.9D - 08	-1.4D - 07
			$BW^{3/4}$ 0.10	0.012288	6.7D - 13	3.7D - 12	0.0D + 00	2.7D - 07	-1.9D - 07
			$BW^{2/3}$ 0.10	0.012288	1.6D - 12	9.1D - 12	0.0D + 00	4.2D - 07	-8.8D - 07
		M&B 0.2	Same 0.80	0.024576	5.6D - 08	1.7D - 07	0.0D + 00	2.0D - 07	-1.3D - 07
			$BW^{3/4}$ 0.10	0.003072	2.2D - 07	6.2D - 07	0.0D + 00	7.3D - 07	-5.4D - 07
			$BW^{2/3}$ 0.10	0.003072	4.1D - 07	9.4D - 07	0.0D + 00	1.1D - 06	-3.8D - 07
	SUBLINEAR (LDL) 0.40	M 0.8	Same 0.80	0.098304	1.8D - 10	8.1D - 10	6.3D - 16	1.3D - 07	-8.4D - 08
			$BW^{3/4}$ 0.10	0.012288	2.1D - 09	1.1D - 08	1.4D - 13	4.1D - 07	-8.5D - 07
			$BW^{2/3}$ 0.10	0.012288	5.1D - 09	2.8D - 08	2.1D - 14	7.3D - 07	-5.1D - 07
		M&B 0.2	Same 0.80	0.024576	9.8D - 08	2.9D - 07	1.5D - 15	3.5D - 07	-1.9D - 07
			$BW^{3/4}$ 0.10	0.003072	3.9D - 07	1.1D - 06	2.8D - 13	1.3D - 06	-6.8D - 07
			$BW^{2/3}$ 0.10	0.003072	7.1D - 07	1.6D - 06	1.8D - 12	2.0D - 06	-7.8D - 07
	LINEAR 0.00	M 0.8	Same 0.80	0.0	4.1D - 07	4.8D - 07	3.4D - 07	4.8D - 07	3.5D - 07
			$BW^{3/4}$ 0.10	0.0	1.5D - 06	1.8D - 06	1.3D - 06	1.8D - 06	1.3D - 06
			$BW^{2/3}$ 0.10	0.0	2.4D - 06	2.8D - 06	2.0D - 06	2.8D - 06	2.0D - 06
		M&B 0.2	Same 0.80	0.0	4.6D - 07	5.2D - 07	3.9D - 07	5.4D - 07	3.9D - 07
			$BW^{3/4}$ 0.10	0.0	1.7D - 06	2.0D - 06	1.5D - 06	2.0D - 06	1.5D - 06
			$BW^{2/3}$ 0.10	0.0	2.7D - 06	3.1D - 06	2.3D - 06	3.1D - 06	2.3D - 06

Legend: See Table 1 for abbreviations. Also, BW = Body Weight; 2.5D - 04 = 2.5×10^{-4};
N/A = Not Applicable. Risk attributes refer to the added risk at one ppb.

Figure 7.4 The Weights, Maximum Likelihood Estimates, 95th and 5th Percentiles of the Nonparametric Bootstrap Distributions, and 95 Percent Upper and Lower Confidence Limits Using the Linearized Multistage Model Procedure for the Paths in the Decision Tree with Mode of Action Having Cell Proliferation Involved but not Genotoxicity.

HUMAN CARCINOGENIC HAZARD	MODE OF ACTION	DOSE SCALE	DOSE-RESPONSE MODEL	EXPERIMENTAL DATA SET	INTERSPECIES EXTRAPOLATION	WEIGHT ON PATH	MAXIMUM LIKELIHOOD ESTIMATE	95TH PERC. OF THE BOOTSTRAP DISTRIBUTION	5TH PERC. OF THE BOOTSTRAP DISTRIBUTION	95TH UPPER CONFIDENCE LIMIT	95TH LOWER CONFIDENCE LIMIT
HUMAN CARCINOGEN 0.8	SEE FIGURE 7 4 0.800										
	GENOTOXICITY INVOLVED BUT NOT CELL PROLIFERATION 0.005	PPM 0.1	THRESHOLD 0.00	M 0.8	Same 0.20	0.0	0.0D + 00	0.0D + 00	0.0D + 00	N/A	N/A
					$BW^{3/4}$ 0.40	0.0	0.0D + 00	0.0D + 00	0.0D + 00	N/A	N/A
					$BW^{2/3}$ 0.40	0.0	0.0D + 00	0.0D + 00	0.0D + 00	N/A	N/A
				M&B 0.2	Same 0.20	0.0	0.0D + 00	0.0D + 00	0.0D + 00	N/A	N/A
					$BW^{3/4}$ 0.40	0.0	0.0D + 00	0.0D + 00	0.0D + 00	N/A	N/A
					$BW^{2/3}$ 0.40	0.0	0.0D + 00	0.0D + 00	0.0D + 00	N/A	N/A
			SUBLINEAR 0.15	M 0.8	Same 0.20	0.000010	5.5D - 18	6.3D - 14	0.0D + 00	2.2D - 06	-2.6D - 05
					$BW^{3/4}$ 0.40	0.000019	1.1D - 15	2.7D - 12	7.6D - 19	8.3D - 06	-8.3D - 05
					$BW^{2/3}$ 0.40	0.000019	3.6D - 14	1.1D - 11	7.7D - 18	1.3D - 05	-6.2D - 05
				M&B 0.2	Same 0.20	0.000002	5.5D - 06	1.2D - 05	0.0D + 00	1.2D - 05	-2.2D - 06
					$BW^{3/4}$ 0.40	0.000005	2.3D - 05	4.4D - 05	3.5D - 18	4.6D - 05	-6.2D - 06
					$BW^{2/3}$ 0.40	0.000005	4.2D - 05	7.1D - 05	4.7D - 15	7.3D - 05	-1.3D - 05
			SUBLINEAR (LDL) 0.50	M 0.8	Same 0.20	0.000032	6.4D - 09	6.5D - 08	1.0D - 09	2.2D - 06	-1.8D - 05
					$BW^{3/4}$ 0.40	0.000064	1.7D - 06	5.7D - 06	7.7D - 07	8.8D - 06	-2.4D - 05
					$BW^{2/3}$ 0.40	0.000064	1.2D - 05	2.8D - 05	7.0D - 06	2.9D - 05	-2.4D - 05
				M&B 0.2	Same 0.20	0.000008	5.5D - 06	1.2D - 05	1.5D - 09	1.2D - 05	-1.6D - 06
					$BW^{3/4}$ 0.40	0.000016	2.4D - 05	4.4D - 05	1.0D - 06	4.6D - 05	-3.8D - 08
					$BW^{2/3}$ 0.40	0.000016	4.8D - 05	7.6D - 05	1.0D - 05	7.7D - 05	6.0D - 06
			LINEAR 0.35	M 0.8	Same 0.20	0.000022	2.9D - 05	3.4D - 05	2.5D - 05	3.4D - 05	2.5D - 05
					$BW^{3/4}$ 0.40	0.000045	1.1D - 04	1.3D - 04	9.4D - 05	1.3D - 04	9.4D - 05
					$BW^{2/3}$ 0.40	0.000045	1.7D - 04	2.0D - 04	1.5D - 04	2.0D - 04	1.5D - 04
				M&B 0.2	Same 0.20	0.000006	3.4D - 05	3.8D - 05	2.9D - 05	3.9D - 05	2.9D - 05
					$BW^{3/4}$ 0.40	0.000011	1.3D - 04	1.4D - 04	1.1D - 04	1.5D - 04	1.1D - 04
					$BW^{2/3}$ 0.40	0.000011	2.0D - 04	2.2D - 04	1.7D - 04	2.3D - 04	1.7D - 04
		INTAKE 0.3	THRESHOLD 0.00	M 0.8	Same 0.50	0.0	0.0D + 00	0.0D + 00	0.0D + 00	N/A	N/A
					$BW^{3/4}$ 0.25	0.0	0.0D + 00	0.0D + 00	0.0D + 00	N/A	N/A
					$BW^{2/3}$ 0.25	0.0	0.0D + 00	0.0D + 00	0.0D + 00	N/A	N/A
				M&B 0.2	Same 0.50	0.0	0.0D + 00	0.0D + 00	0.0D + 00	N/A	N/A
					$BW^{3/4}$ 0.25	0.0	0.0D + 00	0.0D + 00	0.0D + 00	N/A	N/A
					$BW^{2/3}$ 0.25	0.0	0.0D + 00	0.0D + 00	0.0D + 00	N/A	N/A
			SUBLINEAR 0.10	M 0.8	Same 0.50	0.000048	1.9D - 21	3.8D - 14	0.0D + 00	1.2D - 06	-1.5D - 05
					$BW^{3/4}$ 0.25	0.000024	1.4D - 18	1.5D - 13	1.2D - 18	4.5D - 06	-7.2D - 05
					$BW^{2/3}$ 0.25	0.000024	1.3D - 17	2.1D - 13	1.1D - 17	7.0D - 06	-9.5D - 05
				M&B 0.2	Same 0.50	0.000012	2.4D - 06	8.5D - 06	0.0D + 00	9.1D - 06	-3.8D - 06
					$BW^{3/4}$ 0.25	0.000006	9.1D - 06	3.2D - 05	0.0D + 00	3.4D - 05	-2.7D - 04
					$BW^{2/3}$ 0.25	0.000006	1.4D - 05	4.9D - 05	1.0D - 17	5.3D - 05	-1.8D - 04

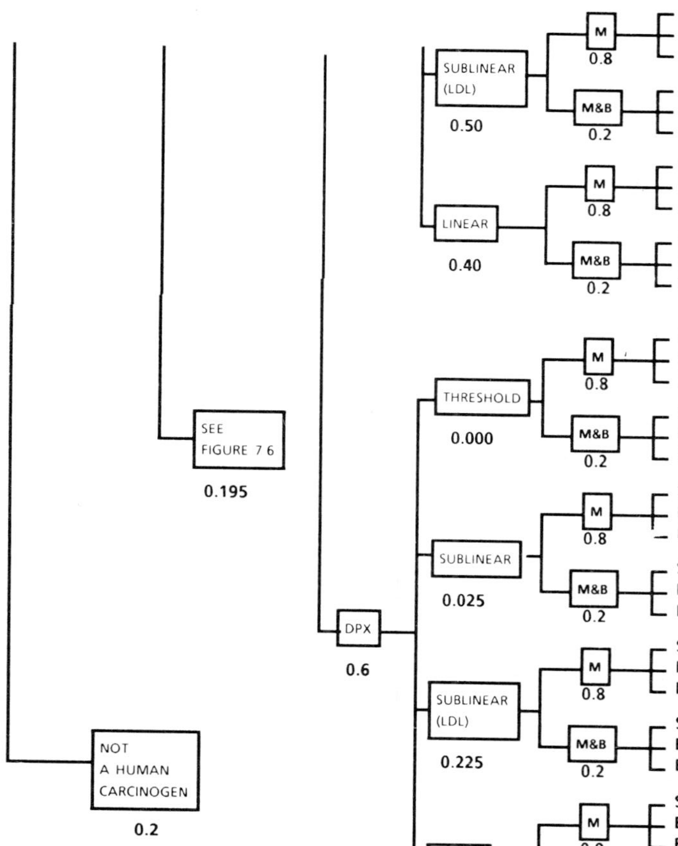

SUBLINEAR (LDL) 0.50	M 0.8	Same	0.50	0.000240	1.9D - 09	2.6D - 09	1.6D - 09	1.2D - 06	-1.4D - 05
		$BW^{3/4}$	0.25	0.000120	1.4D - 06	1.7D - 06	1.2D - 06	5.9D - 06	-3.8D - 05
		$BW^{2/3}$	0.25	0.000120	1.3D - 05	1.6D - 05	1.1D - 05	2.1D - 05	-3.8D - 05
	M&B 0.2	Same	0.50	0.000060	2.4D - 06	8.4D - 06	1.7D - 09	9.0D - 06	-4.2D - 06
		$BW^{3/4}$	0.25	0.000030	1.0D - 05	3.3D - 05	1.2D - 06	3.5D - 05	-1.1D - 05
		$BW^{2/3}$	0.25	0.000030	2.6D - 05	6.1D - 05	1.1D - 05	6.2D - 05	-8.0D - 06
LINEAR 0.40	M 0.8	Same	0.50	0.000192	2.9D - 05	3.4D - 05	2.5D - 05	3.4D - 05	2.5D - 05
		$BW^{3/4}$	0.25	0.000096	1.1D - 04	1.3D - 04	9.5D - 05	1.3D - 04	9.4D - 05
		$BW^{2/3}$	0.25	0.000096	1.7D - 04	2.0D - 04	1.5D - 04	2.0D - 04	1.5D - 04
	M&B 0.2	Same	0.50	0.000048	3.4D - 05	3.8D - 05	2.9D - 05	3.9D - 05	2.9D - 05
		$BW^{3/4}$	0.25	0.000024	1.3D - 04	1.4D - 04	1.1D - 04	1.5D - 04	1.1D - 04
		$BW^{2/3}$	0.25	0.000024	2.0D - 04	2.2D - 04	1.7D - 04	2.3D - 04	1.7D - 04
THRESHOLD 0.000	M 0.8	Same	0.80	0.0	0.0D + 00	0.0D + 00	0.0D + 00	N/A	N/A
		$BW^{3/4}$	0.10	0.0	0.0D + 00	0.0D + 00	0.0D + 00	N/A	N/A
		$BW^{2/3}$	0.10	0.0	0.0D + 00	0.0D + 00	0.0D + 00	N/A	N/A
	M&B 0.2	Same	0.80	0.0	0.0D + 00	0.0D + 00	0.0D + 00	N/A	N/A
		$BW^{3/4}$	0.10	0.0	0.0D + 00	0.0D + 00	0.0D + 00	N/A	N/A
		$BW^{2/3}$	0.10	0.0	0.0D + 00	0.0D + 00	0.0D + 00	N/A	N/A
SUBLINEAR 0.025	M 0.8	Same	0.80	0.000038	5.8D - 14	2.7D - 13	0.0D + 00	6.9D - 08	-1.4D - 07
		$BW^{3/4}$	0.10	0.000005	6.7D - 13	3.7D - 12	0.0D + 00	2.7D - 07	-1.9D - 07
		$BW^{2/3}$	0.10	0.000005	1.6D - 12	9.1D - 12	0.0D + 00	4.2D - 07	-8.8D - 07
	M&B 0.2	Same	0.80	0.000010	5.6D - 08	1.7D - 07	0.0D + 00	2.0D - 07	-1.3D - 07
		$BW^{3/4}$	0.10	0.000001	2.2D - 07	6.2D - 07	0.0D + 00	7.3D - 07	-5.4D - 07
		$BW^{2/3}$	0.10	0.000001	4.1D - 07	9.4D - 07	0.0D + 00	1.1D - 06	-3.8D - 07
SUBLINEAR (LDL) 0.225	M 0.8	Same	0.80	0.000346	1.8D - 10	8.1D - 10	6.3D - 16	1.3D - 07	-8.4D - 08
		$BW^{3/4}$	0.10	0.000043	2.1D - 09	1.1D - 08	1.4D - 13	4.1D - 07	-8.5D - 07
		$BW^{2/3}$	0.10	0.000043	5.1D - 09	2.8D - 08	2.1D - 14	7.3D - 07	-5.1D - 07
	M&B 0.2	Same	0.80	0.000086	9.8D - 08	2.9D - 07	1.5D - 15	3.5D - 07	-1.9D - 07
		$BW^{3/4}$	0.10	0.000011	3.9D - 07	1.1D - 06	2.8D - 13	1.3D - 06	-6.8D - 07
		$BW^{2/3}$	0.10	0.000011	7.1D - 07	1.6D - 06	1.8D - 12	2.0D - 06	-7.8D - 07
LINEAR 0.750	M 0.8	Same	0.80	0.001152	4.1D - 07	4.8D - 07	3.4D - 07	4.8D - 07	3.5D - 07
		$BW^{3/4}$	0.10	0.000144	1.5D - 06	1.8D - 06	1.3D - 06	1.8D - 06	1.3D - 06
		$BW^{2/3}$	0.10	0.000144	2.4D - 06	2.8D - 06	2.0D - 06	2.8D - 06	2.0D - 06
	M&B 0.2	Same	0.80	0.000288	4.6D - 07	5.2D - 07	3.9D - 07	5.4D - 07	3.9D - 07
		$BW^{3/4}$	0.10	0.000036	1.7D - 06	2.0D - 06	1.5D - 06	2.0D - 06	1.5D - 06
		$BW^{2/3}$	0.10	0.000036	2.7D - 06	3.1D - 06	2.3D - 06	3.1D - 06	2.3D - 06

Legend : See Table 1 for abbreviations. Also, BW = Body Weight; 2.5D - 04 = 2.5×10^{-4};
N/A = Not Applicable. Risk attributes refer to the added risk at one ppb.

Figure 7.5 The Weights, Maximum Likelihood Estimates, 95th and 5th Percentiles of the Nonparametric Bootstrap Distributions, and 95 Percent Upper and Lower Confidence Limits Using the Linearized Multistage Model Procedure for the Paths in the Decision Tree with Mode of Action Having Genotoxicity Involved but not Cell Proliferation.

HUMAN CARCINOGENIC HAZARD	MODE OF ACTION	DOSE SCALE	DOSE-RESPONSE MODEL	EXPERIMENTAL DATA SET	INTERSPECIES EXTRAPOLATION	WEIGHT ON PATH	MAXIMUM LIKELIHOOD ESTIMATE	95TH PERC. OF THE BOOTSTRAP DISTRIBUTION	5TH PERC. OF THE BOOTSTRAP DISTRIBUTION	95TH UPPER CONFIDENCE LIMIT	95TH LOWER CONFIDENCE LIMIT
HUMAN CARCINOGEN 0.8	SEE FIGURE 7.4 0.800	PPM 0.1	THRESHOLD 0.00	M 0.8	Same 0.20	0.0	0.0D + 00	0.0D + 00	0.0D + 00	N/A	N/A
					$BW^{3/4}$ 0.40	0.0	0.0D + 00	0.0D + 00	0.0D + 00	N/A	N/A
					$BW^{2/3}$ 0.40	0.0	0.0D + 00	0.0D + 00	0.0D + 00	N/A	N/A
				M&B 0.2	Same 0.20	0.0	0.0D + 00	0.0D + 00	0.0D + 00	N/A	N/A
					$BW^{3/4}$ 0.40	0.0	0.0D + 00	0.0D + 00	0.0D + 00	N/A	N/A
					$BW^{2/3}$ 0.40	0.0	0.0D + 00	0.0D + 00	0.0D + 00	N/A	N/A
			SUBLINEAR 0.50	M 0.8	Same 0.20	0.001248	5.5D - 18	6.3D - 14	0.0D + 00	2.2D - 06	-2.6D - 05
					$BW^{3/4}$ 0.40	0.002496	1.1D - 15	2.7D - 12	7.6D - 19	8.3D - 06	-8.3D - 05
					$BW^{2/3}$ 0.40	0.002496	3.6D - 14	1.1D - 11	7.7D - 18	1.3D - 05	-6.2D - 05
				M&B 0.2	Same 0.20	0.000312	5.5D - 06	1.2D - 05	0.0D + 00	1.2D - 05	-2.2D - 06
					$BW^{3/4}$ 0.40	0.000624	2.3D - 05	4.4D - 05	3.5D - 18	4.6D - 05	-6.2D - 06
					$BW^{2/3}$ 0.40	0.000624	4.2D - 05	7.1D - 05	4.7D - 15	7.3D - 05	-1.3D - 05
			SUBLINEAR (LDL) 0.50	M 0.8	Same 0.20	0.001248	6.4D - 09	6.5D - 08	1.0D - 09	2.2D - 06	-1.8D - 05
					$BW^{3/4}$ 0.40	0.002496	1.7D - 06	5.7D - 06	7.7D - 07	8.8D - 06	-2.4D - 05
					$BW^{2/3}$ 0.40	0.002496	1.2D - 05	2.8D - 05	7.0D - 06	2.9D - 05	-2.4D - 05
				M&B 0.2	Same 0.20	0.000312	5.5D - 06	1.2D - 05	1.5D - 09	1.2D - 05	-1.6D - 06
					$BW^{3/4}$ 0.40	0.000624	2.4D - 05	4.4D - 05	1.0D - 06	4.6D - 05	-3.8D - 08
					$BW^{2/3}$ 0.40	0.000624	4.8D - 05	7.6D - 05	1.0D - 05	7.7D - 05	6.0D - 06
			LINEAR 0.00	M 0.8	Same 0.20	0.0	2.9D - 05	3.4D - 05	2.5D - 05	3.4D - 05	2.5D - 05
					$BW^{3/4}$ 0.40	0.0	1.1D - 04	1.3D - 04	9.4D - 05	1.3D - 04	9.4D - 05
					$BW^{2/3}$ 0.40	0.0	1.7D - 04	2.0D - 04	1.5D - 04	2.0D - 04	1.5D - 04
				M&B 0.2	Same 0.20	0.0	3.4D - 05	3.8D - 05	2.9D - 05	3.9D - 05	2.9D - 05
					$BW^{3/4}$ 0.40	0.0	1.3D - 04	1.4D - 04	1.1D - 04	1.5D - 04	1.1D - 04
					$BW^{2/3}$ 0.40	0.0	2.0D - 04	2.2D - 04	1.7D - 04	2.3D - 04	1.7D - 04
	SEE FIGURE 7.5 0.005	INTAKE 0.3	THRESHOLD 0.00	M 0.8	Same 0.50	0.0	0.0D + 00	0.0D + 00	0.0D + 00	N/A	N/A
					$BW^{3/4}$ 0.25	0.0	0.0D + 00	0.0D + 00	0.0D + 00	N/A	N/A
					$BW^{2/3}$ 0.25	0.0	0.0D + 00	0.0D + 00	0.0D + 00	N/A	N/A
				M&B 0.2	Same 0.50	0.0	0.0D + 00	0.0D + 00	0.0D + 00	N/A	N/A
					$BW^{3/4}$ 0.25	0.0	0.0D + 00	0.0D + 00	0.0D + 00	N/A	N/A
					$BW^{2/3}$ 0.25	0.0	0.0D + 00	0.0D + 00	0.0D + 00	N/A	N/A
			SUBLINEAR 0.40	M 0.8	Same 0.50	0.007488	1.9D - 21	3.8D - 14	0.0D + 00	1.2D - 06	-1.5D - 05
					$BW^{3/4}$ 0.25	0.003744	1.4D - 18	1.5D - 13	1.2D - 18	4.5D - 06	-7.2D - 05
					$BW^{2/3}$ 0.25	0.003744	1.3D - 17	2.1D - 13	1.1D - 17	7.0D - 06	-9.5D - 05
				M&B 0.2	Same 0.50	0.001872	2.4D - 06	8.5D - 06	0.0D + 00	9.1D - 06	-3.8D - 06
					$BW^{3/4}$ 0.25	0.000936	9.1D - 06	3.2D - 05	0.0D + 00	3.4D - 05	-2.7D - 04
					$BW^{2/3}$ 0.25	0.000936	1.4D - 05	4.9D - 05	1.0D - 17	5.3D - 05	-1.8D - 04
				M 0.8	Same 0.50	0.011232	1.9D - 09	2.6D - 09	1.6D - 09	1.2D - 06	-1.4D - 05
					$BW^{3/4}$ 0.25	0.005616	1.4D - 06	1.7D - 06	1.2D - 06	5.9D - 06	-3.8D - 05
					$BW^{2/3}$ 0.25	0.005616	1.3D - 05	1.6D - 05	1.1D - 05	2.1D - 05	-3.8D - 05

NOT A HUMAN CARCINOGEN 0.2									
BOTH CELL PROLIFERATION AND GENOTOXICITY INVOLVED 0.195									
DPX 0.6									
SUBLINEAR (LDL) 0.60	M&B 0.2	Same 0.50	0.002808	2.4D - 06	8.4D - 06	1.7D - 09	9.0D - 06	-4.2D - 06	
		$BW^{3/4}$ 0.25	0.001404	1.0D - 05	3.3D - 05	1.2D - 06	3.5D - 05	-1.1D - 05	
		$BW^{2/3}$ 0.25	0.001404	2.6D - 05	6.1D - 05	1.1D - 05	6.2D - 05	-8.0D - 06	
LINEAR 0.00	M 0.8	Same 0.50	0.0	2.9D - 05	3.4D - 05	2.5D - 05	3.4D - 05	2.5D - 05	
		$BW^{3/4}$ 0.25	0.0	1.1D - 04	1.3D - 04	9.5D - 05	1.3D - 04	9.4D - 05	
		$BW^{2/3}$ 0.25	0.0	1.7D - 04	2.0D - 04	1.5D - 04	2.0D - 04	1.5D - 04	
	M&B 0.2	Same 0.50	0.0	3.4D - 05	3.8D - 05	2.9D - 05	3.9D - 05	2.9D - 05	
		$BW^{3/4}$ 0.25	0.0	1.3D - 04	1.4D - 04	1.1D - 04	1.5D - 04	1.1D - 04	
		$BW^{2/3}$ 0.25	0.0	2.0D - 04	2.2D - 04	1.7D - 04	2.3D - 04	1.7D - 04	
THRESHOLD 0.0000	M 0.8	Same 0.80	0.0	0.0D + 00	0.0D + 00	0.0D + 00	N/A	N/A	
		$BW^{3/4}$ 0.10	0.0	0.0D + 00	0.0D + 00	0.0D + 00	N/A	N/A	
		$BW^{2/3}$ 0.10	0.0	0.0D + 00	0.0D + 00	0.0D + 00	N/A	N/A	
	M&B 0.2	Same 0.80	0.0	0.0D + 00	0.0D + 00	0.0D + 00	N/A	N/A	
		$BW^{3/4}$ 0.10	0.0	0.0D + 00	0.0D + 00	0.0D + 00	N/A	N/A	
		$BW^{2/3}$ 0.10	0.0	0.0D + 00	0.0D + 00	0.0D + 00	N/A	N/A	
SUBLINEAR 0.1875	M 0.8	Same 0.80	0.011322	5.8D - 14	2.7D - 13	0.0D + 00	6.9D - 08	-1.4D - 07	
		$BW^{3/4}$ 0.10	0.001404	6.7D - 13	3.7D - 12	0.0D + 00	2.7D - 07	-1.9D - 07	
		$BW^{2/3}$ 0.10	0.001404	1.6D - 12	9.1D - 12	0.0D + 00	4.2D - 07	-8.8D - 07	
	M&B 0.2	Same 0.80	0.002808	5.6D - 08	1.7D - 07	0.0D + 00	2.0D - 07	-1.3D - 07	
		$BW^{3/4}$ 0.10	0.000351	2.2D - 07	6.2D - 07	0.0D + 00	7.3D - 07	-5.4D - 07	
		$BW^{2/3}$ 0.10	0.000351	4.1D - 07	9.4D - 07	0.0D + 00	1.1D - 06	-3.8D - 07	
SUBLINEAR (LDL) 0.8125	M 0.8	Same 0.80	0.048672	1.8D - 10	8.1D - 10	6.3D - 16	1.3D - 07	-8.4D - 08	
		$BW^{3/4}$ 0.10	0.006084	2.1D - 09	1.1D - 08	1.4D - 13	4.1D - 07	-8.5D - 07	
		$BW^{2/3}$ 0.10	0.006084	5.1D - 09	2.8D - 08	2.1D - 14	7.3D - 07	-5.1D - 07	
	M&B 0.2	Same 0.80	0.012168	9.8D - 08	2.9D - 07	1.5D - 15	3.5D - 07	-1.9D - 07	
		$BW^{3/4}$ 0.10	0.001521	3.9D - 07	1.1D - 06	2.8D - 13	1.3D - 06	-6.8D - 07	
		$BW^{2/3}$ 0.10	0.001521	7.1D - 07	1.6D - 06	1.8D - 12	2.0D - 06	-7.8D - 07	
LINEAR 0.0000	M 0.8	Same 0.80	0.0	4.1D - 07	4.8D - 07	3.4D - 07	4.8D - 07	3.5D - 07	
		$BW^{3/4}$ 0.10	0.0	1.5D - 06	1.8D - 06	1.3D - 06	1.8D - 06	1.3D - 06	
		$BW^{2/3}$ 0.10	0.0	2.4D - 06	2.8D - 06	2.0D - 06	2.8D - 06	2.0D - 06	
	M&B 0.2	Same 0.80	0.0	4.6D - 07	5.2D - 07	3.9D - 07	5.4D - 07	3.9D - 07	
		$BW^{3/4}$ 0.10	0.0	1.7D - 06	2.0D - 06	1.5D - 06	2.0D - 06	1.5D - 06	
		$BW^{2/3}$ 0.10	0.0	2.7D - 06	3.1D - 06	2.3D - 06	3.1D - 06	2.3D - 06	

Legend: See Table 1 for abbreviations. Also, BW = Body Weight; 2.5D - 04 = 2.5×10^{-4}.
N/A = Not Applicable. Risk attributes refer to the added risk at one ppb.

Figure 7.6 The Weights, Maximum Likelihood Estimates, 95th and 5th Percentiles of the Nonparametric Bootstrap Distributions, and 95 Percent Upper and Lower Confidence Limits Using the Linearized Multistage Model Procedure for the Paths in the Decision Tree with Mode of Action Having Both Cell Proliferation and Genotoxicity Involved.

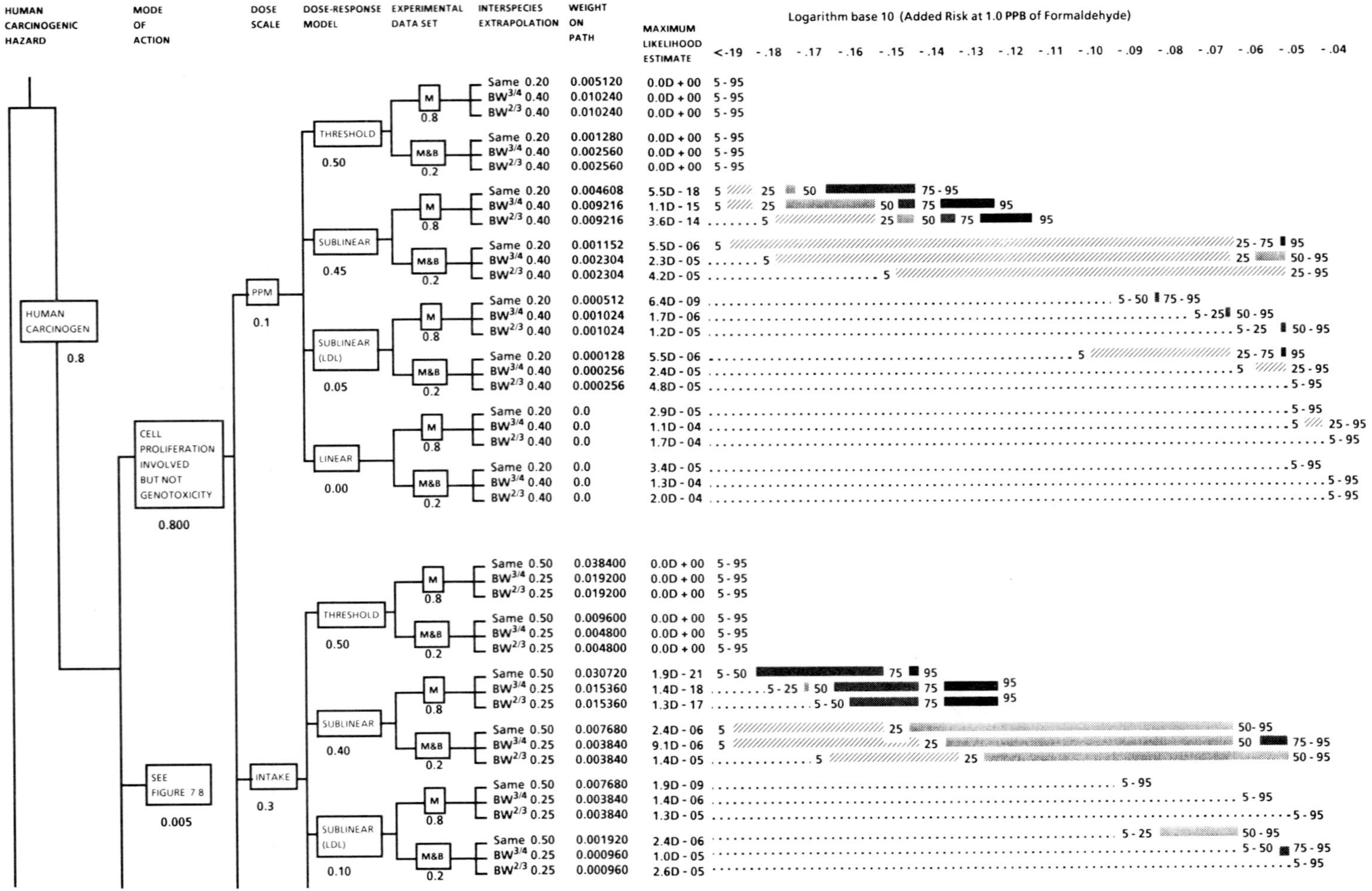
HUMAN CARCINOGENIC HAZARD
MODE OF ACTION
DOSE SCALE
DOSE-RESPONSE MODEL
EXPERIMENTAL DATA SET
INTERSPECIES EXTRAPOLATION
WEIGHT ON PATH
MAXIMUM LIKELIHOOD ESTIMATE
Logarithm base 10 (Added Risk at 1.0 PPB of Formaldehyde)
<-19 -.18 -.17 -.16 -.15 -.14 -.13 -.12 -.11 -.10 -.09 -.08 -.07 -.06 -.05 -.04
HUMAN CARCINOGEN
0.8
CELL PROLIFERATION INVOLVED BUT NOT GENOTOXICITY
0.800
SEE FIGURE 7 8
0.005
PPM
0.1
INTAKE
0.3
THRESHOLD
0.50
SUBLINEAR
0.45
SUBLINEAR (LDL)
0.05
LINEAR
0.00
THRESHOLD
0.50
SUBLINEAR
0.40
SUBLINEAR (LDL)
0.10
M
0.8
M&B
0.2
Same 0.20 0.005120 0.0D+00 5-95
BW3/4 0.40 0.010240 0.0D+00 5-95
BW2/3 0.40 0.010240 0.0D+00 5-95
Same 0.20 0.001280 0.0D+00 5-95
BW3/4 0.40 0.002560 0.0D+00 5-95
BW2/3 0.40 0.002560 0.0D+00 5-95
Same 0.20 0.004608 5.5D-18 5 25 50 75-95
BW3/4 0.40 0.009216 1.1D-15 5 25 50 75 95
BW2/3 0.40 0.009216 3.6D-14 5 25 50 75 95
Same 0.20 0.001152 5.5D-06 5 25-75 95
BW3/4 0.40 0.002304 2.3D-05 5 25 50-95
BW2/3 0.40 0.002304 4.2D-05 5 25-95
Same 0.20 0.000512 6.4D-09 5-50 75-95
BW3/4 0.40 0.001024 1.7D-06 5-25 50-95
BW2/3 0.40 0.001024 1.2D-05 5-25 50-95
Same 0.20 0.000128 5.5D-06 5 25-75 95
BW3/4 0.40 0.000256 2.4D-05 5 25-95
BW2/3 0.40 0.000256 4.8D-05 5-95
Same 0.20 0.0 2.9D-05 5-95
BW3/4 0.40 0.0 1.1D-04 5 25-95
BW2/3 0.40 0.0 1.7D-04 5-95
Same 0.20 0.0 3.4D-05 5-95
BW3/4 0.40 0.0 1.3D-04 5-95
BW2/3 0.40 0.0 2.0D-04 5-95
Same 0.50 0.038400 0.0D+00 5-95
BW3/4 0.25 0.019200 0.0D+00 5-95
BW2/3 0.25 0.019200 0.0D+00 5-95
Same 0.50 0.009600 0.0D+00 5-95
BW3/4 0.25 0.004800 0.0D+00 5-95
BW2/3 0.25 0.004800 0.0D+00 5-95
Same 0.50 0.030720 1.9D-21 5-50 75 95
BW3/4 0.25 0.015360 1.4D-18 5-25 50 75 95
BW2/3 0.25 0.015360 1.3D-17 5-50 75 95
Same 0.50 0.007680 2.4D-06 5 25 50-95
BW3/4 0.25 0.003840 9.1D-06 5 25 50 75-95
BW2/3 0.25 0.003840 1.4D-05 5 25 50-95
Same 0.50 0.007680 1.9D-09 5-95
BW3/4 0.25 0.003840 1.4D-06 5-95
BW2/3 0.25 0.003840 1.3D-05 5-95
Same 0.50 0.001920 2.4D-06 5-25 50-95
BW3/4 0.25 0.000960 1.0D-05 5-50 75-95
BW2/3 0.25 0.000960 2.6D-05 5-95

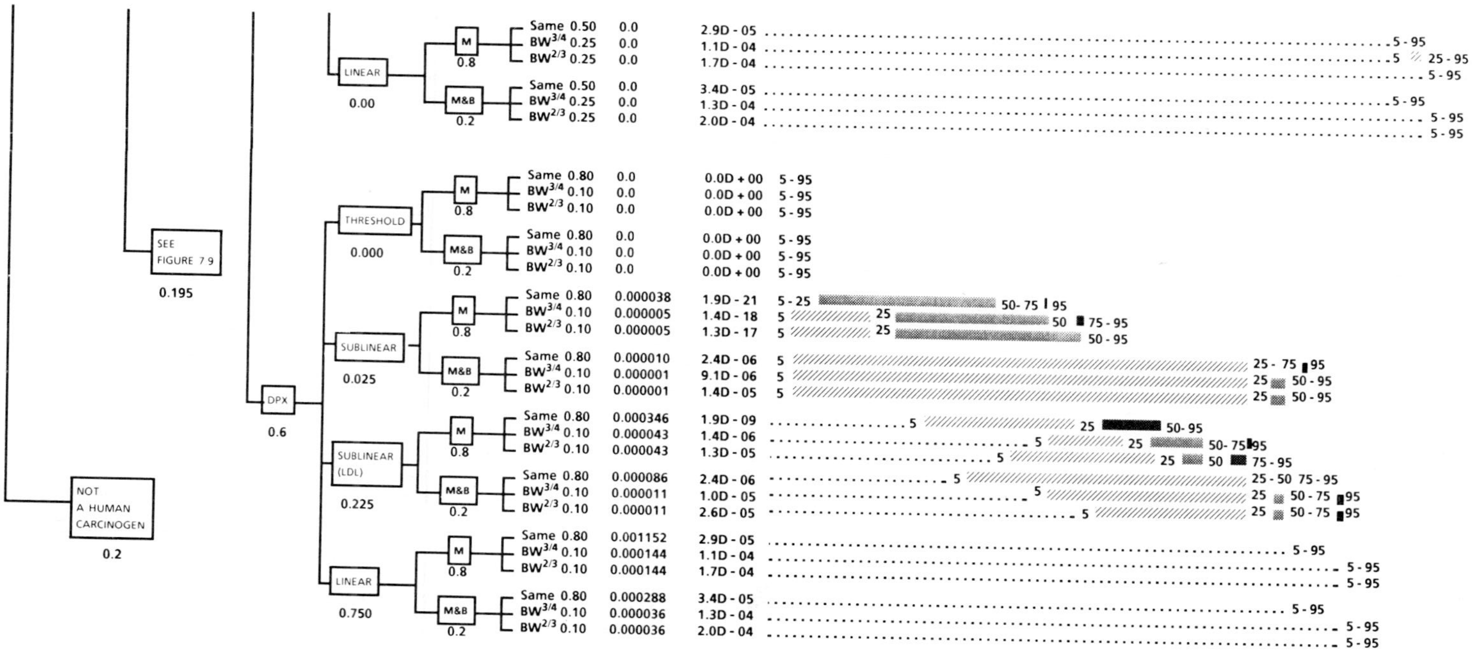

Legend: See Table 1 for abbreviations. Also, BW = Body Weight; 2.5D - 04 = 2.5×10^{-4}.
Risk attributes refer to the added risk at one ppb.

Figure 7.7 The Weights, Maximum Likelihood Estimates, and Percentiles of the Nonparametric Bootstrap Distributions for the Paths in the Decision Tree with Mode of Action Having Cell Proliferation Involved but not Genotoxicity.

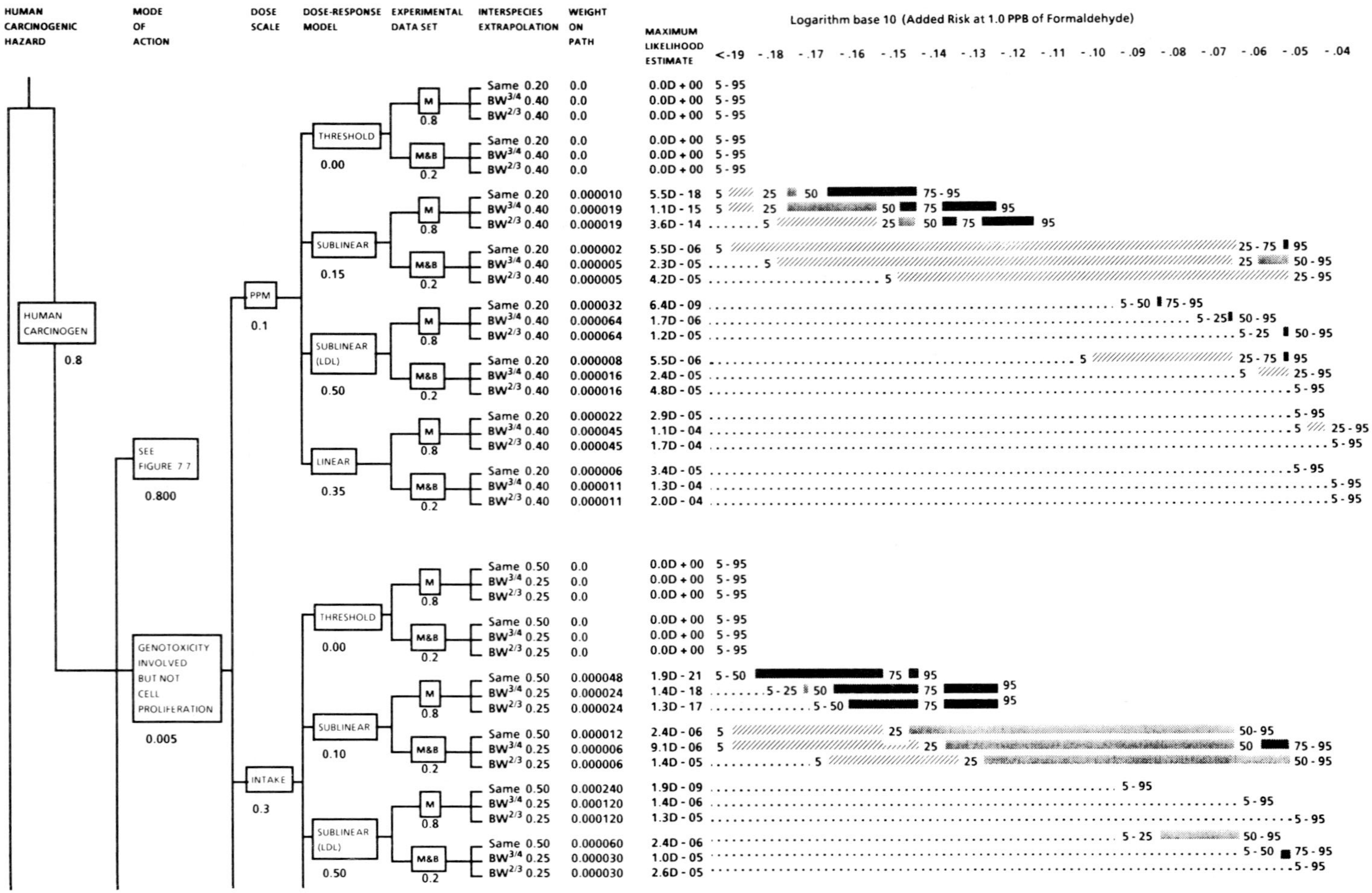

HUMAN CARCINOGENIC HAZARD
MODE OF ACTION
DOSE SCALE
DOSE-RESPONSE MODEL
EXPERIMENTAL DATA SET
INTERSPECIES EXTRAPOLATION
WEIGHT ON PATH
MAXIMUM LIKELIHOOD ESTIMATE
Logarithm base 10 (Added Risk at 1.0 PPB of Formaldehyde)
<-19 -.18 -.17 -.16 -.15 -.14 -.13 -.12 -.11 -.10 -.09 -.08 -.07 -.06 -.05 -.04
HUMAN CARCINOGEN
0.8
SEE FIGURE 7.7
0.800
GENOTOXICITY INVOLVED BUT NOT CELL PROLIFERATION
0.005
PPM
0.1
INTAKE
0.3
THRESHOLD
0.00
SUBLINEAR
0.15
SUBLINEAR (LDL)
0.50
LINEAR
0.35
SUBLINEAR
0.10
M
0.8
M&B
0.2
Same 0.20 0.0 0.0D+00 5-95
BW3/4 0.40 0.0 0.0D+00 5-95
BW2/3 0.40 0.0 0.0D+00 5-95
Same 0.20 0.0 0.0D+00 5-95
BW3/4 0.40 0.0 0.0D+00 5-95
BW2/3 0.40 0.0 0.0D+00 5-95
Same 0.20 0.000010 5.5D-18 5 25 50 75-95
BW3/4 0.40 0.000019 1.1D-15 5 25 50 75 95
BW2/3 0.40 0.000019 3.6D-14 5 25 50 75 95
Same 0.20 0.000002 5.5D-06 5 25-75 95
BW3/4 0.40 0.000005 2.3D-05 5 25 50-95
BW2/3 0.40 0.000005 4.2D-05 5 25-95
Same 0.20 0.000032 6.4D-09 5-50 75-95
BW3/4 0.40 0.000064 1.7D-06 5-25 50-95
BW2/3 0.40 0.000064 1.2D-05 5-25 50-95
Same 0.20 0.000008 5.5D-06 5 25-75 95
BW3/4 0.40 0.000016 2.4D-05 5 25-95
BW2/3 0.40 0.000016 4.8D-05 5-95
Same 0.20 0.000022 2.9D-05 5-95
BW3/4 0.40 0.000045 1.1D-04 5 25-95
BW2/3 0.40 0.000045 1.7D-04 5-95
Same 0.20 0.000006 3.4D-05 5-95
BW3/4 0.40 0.000011 1.3D-04 5-95
BW2/3 0.40 0.000011 2.0D-04 5-95
Same 0.50 0.0 0.0D+00 5-95
BW3/4 0.25 0.0 0.0D+00 5-95
BW2/3 0.25 0.0 0.0D+00 5-95
Same 0.50 0.0 0.0D+00 5-95
BW3/4 0.25 0.0 0.0D+00 5-95
BW2/3 0.25 0.0 0.0D+00 5-95
Same 0.50 0.000048 1.9D-21 5-50 75 95
BW3/4 0.25 0.000024 1.4D-18 5-25 50 75 95
BW2/3 0.25 0.000024 1.3D-17 5-50 75 95
Same 0.50 0.000012 2.4D-06 5 25 50-95
BW3/4 0.25 0.000006 9.1D-06 5 25 50 75-95
BW2/3 0.25 0.000006 1.4D-05 5 25 50-95
Same 0.50 0.000240 1.9D-09 5-95
BW3/4 0.25 0.000120 1.4D-06 5-95
BW2/3 0.25 0.000120 1.3D-05 5-95
Same 0.50 0.000060 2.4D-06 5-25 50-95
BW3/4 0.25 0.000030 1.0D-05 5-50 75-95
BW2/3 0.25 0.000030 2.6D-05 5-95

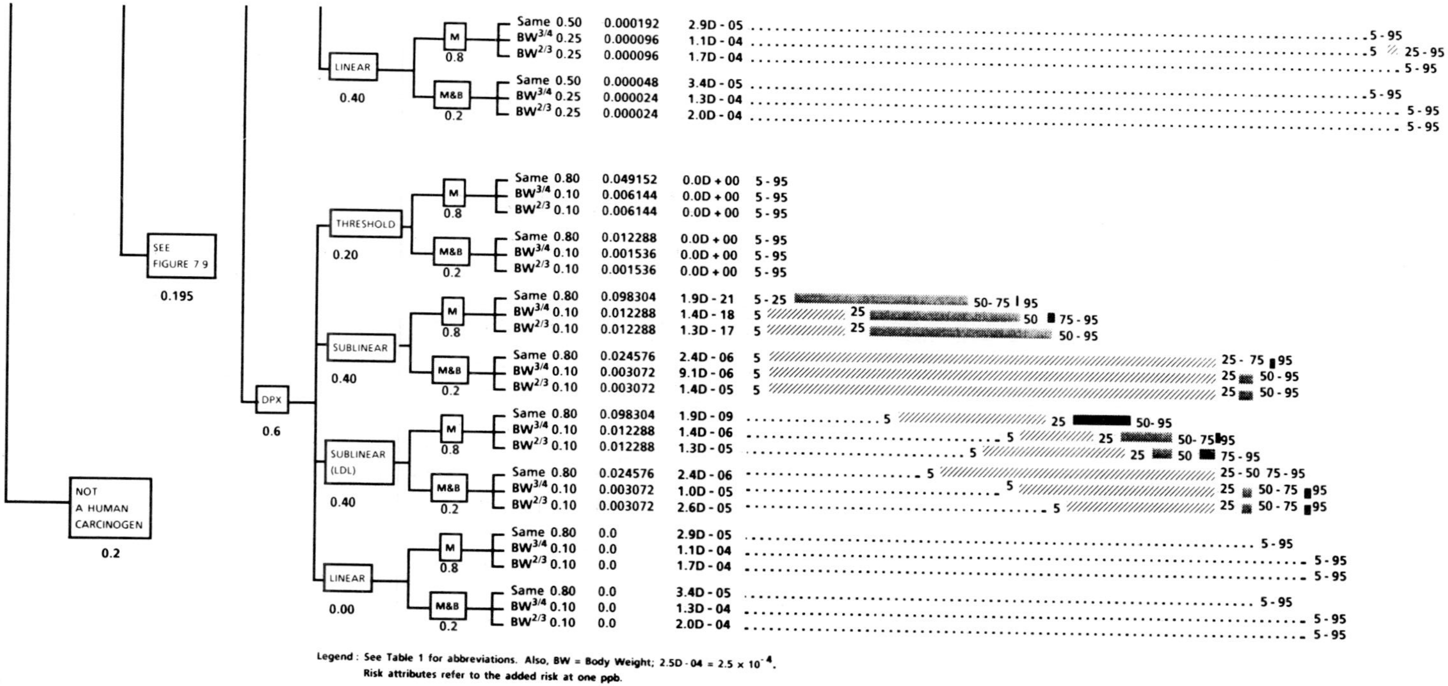

Figure 7.8 The Weights, Maximum Likelihood Estimates, and Percentiles of the Nonparametric Bootstrap Distributions for the Paths in the Decision Tree with Mode of Action Having Genotoxicity Involved but not Cell Proliferation.

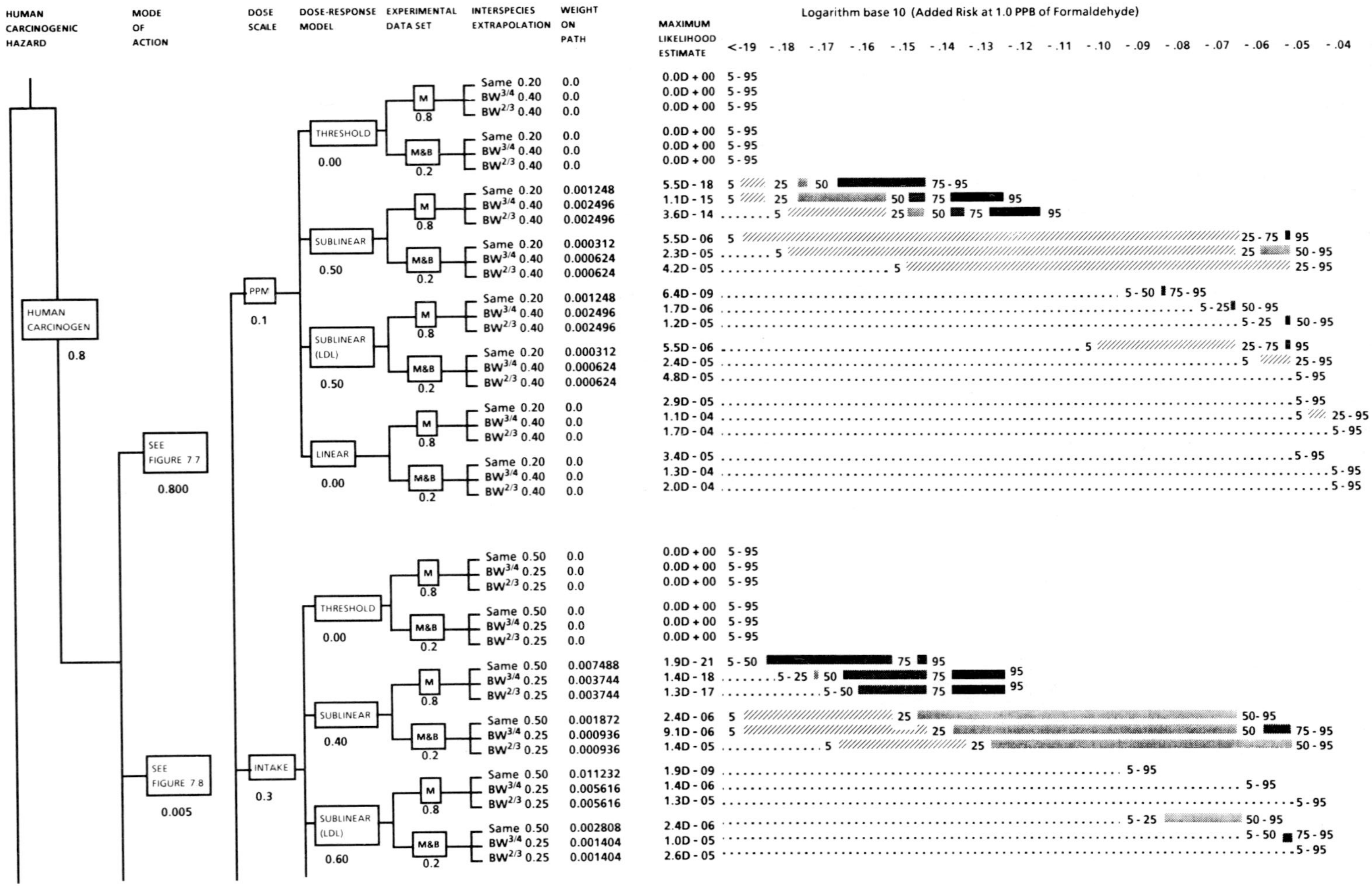
HUMAN CARCINOGENIC HAZARD
MODE OF ACTION
DOSE SCALE
DOSE-RESPONSE MODEL
EXPERIMENTAL DATA SET
INTERSPECIES EXTRAPOLATION
WEIGHT ON PATH
MAXIMUM LIKELIHOOD ESTIMATE
Logarithm base 10 (Added Risk at 1.0 PPB of Formaldehyde)
<-19 -.18 -.17 -.16 -.15 -.14 -.13 -.12 -.11 -.10 -.09 -.08 -.07 -.06 -.05 -.04
HUMAN CARCINOGEN
0.8
SEE FIGURE 7 7
0.800
SEE FIGURE 7 8
0.005
PPM
0.1
INTAKE
0.3
THRESHOLD
0.00
SUBLINEAR
0.50
SUBLINEAR (LDL)
0.50
LINEAR
0.00
THRESHOLD
0.00
SUBLINEAR
0.40
SUBLINEAR (LDL)
0.60
M
0.8
M&B
0.2
Same 0.20
BW3/4 0.40
BW2/3 0.40
Same 0.50
BW3/4 0.25
BW2/3 0.25
0.0
0.001248
0.002496
0.000312
0.000624
0.007488
0.003744
0.001872
0.000936
0.011232
0.005616
0.002808
0.001404
0.0D+00
5.5D-18
1.1D-15
3.6D-14
5.5D-06
2.3D-05
4.2D-05
6.4D-09
1.7D-06
1.2D-05
2.4D-05
4.8D-05
2.9D-05
1.1D-04
1.7D-04
3.4D-05
1.3D-04
2.0D-04
1.9D-21
1.4D-18
1.3D-17
2.4D-06
9.1D-06
1.4D-05
1.9D-09
1.4D-06
1.3D-05
1.0D-05
2.6D-05

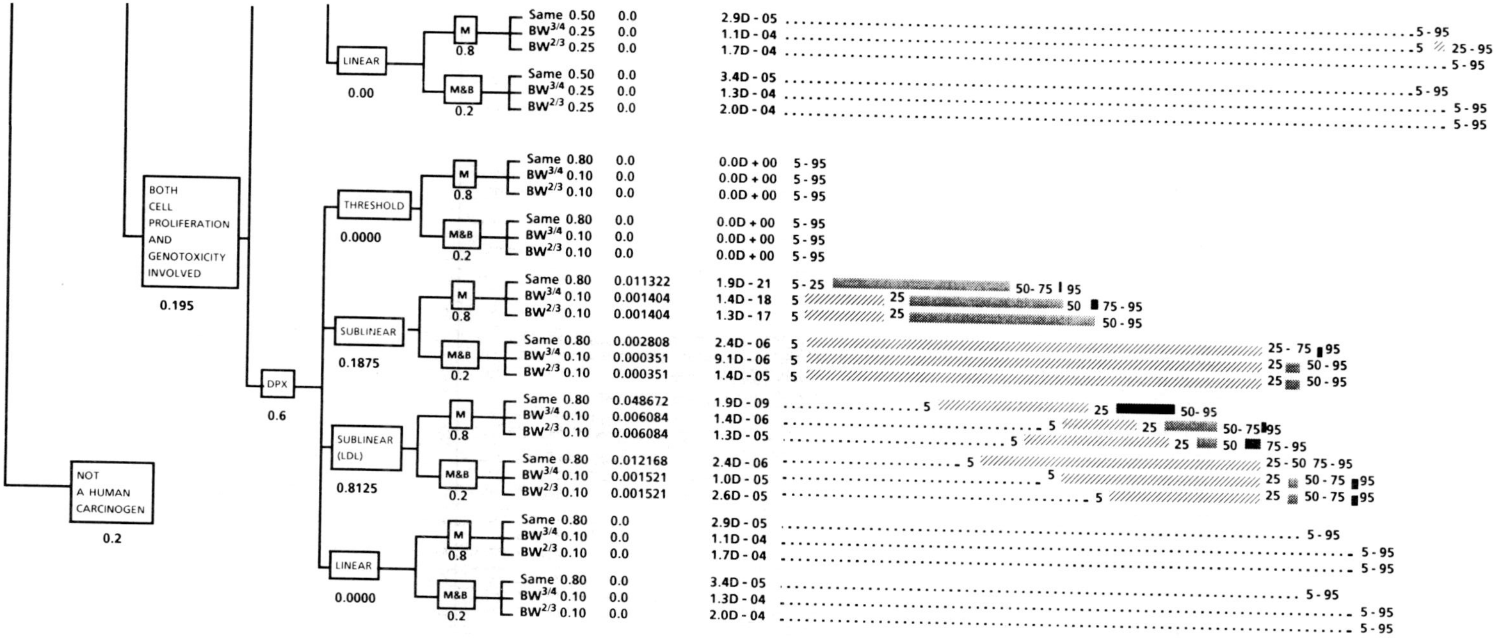

Legend: See Table 1 for abbreviations. Also, BW = Body Weight; 2.5D - 04 = 2.5×10^{-4}
Risk attributes refer to the added risk at one ppb.

Figure 7.9 The Weights, Maximum Likelihood Estimates, and Percentiles of the Nonparametric Bootstrap Distributions for the Paths in the Decision Tree with Mode of Having Both Cell Proliferation and Genotoxicity Involved.

threshold like shapes. The five-stage multistage model is used to describe sublinear shapes (convex curves). Sublinear shapes that are modified to be low-dose linear are referred to herein as *sublinear and low-dose linear* or *sublinear (LDL)* and are described by the five-stage multistage model shape above 1 *ppm* and a straight line interpolation between the response rates at 1 *ppm* and 0 *ppm*. The one-hit model (or, equivalently, the one-stage multistage model) is used to dose-response relationships that are essentially linear at all doses.

Each of these four alternative dose-response models is considered in conjunction with each combination of the three modes of action and the three alternative dose scales.

Factor 5. Experimental Data Set

As indicated in Section 7.4, the bioassay data used explicitly in this information analysis to quantify the human dose-response relationship are the CIIT rat formaldehyde inhalation study data. The responses in that study that have been analyzed in the context of human formaldehyde inhalation exposures are (1) malignant squamous cell carcinoma and (2) malignant squamous cell carcinoma or benign polypoid adenoma. These two responses in the rat nasal cavity are the two alternatives for the *specified carcinogenic response* in the dose-response model of the probability of a *specified carcinogenic response*. (There has been considerable debate about the appropriateness of considering the benign polypoid adenomas, but that debate will not be explicitly explored here.[47,48,63,64])

Each of these two alternative experimental data sets is evaluated for each combination of the alternatives for mode of action, dose scale, and dose-response model.

Factor 6. Interspecies Extrapolation

When formaldehyde is assumed to be a human carcinogen and a particular combination of mode of action, dose scale, dose-response model, and experimental data set is being evaluated, three methods of extrapolating the dose-response relationship in rats to a dose-response relationship in humans have been predominantly discussed. These methods of interspecies extrapolation attempt to reflect interspecies differences not already captured in the dose scale being used for dose-response modeling. One method is to assume that the probability of a carcinogenic response in humans at a specified dose is the same as it is in rats at that same dose. The other two methods of interspecies extrapolation that have been considered are *default* methods that assume the human and rat response probabilities are equal when the dose in humans is $\{[\text{rat body weight}]/[\text{human body weight}]\}^{1/4}$ times the dose in rats or equal when the dose in humans is $\{[\text{rat body weight}]/[\text{human body weight}]\}^{1/3}$ times the dose in rats. The former method is sometimes described as the best (default) regression estimate or $BW^{3/4}$ ($[\text{body weight}]^{3/4}$) equivalence. The latter method is usually described as surface area equivalence or $BW^{2/3}$($[\text{body weight}]^{2/3}$) equivalence.

Each of these three alternative methods of interspecies extrapolation is evaluated for each combination of the alternatives for mode of action, dose scale, dose-response model, and experimental data set.

7.4.2 Risk Attribute

When each combination of alternatives for the six major Factors in the formaldehyde dose-response characterization is evaluated, the specified dose-response feature (the increased risk at a particular dose or the slope of a straight line extrapolation from the risk at a particular starting dose back to the risk at dose zero) can be described in several alternative ways. These alternative descriptions are referred to as *risk attributes*.[26] Alternative risk attributes include maximum likelihood estimates, upper bounds, lower bounds, ranges, and bootstrap distributions. Examples of these risk attributes are given in Figures 7.4 through 7.9.

Maximum likelihood estimates can be generated for any dose-response model (Figures 7.4 through 7.6).

Upper bounds for the multistage model can be determined using a linearized multistage model (Figures 7.4 through 7.6). A technique analogous to that used to determine the upper bounds in the linearized multistage model can be used to determine lower bounds on the risk for the multistage model (Figures 7.4 through 7.6) as described below Equation (3.31) of Chapter 3. These bounds are usually determined to be 95 percent confidence limits. Confidence levels other than 95 percent are seldom used but could be. Several confidence limit procedures have been suggested for quantal response models other than the multistage model. However, none of these confidence limit procedures has been universally adopted.

Nonparametric bootstrap procedures (described in Chapter 3) can be used to describe the impact of experimental variability on the maximum likelihood estimation procedure for any dose-response model. In Figures 7.4 through 7.6 the 95th and 5th percentiles of a nonparametric bootstrap procedure are used as upper and lower bounds on risk and provide a range of estimates. However, the entire nonparametric bootstrap distribution provides more information than its 95th percentile, 5th percentile, or resultant range because the entire distribution indicates the relative likelihoods of the different risk values including the values in the range between the percentile bounds. Figures 7.7 through 7.9 indicate the maximum likelihood estimate and the 5, 25, 50, 75, and 95th percentiles of the nonparametric bootstrap distribution for each path in the decision tree. For example, for any mode of action, if the dose scale is *ppm*, the dose-response model is sublinear and modified to be low-dose linear, the experimental data set is malignant squamous cell carcinomas, and the method of interspecies extrapolation is to assume the same dose-response relationship in rats and humans, then the maximum likelihood estimate of the added risk at 1 *ppb* is 6.4×10^{-9} and the 5, 25, and 50th percentiles of the bootstrap distribution of the added risk at 1 *ppb* of formaldehyde are between 10^{-9} and 10^{-8} while the 75 and 95th percentiles are between 10^{-8} and 10^{-7}.

Starting Point for Linear Extrapolation

It would be most appropriate to evaluate and present the risk attributes for each specific dose level of interest. For example, if 0.001 *ppm*, 0.01 *ppm*, 0.1 *ppm*, and 1.0 were all of interest, then the risk attributes in the decision tree should be evaluated and reported separately for each of these four concentration levels. Unfortunately, instead of characterizing the dose-response information separately for dose levels of different magnitudes, it frequently happens that the characterization of the dose-response relationship is oversimplified, and the only aspect of the dose-response relationship that is characterized is the *slope* of the straight line between the probability of the specified carcinogenic response at dose zero and the probability at some other specified dose.

This slope is commonly referred to as the *cancer potency* and is interpreted as an upper bound on the added cancer risk (or, sometimes, extra risk) per unit concentration.

The current emphasis on the *slope* of the added risk is a (much debated) holdover from the early assumption that all cancer dose-response relationships are linear in the low-dose region, or that a straight line provides an upper bound on the low-dose risk that is sufficient for risk assessment purposes.

The *other specified dose* in the definition of the slope or cancer potency is usually referred to as the *starting point for linear extrapolation.* (Technically, the phenomenon is usually linear *interpolation* as opposed to linear *extrapolation* because the zero dose or control level is included in the experiment.)

The starting point for any linear extrapolation should be near the exposure levels at which inferences are to be made. Herein, the example decision tree refers to 1 *ppb*. In Figures 7.4 through 7.9, the characterizations of the added cancer risk at 1 *ppb* are also characterizations of the cancer slope or cancer potency when the starting point for the linear extrapolation is 1 *ppb*. These characterizations pertain only to doses near 1 *ppb* and do *not* necessarily apply to doses much smaller or larger than 1 *ppb*.

In the decision tree for formaldehyde, one alternative for the dose-response model is a five-stage multistage model that is modified to be linear below 1 *ppm*. The choice of a starting point (1 *ppm* in the decision tree) for an assumed linear portion of a dose-response model is different than the choice of 1 *ppb* as the dose level for dose-response characterization. The former choice is based on an interpretation of the underlying carcinogenic mechanisms potentially associated with formaldehyde and the concentration level at which those mechanisms might lead to a linear dose-response relationship. The latter choice is based on the desire to characterize the risks when the exposure concentrations are near 0.001 *ppm*. If, in addition, the risks for concentrations near 0.1 *ppm* were also to be quantified, then a separate evaluation and presentation of the risk attributes for 0.1 *ppm* would have also been presented.

7.4.3 Weighted Frequencies of Decision Tree Outcomes

The state of knowledge concerning the added cancer risk at 1 *ppb* of formaldehyde can be communicated in at least two ways. One form of communication is to present the individual quantitative outcomes of the combinations of alternatives for the dose-response Factors. These outcomes can be explicitly presented in any one of several convenient formats such as in Figures 7.4 through 7.9. Another presentation format is a user-friendly display on a personal computer.

A second means of communicating the state of knowledge concerning the added risk at 1 *ppb* of formaldehyde is the weighted frequencies of the decision tree outcomes. This is generally the primary and most convenient information-analysis based dose-response characterization.

A very simple example of this form of communication is given in Figure 7.10. In this example, a horse racing fan is considering a \$2 bet on a horse with four-to-one odds in a race. The fan decides that his strategy is to flip a coin. If the coin lands tails up, then he will bet, and, if the coin lands heads up, then he will not bet. If the probability that the horse wins is really 0.2 and loses is 0.8, then the decision tree is as shown in Figure 7.10. The three possible decision tree outcomes are as follows:

1. Bet and horse wins with combined probability 0.1 (0.5×0.2) and outcome \$8 in his pocket.
2. Bet and horse loses with combined probability 0.4 (0.5×0.8) and outcome \$0 in his pocket.
3. No bet with probability 0.5 and outcome \$2 in his pocket.

The probability distribution of the decision tree outcomes is also shown in Figure 7.10. The probability density function (pdf) indicates the probability that the outcome has a particular value, and the cumulative distribution function (cdf) indicates the probability that the outcome does not exceed a particular value. For example, the pdf at \$2 is 0.5, and the cdf at \$2 is 0.9 ($0.5 + 0.4$). The pdf and cdf both convey the same information but in different formats.

An example is presented in Figure 7.11 of the formaldehyde dose-response characterization consisting of the probability distribution on the added cancer risk at 1 *ppb* corresponding to the weighted frequencies of the decision tree outcomes. In Figure 7.11, the risk attribute describing the outcome of each path in the decision tree is the maximum likelihood estimate. The probability distribution is shown in both a probability density function (pdf) form and a cumulative distribution function (cdf) form. For example, in the top portion of the figure, the pdf indicates that the probability that the added risk at 1 ppb is between 0.0000001 (1×10^{-7}) and 0.000001 (1×10^{-6}) is 0.0175 (1.75 percent of the total weight is on maximum likelihood estimates between 0.0000001 and 0.000001). In the bottom portion of the figure, the cdf indicates that the probability that the added risk at 1 *ppb* is less

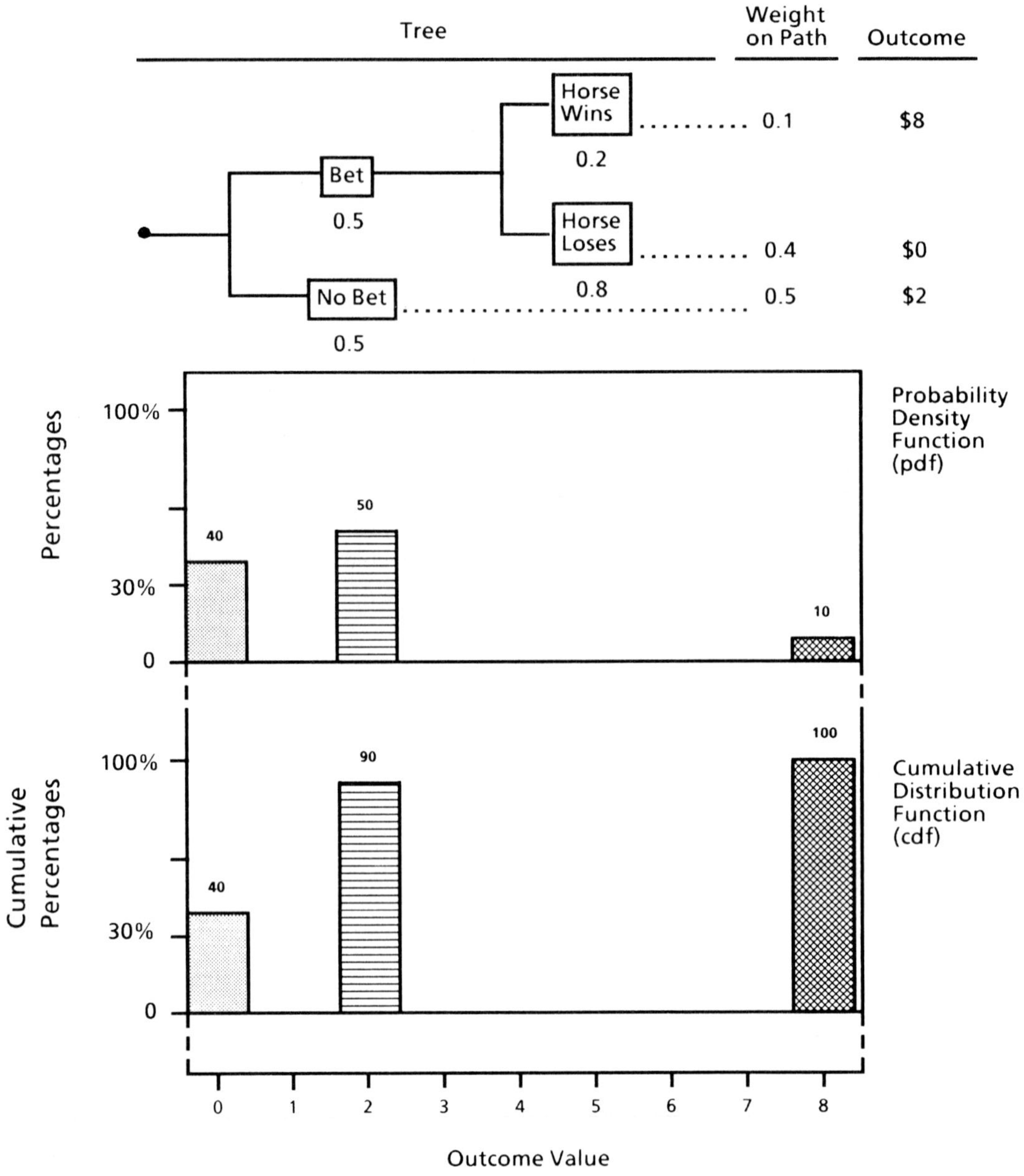

Figure 7.10 A Simple Example of a Decision Tree, the Weights on its Paths, the Outcome of Each Path, and the Outcome's Probability Density Function (pdf) and Cumulative Distribution Function (cdf).

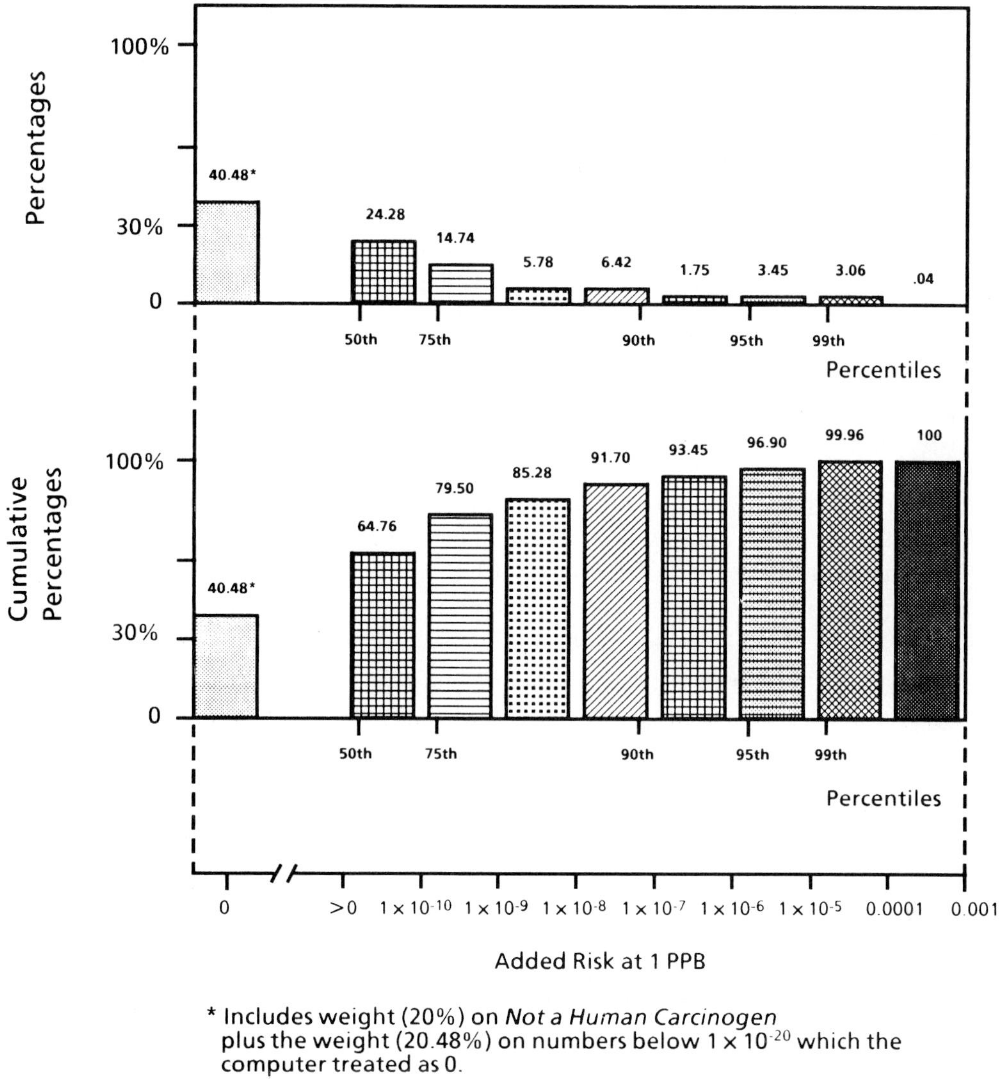

Figure 7.11 Weighted Frequencies of the Maximum Likelihood Estimates from the Decision Tree for Added Risk at one *ppb* for Formaldehyde.

than 0.000001 (1 in a million) is 0.9345 (93.45 percent of the total weight is on maximum likelihood estimates less than 0.000001). Both the pdf and cdf have equivalent information content. The sensitivity of the probability distribution to the decision tree weights and the risk attribute is discussed in Section 7.4.5

The information-analysis distribution exemplified in Figure 7.11 reflects each decision tree outcome. Because the different alternatives for the dose-response Factors may not be equally relevant or have the same scientific support, the decision tree outcomes are weighted with the combinations of alternatives having more scientific support being given more weight. Thus, the information-analysis distribution is a quantitative weight-of-evidence dose-response characterization.

For a particular set of weights, the information-analysis distribution is determined as follows. The range of possible dose-response characteristics is partitioned into convenient nonoverlapping intervals. For example, in Figure 7.11, the range of added cancer risks is partitioned into the following nine intervals:

1. ≤ 0; that is, outcomes indicating that formaldehyde is not a human carcinogen at the doses to which humans are expected to be exposed and outcomes where the added risk is characterized as less than 1×10^{-20} which the computer treated as zero.
2. $(0, 1 \times 10^{-10}]$; that is, outcomes indicating the added risk to be greater than zero (1×10^{-20}) and less than or equal to 1×10^{-10}.
3. $(1 \times 10^{-10}, 1 \times 10^{-9}]$; that is, outcomes indicating the added risk to be greater than 0.0000000001 and less than or equal to 0.000000001.
4. $(1 \times 10^{-9}, 1 \times 10^{-8}]$; that is, outcomes indicating the added risk to be greater than 0.000000001 and less than or equal to 0.00000001.
5. $(1 \times 10^{-8}, 1 \times 10^{-7}]$; that is, outcomes indicating the added risk to be greater than 0.00000001 and less than or equal to 0.0000001.
6. $(1 \times 10^{-7}, 1 \times 10^{-6}]$; that is, outcomes indicating the added risk to be greater than 0.0000001 and less than or equal to 0.000001.
7. $(1 \times 10^{-6}, 1 \times 10^{-5}]$; that is, outcomes indicating the added risk to be greater than 0.000001 and less than or equal to 0.00001.
8. $(1 \times 10^{-5}, 1 \times 10^{-4}]$; that is, outcomes indicating the added risk to be greater than 0.00001 and less than or equal to 0.0001.
9. $(1 \times 10^{-4}, 1 \times 10^{-3}]$; that is, outcomes indicating the added risk to be greater than 0.0001 and less than or equal to 0.001.

The sum of the weights associated with decision tree outcomes in each interval is calculated. In Figure 7.11, these sums are expressed as a percentage of the total weight. Because the total weight for all decision tree outcomes equals 1.0, the sum of weights associated with decision tree outcomes in an interval can be interpreted as the probability that the dose-response characteristic is in that interval. Thus, the information-analysis distribution determined by these sums indicates the relative likelihood under the current state of knowledge that the dose-response characteristic is in different intervals.

7.4.4 Weights

The most difficult part of evaluating multiple pieces of information is determining the relative emphasis or weight that should be associated with each piece of information.[41] Even though this determination is generally not easy, it is inescapable, and there are scientific methods for making this determination[35,41,42,50,65–67]. However, most importantly, weighting provides an opportunity to reflect the current state of knowledge in the quantitative dose-response characterization.

The weights in a decision tree are intended to reflect the relative level of scientific support or relevance associated with each alternative. The weights for the different alternatives of a dose-response Factor are non-negative and sum to one. Hence, the weights represent a partitioning of emphasis between the alternatives.

Examples

The role and properties of the weights in an information analysis are illustrated in the formaldehyde example. Figure 7.3 indicates the entire decision tree, but there is not enough room in that figure to explicitly indicate the weights for each branch in the tree. For convenience, the decision tree in Figure 7.3 is divided into three parts and the weights for each branch explicitly indicated in Figures 7.4 through 7.6. In each of these three figures, the two alternatives for the first Factor, *Human Carcinogenic Response*, are shown. The weight judged to be applicable to the alternative *Human Carcinogen* is 0.8, and the weight for *Not a Human Carcinogen* is 0.2. These weights appear in *The Likelihood of Alternative Potencies: Uncertainty Analysis of Formaldehyde*, Evans et al.[13] and reflect the authors' judgments of the current state of knowledge with respect to the human carcinogenicity of formaldehyde.[13] These two weights for the alternatives for the first Factor bear the common characteristics of all weights in that they are non-negative and sum to 1.0. These weights indicate that 80 percent of the probability distribution characterization of formaldehyde's dose-response relationship corresponds to paths in the decision tree which contain the alternative *Human Carcinogen* for Factor 1. The other 20 percent of the information-analysis distribution corresponds to the path containing the alternative *Not a Human Carcinogen*.

The weights for the portion of the decision tree corresponding to formaldehyde's mode of action being *Cell Proliferation Involved but not Genotoxicity* are shown in Figure 7.4. The weight on this alternative for Factor 2, mode of action, is 0.8 while the weights on the other two alternatives for Factor 2 are 0.005 and 0.195. As always, the weights on the alternatives for a Factor sum to 1.0. The combined weight in the probability distribution characterization of formaldehyde's dose-response relationship corresponding to the combination of alternatives for the first two Factors being *Human Carcinogen* and *Cell Proliferation Involved But Not Genotoxicity* is $(0.8)(0.8) = 0.64$. Thus, the total weight on all of the paths in Figure 7.4 stemming from the node identified as *Cell Proliferation Involved But Not Genotoxicity* under the node for *Human Carcinogen* is 0.64. In Figure 7.5, the total weight on all of the paths stemming from the node identified as *Genotoxicity Involved but not Cell Proliferation* under the node for *Human Carcinogen* is $(0.8)(0.005) = 0.004$. Finally, in Figure 7.6, the total weight on all of the paths stemming from the node identified as *Both Cell Proliferation and Genotoxicity Involved* under the node for *Human Carcinogen* is $(0.8)(0.195) = 0.156$. Thus, the 80 percent weight for *Human Carcinogen* is subdivided among the three modes of action with relative weights 0.8, 0.005, and 0.195 and combined weights 0.64, 0.004, and 0.156 which sum to 0.80 (i.e., $0.64 + 0.004 + 0.156 = 0.80$).

The weight on the outcome at the end of path in the decision tree is equal to the product of the weights along that path. For example, in Figure 7.4, the weight on the top most outcome is 0.00512 which equals the product (0.8)(0.8)(0.1)(0.5)(0.8)(0.2). Similarly, the weight on the path which is second from the top (which does interspecies extrapolation on the basis of $BW^{3/4}$ instead of equal sensitivity across species on the *"PPM"* dose scale as in the top most path) is 0.01024 which equals the product (0.8)(0.8)(0.1)(0.5)(0.8)(0.4).

Determination of Weights

The weights in an information analysis can be determined by several different methods. Sometimes, objective statistical analyses of the historical performance or empirical behavior of the alternatives can be used to determine the weights. For example, the relative mean square errors of different numerical procedures would imply one set of relative weights for those procedures. More often, consensus evaluation or expert judgment will be needed to determine the weights. In general, the weights are not determined by the risk assessor but are determined by the current state of knowledge in the relevant scientific community. An information-analysis based dose-response characterization should include an indication of the weights utilized and their method of determination. An evaluation of the appropriateness of the weights would normally be expected to be part of the evaluation of the database for the dose-response characterization.

Illustrative Weights

The example information-analysis distribution in Figure 7.11 utilizes the weights proposed in *The Likelihood of Alternative Potencies: Uncertainty Analysis of Formaldehyde*, Evans et al.[13] The weights were based on those authors' reading of the scientific literature and their participation in the risk characterization of formaldehyde. Although the authors did perform some interviews with scientists[18,19,42,65], the weights were developed by the authors and were not formally elicited from recognized experts in toxicology, epidemiology, pathology, biochemistry, and cancer biology. Hence, the weights should be considered illustrative of the kinds of information that need to be elicited from the relevant scientific communities if the weight-of-evidence approach is to be fully implemented.

The Necessity for Weights

Weights are inescapable because any method of evaluating multiple pieces of information involves some weighting. For example, choosing the maximum value implies assigning weight 1.0 to the piece of information corresponding to the maximum value and weight 0.0 to all other pieces of information. Of course, averaging the pieces of information implies assigning equal weights to all pieces of information. Equal weights reflect a judgment that all alternatives are equally relevant and do not imply that no judgment has been made. Equal weights are not unbiased unless equal emphasis accurately reflects the current state of knowledge.

Any use of the data implies some judgment. All current risk assessment procedures include some judgment. If that judgment is determined by legislation, then, hopefully, the legislated weights will evolve as the state of knowledge evolves. Information analysis makes the use of weights explicit and facilitates their evolution.

The Utility of Weights

Weighting provides an opportunity for the quantitative characterization to reflect more of the available qualitative toxicological and biological information. For example, if a monkey study is more relevant than a rat study to the human inference situation, then the monkey study can be given more weight than the rat study. If an inhalation study is more relevant than a gavage study, the inhalation study can receive more weight. If 80 percent of the scientific community thinks that one dose scale should be used and 20 percent thinks that another dose scale should be used, then the results using the two different dose scales could be weighted 80 percent and 20 percent (that is, 0.8 and 0.2), respectively. In a world with few absolutes and insufficient data to know for sure what the correct answer is, weights are a useful tool in reflecting the current state of knowledge.

The use of weights in the dose-response characterization actually promotes research and data collection.[68,69] In contrast to the use of fixed defaults for the values of the dose-response Factors or the use of strength-of-evidence procedures, new data that are relevant always impact weight-of-evidence approaches. New data are weighted on the basis of their merits. That is, new data do not have to disprove a default value or replace older data; instead, all of the data is weighed together. New data can also change old weights.

Obviously, the weights can have a significant impact on the information-analysis based dose-response characterization. Hence, a dose-response assessment will generally benefit from a sensitivity analysis on the impact of the weights.

Also, obviously, this chapter cannot be an exhaustive treatment of the use of weights in risk assessment or even dose-response characterization. However, this chapter will hopefully introduce an important approach that should see increasing and evolving use in the future.

7.4.5 Sensitivity Analyses

The probability distribution characterization of the dose-response relationship for formaldehyde in Figure 7.11 reflects the combined effects of all of dose-response Factors and all of the alternatives for each Factor. Sensitivity analyses can provide information on the relative quantitative impacts of the different Factors and alternatives in the decision tree on the location and shape of that distribution. This information can identify which dose-response Factors and alternatives most strongly affect the distribution. Such knowledge helps to prioritize and focus research, data collection, discussion, and critical review onto the Factors and weights with the most significant impacts on the dose-response characterization.

For example, Figure 7.12 shows the quantitative impact of the assumed mode of action for formaldehyde. In Figure 7.12, the three probability distributions on the added risk at 1 *ppb* (the slope factor at 1 *ppb*) have been computed from Figures 7.4 through 7.6 by changing the weights on the three modes of action from (0.800, 0.005, 0.195) to (1.0, 0.0, 0.0), (0.0, 1.0, 0.0), and (0.0, 0.0, 1.0) for the top, middle, and bottom distributions, respectively. Thus, the top probability distribution corresponds to a weight-of-evidence evaluation that assumed that cell proliferation is involved but not genotoxicity. The differences between these three distributions gives a quantitative indication of the impact of the assumption (or, equivalently, the weighting) concerning formaldehyde's mode of action. For example, the 95th percentile of the distribution of maximum likelihood estimates of the added risk at one ppb is two or three orders of magnitude less if formaldehyde's mode of action does not include genotoxicity. Hence, this Factor is an important one for formaldehyde.

The probability distributions in Figures 7.11 and 7.12 are determined by a weight-of-evidence based combination of the risk attributes from multiple different paths through the tree (that is, multiple different individual analyses). Hence, the differences in Figure 7.12 between the distributions for the three different alternative modes of action are the differences between the *overall* effects of the mode of action on the set of all combinations of all of the other Factors and their alternatives.

In addition to the overall effects of a Factor's alternatives on the risk attributes, the *interactive* effects of a Factor's alternatives on each individual path (combination of the other Factors' alternatives) are often also of interest. For example, Figures 7.7 through 7.9 show the percentiles of the nonparametric bootstrap distribution of maximum likelihood estimates of the added risk at one *ppb for each individual combination of Factor alternatives*. Therefore, in these figures it can be seen that, for instance, the difference between using a threshold model dose-response model and a non-threshold model is a lot greater when the dose scale is *ppm* than when the dose scale is DPX. Hence, there is an interactive effect between the dose scale and the dose-response model. In fact, there are interactive effects among four of the Factors, namely, the dose scale, dose-response model, experimental data set, and method of interspecies extrapolation. However, Figures 7.4 through 7.9 also indicate that the mode of action only influences the weight on a path and not the numerical value of the paths' risk attributes. Hence, there is no interaction between

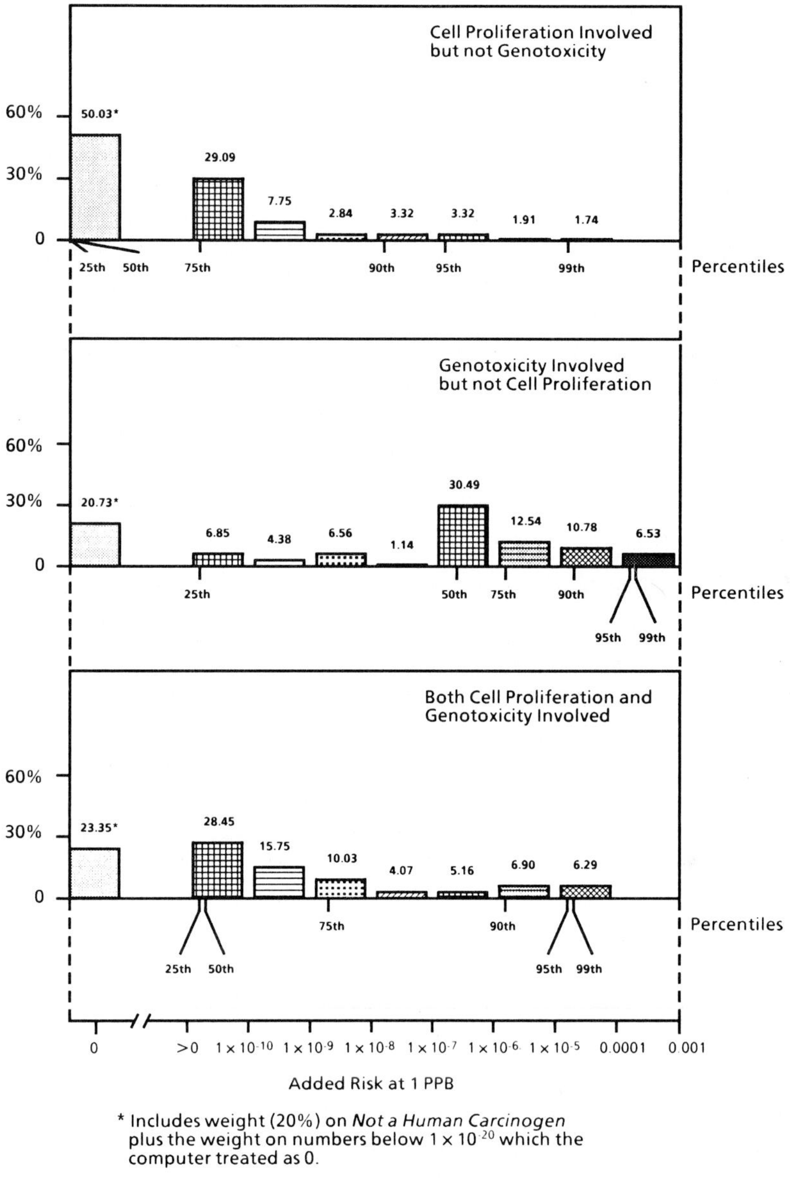

Figure 7.12 The Quantitative Impact of Alternative Modes of Action on the Dose-Response Characterization of the Added Risk of One *ppb* Formaldehyde.

the mode of action and the numerical value of the risk attribute determined by the rest of the Factors on a path.

Often, the easiest way to visualize the overall and interactive effects of the alternatives for the different Factors is to reorder the Factors as in Figure 7.13. There the Factor (dose-response model) with the largest overall effect is first; the Factor (experimental data set) with the second largest effect second; etc. Because all of the distinct methods of analysis are explicitly included in Figure 7.13, they can be ordered in any convenient manner during sensitivity analyses. (On the other hand, in the decision tree itself, the Factors are usually ordered in a logical decomposition sequence that facilitates the specification of weights by nesting Factors appropriately.)

In Figures 7.7 through 7.13, the risk attribute is the maximum likelihood estimate or its nonparametric bootstrap distribution. Figure 7.14 concerns alternative risk attributes. The issues here deserve special attention. The statistical functions of these attributes in describing a specified dose-response characteristic (the added risk at one *ppb* in this example) are as follows:

1. the maximum likelihood estimate (the dose-response model's best estimate),
2. the nonparametric bootstrap distribution (reflecting the impact of experimental variability about the observed experimental outcome on the maximum likelihood estimation procedure),
3. the 95th percentile of the bootstrap distribution (an upper bound associated with experimental variability about the observed experimental outcome),
4. the 5th percentile of the bootstrap distribution (a lower bound associated with experimental variability about the observed experimental outcome),
5. the linearized multistage model's 95% upper confidence limit (an upper bound whose confidence level is unknown for the underlying dose-response relationship but is at least 95% for any dose-response relationship), and
6. the linearized multistage model's 95% lower confidence limit (a lower bound indicating the range of possibilities consistent with the confidence limit procedure used to generate the linearized multistage model upper bound).

The frequency distribution for each of these attributes is shown in Figure 7.14. The functions of the six risk attributes, as described in items 1 through 6 above, indicate that these risk attributes are calculated for very different specific purposes, even though each risk attribute contributes some information about the target dose-response feature. The maximum likelihood estimates indicate where the target is most likely to be. The bootstrap distribution reflects the relative likelihood of different target values if the observed experimental outcome is a good indication of the true dose-response relationship. The bootstrap bounds reflect the impact of experimental variability on the range of likely values if the observed experimental outcome is a good indication of the true dose-response

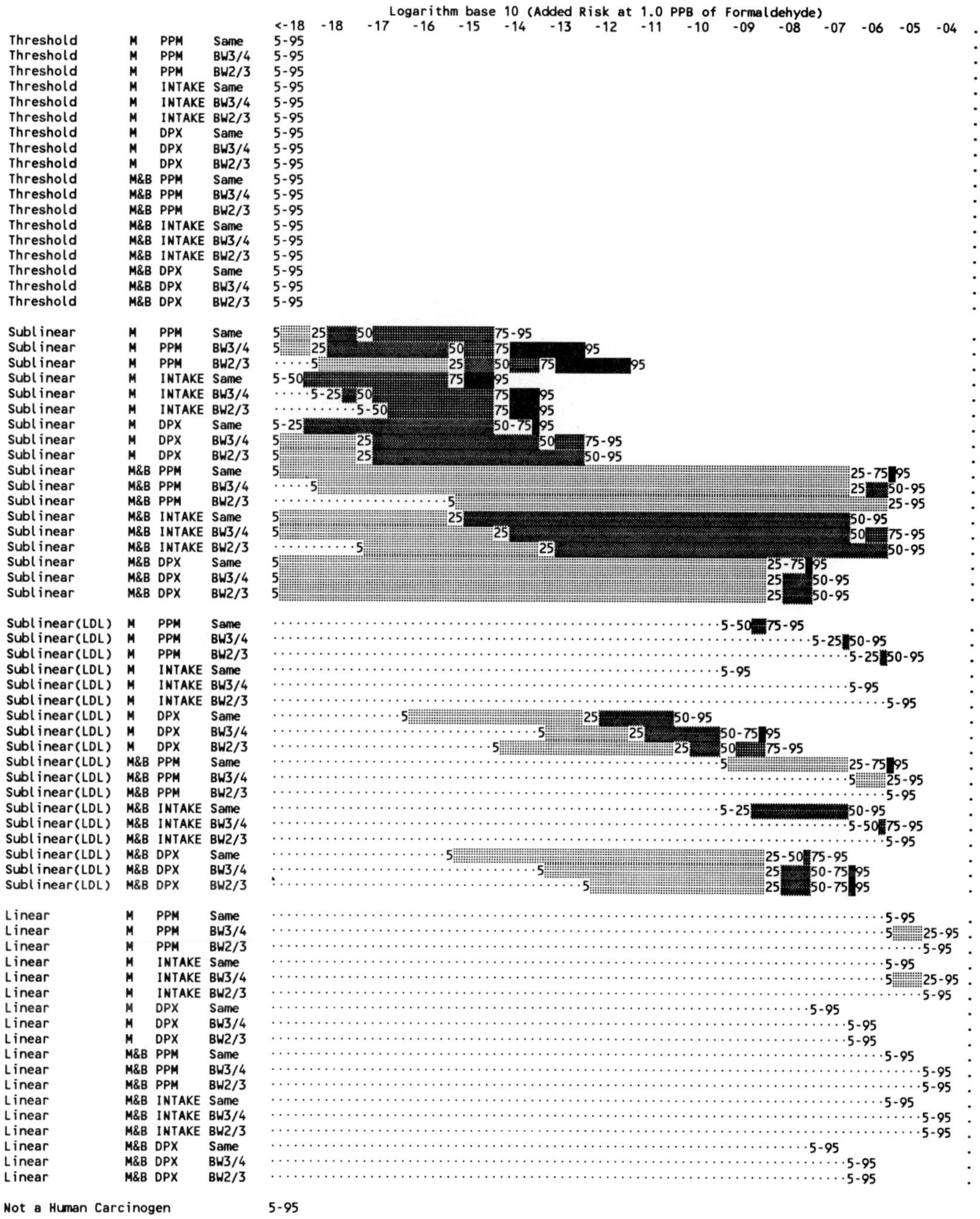

Figure 7.13 The Interactive Effects of the Factor Alternative on the Nonparamteric Bootstrap Distribution Characterization of the Added Risk at One *ppb* of Formaldehyde.

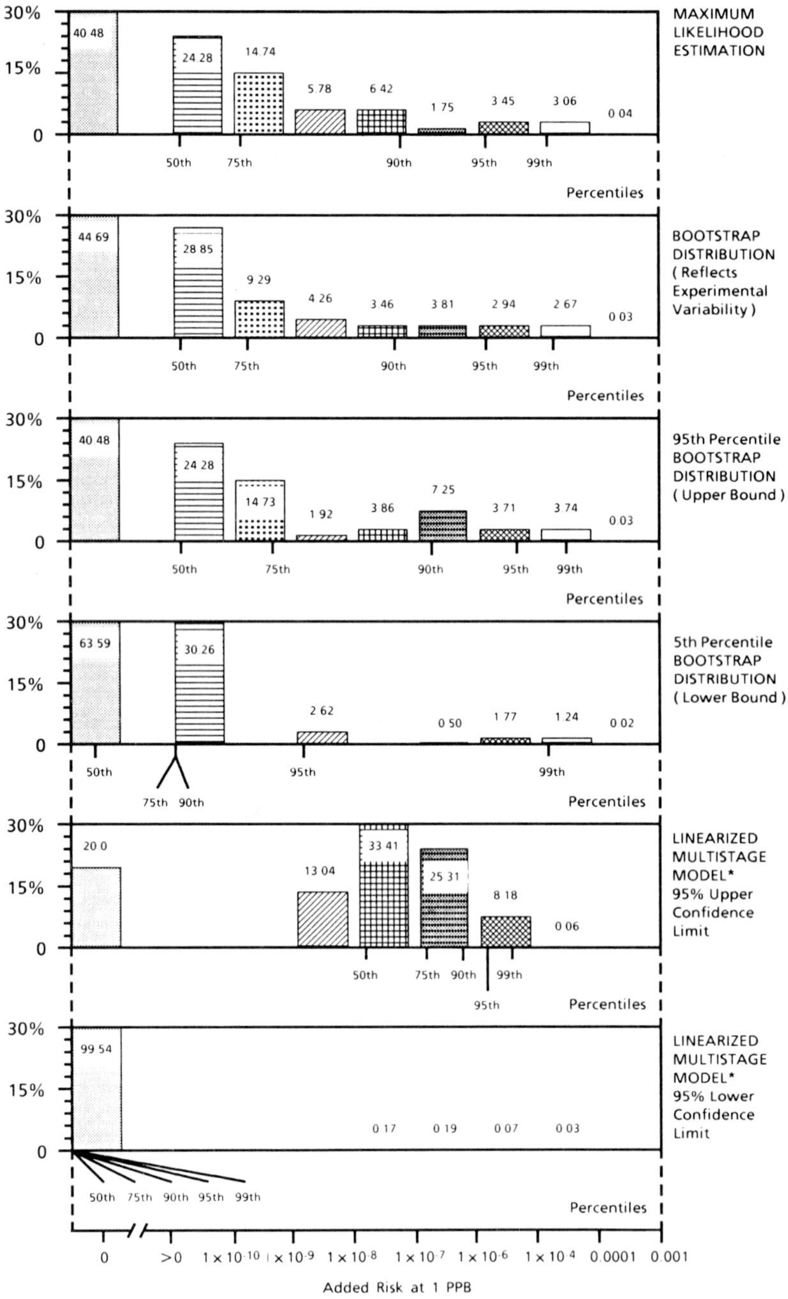

* Because the probit model is not a multistage model, the histograms for the linearized multistage model confidence limits were constructed ignoring the probit model. That is, the weights on the one-hit, multistage, and multistage low-dose linear models were normalized to add up to one.

Figure 7.14 The Quantitative Impact of Alternative RISK ATTRIBUTES on the Dose-Response Characterization of Added Risk at One *ppb* Formaldehyde.

relationship. The linearized multistage model bounds are extreme enough to be bounds at least 95 percent of the time even if the experimental outcome is not a good indication of the true dose-response relationship.

In Figure 7.14, it is clear that the linearized multistage models' 95 percent upper confidence limits place much greater emphasis on the more extreme possibilities than the bootstrap distributions' 95th percentiles do. This is consistent with the lesser emphasis on the observed experimental data in the linearized multistage model procedure than in the bootstrap procedure. Another interesting characteristic in Figure 7.14 is the similarity between the distribution of maximum likelihood estimates and the distributions reflecting both the maximum likelihood estimates and the bootstrap replicates. The bootstrap distributions' reflection of experimental variability primarily just smoothes out the distribution of maximum likelihood estimates.

Because the different risk attributes serve different functions, their emphasis in an information analysis is very dependent upon the intended use of the resulting characterization. If the dose-response characterization is intended to indicate the most likely value of the cancer potency, then the maximum likelihood estimates should receive the most emphasis. If the dose-response characterization is intended to include the portion of uncertainty associated with the variability in the maximum likelihood estimate in response to experimental variability under the assumption that the observed experimental outcome is a good indication of the true dose-response relationship, then the bootstrap distribution should receive the most emphasis. The bootstrap distribution should also receive substantial emphasis if the relative likelihood of the different values in the range of possible values is important. In this last case, both the maximum likelihood estimates and the bootstrap distribution might receive emphasis. In this way, emphasis is given to the observed experimental outcome as well as the simulated outcomes associated with experimental variability. (The bootstrap distribution gives the same weight to the one observed outcome and each one of the simulated outcomes.) If only the range of possible values and not the relative likelihood of the different values within that range is important, then the bootstrap upper and lower bounds (e.g., the 95th and 5th percentiles of the bootstrap distribution) should receive emphasis. If the observed experimental outcomes are not necessarily believed to be good indications of the true underlying dose-response relationship, and there is a conscious desire to emphasize the most extreme dose-response relationships that can not be shown to be statistically, significantly inconsistent with the observed experimental outcomes, then emphasizing the linearized multistage model upper and lower bounds is appropriate.

The preceding sensitivity analyses have focused on the relative significance of the alternatives for the dose-response Factors. In general, such analyses would incorporate weights which reflect either individual experts or the composite current state of knowledge in the entire relevant community of experts.

There are additional sensitivity analyses which can reflect the impacts on the information-analysis probability distribution characterization of the dose-response relationship of *variability in expert judgment weights and variability in the assessment of expert judgment weights.*

For example, weights on the alternatives for the dose scale used for dose-response modeling have been solicited from the portion of the scientific community capable of evaluating the issues associated with the biologically effective dose for formaldehyde.[35,42] Eight such experts were selected, and their judgments quantified. These eight experts each made different judgments. As part of the sensitivity analyses, the probability distribution characterization of the added risk at one *ppb* could be determined separately eight times using each individual expert's weights on the alternative dose scales. The eight distributions would provide an indication of the impact of differences between individual experts.

In addition, the impact of sampling variability in the assessment of expert judgments could also be characterized as part of the sensitivity analyses. For example, the probability distribution on the added risk of one *ppb* formaldehyde using the combined weights from the original eight experts could be compared with not only the eight probability distributions determined separately for each expert but also one or more probability distribution characterizations obtained using the combined weights from one or more *random samples of eight such experts*. In some cases, pseudo-random samples from the expert community could be created by randomly sampling with replacement the original set of selected experts.

7.4.6 Risk Characterizations for Specific Populations

The characterization of the risk for a population with a specified exposure can incorporate an information-analysis based dose-response characterization. For example, Figure 7.15 displays the probability distribution characterizing the expected number of increased cancer cases in the lifetimes of a population of 100,000,000 people exposed to 1.0 *ppb* for 30 hours per week starting at age four and continuing throughout their lifetimes. Here, increased cancer cases means the number of cancer cases in addition to the number expected at the background dose level. This probability distribution is calculated simply by multiplying the information-analysis distribution for the added cancer risk at 1.0 *ppb* shown in Figure 7.11 by 100,000,000. Thus, the distribution in Figure 7.15 is based on the maximum likelihood estimates of added risk and the weight-of-evidence analysis depicted in Figures 7.4 through 7.6.

The probability distribution in Figure 7.15 refers to a *temporal exposure pattern* (that is, a constant exposure for 30 hours per week starting at age four and continuing throughout the lifetime) that is comparable to that used in the CIIT study upon which the maximum likelihood estimates of added risk were based. (This temporal exposure pattern is comparable to the exposure pattern that the rats had in the CIIT study under the assumption that an initial exposure at age 4 in an expected 70 year human lifetime is comparable to an initial exposure at age 1.5 months in a 25.5 month rat lifetime, $4/70 = 1.5/(1.5 + 24)$ approximately). This temporal exposure pattern has been implicitly assumed in all of the figures related to formaldehyde herein. This implicit assumption manifests itself in the values of the doses used in the dose-response modeling of the CIIT data set. In particular, the experimental dose levels of 0, 2, 5.6, and 14.3 ppm refer to the concentration during 30

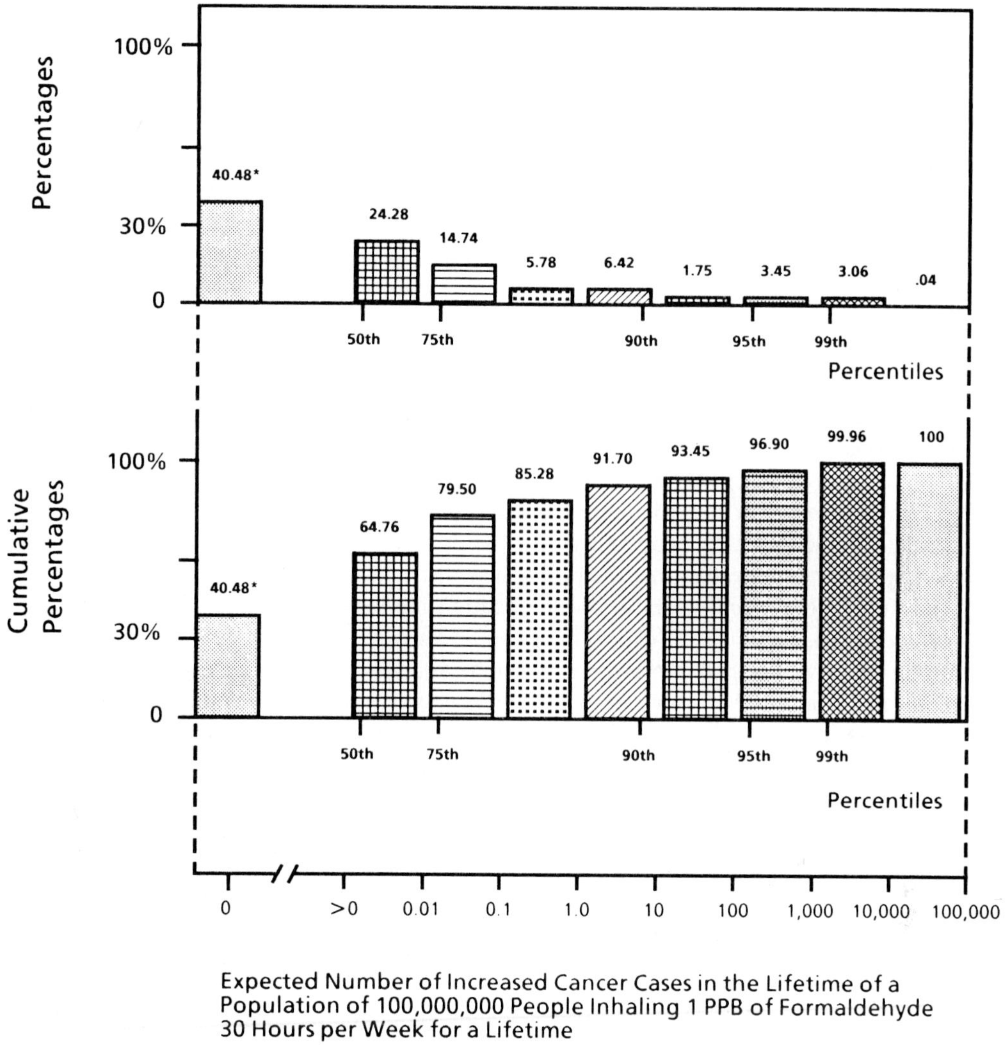

Figure 7.15 Information-Analysis based Risk Characterization for a Population.

hours of exposure per week. Similarly, the values of dose calculated using the *intake* and *DPX* dose scales are the dose received during a minute and hour, respectively, of exposure during 30 hours per week of exposure to a constant formaldehyde concentration level.

If the risk is to be characterized for a population with a different temporal exposure pattern than that in the experimental data or the temporal exposure patterns in different experimental data sets are different, then an assumption must be made concerning the *relevant dose measure* in a temporal exposure pattern. The average daily dose in a lifetime and the total dose in a lifetime are examples of commonly used alternatives for the relevant dose measure. (However, dose rate is often important too.) If the relationship between the administered dose and a particular dose scale is nonlinear, then a dose measure like lifetime average daily dose must be computed as a time weighted average of the different dose scale values for the different administered dose levels. For example, for formaldehyde, DPX is a nonlinear function of the concentration; hence, the lifetime average daily amount of DPX must be computed as a time weighted average of the DPX values corresponding to the different exposure concentrations in a lifetime. In this example, the nonlinearity would make it *incorrect* to simply compute the lifetime average daily amount of DPX formed as the amount of DPX formed during a lifetime of exposure to the lifetime average daily concentration level.

If there is more than one potentially reasonable assumption about the relevant dose measure corresponding to varying temporal exposure patterns, then the *relevant dose measure* can be another factor in the decision tree.

Although the example in Figure 7.15 is for a population with the same exposure level for each member of the population, an information-analysis based risk characterization could also incorporate a probability distribution of exposure levels within the population. This would require either that the probability distribution of added risk be known at each exposure level or, equivalently, that the relationship between the probability distributions of added risks at different exposure levels be known. An example of the latter case is when the simplifying assumption is made that, at the exposure levels of interest, the added risks are linear functions of the exposure level in which case the probability distribution on added risk at one exposure level is the same as the probability distribution on added risk at any other exposure level of interest except that its location is shifted proportionally.

7.5 RISK COMMUNICATION: ADVANTAGES OF INFORMATION-ANALYSIS BASED DOSE-RESPONSE CHARACTERIZATIONS

A major advantage of the information-analysis based dose-response characterization is its incorporation of all of the available relevant information and its explicit quantitative representation of the current state of knowledge including its uncertainty.

The most common alternative to the weight-of-evidence based distributional characterization of the dose-response relationship is to characterize that relationship by the single value that corresponds to considering only the most conservative alternative for each Factor in the decision tree. For example, in the decision tree in Figures 7.4 through 7.6, if the only path that is considered is the one which assumes that formaldehyde's mode of action is genotoxicity, the dose scale is *ppm*, the dose-response model is linear, the only relevant experimental data are the combined malignant and benign responses, and interspecies extrapolation should be done on a body surface area basis, then the maximum likelihood estimate of the added risk at one *ppb* is $2.0D{-}04$ (or 2×10^{-4}). This value combines the conservatism in the selection of the most conservative mode of action, with the conservatism in the selection of the most conservative dose scale, with the conservatism in the selection of the most conservative dose-response model, with the conservatism in the selection of the most conservative experimental data set, with the conservatism in the selection of the most conservative interspecies extrapolation. Without a weight-of-evidence analysis such as that shown in Figures 7.4 through 7.6 and summarized in Figure 7.11, the quantitative effect of these multiple conservatisms would be unknown. With the weight-of- evidence analysis it can be determined that 2×10^{-4} exceeds the 99.96th percentile of the distribution of maximum likelihood estimates; so that, less than 0.04 percent of the evidence is on added risks as high as 2×10^{-4}.

There is considerably more information in the available data than just a single maximum likelihood estimate or a single upper bound. The information-analysis based distributional characterization communicates that information.

As new data become available, the updating of weight-of-evidence based distributional characterizations can be more believably communicated than the updating of single number characterizations. It is hard to expect a risk manager to be very comfortable with a characterization procedure that last year proclaimed that only one value for added risk was relevant and this year proclaims that a different value for added risk is the only relevant value. It seems to be a lot more believable to include variability and uncertainty in the characterization of the current state of knowledge; so that, when new evidence becomes available, it is natural for the weight of evidence to change. Because distributional characterizations assign nonzero weight to a range of possibilities, new data merely shift the emphasis from some possibilities to others rather than shifting the characterization of a value from totally irrelevant to all important. Figure 7.16 illustrates these points.

7.6 RISK: A FUNCTION OF BOTH THE DOSE-RESPONSE RELATIONSHIP AND EXPOSURE

Risk depends on exposure as well as the dose-response relationship. Hence, risk characterization must combine the exposure and dose-response characterizations. This also means that the usefulness of a dose-response characterization depends not only on its ability to adequately characterize the dose-response relationship itself, but also on how well the dose-response characterization can be combined with exposure characterizations to generate informative risk characterizations.

7.6.1 Exposure Characterizations

The most recent advances in exposure assessment are leading to exposure characterizations in form of probability distributions.[16,70,71] In such characterizations, an individual or population's exposure is described by the different probabilities of the exposure being different levels rather than the exposure being described as a single number. The probability distribution describes how probability is distributed over the different possible exposure values.

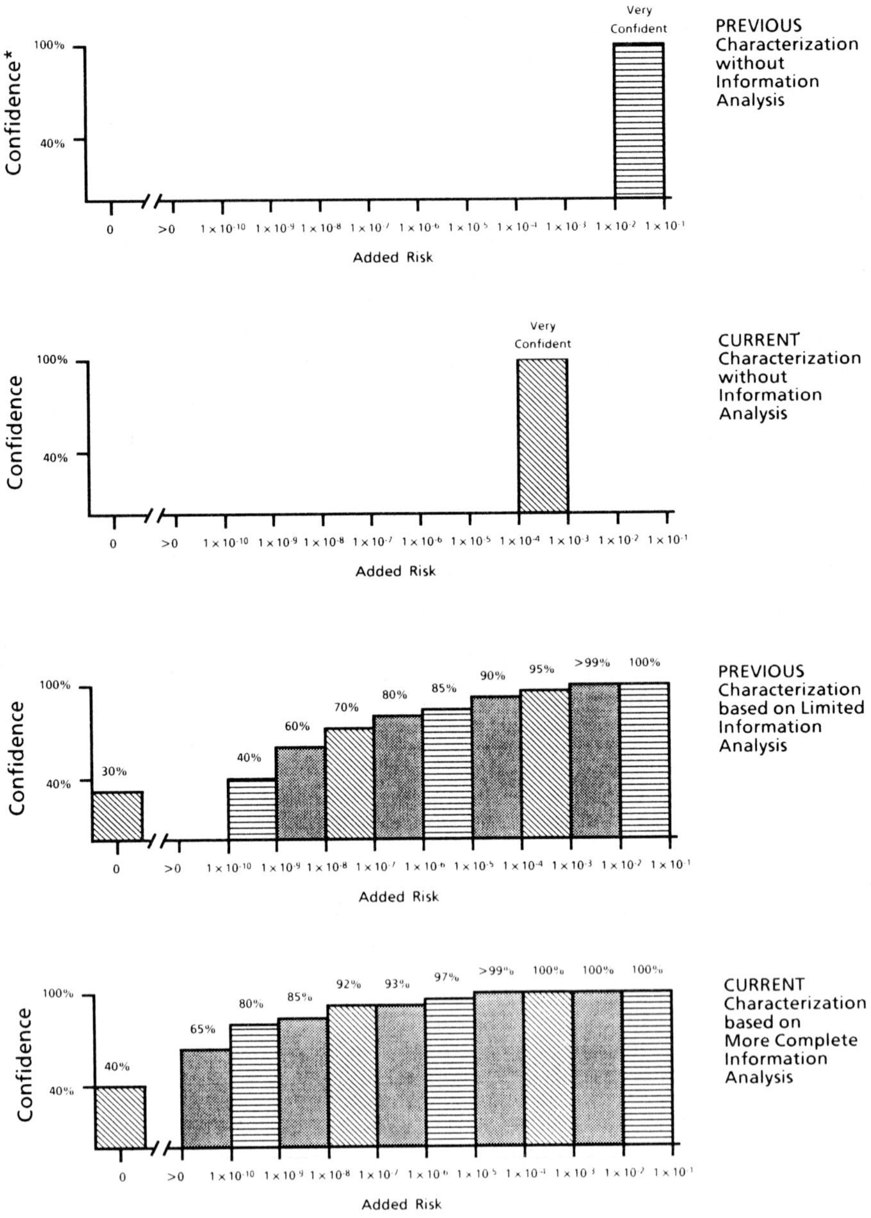

*Confidence that the true added risk at one ppb does not exceed the specified value on the added risk axis

Figure 7.16 Information-Analysis Based Characterizations Change in a More Believable Manner with New Information than Single Number Characterizations.

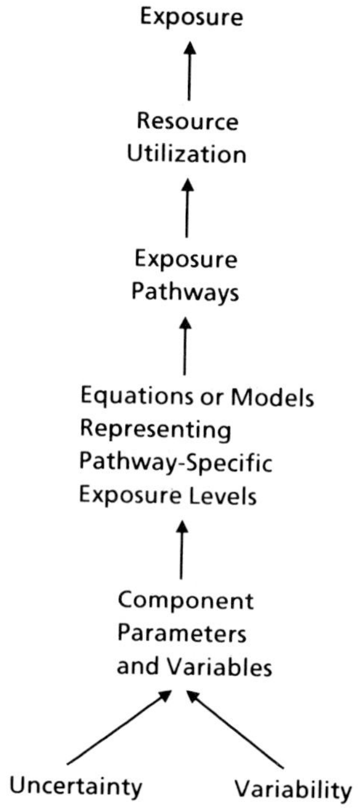

Figure 7.17 Overview of Factors Affecting the Quantitative Characterization of Exposure.

Probability distributions are being used to incorporate both variability and uncertainty into exposure characterizations. Variability arises because exposure generally varies from individual to individual in a population and from time to time for a particular individual. This variability is frequently due to differences in lifestyles, activity patterns, and occupations. Variability also can be due to different chemical concentrations in different foods or work environments, the amount of dermal contact with a chemical during a certain activity, etc. Uncertainty enters into the exposure characterization in several ways. The difference between variability and uncertainty is illustrated in the following example. A chemical's concentration in a drinking water supply may vary from day to day. On a particular day, the actual value of the concentration is uncertain because of measurement errors and sampling variation. Because probability distributions usually reflect the combined effects of uncertainty and variability, it is often useful to present sensitivity analyses indicating the individual impacts of variability and uncertainty as well as the individual impacts of each of the components of variability and uncertainty.[72]

An overview of the factors affecting exposure is given in Figure 7.17. In general, exposure depends on the how resources (such as land and water) are utilized. For example, exposure would usually be different if a former superfund site were to be utilized as a wildlife refuge, a recreational facility, or an industrial site. For a given resource utilization, exposure occurs via one or more exposure pathways (e.g., soil ingestion, dermal absorption,

Simple Example:

Pathway: Inhalation

Media: Ambient Air

Exposure = [Amount of Chemical in Ambient Air (mg / m^3)*]
×
[Inhalation Rate (m3 / day)]
×
[Fraction of Day Exposed: (Exposure Hours / Day) / (24 Hours / Day)]
×
[Fraction of Year Exposed: (Exposure Days / Year) / (365 Days / Year)]
×
[Fraction of Lifetime Exposed: (Exposure Years / Lifetime) / (Lifetime in Years)]
×
[1 / Body Weight (kg)]

*If the chemical is a gas and the concentration is # ppm by volume, then

#mg / m^3 = [(# ppm Molecules of Chemical) / (1 × 10^6 Molecules of Air)]
× (Gram Molecular Weight of Chemical in mg)
/ (Volume of One Gram Molecular Weight of Chemical: 0.0245 m^3)]

= (# ppm) × (Density of Air: 1.2 mg / m^3)
× (Gram Molecular Weight of Chemical in g)
/ (Gram Molecular Weight of Air: 29g)

with volumes and densities at 25° C and one atmospheric absolute pressure.

Figure 7.18 Exposure Parameters Determine the Exposure (*mg/kg/day*) through an Exposure Equation or Model.

and inhalation). Pathway-specific exposure levels are described in terms of equations or models. These equations or models involve component parameters or variables. For example, in the simple example shown in Figure 7.18, the average daily exposure to a chemical via the inhalation pathway is represented by an equation with components equal to the chemical concentration in the ambient air, the inhalation rate, the hours/day, days/year, and years of exposure to ambient air, the averaging time, and the body weight. Some of these components may be constants, but most have probability distributions because of variability and uncertainty. Even with the components being a mixture of constants and different probability distributions, a probability distribution, such as that shown in Figure 7.19, for the associated exposure can be determined using simulation techniques (e.g., *Monte Carlo* or *Latin Hypercube Sampling* techniques). Furthermore, these probability distributions can also incorporate multiple exposure media (e.g., soil, vegetables, and ground water) and, when biologically appropriate, can combine probability distributions for different routes of exposure.

7.6.2 Implications for Dose-Response Characterization

The use of probability distributions to characterize exposure has significant practical implications for dose-response characterization. The recognition of the importance of reflecting the variability and uncertainty in the characterization of exposure suggests that the same recognition can not be too far behind with respect to the reflection of the variability and uncertainty in the dose-response characterization. As suggested in Figure 7.20, whenever a probability distribution is used to characterize the exposure, the risk characterization will also be a probability distribution regardless of whether the dose-response characterization is restricted to being a single number or is more fully characterized as a probability distribution. Thus, the ultimate risk characterization is *not* simplified by forcing the dose-response characterization to be a single number. The real consequence of forcing the dose-response characterization to be a single number is a loss of information. A loss that can be avoided by characterizing the dose-response relationship in terms of a probability distribution that reflects the current state of knowledge including both variability and uncertainty.

Combining a single number dose-response characterization with an exposure characterization may *not* provide a meaningful result. However, distributional dose-response characterizations can be meaningfully combined with exposure characterizations. For instance, consider the simplest case in which the dose-response relationship is linear and

$$\text{added risk} = \text{cancer potency} \times \text{dose}$$

and the relationship between exposure and dose is known with certainty. Suppose, for example, 0.01 is a 95 percent upper confidence limit on the cancer potency and 5 is a 95 percent upper confidence limit on dose, then

$$0.01 \times 5 = 0.05$$

may not be a 95 percent upper confidence limit on the added risk. In fact, depending upon the shape of the distributions of cancer potency and dose, 0.05 may be either greater than or less than the 95th percentile of added risk (see Problem 1 for some related numerical examples). Therefore, combining 95 percent upper confidence limits does not result in a 95 percent confidence limit. Because the result is not necessarily above or below the 95th percentile, the result is not meaningful. However, if the entire distribution of the cancer potency is known instead of just its 95th percentile or some other upper bound and the entire exposure distribution is known, then the distribution of added risk (including its 95th

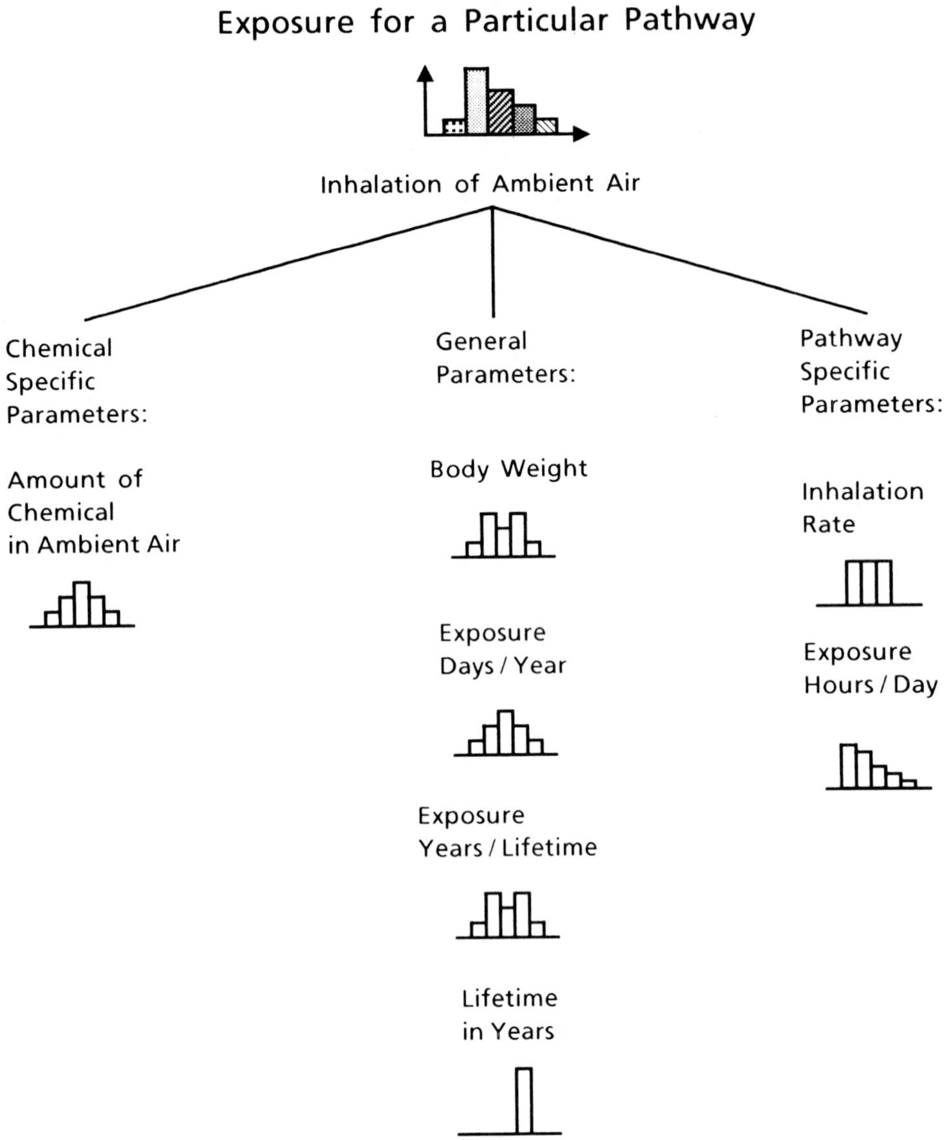

Figure 7.19 A Probability Distribution Characterization of Exposure Can Reflect the Variablility and Uncertainty in an Exposure Pathway's Components.

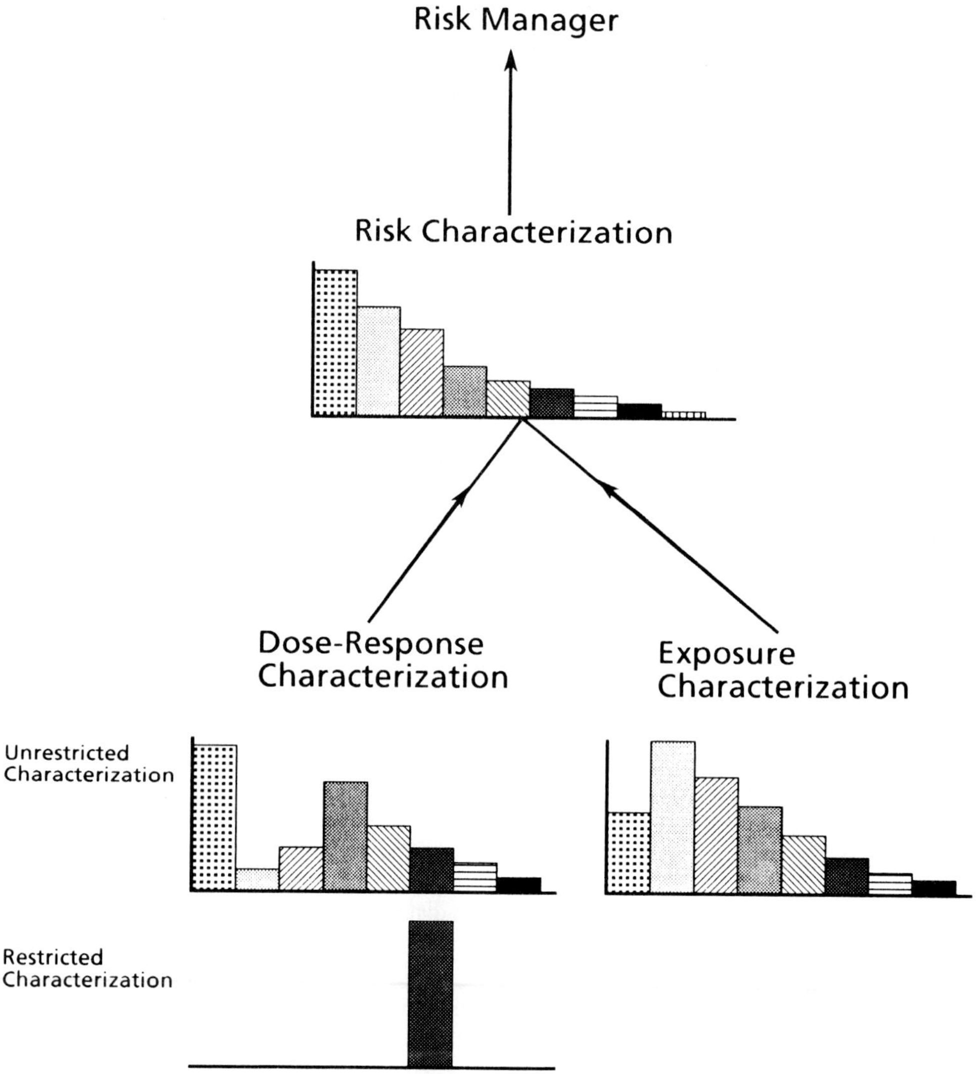

Figure 7.20 Risk Characterization Combines Both Dose-Response Characterization and Exposure Characterization.

percentile and any other percentile) can be determined. Hence, if information on the risk distribution or an upper confidence limit on risk is desired, then it is necessary to determine the cancer potency distribution and the exposure distribution.

In order for the risk distribution to be communicated to the risk manager, the dose-response and exposure distributions must be determined.

In the above example, added risk was assumed to be linearly related to dose. In some important cases, such a simple dose-response relationship is not likely to be the true dose-response relationship. In such cases, a separate distributional characterization for each dose or range of doses needs to be determined. These distributional characterizations can be combined with a distributional characterization of exposure in the manner suggested in Figure 7.21.

7.6.3 Example

Some of the advantages of distributional characterizations are illustrated in the following example concerning site remediation. The risk assessment objective in this example is to characterize a chemical's concentration in a particular media (e.g., soil or ground water) that would be consistent with specified public health objectives (e.g., a lifetime cancer risk not exceeding a specified level like 1/10,000). Thus, the objective here is a *concentration* characterization rather than a *risk* characterization. The components of the concentration characterization for a specified site utilization option are depicted in Figure 7.22.

In Figure 7.22, the exposure characterization is a probability distribution for an individual's daily intake dose (*mg chemical/ kg body weight/day*) per unit media concentration. The dose-response characterization is a probability distribution (among individuals in a specified population) for the *Lifetime Average Daily Dose* (LADD, *mg chemical/kg body weight/day*) corresponding to a specified risk level. This latter probability distribution could have been obtained in either of the following two ways:

1. Determine the information-analysis based distributional characterization of the cancer potency or slope. Here, the decision tree outcomes are a slope. Then, *assuming that the dose-response relationship is linear in the dose region of interest,* the LADD corresponding to a specified risk level and a particular decision tree slope value is

   $$\text{specified risk level}/\text{slope}$$

   The probability distribution for the LADD corresponding to a specified risk level is assumed to be the distribution of this ratio.

2. In the decision tree, when a particular combination of alternatives for the dose-response Factors is being considered, calculate the dose corresponding to the specified risk level. That is, let the decision tree outcome be this dose instead of a slope or an added risk. The corresponding information-analysis distribution is the desired probability distribution for the LADD corresponding to a specified risk level instead of a probability distribution for an approximate low-dose slope.

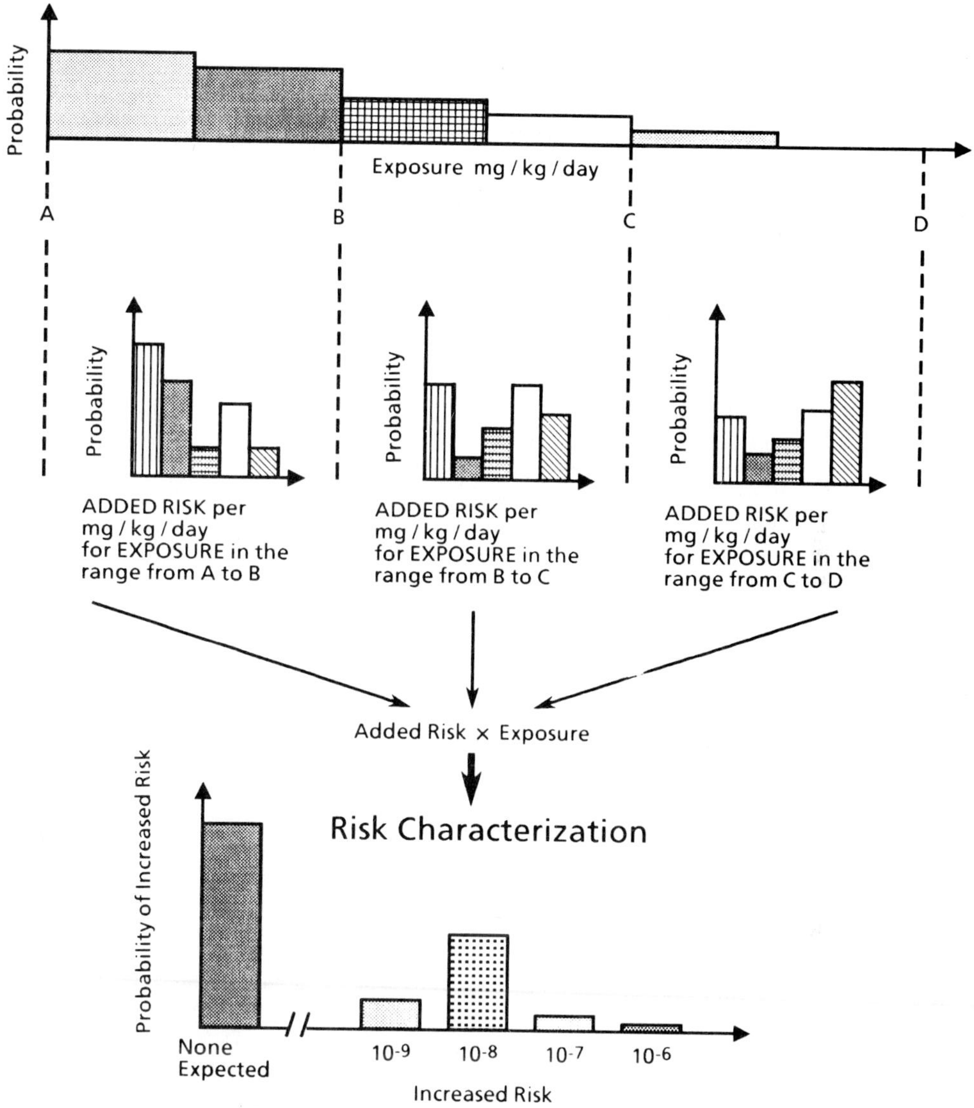

Figure 7.21 Combining Weight-of-Evidence Evaluations of Dose-Response and Exposure when a Chemical Has Different Cancer Potencies in Different Exposure Ranges.

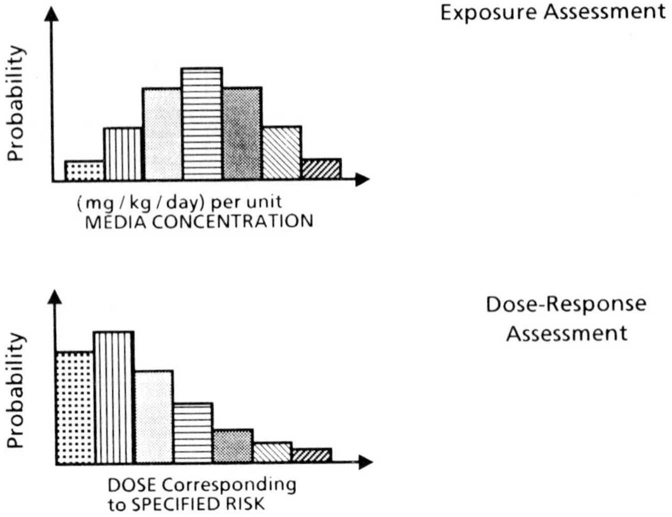

$$\textbf{Media Concentration Standard} = \frac{\textbf{Dose Corresponding to Specified Risk}}{\textbf{Dose per unit Media Concentration}}$$

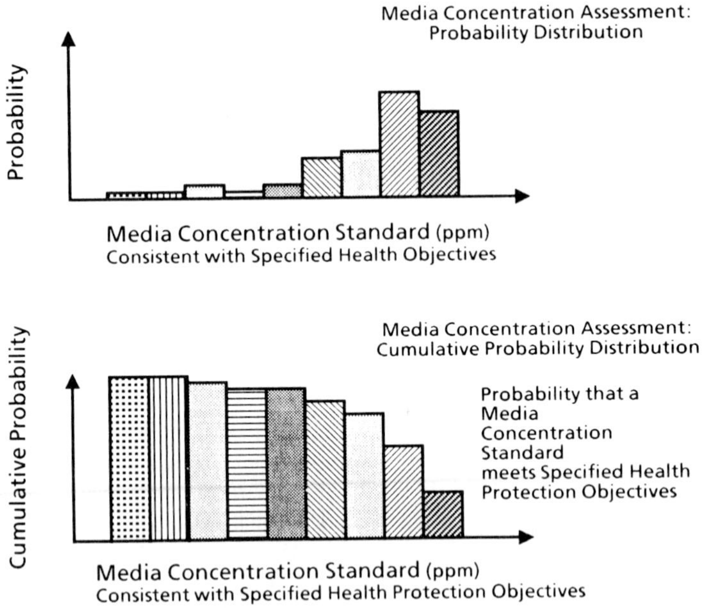

Figure 7.22 Information-Analysis Based Characterization of the Media Concentration of a Chemical Consistent with Specified Health Protection Objectives.

The advantage to the first approach is convenience or simplicity in that one information-analysis distribution for the slope can be developed and used in different situations involving different specified risk levels under the assumption that the dose-response relationship is linear in the dose region of interest and that the slope of the linear relationship is well characterized by the slopes in the decision tree. The advantage to the second approach is that the information-analysis distribution incorporates the *actual shape* of the dose-response relationship between dose zero and the target LADD (not a linear approximation between zero and some fixed dose level which might not be particularly relevant to the target LADD).

The media concentration corresponding to a LADD with risk not exceeding the specified risk level equals

$$\frac{\text{(dose corresponding to specified risk)}}{\text{(dose per unit media concentration)}}$$

The probability distribution for the media concentration standard is determined by the probability distribution for this ratio which can be calculated from the probability distributions for the numerator (the distributional dose-response characterization) and for the denominator (the distributional exposure characterization).

In Figure 7.22, the probability distribution for the media concentration standard is depicted as a histogram analogous to a probability density function. In this histogram, the height of each rectangle (or bar) indicates the probability that the media concentration standard is in the interval corresponding to the base of the rectangle. The cumulative distribution function for the media concentration standard would cumulate the probabilities associated with the rectangles starting from the left. In this application, it is more convenient to cumulate the probabilities starting from the right; so that, the cumulated total at any standard represents the probability that the standard is sufficiently small to be consistent with the specified health protection objectives. Of course, figures analogous to Figure 7.22 could be prepared and presented for each different potential health protection objective.

7.6.4 Example Communications

Information-analysis based distributional characterizations of risk or a media concentration standard provide useful information for risk managers (including the public) for evaluating alternative remediation strategies.[5,15] For example, in Figure 7.23, the distributional characterization of a media concentration standard reflects the variability in the concentration required to meet specified health protection objectives as well as the uncertainty in the current state of knowledge. The distribution quantifies the level of confidence associated with each alternative remediation strategy for meeting specified health protection objectives. In this example, the confidence level increases from 30 percent to 75 percent to 97 percent to almost 100 percent as the remediation strategy moves from strategy A to B to C to D. If, for example, the specified health protection objective was to have the cancer risk not exceed 1/100,000, then strategy A would have a 30 percent chance of meeting

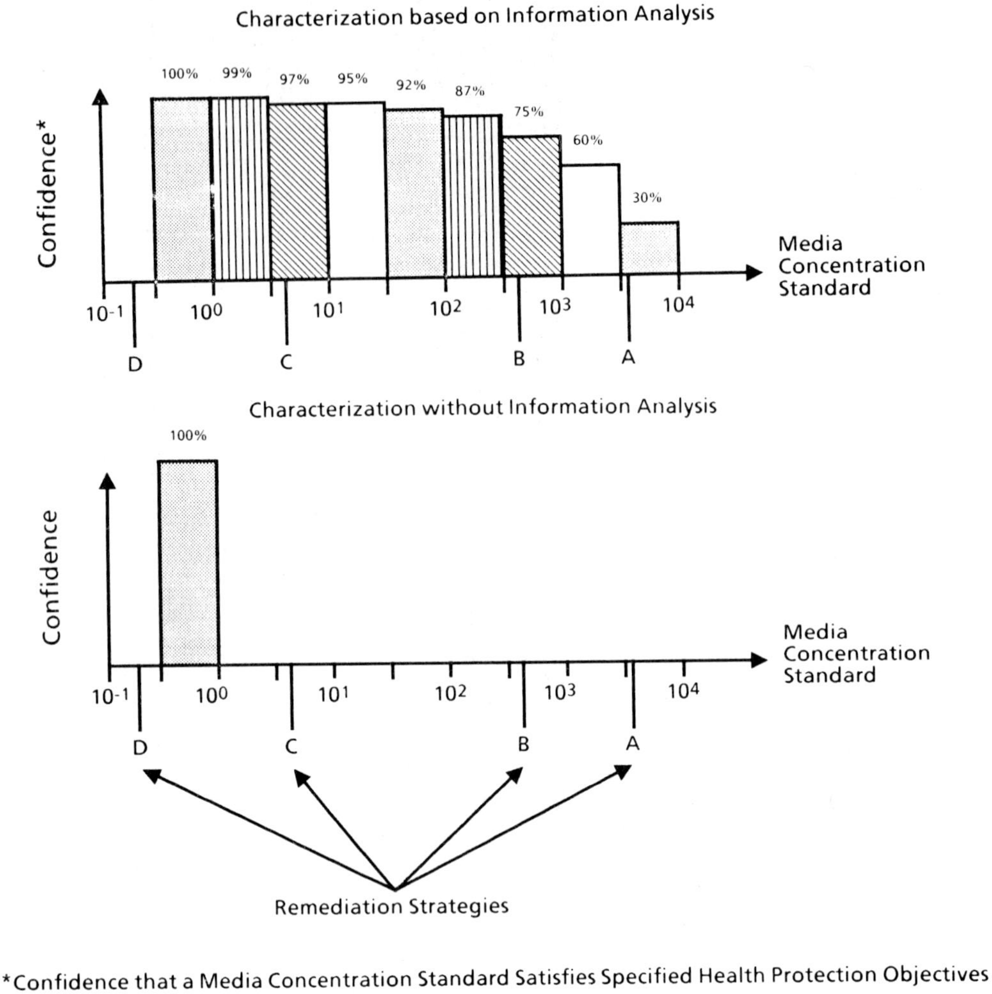

Figure 7.23 Information-Analysis Based Characterizations of the Media Concentration Standard Provide Useful Information for Risk Managers Evaluating Alternative Remediation Strategies.

that objective, strategy B a 75 percent, etc. The difference between remediation strategies is reflected by the differences in the corresponding confidence levels. The difference between remediation strategies is not, generally, the difference between risk and safety or the difference between definitely meeting the health protection objectives and definitely failing to meet those objectives. The differences between remediation strategies are much less dramatic than black versus white. On the other hand, if, as suggested in the bottom part of Figure 7.23, the sole characterization is a single number such as a simple bound, then the differences between remediation strategies is falsely indicated to be like black versus white. Furthermore, with these simplistic single number characterizations, there is no indication of what the differences are between remediation strategies A, B, and C except the false impression that they will definitely not meet the specified health protection objectives. Roughly speaking, distributional characterizations give a much better quantitative indication of the trade-offs between remediation strategies than single number characterizations do. Of course, distributional characterizations do not make remediation decisions, but distributional characterizations do provide more information with which to make that decision.

By quantifying the differences between remediation alternatives, distributional characterizations facilitate cost-benefit analyses and risk management evaluations of trade-offs. Figure 7.24 illustrates the differences between single number characterizations and distributional characterizations in this regard. Figure 7.24 is also a hint of analyses in which the adverse health impacts to remediation personnel are incorporated as well as the adverse health effects of negative economic impacts on a population. Figure 7.25 shows an example of the trade-off between remediation cost in monetary terms and shifting the probability distribution on the residual risk by changing the media concentration standard. In Figure 7.25, for example, the gain from decreasing the media concentration from 1 to 1/2 to 1/10 is that the probability of the residual risk being less than 1/1,000,000 increases from 0.75 to 0.88 to 0.95 with the indicated relative increases in monetary cost.

7.6.5 Future

Probabilistic exposure characterizations are leading the way into an age of probabilistic health risk characterizations. There are many benefits of such characterizations. Some of these benefits have been discussed and illustrated in this section. Among those benefits, is the ability to reflect the current state of knowledge (including variability and uncertainty) concerning both exposure and dose-response in the risk characterization. In the future, risk management decisions, regulations and standards may still be frequently formulated and communicated in terms of single numbers, but those single numbers are expected to be based more and more frequently on probability distributions that reflect all of the available, relevant information.

7.7 SUMMARY

Information analysis identifies the Factors entering into the extrapolation of risks. Then it identifies each relevant alternative for each Factor. Each combination of alternatives for the Factors is explicitly evaluated and its quantitative dose-response attribute computed. These quantitative attributes are reported individually and then summarized in the form of a weighted frequency distributions indicating the proportion of scientific support for each combination of Factor alternatives. Weights can reflect sample sizes, statistical

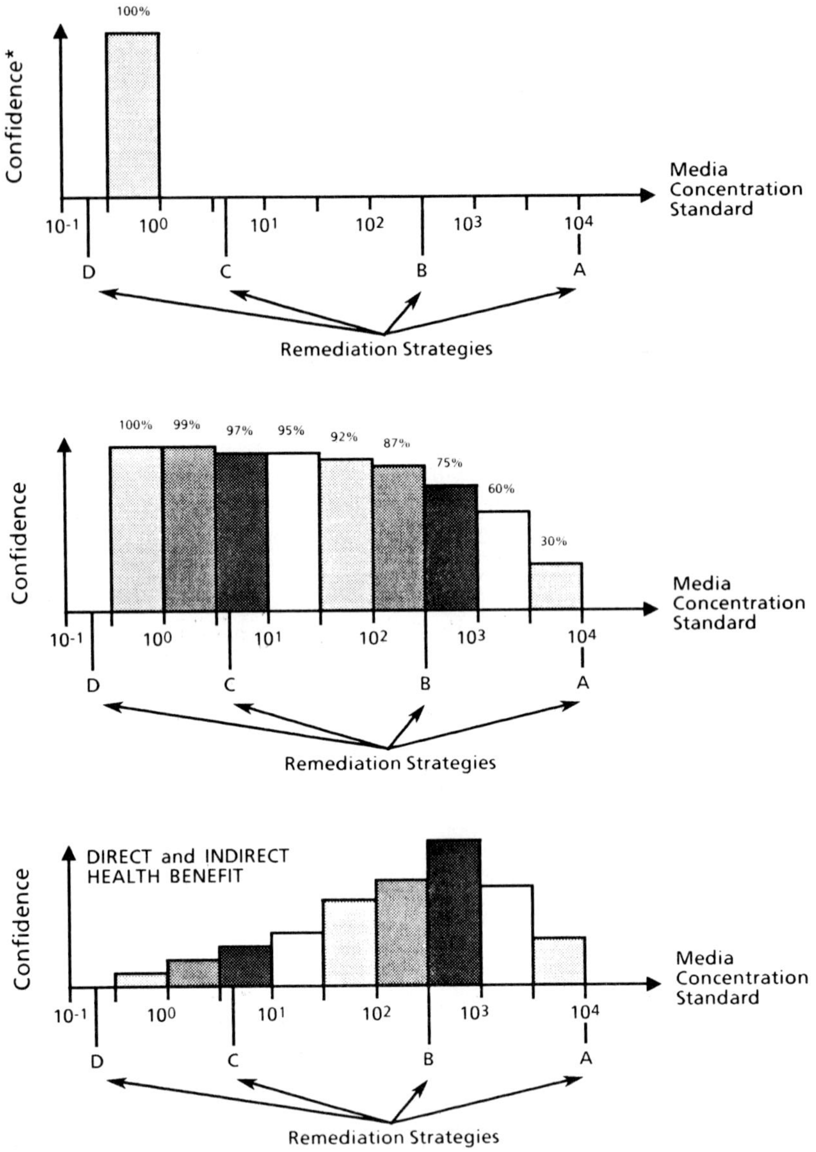

*Confidence that a Media Concentration Standard Satisfies Specified Health Protection Objectives

Figure 7.24 Information for Risk Managers Evaluating Alternative Remediation Strategies.

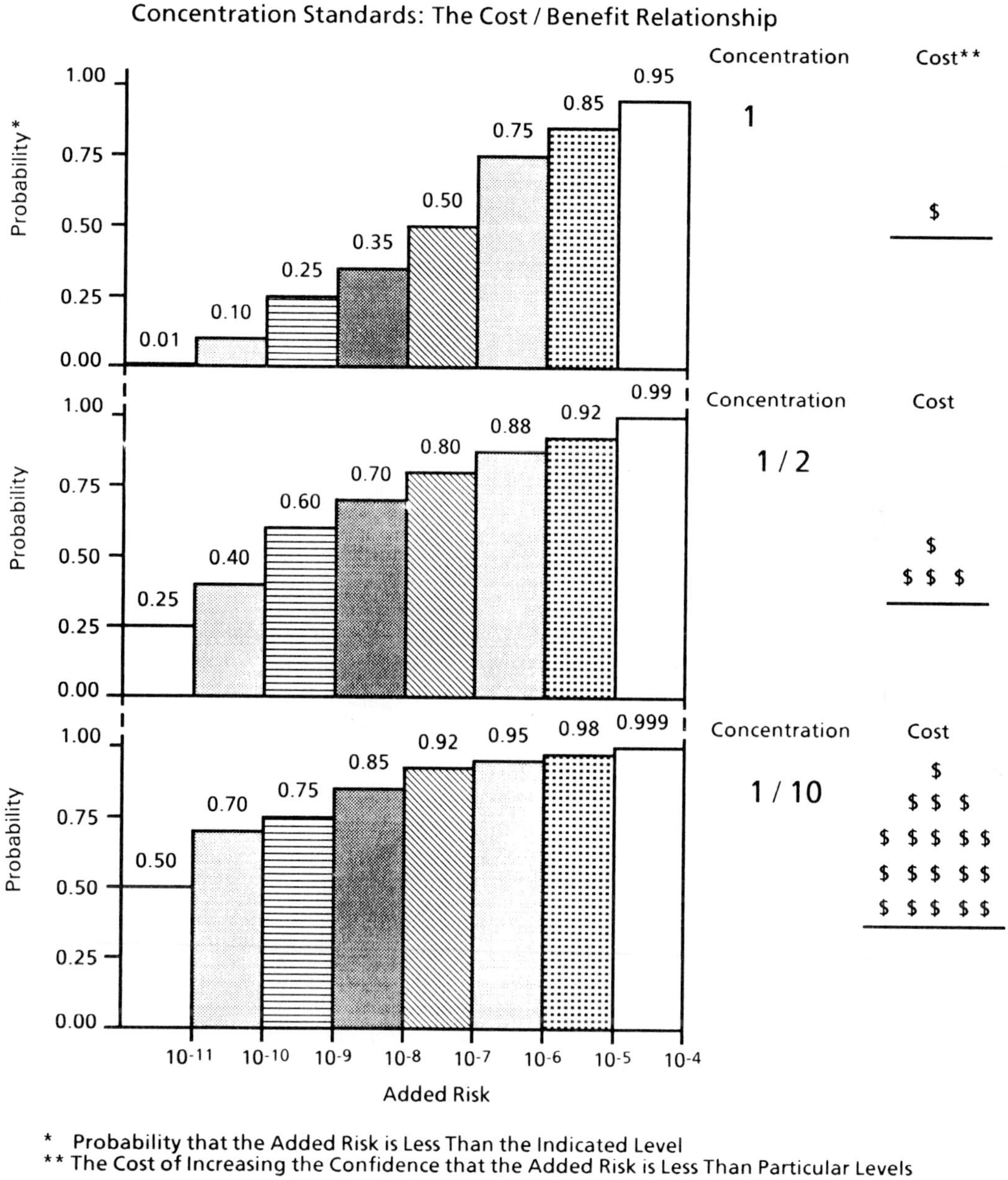

Figure 7.25 The Trade-off between Monetary Cost and Shifting the Probability Distribution on Residual Risk by Changing the Media Concentration Standard.

analyses, or expert judgments of the appropriateness of particular alternatives. Weighting allows relevant alternatives to be evaluated without requiring unattainable proof that a default method is *wrong*. In this manner information analyses also encourage additional data collection and stimulate research. Sensitivity analyses using alternative weights can identify the critical Factors in the quantitative assessment and, thereby, help prioritize and direct research as well as focusing discussions.

A key feature of information analysis as a tool is its focus on defining the problem, its major components, and the alternatives within these components. Decision trees are helpful tools for visualizing this structure. The *divide and conquer* strategy is another key feature of information analysis. By subdividing the problem into comprehensible and manageable pieces, information analysis enables biologists, toxicologists, and other experts to identify the pieces to which they can contribute.[50] This not only encourages broader participation in risk assessment but also helps identify places where additional expertise or more research would be particularly useful.[14,68,69] A third important feature of information analysis is that it encourages the explicit evaluation and presentation of each relevant combination of possibilities or analytical methodologies. This feature encourages the explicit evaluation of alternative approaches as well as default approaches.

An important advantage of the information-analysis based dose-response characterization is its capability of being effectively combined with distributional characterizations of exposure to yield risk characterizations that reflect the variability and uncertainty inherent in both exposure and dose-response relationships as well as the states of knowledge about them. Probability distributions characterizing exposure and dose-response can be combined into a probability distribution for risk that can be effectively communicated, facilitate risk management analyses, readily incorporate new data, and be meaningfully interpreted both statistically and logically.

Information analysis provides a weight-of-evidence approach to quantitative cancer risk assessment.

PROBLEMS

1. For a specified exposure and its corresponding dose, the probability of a carcinogenic response is obtained by evaluating the dose-response model at that dose. Often, this evaluation is roughly approximated by simply multiplying the dose by a cancer potency factor corresponding to the slope in a linear approximation of the dose-response relationship in the low-dose region. This risk characterization is often further simplified by replacing the information-analysis based distributional characterizations of dose and potency by single-number upper bounds, usually the 95th percentiles of the distributions or 95 percent upper confidence limits. The product of these bounds on dose and potency can be either above or below the true 95th percentile of the product. The risk manager can avoid this unnecessary uncertainty by evaluating the distribution (and its 95th percentile) of the product from the distributions of dose and potency.

(a) Assume that the probability distributions for dose and potency are independent and

$$P(\text{dose} = 0\ ppm) = 0.94$$
$$P(\text{dose} = 10\ ppm) = 0.01$$
$$P(\text{dose} = 100\ ppm) = 0.05$$

$$P(\text{cancer potency} = 0.00000 \text{ per } ppm) = 0.94$$
$$P(\text{cancer potency} = 0.00010 \text{ per } ppm) = 0.01$$
$$P(\text{cancer potency} = 0.00100 \text{ per } ppm) = 0.05$$

Find the probability distribution of the product of dose and cancer potency. Compare the 95th percentile of this distribution with the product of the 95th percentile of dose and the 95th percentile of cancer potency.

Answer: 95th percentile of distribution of products = 0.0.
Product of 95th percentile of potency and 95th percentile of dose = 0.001.

(b) Repeat part (a) with

$$P(\text{dose} = 9\ ppm) = 0.94$$
$$P(\text{dose} = 10\ ppm) = 0.01$$
$$P(\text{dose} = 100\ ppm) = 0.05$$

$$P(\text{cancer potency} = 0.00009 \text{ per } ppm) = 0.94$$
$$P(\text{cancer potency} = 0.00010 \text{ per } ppm) = 0.01$$
$$P(\text{cancer potency} = 0.00100 \text{ per } ppm) = 0.05$$

Answer: 95th percentile of distribution of products = 0.009.
Product of 95th percentile of potency and 95th percentile of dose = 0.001.

2. The information-analysis based probability distributions for risk can be combined to describe the aggregate risk from multiple independently acting chemicals. Combining only the 95th percentiles from each distribution can either overstate or understate the true 95th percentile of the aggregate risk. In (a) and (b) find the probability distribution of the combined risk from chemicals X and Y which act independently. Compare the 95th percentile of the combined risk with the sum of the 95th percentiles from the individual chemical risk distributions.

(a)

$$P(\text{risk} = 0 \text{ for chemical X}) = .94$$

$$P(\text{risk} = 50 \times 10^{-8} \text{ for chemical X}) = .01$$

$$P(\text{risk} = 51 \times 10^{-8} \text{ for chemical X}) = .05$$

$$P(\text{risk} = 0 \text{ for chemical Y}) = .94$$

$$P(\text{risk} = 50 \times 10^{-8} \text{ for chemical Y}) = .01$$

$$P(\text{risk} = 51 \times 10^{-8} \text{ for chemical Y}) = .05$$

Answer: 95th percentile of distribution of combined risk = 51×10^{-8}.
Sum of 95th percentile for chemical X and 95th percentile for chemical Y = 100×10^{-8}.

(b)

$$P(\text{risk} = 49 \times 10^{-8} \text{ for chemical X}) = .94$$

$$P(\text{risk} = 50 \times 10^{-8} \text{ for chemical X}) = .01$$

$$P(\text{risk} = 100 \times 10^{-8} \text{ for chemical X}) = .05$$

$$P(\text{risk} = 49 \times 10^{-8} \text{ for chemical Y}) = .94$$

$$P(\text{risk} = 50 \times 10^{-8} \text{ for chemical Y}) = .01$$

$$P(\text{risk} = 100 \times 10^{-8} \text{ for chemical Y}) = .05$$

Answer: 95th percentile of distribution of combined risk = 149×10^{-8}.
Sum of 95th percentile for chemical X and 95th percentile for chemical Y = 100×10^{-8}.

3. Given the following decision tree, compute the weights for all the branches (t, u, v) and paths (w, x, y, z) that do not have a weight assigned.

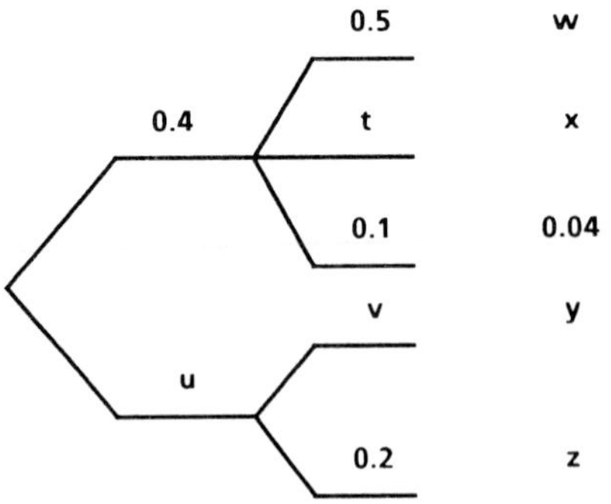

Answer: $t = 0.4$, $u = 0.6$, $v = 0.8$, $w = 0.2$, $x = 0.16$, $y = 0.48$, $z = 0.12$.

4. Given the following decision tree, compute the weights for all the branches $(n, p, q, r, s, t, u, v, w)$ and paths (x, y, z) that do not have a weight assigned. The weights at the end of the tree are the product of the weights on the corresponding path.

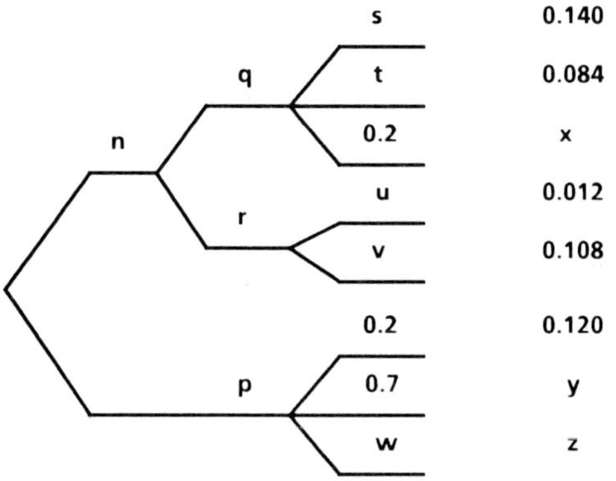

Answer: $n = 0.4, p = 0.6, q = 0.7, r = 0.3, s = 0.5, t = 0.3, u = 0.1, v = 0.9, w = 0.1, x = 0.056, y = 0.42, z = 0.06$.

5. Very often the weights for different alternatives for a Factor are obtained from professional judgment obtained from different leading experts in the field. The judgments expressed by experts may differ as to what weights to assign to the different alternatives for a Factor. In other words, in cancer risk assessment experts frequently have different opinions about different issues. Given the table below with the weights of four experts assigned to four alternatives for a Factor, describe at least three different ways in which the weights for the different alternatives could be derived from the set of weights of the experts.

	Alternatives			
Expert	1	2	3	4
A	0.80	0.00	0.10	0.10
B	0.25	0.25	0.25	0.25
C	0.70	0.15	0.10	0.05
D	0.50	0.30	0.00	0.20

Answer: 1. Select an expert randomly. 2. Assign weights to each expert and compute a weighted average. 3. Use a random sample of more than one expert.

6. In the previous problem the experts had different constant weights assigned to each alternatives for a Factor. A constant weight to each alternative for a Factor is a simplification of what most experts really believe. That is, experts normally have excellent "ball-park" weights of the different alternatives, but not an exact weight. This, in turn, creates a conflict as to what the experts weights ought to be when the weights for an alternative is expressed as a distribution rather than as constant. The following table shows the professional judgment of two experts on the three alternatives for a Factor.

	Alternatives		
Expert	1	2	3
A	$U(0.3, 0.5)$	$N(0.1, 0.1^2)$	$N(0.6, 0.1^2)$
B	0.3	$U(0.1, 0.3)$	$U(0.2, 0.8)$

where, $U(a, b)$ = Uniform distribution between a and b, and $N(a, b^2)$ = Normal distribution truncated between 0 and 1, with mean a and variance b^2. Using the table given above describe different ways in which weights valid for a decision tree could be derived. Remember that the sum of the weights for the different alternatives must be equal to 1.

Answer: 1. Replace each weight distribution by its mean weight and then normalize so that they add up to one. 2. Select a random sample from each distribution and normalize the weights so that they add up to one. 3. Generalize the ideas from the previous problem.

7. Given the following description of existing data, construct the decision tree that represents the relationship among the different factors and alternatives. There are two species analyzed, rat and mouse. There are two sexes within each species, male and female. The responses of interest are kidney carcinomas in all species and sexes, liver carcinomas in male and female rats, and ovarian tumors in female rats and mice. The data is analyzed using the Weibull and the multistage quantal response models. Humans and animals are assumed to be equally sensitive to the same dose levels.

8. Use the following tree, weights, and risk attribute.

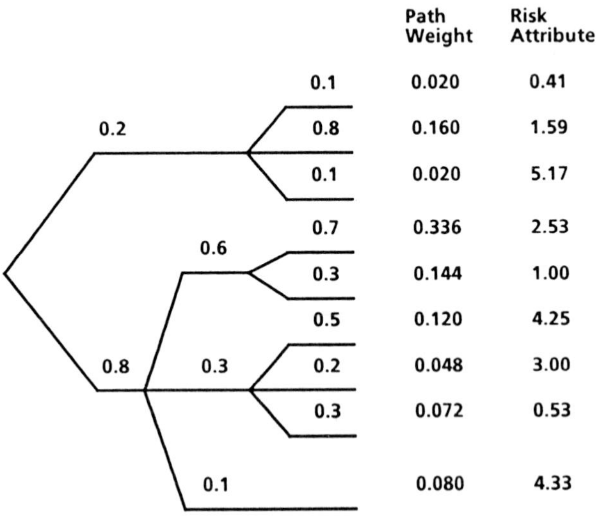

Use the following histogram grid:
0, 1, 2, 3, 4, 5, 6, where the grid defines intervals closed on the right; that is, if $x = 2.0$ then the weight of x belongs in the interval from 1 to 2

(a) Construct the histogram of risk attributes.

(b) Construct the cumulative histogram of risk attributes.

(c) Using linear interpolation and the cumulative histogram from part (b), find the 95th percentile of risk attributes.

(d) Using the risk attribute values, find the 95th percentile of risk attributes; that is, find $x =$ smallest risk attribute such that 95% or more risk attributes are less than or equal to x.

9. Use the results shown in Figures 7.4 through 7.6 on the maximum likelihood estimates of the added risk at one *ppb* and the following information on weights. Note that the maximum likelihood estimates in Figure 7.4 are the same as in Figures 7.5 and 7.6, only the weights are different for different modes of action. For simplicity, assume that the weights given below apply to all three modes of action; so that, effectively the mode of action can be ignored in this problem.

Alternatives:	Weights:
Human Carcinogen	= 0.8
Not a Human Carcinogen	= 0.2
Malignant (M)	= 0.8
Malignant and Benign (M&B)	= 0.2
PPM	= 0.1
INTAKE	= 0.3
DPX	= 0.6
When Dose Scale = PPM	
Same Dose Scale	= 0.2
$BW^{3/4}$	= 0.4
$BW^{2/3}$	= 0.4
THRESHOLD	= 0.4
SUBLINEAR	= 0.4
SUBLINEAR (LDL)	= 0.1
LINEAR	= 0.1
When Dose Scale = INTAKE	
Same Dose Scale	= 0.50
$BW^{3/4}$	= 0.25
$BW^{2/3}$	= 0.25
THRESHOLD	= 0.4
SUBLINEAR	= 0.4
SUBLINEAR (LDL)	= 0.1

LINEAR	= 0.1
When Dose Scale = DPX	
Same Dose Scale	= 0.8
$BW^{3/4}$	= 0.1
$BW^{2/3}$	= 0.1
THRESHOLD	= 0.2
SUBLINEAR	= 0.3
SUBLINEAR (LDL)	= 0.4
LINEAR	= 0.1

Use the following histogram grid:

$$0,\ 1 \times 10^{-20},\ 0.0000000001,\ 0.000000001,\ 0.00000001,\ 0.0000001,\ 0.000001,$$

$$0.00001,\ 0.0001,\ 0.001$$

where the grid defines intervals closed on the right; that is, if $x = 0.00001$ then the weight of x belongs in the interval from 0.000001 to 0.00001

(a) Construct the histogram of maximum likelihood estimates of the added risk at one *ppb*.

(b) Construct the cumulative histogram of maximum likelihood estimates of the added risk at one *ppb*.

(c) Using linear interpolation and the cumulative histogram from part (b), find the 95th percentile of maximum likelihood estimates of the added risk at one *ppb*.

(d) Using the data in Figures 7.4 through 7.6, find the 95th percentile of maximum likelihood estimates of the added risk at one *ppb*; that is, find x=smallest maximum likelihood estimate of the added risk at one *ppb* such that 95 percent or more estimates are less than or equal to x.

10. Using the results shown in Figures 7.4 through 7.6, and the weights and grid for the histogram from problem 9, perform a sensitivity analysis on the dose scale being used. In other words, construct three histograms that show the impact on the added risk distribution of different assumptions regarding the dose scale.
Answer: Construct one histogram for each dose scale, assigning weight 1 to the dose scale being analyzed.

11. Using the results shown in Figures 7.4 through 7.6, and the weights and grid for the histogram from problem 9, perform a sensitivity analysis on the interspecies extrapolation method being used. In other words, construct three histograms that show the impact on the added risk distribution of different assumptions regarding the method of adjusting dose scales to account for interspecies differences.
Answer: Construct one histogram for each interspecies extrapolation method, assigning weight 1 to the interspecies extrapolation method being analyzed.

12. Using the results shown in Figures 7.4 through 7.6 for the 95 percent upper confidence limit on the added risk at one *ppb* and the weights and grid for the histograms from problem 9,

(a) Construct the histogram of 95 percent upper confidence limits on the added risk at one *ppb*.

(b) Construct the cumulative histogram of 95 percent upper confidence limits on the added risk at one *ppb*.

(c) Using linear interpolation and the cumulative histogram from part (b), find the approximate 95th percentile of 95 percent upper confidence limits on the added risk at one *ppb*.

(d) Using the data in Figures 7.4 through 7.6 find the 95th percentile of 95 percent upper confidence limits on the added risk at one *ppb*; that is, find x=smallest 95 percent upper confidence limit on the added risk at one *ppb* such that 95 percent or more of the 95 percent upper confidence limits are less than or equal to x.

13. In previous problems we have seen the impact that different assumptions have on the distributions of added cancer risks at one *ppb*. Figures 7.7 through 7.9 show the percentiles of the different combinations of possibilities when bootstrap samples are simulated to determine a distribution of the maximum likelihood estimate of the added risk at one *ppb*. By eyeballing Figures 7.7 through 7.9, discuss which factors seem to impact the distribution of the added risks the most and therefore are most worthy of further research. In other words, assume the risk manager wants a ranking of the different areas where limited research funds should be spent in order to reduce risk and uncertainty.

14. There may be more than one temporal exposure pattern of interest. Either the temporal exposure pattern must be explicitly included in the dose-response modeling, or a relevant dose measure, such as lifetime average daily dose, must be evaluated. In the CIIT formaldehyde inhalation study, rats were exposed beginning at age 1.5 months and continuing for the next 24 months or until death. The exposure concentrations for 6 hours per day and 5 days per week were 0, 2, 5.6 and 14.3 *ppm*.

(a) Determine the lifetime average daily formaldehyde concentration.

(b) The amount of DPX formed in the respiratory tract per hour of exposure has been estimated by Casanova *et al.*[61] to be

$$C_{\mathrm{DPX}} = 0.5\left\{QC_e - \frac{P(1+R)}{R}\sqrt{\left[\frac{P(1+R)}{R} - QC_e\right]^2 \frac{4PQC_e}{R}}\right\}$$

where

C_e = is the exposure concentration of formaldehyde, *ppm*

C_{DPX} = DPX formed in the respiratory tract, *p mol* of *DPX/mg DNA/hr* [One *picomole (p mol)* is equal to one trillionth of a gram mole.]

$P = 30.7$ *p mol/mg DNA/hr*

$R = 8.1$ (dimensionless)

$Q = 7.3$ *p mol/mg DNA/hr/ppm*

for rats, and for humans

$P = 1.3$ *p mol/mg DNA/hr*

$R = 11.5$ (dimensionless)

$Q = 0.7\ p\ mol/mg\ DNA/hr/ppm.$

Determine the lifetime average daily amount of DPX formed in the experimental rats.

(c) Show that the lifetime average daily amount of DPX formed in the experimental rats at 2 *ppm* is not equal to the lifetime average daily amount of DPX formed in rats if they had been exposed continuously to the lifetime average daily concentration determined in (a) corresponding to the 2 *ppm* dose group.

(d) Using the equation for the concentration of DPX in (b), determine the lifetime average daily amount of DPX formed in the respiratory tract of humans exposed to one ppb for 8 hours per day, 5 days per week, 50 weeks per year and 40 years per lifetime in a 70-year lifetime. [If the risk is to be characterized for these people and the lifetime average daily dose is assumed to be the relevant dose measure, then the maximum likelihood estimates in the decision tree in Figures 7.4 through 7.6 should be recalculated using lifetime average daily dose instead of dose during exposure and the probability distribution in Figure 7.11 recomputed.]

REFERENCES

1. Paustenbach, D.J., "Health Risk Assessments: Opportunities and Pitfalls," *Columbia Journal of Environmental Law*, **14**, 411 (1989).
2. Finkel, A.M., "Is Risk Assessment Really Too Conservative? Revising the Revisionists," *Columbia Journal of Environmental Law*, **14**, 427 (1989).
3. Nichols, A.L., and R.J. Zeckhauser, "The Perils of Prudence: How Conservative Risk Assessments Distort Regulation," *Regulatory Toxicology and Pharmacology*, **8**, 61 (1988).
4. Sielken, R.L. Jr., "Useful Tools for Evaluating and Presenting More Science in Quantitative Cancer Risk Assessments," *Toxic Substances Journal*, **9**, 353 (1989).
5. Habicht II, F.H., "Guidance on Risk Characterization for Risk Managers and Risk Assessors," Office of the Administrator, U.S. Environmental Protection Agency, Washington, D.C., February, 26 (1992).
6. North, W., "Representing Uncertainty Explicitly in Environmental Risk Management: An Example from Acid Deposition Policy Analysis," *Proceedings of the Specialty Conference on Environmental Risk Management*, "Is Analysis Useful?" Air Pollution Control Association, Chicago, IL, April (1986).
7. Richmond, H.R., "Development of Probabilistic Health Risk Assessment for National Ambient Air Quality Standards," Presented at APCA International Specialty Conference on Regulatory Approaches for Control of Air Pollution, Atlanta, GA, February 17-20 (1987).
8. Whitfield, R.G., T.S. Wallsten, R.L. Winkler, and H.M. Richmond, *Assessing the Risk of Chronic Lung Injury Attributable to Ozone Exposure*, Argonne National Laboratory, Argonne, IL, August (1990).
9. Whitfield, R.G. and T.S. Wallsten, "A Risk Assessment for Selected Lead-Induced Health Effects: An Example of a General Methodology," *Risk Analysis*, **9**, 197 (1989).
10. Hammit, J.K., "Subjective-Probability-Based Scenarios for Uncertain Input Parameters: Stratospheric Ozone Depletion," *Risk Analysis*, **10**, 93 (1990).

11. Harris, R.H. and D.E. Burmaster, "Restoring Science to Superfund Risk Assessment," *Toxics Law Reporter*, 1318 (1992).
12. Thompson, K.M., D.E. Burmaster, and E. Crouch, "Monte Carlo Techniques for Quantitative Uncertainty Analysis in Public Health Risk Assessments," *Risk Analysis*, **12**, 53 (1992).
13. Evans, J.S., J.D. Graham, G.M. Gray, and R.L. Sielken, Jr., "The Likelihood of Alternative Carcinogenic Potencies: Uncertainty Analysis of Formaldehyde," Cancer Dose-Response Working Group, Workshop # 3, Characterization of Cancer Dose-Response, ILSI Risk Science Institute, Washington, D.C., March 23-24 (1992).
14. Evans, J.S., J.D. Graham, G.M. Gray, A. Hollis, B. Ryan, A. Smith, M. Smith, and A. Taylor, "Summary of Workshop to Review an OMB Report on Risk Assessment and Management," *Risk: Issues in Health and Safety*, **3**, 71 (1992).
15. Report of an Ad Hoc Study Group on Risk Assessment Presentation, *Presentation of Risk Assessments of Carcinogens*, American Industrial Health Council, Washington, D.C., July (1989).
16. Paustenbach, D.J., "Important Recent Advances in the Practice of Health Risk Assessment: Implications for the 1990s," *Regulatory Toxicology and Pharmacology*, **10**, 204 (1989).
17. Graham, J.D., L. Green, and M. Roberts, *In Search of Safety: Chemicals and Cancer Risk*, Cambridge, MA, Harvard University Press (1988).
18. Gray, G.M. and J.D. Graham, "The Challenge of Risk Characterization: Illustrations Using Unleaded Gasoline and Formaldehyde," in *Environmental Health Perspectives*, in press.
19. Graham, J.D. and G.M. Gray, "Air Toxics: Characterizing the Risks," *Journal of the Air and Waste Management Association*, in press.
20. Sielken, R.L. Jr., "Some Capabilities, Limitations, and Pitfalls in the Quantitative Risk Assessment of Formaldehyde," *Risk Analysis in the Chemical Industry*, Chemical Manufacturers Association, Washington, D.C. (1985).
21. Sielken, R.L. Jr., "The Capabilities, Sensitivity, Pitfalls and Future of Quantitative Risk Assessment," in *Environmental Health Risks: Assessment and Management*, McColl, R.S., Ed., University of Waterloo Press, Waterloo, Ontario (1987).
22. Rusch, G.M., H.F. Bolte, and W.E. Rinehart, "A 26-Week Inhalation Toxicity Study with Formaldehyde in the Monkey, Rat, and Hamster," in *Formaldehyde Toxicity*, Gibson, J.E., Ed., Hemisphere Publishing Corporation, New York, 98 (1983).
23. Clary, J.J., "Risk Assessment for Exposure to Formaldehyde," in *Formaldehyde Toxicity*, Gibson, J.E., Ed., Hemisphere Publishing Corporation, New York, 284 (1983).
24. Battelle Columbus Laboratories, "Final Report on A Chronic Inhalation Toxicity Study in Rats and Mice Exposed to Formaldehyde to Chemical Industry Institute of Toxicology, submitted September 18, 1981; revised December 31, 1981," Battelle Columbus Laboratories, Columbus, Ohio [Chemical Industry Institute of Toxicology (CIIT) Docket # 10922, 1982].
25. Kerns, W.D., K.L. Pavkov, D.J. Donofrio, and J.A. Swenberg, "Carcinogenicity of Formaldehyde in Rats and Mice After Long-term Inhalation Exposure," *Cancer Research*, **43**, 4382 (1983).
26. Lu, F.C. and R.L. Sielken, Jr., "Assessment of Safety/Risk of Chemicals: Inception and Evolution of the ADI and Dose-Response Modeling Procedures," *Toxicology Letters*, **59**, 5 (1991).

27. Finkel, A.M. "Confronting Uncertainty in Risk Management: A Guide for Decision-Makers," Report prepared by Center for Risk Management, Resources for the Future, Washington, D.C. (1990).
28. Morgan, M.G. and M. Henrion, *Uncertainty: A Guide to Dealing with Uncertainty in Risk and Policy Analysis*, Cambridge University Press, New York, N.Y. (1990).
29. Bogen, K.T., *Uncertainty in Environmental Health Risk Assessment*, Garland Publishing Inc., New York, N.Y. (1990).
30. Hattis, D., "Three Candidate 'Laws' of Uncertainty Analysis," *Risk Analysis*, **10**, 11 (1990).
31. Morgan, M.G., "Uncertainty and Quantitative Assessment in Risk Management," in *Assessment and Management of Chemical Risks*, Rodricks, J.V. and R.G. Tardiff, Eds., American Chemical Society, Washington, D.C., 113 (1984).
32. Park, C.N., "Mathematical Models in Quantitative Assessment of Carcinogenic Risk," *Regulatory Toxicology and Pharmacology*, **9**, 236 (1989).
33. Sielken, R.L. Jr., "A Weight-of-Evidence Approach to Quantitative Cancer Risk Assessment: Information Analysis," in *Proceedings of the Satellite Symposium on Risk Assessment in Chemical Carcinogenesis*, Schettler, G., D. Schmähl, and T. Klenner, Eds., Springer-Verlag, New York, 64 (1991).
34. Sielken, R.L. Jr., "New Approaches and Tools for Quantitative Cancer Risk Assessment," *The Analysis, Communication, and Perception of Risk*, Plenum Publishing Corporation, New York, 677 (1991).
35. Graham, J.D., N.C. Hawkins, and M.J. Roberts, "Expert Scientific Judgment in Quantitative Risk Assessment," *Carcinogen Risk Assessment: New Directions in the Qualitative and Quantitative Aspects* [Banbury Report 31], R.W. Hart and F.D. Hoerger, Eds., Cold Spring Harbor Laboratory, Cold Spring Harbor, New York, 231 (1988).
36. Brown, K.G., "Risk Assessment of Laboratory Rats and Mice Chronically Exposed to Formaldehyde Vapors," *Risk Analysis*, **5**, 171 (1985).
37. Starr, T.B., "Quantitative Cancer Risk Estimation for Formaldehyde," *Risk Analysis*, **10**, 85 (1990).
38. Finkel, A.M., "Edifying Presentation of Risk Estimates: Not As Easy As It Seems," *Journal of Policy Analysis and Management*, **10**, 296 (1991).
39. Zeckhauser, R.J. and W.K. Viscusi, "Risk Within Reason," *Science*, **238**, 559 (1990).
40. Spetzler, C.S. and C.S. von Holstein, "Probability Encoding in Decision Analysis," *Management Science*, **22**, 340 (1975).
41. Morgan, M.G., M. Henrion, and S.C. Morrise, "Expert Judgments for Policy Analysis," BNL 51358 UC-13, Brookhaven National Laboratory, Upton, New York (1980).
42. Hawkins, N.C. and J.D. Graham, "Expert Scientific Judgment and Cancer Risk Assessment: A Pilot Study of Pharmacokinetic Data," *Risk Analysis*, **8**, 615 (1988).
43. Morgan, M.G., M. Henrion, S.C. Morris, and D.A.L. Amaral, "Uncertainty in Risk Assessment," *Environmental Science and Technology*, **19**, 662 (1985).
44. Sielken, R.L. Jr. and D.E. Stevenson, "Comparisons of Human Cancer Potency Projections for Dieldrin Based on Human Data with those Based on Animal Data," *Relevance of Animal Studies to the Evaluation of Human Cancer Risk*, D'Amato, R., T.J. Slaga, W.H. Farland,

and C. Henry, Eds., Wiley-LISS, New York, N.Y. 295 (1992).

45. Environmental Protection Agency (EPA), "Formaldehyde Risk Assessment Update, June 11, 1991," Office of Toxic Substances, U.S. EPA, Washington, D.C. (1991).
46. Environmental Protection Agency (EPA), *Cancer Risk from Outdoor Exposure to Air Toxics*, U.S. EPA, Washington, D.C., EPA-450/89 (1990).
47. Report on the Consensus Conference on Formaldehyde, *Environmental Health Perspectives*, **58**, 334 (1984).
48. Swenberg, J.A. and C.J. Boreiko, "Appropriateness of Polypoid Adenoma Data for Quantitative Risk Assessment," Chemical Industry Institute of Toxicology, Research Triangle Park, NC (1985).
49. University Associated for Research and Education in Pathology Inc., "Epidemiology of Chronic Exposure to Formaldehyde, Report of the Ad Hoc Panel on Health Aspects of Formaldehyde," *Toxicology and Industrial Health*, **4**, 77 (1988).
50. Bonano, E.J., S.C. Hora, R.L. Keeney, and D. von Winterfeldt, *Elicitation and Use of Expert Judgment in Performance Assessment for High-Level Radioactive Waste Repositories*, Sandia National Laboratories, Albuquerque, NM, SAND89-1821, May 1990.
51. Environmental Protection Agency (EPA), "Guidelines for Carcinogenic Risk Assessment," Federal Register, **51**, 33993 (1986).
52. Monticello, T.M., F.J. Miller, J.A. Swenberg, T.B. Starr, and J.E. Gibson, "Association of Enhanced Cell Proliferation and Nasal Cancer in Rats Exposed to Formaldehyde," Chemical Industry Institute of Toxicology, Research Triangle Park, NC, *The Toxicologist*, **12**, 1017 (1992).
53. Goldmacher, V.S. and W.G. Thilly, "Formaldehyde is Mutagenic for Cultured Human Cells," *Mutation Research*, **116**, 417 (1983).
54. Conolly, R.B. and M.E. Andersen, "Biologically Based Pharmacodynamic Models: Tools for Toxicological Research and Risk Assessment," *Annual Review of Pharmacology and Toxicology*, **31**, 503 (1991).
55. Starr, T.B., "Quantitative Cancer Risk Estimation for Formaldehyde," in *Nasal Carcinogenesis in Rodents: Relevance to Human Health Risks*, Feron, V.J., and M.C. Bosland, Eds., Pudoc, Wageningen, The Netherlands, 179 (1989).
56. Starr, T.B., and R.D. Buck, "The Importance of Delivered Dose in Estimating Low-Dose Risk from Inhalation Exposure to Formaldehyde," *Fundamental and Applied Toxicology*, **4**, 740 (1984).
57. Hoel, D.G., N.L. Kaplan, and M.W. Anderson, "Implication of Nonlinear Kinetics on Risk Estimation in Carcinogenesis," *Science*, **219**, 1032 (1983).
58. Chang, J.C., E.A. Gross, J. Martin, and J.A. Popp, "Nasal Cavity Deposition, Histopathology and Cell Proliferation Following Single or Repeated Formaldehyde Exposures in B6C3F1 mice and F-344 Rats," *Toxicology and Applied Pharmacology*, **68**, 161 (1983).
59. Chang, J.C., W.H. Steinhagen, and C.S. Barrow, "Effect of Single or Repeated Formaldehyde Exposure on Minute Volume of B6C3F mice and F-344 Rats," *Toxicology and Applied Pharmacology*, **61**, 451 (1981).
60. Casanova, M., D.F. Deyo, and H. d'A. Heck, "Covalent Binding of Inhaled Formaldehyde

to DNA in Nasal Mucosa of Fischer 344 Rats: Analysis of Formaldehyde and DNA by High-Performance Liquid Chromatography and Provisional Pharmacokinetic Interpretation," *Fundamental and Applied Toxicology*, **12**, 397 (1989).

61. Casanova, M., K.T. Morgan, W.H. Steinhagen, J.I. Everitt, J.A. Popp, and H. d'A. Heck, "Covalent Binding of Inhaled Formaldehyde to DNA in the Respiratory Tract of Rhesus Monkeys: Pharmacokinetics, Rat-to-Monkey Interspecies Scaling, and Extrapolation to Man," *Fundamental and Applied Toxicology*, **17**, 409 (1991).
62. Casanova, M. and H. d'A. Heck, "The Impact of DNA-Protein Cross- Linking Studies on Quantitative Risk Assessments of Formaldehyde," *CIIT Activities*, **11**, 1, August (1991).
63. Albert, R.E., A.R. Sellakumar, S. Laskin, M. Kuschner, N. Nelson, and C.A. Snyder, "Gaseous Formaldehyde and Hydrogen Chloride Induction of Nasal Cancer in the Rat," *Journal of the National Cancer Institute*, **68**, 597 (1982).
64. Sellakumar, A.R., C.A. Snyder, J.J. Solomon, and R.E. Albert, "Carcinogenicity of Formaldehyde and Hydrogen Chloride in Rats," *Toxicology and Applied Pharmacology*, **81**, 401 (1985).
65. Wolff, S.K., N.C. Hawkins, S.M. Kennedy, and J.D. Graham, "Selecting Experimental Data for Use in Quantitative Risk Assessment: An Expert-Judgment Approach," *Toxicology and Industrial Health*, **6**, 275 (1990).
66. Otway, H. and D. von Winterfledt, "Expert Judgment in Risk Analysis and Management: Process, Context, and Pitfalls," *Risk Analysis*, **12**, 83 (1992).
67. Kahneman, D., P. Slovic, and A. Tversky, *Judgment Under Uncertainty: Heuristics and Biases*, Cambridge University Press, New York, N.Y. (1982).
68. Hammit, J.K. and J.A. Cave, *Research Planning for Food Safety: A Value-of-Information Approach*, Santa Monica, CA, Rand Corporation, R-3946-ASPE/NCTR (1991).
69. Environmental Protection Agency (EPA), "Research to Improve Health Risk Assessments Program," U.S. EPA, Washington, D.C., June (1990).
70. Paustenbach, D.J., Ed., *The Risk Assessment of Environmental and Human Health Hazards: A Textbook of Case Studies*, John Wiley & Sons (1989).
71. Environmental Protection Agency, *Exposure Factors Handbook*, EPA/600/8-89/043, Office of Health and Environmental Assessment, U.S. EPA, Washington, D.C. (1989).
72. Bogen, K.T. and R.C. Spear, "Integrating Uncertainty and Interindividual Variability in Environmental Risk Assessment," *Risk Analysis*, **7**, 427 (1987).

I

Calculation of Age-Standardized Rates

The term *age-standardized* death rates as used by Doll and Peto[1] and most other authors is defined as the weighted average of the 18 separate *age-specific rates*. The age-specific death rate is defined as the death rate from some particular type of cancer (say, lung cancer) in a particular population (say U.S. males) in a particular narrow range of ages. That is, let $d_{i,1978}$ denote the number of deaths from a particular type of cancer for a population in the age range i (say 60–64 years) for the year 1978, and let $n_{i,1978}$ denote the total population in age range i. Then

$$\textit{Age-specific death rate for a particular type of cancer} = \frac{d_{i,1978}}{n_{i,1978}}$$

The 18 *five year age ranges* used by Doll and Peto are: 0–4, 5–9, 10–14, 15–19, . . ., 75–79, 80–84, and 85 and over.

The age-standardized rate obviously depends on the weights selected. For example, consider the case of stomach cancer rates for U.S. males. If positive weights were assigned to the first 13 age-specific cancer rates (those for 0–4, 5–9, . . ., 60–64) and zero weights for the last five ranges (65–69, 70–74, . . ., 80–84, and 85 and over), then one would obtain the age-standardized stomach cancer rates among men under 65 years of age. To demonstrate the age-standardization procedure, the male cancer rates for the year 1977 are age-standardized to the U.S. 1970 population. The U.S. male cancer deaths for each age group for 1977, the male population for 1977, and the 1970 population distribution per $1,000,000$ people (all taken from the U.S. census) is shown in Table I.1.

From column 3 of Table I.1, it is evident that for any age range i, the 1977 male cancer death rate is age-adjusted to the 1970 census (per 100 million people) as follows:

$$\bar{d}_{i,1977} = \left(\frac{d_{i,1977}}{n_{i,1977}}\right) w_{i,1970}$$

where

$d_{i,1977}$ = number of U.S. male cancer deaths in range i in 1977.

$\bar{d}_{i,1977}$ = number of U.S. male cancer deaths in age range i in 1977 after age-adjusting to the 1970 U.S. census (per 100 million people).

$n_{i,1977}$ = number of U.S. males in age range i in 1977.

$w_{i,1977}$ = weight for range i = number of people in range i per 100 million population.

The total U.S. male deaths due to lung cancer in 1977 [age-adjusted to 1970 per 100 million people] is the sum of the entries of column 3 of Table I.1, or the sum of the $\bar{d}_{i,1977}$'s. Since there are approximately 100 million males and 110 million females in the United States (with 10 million of each being over 65), the basis of 100 million people for the 1970 weight factor is a convenient basis because the resulting weighed cancer deaths are approximately equal to the actual number of cancer deaths.

The age-adjustment of the deaths for different years relative to one particular year, such as 1970 makes the comparison of trends more meaningful as discussed by Doll and Peto. Cancer mortality rates are commonly expressed as deaths per 100,000 population. The rates presented in Table I.1 may be expressed on this basis. For example, the weighted sum of 68,643.9 cancer deaths for men for the year 1977 per 100 million population may be expressed in deaths per 100,000; that is,

$$68,643.9\left(\frac{deaths}{100\ million}\right) = 68.6439\left(\frac{deaths}{100,000}\right)$$

REFERENCES

1. Doll, R., and R. Peto, "The Causes of Cancer: Quantitative Estimates of Avoidable Risks of Cancer in the United States Today," *JNCI*, **66**(6), 1191 (1981).

Table I.1 Calculation of the 1977 U.S. Male Cancer Deaths, Age-adjusted to the 1970 U.S. Census.

	Age Range	Column 1 U.S. Male, Lung Cancer Deaths in 1977	Column 2 U.S. Male Population in 1977	Column 3 U.S. Census per 100 Million People, 1970	Column 4* 1977, Deaths per 100 Million Age-adjusted to 1970
No.	Years				
1	0–4	2	8.090×10^6	8.4416×10^6	2.1
2	5–9	5	9.051×10^6	9.8204×10^6	5.4
3	10–14	2	9.922×10^6	10.2304×10^6	2.1
4	15–19	10	10.896×10^6	9.3845×10^6	8.6
5	20–24	23	10.404×10^6	8.0561×10^6	18.6
6	25–29	55	9.378×10^6	6.6320×10^6	38.9
7	30–34	147	8.016×10^6	5.6249×10^6	103.2
8	35–39	423	6.397×10^6	5.4656×10^6	361.4
9	40–44	1,119	5.740×10^6	5.8958×10^6	1,149.4
10	45–49	2,921	5.879×10^6	5.9622×10^6	2,962.3
11	50–54	5,780	5.863×10^6	5.4643×10^6	5,386.9
12	55–59	8,607	5.425×10^6	4.9077×10^6	7,786.3
13	60–64	11,495	4.500×10^6	4.2403×10^6	10,831.6
14	65–69	12,987	3.704×10^6	3.4406×10^6	12,063.8
15	70–74	11,479	2.592×10^6	2.6789×10^6	11,863.8
16	75–79	7,972	1.648×10^6	1.8871×10^6	9,128.6
17	80–84	4,241	1.018×10^6	1.1241×10^6	4,683.0
18	85+	2,038	0.674×10^6	0.7435×10^6	2,248.1
	Totals	69,307	109.197×10^6	100.000×10^6	68,643.9

* Column 4 equals (Column 1/Column 2) $\times$ Column 3

II

Theorems

A small number of well-known definitions and theorems are used repeatedly throughout the development. Although these definitions and theorems are to be found in most texts dealing with functional analysis, they are repeated here for the convenience of the reader.

Definition II.1 *Continuity of $f(x)$ at x_0: The function $f(x)$ is said to be continuous at the point x_0 if, for every positive number ϵ, there exists a δ_ϵ depending upon ϵ such that for all x of the domain for which*

$$|x - x_0| < \delta_\epsilon$$

then

$$|f(x) - f(x_0)| < \epsilon$$

Definition II.2 *Continuity of $f(x)$ in an interval: A function which is continuous at each point in an interval is said to be continuous in the interval.*

Theorem II.1 (Mean Value Theorem of Differential Calculus) *If the function $f(x)$ is continuous in the interval $a \leq x \leq b$ and differentiable at every point of the interval $a < x < b$, then there exists at least one value ξ such that*

$$f(b) = f(a) + (b - a)f'[a + \xi(b - a)]$$

where $0 < \xi < 1$.

Theorem II.2 (Mean Value Theorem of Integral Calculus) *If the function $f(x)$ is continuous in the interval $a \leq x \leq b$, then*

$$\int_a^b f(x)\,dx = f(\xi)(b - a)$$

where $a \leq \xi \leq b$.

Theorem II.3 (Generalized Theorem of Integral Calculus) *If $f(x)$ and $g(x)$ are continuous functions in the interval $a \leq x \leq b$, and $g(x) \geq 0$, then*

$$\int_a^b f(x)g(x)\,dx = f(\xi)\int_a^b g(x)\,dx$$

where $a \leq \xi \leq b$.

Theorem II.4 (Taylor's Theorem) *If the functions $f(x), f'(x), \ldots, f^{(n)}(x)$ are continuous for each x in the interval $a \leq x \leq b$, and $f^{(n+1)}(x)$ exists for each x in the interval $a < x < b$, then there exists a ξ in the interval $a < x < b$ such that*

$$f(a + h) = f(a) + hf'(a) + \frac{h^2}{2!}f^{(2)}(a) + \frac{h^3}{3!}f^{(3)}(a) + \cdots + \frac{h^n}{n!}f^{(n)}(a) + R_n$$

where $h = b - a$, and the remainder R_n is given by the formula

$$R_n = \frac{h^{n+1}}{(n+1)!}f^{(n+1)}(\xi), \qquad (a < \xi < b)$$

III

Binomial Probabilities

TABLES

Table III.1 Binomial Probabilities, $P(X = x) = \left(\frac{n!}{x!(n-x)!}\right)(p^x)(1-p)^{(n-x)}$

						p						
n	x	0.0010	0.0025	0.0050	0.0075	0.0100	0.0250	0.0500	0.0750	0.1000		
1	0	0.9990	0.9975	0.9950	0.9925	0.9900	0.9750	0.9500	0.9250	0.9000	1	1
1	1	0.0010	0.0025	0.0050	0.0075	0.0100	0.0250	0.0500	0.0750	0.1000	0	1
2	0	0.9980	0.9950	0.9900	0.9851	0.9801	0.9506	0.9025	0.8556	0.8100	2	2
2	1	0.0020	0.0050	0.0099	0.0149	0.0198	0.0488	0.0950	0.1388	0.1800	1	2
2	2	0.0000	0.0000	0.0000	0.0001	0.0001	0.0006	0.0025	0.0056	0.0100	0	2
3	0	0.9970	0.9925	0.9851	0.9777	0.9703	0.9269	0.8574	0.7915	0.7290	3	3
3	1	0.0030	0.0075	0.0149	0.0222	0.0294	0.0713	0.1354	0.1925	0.2430	2	3
3	2	0.0000	0.0000	0.0001	0.0002	0.0003	0.0018	0.0071	0.0156	0.0270	1	3
3	3	0.0000	0.0000	0.0000	0.0000	0.0000	0.0000	0.0001	0.0004	0.0010	0	3
4	0	0.9960	0.9900	0.9801	0.9703	0.9606	0.9037	0.8145	0.7321	0.6561	4	4
4	1	0.0040	0.0099	0.0197	0.0293	0.0388	0.0927	0.1715	0.2374	0.2916	3	4
4	2	0.0000	0.0000	0.0001	0.0003	0.0006	0.0036	0.0135	0.0289	0.0486	2	4
4	3	0.0000	0.0000	0.0000	0.0000	0.0000	0.0001	0.0005	0.0016	0.0036	1	4
4	4	0.0000	0.0000	0.0000	0.0000	0.0000	0.0000	0.0000	0.0000	0.0001	0	4
5	0	0.9950	0.9876	0.9752	0.9631	0.9510	0.8811	0.7738	0.6772	0.5905	5	5
5	1	0.0050	0.0124	0.0245	0.0364	0.0480	0.1130	0.2036	0.2745	0.3281	4	5
5	2	0.0000	0.0001	0.0002	0.0005	0.0010	0.0058	0.0214	0.0445	0.0729	3	5
5	3	0.0000	0.0000	0.0000	0.0000	0.0000	0.0001	0.0011	0.0036	0.0081	2	5
5	4	0.0000	0.0000	0.0000	0.0000	0.0000	0.0000	0.0000	0.0001	0.0005	1	5
5	5	0.0000	0.0000	0.0000	0.0000	0.0000	0.0000	0.0000	0.0000	0.0000	0	5
6	0	0.9940	0.9851	0.9704	0.9558	0.9415	0.8591	0.7351	0.6264	0.5314	6	6
6	1	0.0060	0.0148	0.0293	0.0433	0.0571	0.1322	0.2321	0.3047	0.3543	5	6
6	2	0.0000	0.0001	0.0004	0.0008	0.0014	0.0085	0.0305	0.0618	0.0984	4	6
6	3	0.0000	0.0000	0.0000	0.0000	0.0000	0.0003	0.0021	0.0067	0.0146	3	6
6	4	0.0000	0.0000	0.0000	0.0000	0.0000	0.0000	0.0001	0.0004	0.0012	2	6
6	5	0.0000	0.0000	0.0000	0.0000	0.0000	0.0000	0.0000	0.0000	0.0001	1	6
6	6	0.0000	0.0000	0.0000	0.0000	0.0000	0.0000	0.0000	0.0000	0.0000	0	6
7	0	0.9930	0.9826	0.9655	0.9487	0.9321	0.8376	0.6983	0.5794	0.4783	7	7
7	1	0.0070	0.0172	0.0340	0.0502	0.0659	0.1503	0.2573	0.3289	0.3720	6	7
7	2	0.0000	0.0001	0.0005	0.0011	0.0020	0.0116	0.0406	0.0800	0.1240	5	7
7	3	0.0000	0.0000	0.0000	0.0000	0.0000	0.0005	0.0036	0.0108	0.0230	4	7
7	4	0.0000	0.0000	0.0000	0.0000	0.0000	0.0000	0.0002	0.0009	0.0026	3	7
7	5	0.0000	0.0000	0.0000	0.0000	0.0000	0.0000	0.0000	0.0000	0.0002	2	7
7	6	0.0000	0.0000	0.0000	0.0000	0.0000	0.0000	0.0000	0.0000	0.0000	1	7
7	7	0.0000	0.0000	0.0000	0.0000	0.0000	0.0000	0.0000	0.0000	0.0000	0	7
8	0	0.9920	0.9802	0.9607	0.9416	0.9227	0.8167	0.6634	0.5360	0.4305	8	8
8	1	0.0079	0.0197	0.0386	0.0569	0.0746	0.1675	0.2793	0.3477	0.3826	7	8
8	2	0.0000	0.0002	0.0007	0.0015	0.0026	0.0150	0.0515	0.0987	0.1488	6	8
8	3	0.0000	0.0000	0.0000	0.0000	0.0001	0.0008	0.0054	0.0160	0.0331	5	8
8	4	0.0000	0.0000	0.0000	0.0000	0.0000	0.0000	0.0004	0.0016	0.0046	4	8
8	5	0.0000	0.0000	0.0000	0.0000	0.0000	0.0000	0.0000	0.0001	0.0004	3	8
8	6	0.0000	0.0000	0.0000	0.0000	0.0000	0.0000	0.0000	0.0000	0.0000	2	8
8	7	0.0000	0.0000	0.0000	0.0000	0.0000	0.0000	0.0000	0.0000	0.0000	1	8
8	8	0.0000	0.0000	0.0000	0.0000	0.0000	0.0000	0.0000	0.0000	0.0000	0	8
		0.9990	0.9975	0.9950	0.9925	0.9900	0.9750	0.9500	0.9250	0.9000	x	n
						p						

For example, $P[X = 2;\ n = 3,\ p = 0.1] = 0.0270 = P[X = 1;\ n = 3,\ p = 0.9]$.

Table III.1 (cont'd) Binomial Probabilities, $P(X = x) = \left(\frac{n!}{x!(n-x)!}\right)(p^x)(1-p)^{(n-x)}$

		p										
n	*x*	0.1250	0.1500	0.2000	0.2500	0.3000	0.3500	0.4000	0.4500	0.5000		
1	0	0.8750	0.8500	0.8000	0.7500	0.7000	0.6500	0.6000	0.5500	0.5000	1	1
1	1	0.1250	0.1500	0.2000	0.2500	0.3000	0.3500	0.4000	0.4500	0.5000	0	1
2	0	0.7656	0.7225	0.6400	0.5625	0.4900	0.4225	0.3600	0.3025	0.2500	2	2
2	1	0.2188	0.2550	0.3200	0.3750	0.4200	0.4550	0.4800	0.4950	0.5000	1	2
2	2	0.0156	0.0225	0.0400	0.0625	0.0900	0.1225	0.1600	0.2025	0.2500	0	2
3	0	0.6699	0.6141	0.5120	0.4219	0.3430	0.2746	0.2160	0.1664	0.1250	3	3
3	1	0.2871	0.3251	0.3840	0.4219	0.4410	0.4436	0.4320	0.4084	0.3750	2	3
3	2	0.0410	0.0574	0.0960	0.1406	0.1890	0.2389	0.2880	0.3341	0.3750	1	3
3	3	0.0020	0.0034	0.0080	0.0156	0.0270	0.0429	0.0640	0.0911	0.1250	0	3
4	0	0.5862	0.5220	0.4096	0.3164	0.2401	0.1785	0.1296	0.0915	0.0625	4	4
4	1	0.3350	0.3685	0.4096	0.4219	0.4116	0.3845	0.3456	0.2995	0.2500	3	4
4	2	0.0718	0.0975	0.1536	0.2109	0.2646	0.3105	0.3456	0.3675	0.3750	2	4
4	3	0.0068	0.0115	0.0256	0.0469	0.0756	0.1115	0.1536	0.2005	0.2500	1	4
4	4	0.0002	0.0005	0.0016	0.0039	0.0081	0.0150	0.0256	0.0410	0.0625	0	4
5	0	0.5129	0.4437	0.3277	0.2373	0.1681	0.1160	0.0778	0.0503	0.0313	5	5
5	1	0.3664	0.3915	0.4096	0.3955	0.3601	0.3124	0.2592	0.2059	0.1563	4	5
5	2	0.1047	0.1382	0.2048	0.2637	0.3087	0.3364	0.3456	0.3369	0.3125	3	5
5	3	0.0150	0.0244	0.0512	0.0879	0.1323	0.1811	0.2304	0.2757	0.3125	2	5
5	4	0.0011	0.0022	0.0064	0.0146	0.0284	0.0488	0.0768	0.1128	0.1563	1	5
5	5	0.0000	0.0001	0.0003	0.0010	0.0024	0.0053	0.0102	0.0185	0.0313	0	5
6	0	0.4488	0.3771	0.2621	0.1780	0.1176	0.0754	0.0467	0.0277	0.0156	6	6
6	1	0.3847	0.3993	0.3932	0.3560	0.3025	0.2437	0.1866	0.1359	0.0938	5	6
6	2	0.1374	0.1762	0.2458	0.2966	0.3241	0.3280	0.3110	0.2780	0.2344	4	6
6	3	0.0262	0.0415	0.0819	0.1318	0.1852	0.2355	0.2765	0.3032	0.3125	3	6
6	4	0.0028	0.0055	0.0154	0.0330	0.0595	0.0951	0.1382	0.1861	0.2344	2	6
6	5	0.0002	0.0004	0.0015	0.0044	0.0102	0.0205	0.0369	0.0609	0.0938	1	6
6	6	0.0000	0.0000	0.0001	0.0002	0.0007	0.0018	0.0041	0.0083	0.0156	0	6
7	0	0.3927	0.3206	0.2097	0.1335	0.0824	0.0490	0.0280	0.0152	0.0078	7	7
7	1	0.3927	0.3960	0.3670	0.3115	0.2471	0.1848	0.1306	0.0872	0.0547	6	7
7	2	0.1683	0.2097	0.2753	0.3115	0.3177	0.2985	0.2613	0.2140	0.1641	5	7
7	3	0.0401	0.0617	0.1147	0.1730	0.2269	0.2679	0.2903	0.2918	0.2734	4	7
7	4	0.0057	0.0109	0.0287	0.0577	0.0972	0.1442	0.1935	0.2388	0.2734	3	7
7	5	0.0005	0.0012	0.0043	0.0115	0.0250	0.0466	0.0774	0.1172	0.1641	2	7
7	6	0.0000	0.0001	0.0004	0.0013	0.0036	0.0084	0.0172	0.0320	0.0547	1	7
7	7	0.0000	0.0000	0.0000	0.0001	0.0002	0.0006	0.0016	0.0037	0.0078	0	7
8	0	0.3436	0.2725	0.1678	0.1001	0.0576	0.0319	0.0168	0.0084	0.0039	8	8
8	1	0.3927	0.3847	0.3355	0.2670	0.1977	0.1373	0.0896	0.0548	0.0313	7	8
8	2	0.1963	0.2376	0.2936	0.3115	0.2965	0.2587	0.2090	0.1569	0.1094	6	8
8	3	0.0561	0.0839	0.1468	0.2076	0.2541	0.2786	0.2787	0.2568	0.2188	5	8
8	4	0.0100	0.0185	0.0459	0.0865	0.1361	0.1875	0.2322	0.2627	0.2734	4	8
8	5	0.0011	0.0026	0.0092	0.0231	0.0467	0.0808	0.1239	0.1719	0.2188	3	8
8	6	0.0001	0.0002	0.0011	0.0038	0.0100	0.0217	0.0413	0.0703	0.1094	2	8
8	7	0.0000	0.0000	0.0001	0.0004	0.0012	0.0033	0.0079	0.0164	0.0313	1	8
8	8	0.0000	0.0000	0.0000	0.0000	0.0001	0.0002	0.0007	0.0017	0.0039	0	8
		0.8750	0.8500	0.8000	0.7500	0.7000	0.6500	0.6000	0.5500	0.5000	*x*	*n*
		p										

Table III.1 (cont'd) Binomial Probabilities, $P(X = x) = \left(\frac{n!}{x!(n-x)!}\right)(p^x)(1-p)^{(n-x)}$

		p										
n	*x*	0.0010	0.0025	0.0050	0.0075	0.0100	0.0250	0.0500	0.0750	0.1000		
9	0	0.9910	0.9777	0.9559	0.9345	0.9135	0.7962	0.6302	0.4958	0.3874	9	9
9	1	0.0089	0.0221	0.0432	0.0636	0.0830	0.1837	0.2985	0.3618	0.3874	8	9
9	2	0.0000	0.0002	0.0009	0.0019	0.0034	0.0188	0.0629	0.1173	0.1722	7	9
9	3	0.0000	0.0000	0.0000	0.0000	0.0001	0.0011	0.0077	0.0222	0.0446	6	9
9	4	0.0000	0.0000	0.0000	0.0000	0.0000	0.0000	0.0006	0.0027	0.0074	5	9
9	5	0.0000	0.0000	0.0000	0.0000	0.0000	0.0000	0.0000	0.0002	0.0008	4	9
9	6	0.0000	0.0000	0.0000	0.0000	0.0000	0.0000	0.0000	0.0000	0.0001	3	9
9	7	0.0000	0.0000	0.0000	0.0000	0.0000	0.0000	0.0000	0.0000	0.0000	2	9
9	8	0.0000	0.0000	0.0000	0.0000	0.0000	0.0000	0.0000	0.0000	0.0000	1	9
9	9	0.0000	0.0000	0.0000	0.0000	0.0000	0.0000	0.0000	0.0000	0.0000	0	9
10	0	0.9900	0.9753	0.9511	0.9275	0.9044	0.7763	0.5987	0.4586	0.3487	10	10
10	1	0.0099	0.0244	0.0478	0.0701	0.0914	0.1991	0.3151	0.3718	0.3874	9	10
10	2	0.0000	0.0003	0.0011	0.0024	0.0042	0.0230	0.0746	0.1357	0.1937	8	10
10	3	0.0000	0.0000	0.0000	0.0000	0.0001	0.0016	0.0105	0.0293	0.0574	7	10
10	4	0.0000	0.0000	0.0000	0.0000	0.0000	0.0001	0.0010	0.0042	0.0112	6	10
10	5	0.0000	0.0000	0.0000	0.0000	0.0000	0.0000	0.0001	0.0004	0.0015	5	10
10	6	0.0000	0.0000	0.0000	0.0000	0.0000	0.0000	0.0000	0.0000	0.0001	4	10
10	7	0.0000	0.0000	0.0000	0.0000	0.0000	0.0000	0.0000	0.0000	0.0000	3	10
10	8	0.0000	0.0000	0.0000	0.0000	0.0000	0.0000	0.0000	0.0000	0.0000	2	10
10	9	0.0000	0.0000	0.0000	0.0000	0.0000	0.0000	0.0000	0.0000	0.0000	1	10
10	10	0.0000	0.0000	0.0000	0.0000	0.0000	0.0000	0.0000	0.0000	0.0000	0	10
12	0	0.9881	0.9704	0.9416	0.9136	0.8864	0.7380	0.5404	0.3924	0.2824	12	12
12	1	0.0119	0.0292	0.0568	0.0828	0.1074	0.2271	0.3413	0.3818	0.3766	11	12
12	2	0.0001	0.0004	0.0016	0.0034	0.0060	0.0320	0.0988	0.1702	0.2301	10	12
12	3	0.0000	0.0000	0.0000	0.0001	0.0002	0.0027	0.0173	0.0460	0.0852	9	12
12	4	0.0000	0.0000	0.0000	0.0000	0.0000	0.0002	0.0021	0.0084	0.0213	8	12
12	5	0.0000	0.0000	0.0000	0.0000	0.0000	0.0000	0.0002	0.0011	0.0038	7	12
12	6	0.0000	0.0000	0.0000	0.0000	0.0000	0.0000	0.0000	0.0001	0.0005	6	12
12	7	0.0000	0.0000	0.0000	0.0000	0.0000	0.0000	0.0000	0.0000	0.0000	5	12
12	8	0.0000	0.0000	0.0000	0.0000	0.0000	0.0000	0.0000	0.0000	0.0000	4	12
12	9	0.0000	0.0000	0.0000	0.0000	0.0000	0.0000	0.0000	0.0000	0.0000	3	12
12	10	0.0000	0.0000	0.0000	0.0000	0.0000	0.0000	0.0000	0.0000	0.0000	2	12
12	11	0.0000	0.0000	0.0000	0.0000	0.0000	0.0000	0.0000	0.0000	0.0000	1	12
12	12	0.0000	0.0000	0.0000	0.0000	0.0000	0.0000	0.0000	0.0000	0.0000	0	12
15	0	0.9851	0.9631	0.9276	0.8932	0.8601	0.6840	0.4633	0.3105	0.2059	15	15
15	1	0.0148	0.0362	0.0699	0.1012	0.1303	0.2631	0.3658	0.3777	0.3432	14	15
15	2	0.0001	0.0006	0.0025	0.0054	0.0092	0.0472	0.1348	0.2144	0.2669	13	15
15	3	0.0000	0.0000	0.0001	0.0002	0.0004	0.0052	0.0307	0.0753	0.1285	12	15
15	4	0.0000	0.0000	0.0000	0.0000	0.0000	0.0004	0.0049	0.0183	0.0428	11	15
15	5	0.0000	0.0000	0.0000	0.0000	0.0000	0.0000	0.0006	0.0033	0.0105	10	15
15	6	0.0000	0.0000	0.0000	0.0000	0.0000	0.0000	0.0000	0.0004	0.0019	9	15
15	7	0.0000	0.0000	0.0000	0.0000	0.0000	0.0000	0.0000	0.0000	0.0003	8	15
15	8	0.0000	0.0000	0.0000	0.0000	0.0000	0.0000	0.0000	0.0000	0.0000	7	15
15	9	0.0000	0.0000	0.0000	0.0000	0.0000	0.0000	0.0000	0.0000	0.0000	6	15
15	10	0.0000	0.0000	0.0000	0.0000	0.0000	0.0000	0.0000	0.0000	0.0000	5	15
15	11	0.0000	0.0000	0.0000	0.0000	0.0000	0.0000	0.0000	0.0000	0.0000	4	15
15	12	0.0000	0.0000	0.0000	0.0000	0.0000	0.0000	0.0000	0.0000	0.0000	3	15
15	13	0.0000	0.0000	0.0000	0.0000	0.0000	0.0000	0.0000	0.0000	0.0000	2	15
15	14	0.0000	0.0000	0.0000	0.0000	0.0000	0.0000	0.0000	0.0000	0.0000	1	15
15	15	0.0000	0.0000	0.0000	0.0000	0.0000	0.0000	0.0000	0.0000	0.0000	0	15
		0.9990	0.9975	0.9950	0.9925	0.9900	0.9750	0.9500	0.9250	0.9000	*x*	*n*
		p										

Table III.1 (cont'd) Binomial Probabilities, $P(X = x) = \left(\frac{n!}{x!(n-x)!}\right)(p^x)(1-p)^{(n-x)}$

		p										
n	*x*	0.1250	0.1500	0.2000	0.2500	0.3000	0.3500	0.4000	0.4500	0.5000		
9	0	0.3007	0.2316	0.1342	0.0751	0.0404	0.0207	0.0101	0.0046	0.0020	9	9
9	1	0.3866	0.3679	0.3020	0.2253	0.1556	0.1004	0.0605	0.0339	0.0176	8	9
9	2	0.2209	0.2597	0.3020	0.3003	0.2668	0.2162	0.1612	0.1110	0.0703	7	9
9	3	0.0736	0.1069	0.1762	0.2336	0.2668	0.2716	0.2508	0.2119	0.1641	6	9
9	4	0.0158	0.0283	0.0661	0.1168	0.1715	0.2194	0.2508	0.2600	0.2461	5	9
9	5	0.0023	0.0050	0.0165	0.0389	0.0735	0.1181	0.1672	0.2128	0.2461	4	9
9	6	0.0002	0.0006	0.0028	0.0087	0.0210	0.0424	0.0743	0.1160	0.1641	3	9
9	7	0.0000	0.0000	0.0003	0.0012	0.0039	0.0098	0.0212	0.0407	0.0703	2	9
9	8	0.0000	0.0000	0.0000	0.0001	0.0004	0.0013	0.0035	0.0083	0.0176	1	9
9	9	0.0000	0.0000	0.0000	0.0000	0.0000	0.0001	0.0003	0.0008	0.0020	0	9
10	0	0.2631	0.1969	0.1074	0.0563	0.0282	0.0135	0.0060	0.0025	0.0010	10	10
10	1	0.3758	0.3474	0.2684	0.1877	0.1211	0.0725	0.0403	0.0207	0.0098	9	10
10	2	0.2416	0.2759	0.3020	0.2816	0.2335	0.1757	0.1209	0.0763	0.0439	8	10
10	3	0.0920	0.1298	0.2013	0.2503	0.2668	0.2522	0.2150	0.1665	0.1172	7	10
10	4	0.0230	0.0401	0.0881	0.1460	0.2001	0.2377	0.2508	0.2384	0.2051	6	10
10	5	0.0039	0.0085	0.0264	0.0584	0.1029	0.1536	0.2007	0.2340	0.2461	5	10
10	6	0.0005	0.0012	0.0055	0.0162	0.0368	0.0689	0.1115	0.1596	0.2051	4	10
10	7	0.0000	0.0001	0.0008	0.0031	0.0090	0.0212	0.0425	0.0746	0.1172	3	10
10	8	0.0000	0.0000	0.0001	0.0004	0.0014	0.0043	0.0106	0.0229	0.0439	2	10
10	9	0.0000	0.0000	0.0000	0.0000	0.0001	0.0005	0.0016	0.0042	0.0098	1	10
10	10	0.0000	0.0000	0.0000	0.0000	0.0000	0.0000	0.0001	0.0003	0.0010	0	10
12	0	0.2014	0.1422	0.0687	0.0317	0.0138	0.0057	0.0022	0.0008	0.0002	12	12
12	1	0.3453	0.3012	0.2062	0.1267	0.0712	0.0368	0.0174	0.0075	0.0029	11	12
12	2	0.2713	0.2924	0.2835	0.2323	0.1678	0.1088	0.0639	0.0339	0.0161	10	12
12	3	0.1292	0.1720	0.2362	0.2581	0.2397	0.1954	0.1419	0.0923	0.0537	9	12
12	4	0.0415	0.0683	0.1329	0.1936	0.2311	0.2367	0.2128	0.1700	0.1208	8	12
12	5	0.0095	0.0193	0.0532	0.1032	0.1585	0.2039	0.2270	0.2225	0.1934	7	12
12	6	0.0016	0.0040	0.0155	0.0401	0.0792	0.1281	0.1766	0.2124	0.2256	6	12
12	7	0.0002	0.0006	0.0033	0.0115	0.0291	0.0591	0.1009	0.1489	0.1934	5	12
12	8	0.0000	0.0001	0.0005	0.0024	0.0078	0.0199	0.0420	0.0762	0.1208	4	12
12	9	0.0000	0.0000	0.0001	0.0004	0.0015	0.0048	0.0125	0.0277	0.0537	3	12
12	10	0.0000	0.0000	0.0000	0.0000	0.0002	0.0008	0.0025	0.0068	0.0161	2	12
12	11	0.0000	0.0000	0.0000	0.0000	0.0000	0.0001	0.0003	0.0010	0.0029	1	12
12	12	0.0000	0.0000	0.0000	0.0000	0.0000	0.0000	0.0000	0.0001	0.0002	0	12
15	0	0.1349	0.0874	0.0352	0.0134	0.0047	0.0016	0.0005	0.0001	0.0000	15	15
15	1	0.2891	0.2312	0.1319	0.0668	0.0305	0.0126	0.0047	0.0016	0.0005	14	15
15	2	0.2891	0.2856	0.2309	0.1559	0.0916	0.0476	0.0219	0.0090	0.0032	13	15
15	3	0.1790	0.2184	0.2501	0.2252	0.1700	0.1110	0.0634	0.0318	0.0139	12	15
15	4	0.0767	0.1156	0.1876	0.2252	0.2186	0.1792	0.1268	0.0780	0.0417	11	15
15	5	0.0241	0.0449	0.1032	0.1651	0.2061	0.2123	0.1859	0.1404	0.0916	10	15
15	6	0.0057	0.0132	0.0430	0.0917	0.1472	0.1906	0.2066	0.1914	0.1527	9	15
15	7	0.0011	0.0030	0.0138	0.0393	0.0811	0.1319	0.1771	0.2013	0.1964	8	15
15	8	0.0002	0.0005	0.0035	0.0131	0.0348	0.0710	0.1181	0.1647	0.1964	7	15
15	9	0.0000	0.0001	0.0007	0.0034	0.0116	0.0298	0.0612	0.1048	0.1527	6	15
15	10	0.0000	0.0000	0.0001	0.0007	0.0030	0.0096	0.0245	0.0515	0.0916	5	15
15	11	0.0000	0.0000	0.0000	0.0001	0.0006	0.0024	0.0074	0.0191	0.0417	4	15
15	12	0.0000	0.0000	0.0000	0.0000	0.0001	0.0004	0.0016	0.0052	0.0139	3	15
15	13	0.0000	0.0000	0.0000	0.0000	0.0000	0.0001	0.0003	0.0010	0.0032	2	15
15	14	0.0000	0.0000	0.0000	0.0000	0.0000	0.0000	0.0000	0.0001	0.0005	1	15
15	15	0.0000	0.0000	0.0000	0.0000	0.0000	0.0000	0.0000	0.0000	0.0000	0	15
		0.8750	0.8500	0.8000	0.7500	0.7000	0.6500	0.6000	0.5500	0.5000	*x*	*n*
		p										

Table III.1 (cont'd) Binomial Probabilities, $P(X = x) = \left(\frac{n!}{x!(n-x)!}\right)(p^x)(1-p)^{(n-x)}$

		p										
n	*x*	0.0010	0.0025	0.0050	0.0075	0.0100	0.0250	0.0500	0.0750	0.1000		
20	0	0.9802	0.9512	0.9046	0.8602	0.8179	0.6027	0.3585	0.2103	0.1216	20	20
20	1	0.0196	0.0477	0.0909	0.1300	0.1652	0.3091	0.3774	0.3410	0.2702	19	20
20	2	0.0002	0.0011	0.0043	0.0093	0.0159	0.0753	0.1887	0.2627	0.2852	18	20
20	3	0.0000	0.0000	0.0001	0.0004	0.0010	0.0116	0.0596	0.1278	0.1901	17	20
20	4	0.0000	0.0000	0.0000	0.0000	0.0000	0.0013	0.0133	0.0440	0.0898	16	20
20	5	0.0000	0.0000	0.0000	0.0000	0.0000	0.0001	0.0022	0.0114	0.0319	15	20
20	6	0.0000	0.0000	0.0000	0.0000	0.0000	0.0000	0.0003	0.0023	0.0089	14	20
20	7	0.0000	0.0000	0.0000	0.0000	0.0000	0.0000	0.0000	0.0004	0.0020	13	20
20	8	0.0000	0.0000	0.0000	0.0000	0.0000	0.0000	0.0000	0.0000	0.0004	12	20
20	9	0.0000	0.0000	0.0000	0.0000	0.0000	0.0000	0.0000	0.0000	0.0001	11	20
20	10	0.0000	0.0000	0.0000	0.0000	0.0000	0.0000	0.0000	0.0000	0.0000	10	20
20	11	0.0000	0.0000	0.0000	0.0000	0.0000	0.0000	0.0000	0.0000	0.0000	9	20
20	12	0.0000	0.0000	0.0000	0.0000	0.0000	0.0000	0.0000	0.0000	0.0000	8	20
20	13	0.0000	0.0000	0.0000	0.0000	0.0000	0.0000	0.0000	0.0000	0.0000	7	20
20	14	0.0000	0.0000	0.0000	0.0000	0.0000	0.0000	0.0000	0.0000	0.0000	6	20
20	15	0.0000	0.0000	0.0000	0.0000	0.0000	0.0000	0.0000	0.0000	0.0000	5	20
20	16	0.0000	0.0000	0.0000	0.0000	0.0000	0.0000	0.0000	0.0000	0.0000	4	20
20	17	0.0000	0.0000	0.0000	0.0000	0.0000	0.0000	0.0000	0.0000	0.0000	3	20
20	18	0.0000	0.0000	0.0000	0.0000	0.0000	0.0000	0.0000	0.0000	0.0000	2	20
20	19	0.0000	0.0000	0.0000	0.0000	0.0000	0.0000	0.0000	0.0000	0.0000	1	20
20	20	0.0000	0.0000	0.0000	0.0000	0.0000	0.0000	0.0000	0.0000	0.0000	0	20
25	0	0.9753	0.9393	0.8822	0.8284	0.7778	0.5310	0.2774	0.1424	0.0718	25	25
25	1	0.0244	0.0589	0.1108	0.1565	0.1964	0.3404	0.3650	0.2887	0.1994	24	25
25	2	0.0003	0.0018	0.0067	0.0142	0.0238	0.1047	0.2305	0.2809	0.2659	23	25
25	3	0.0000	0.0000	0.0003	0.0008	0.0018	0.0206	0.0930	0.1746	0.2265	22	25
25	4	0.0000	0.0000	0.0000	0.0000	0.0001	0.0029	0.0269	0.0779	0.1384	21	25
25	5	0.0000	0.0000	0.0000	0.0000	0.0000	0.0003	0.0060	0.0265	0.0646	20	25
25	6	0.0000	0.0000	0.0000	0.0000	0.0000	0.0000	0.0010	0.0072	0.0239	19	25
25	7	0.0000	0.0000	0.0000	0.0000	0.0000	0.0000	0.0001	0.0016	0.0072	18	25
25	8	0.0000	0.0000	0.0000	0.0000	0.0000	0.0000	0.0000	0.0003	0.0018	17	25
25	9	0.0000	0.0000	0.0000	0.0000	0.0000	0.0000	0.0000	0.0000	0.0004	16	25
25	10	0.0000	0.0000	0.0000	0.0000	0.0000	0.0000	0.0000	0.0000	0.0001	15	25
25	11	0.0000	0.0000	0.0000	0.0000	0.0000	0.0000	0.0000	0.0000	0.0000	14	25
25	12	0.0000	0.0000	0.0000	0.0000	0.0000	0.0000	0.0000	0.0000	0.0000	13	25
25	13	0.0000	0.0000	0.0000	0.0000	0.0000	0.0000	0.0000	0.0000	0.0000	12	25
25	14	0.0000	0.0000	0.0000	0.0000	0.0000	0.0000	0.0000	0.0000	0.0000	11	25
25	15	0.0000	0.0000	0.0000	0.0000	0.0000	0.0000	0.0000	0.0000	0.0000	10	25
25	16	0.0000	0.0000	0.0000	0.0000	0.0000	0.0000	0.0000	0.0000	0.0000	9	25
25	17	0.0000	0.0000	0.0000	0.0000	0.0000	0.0000	0.0000	0.0000	0.0000	8	25
25	18	0.0000	0.0000	0.0000	0.0000	0.0000	0.0000	0.0000	0.0000	0.0000	7	25
25	19	0.0000	0.0000	0.0000	0.0000	0.0000	0.0000	0.0000	0.0000	0.0000	6	25
25	20	0.0000	0.0000	0.0000	0.0000	0.0000	0.0000	0.0000	0.0000	0.0000	5	25
25	21	0.0000	0.0000	0.0000	0.0000	0.0000	0.0000	0.0000	0.0000	0.0000	4	25
25	22	0.0000	0.0000	0.0000	0.0000	0.0000	0.0000	0.0000	0.0000	0.0000	3	25
25	23	0.0000	0.0000	0.0000	0.0000	0.0000	0.0000	0.0000	0.0000	0.0000	2	25
25	24	0.0000	0.0000	0.0000	0.0000	0.0000	0.0000	0.0000	0.0000	0.0000	1	25
25	25	0.0000	0.0000	0.0000	0.0000	0.0000	0.0000	0.0000	0.0000	0.0000	0	25
		0.9990	0.9975	0.9950	0.9925	0.9900	0.9750	0.9500	0.9250	0.9000	*x*	*n*
		p										

Table III.1 (cont'd) Binomial Probabilities, $P(X = x) = \left(\frac{n!}{x!(n-x)!}\right)(p^x)(1-p)^{(n-x)}$

		p										
n	x	0.1250	0.1500	0.2000	0.2500	0.3000	0.3500	0.4000	0.4500	0.5000		
20	0	0.0692	0.0388	0.0115	0.0032	0.0008	0.0002	0.0000	0.0000	0.0000	20	20
20	1	0.1977	0.1368	0.0576	0.0211	0.0068	0.0020	0.0005	0.0001	0.0000	19	20
20	2	0.2684	0.2293	0.1369	0.0669	0.0278	0.0100	0.0031	0.0008	0.0002	18	20
20	3	0.2300	0.2428	0.2054	0.1339	0.0716	0.0323	0.0123	0.0040	0.0011	17	20
20	4	0.1397	0.1821	0.2182	0.1897	0.1304	0.0738	0.0350	0.0139	0.0046	16	20
20	5	0.0638	0.1028	0.1746	0.2023	0.1789	0.1272	0.0746	0.0365	0.0148	15	20
20	6	0.0228	0.0454	0.1091	0.1686	0.1916	0.1712	0.1244	0.0746	0.0370	14	20
20	7	0.0065	0.0160	0.0545	0.1124	0.1643	0.1844	0.1659	0.1221	0.0739	13	20
20	8	0.0015	0.0046	0.0222	0.0609	0.1144	0.1614	0.1797	0.1623	0.1201	12	20
20	9	0.0003	0.0011	0.0074	0.0271	0.0654	0.1158	0.1597	0.1771	0.1602	11	20
20	10	0.0000	0.0002	0.0020	0.0099	0.0308	0.0686	0.1171	0.1593	0.1762	10	20
20	11	0.0000	0.0000	0.0005	0.0030	0.0120	0.0336	0.0710	0.1185	0.1602	9	20
20	12	0.0000	0.0000	0.0001	0.0008	0.0039	0.0136	0.0355	0.0727	0.1201	8	20
20	13	0.0000	0.0000	0.0000	0.0002	0.0010	0.0045	0.0146	0.0366	0.0739	7	20
20	14	0.0000	0.0000	0.0000	0.0000	0.0002	0.0012	0.0049	0.0150	0.0370	6	20
20	15	0.0000	0.0000	0.0000	0.0000	0.0000	0.0003	0.0013	0.0049	0.0148	5	20
20	16	0.0000	0.0000	0.0000	0.0000	0.0000	0.0000	0.0003	0.0013	0.0046	4	20
20	17	0.0000	0.0000	0.0000	0.0000	0.0000	0.0000	0.0000	0.0002	0.0011	3	20
20	18	0.0000	0.0000	0.0000	0.0000	0.0000	0.0000	0.0000	0.0000	0.0002	2	20
20	19	0.0000	0.0000	0.0000	0.0000	0.0000	0.0000	0.0000	0.0000	0.0000	1	20
20	20	0.0000	0.0000	0.0000	0.0000	0.0000	0.0000	0.0000	0.0000	0.0000	0	20
25	0	0.0355	0.0172	0.0038	0.0008	0.0001	0.0000	0.0000	0.0000	0.0000	25	25
25	1	0.1268	0.0759	0.0236	0.0063	0.0014	0.0003	0.0000	0.0000	0.0000	24	25
25	2	0.2173	0.1607	0.0708	0.0251	0.0074	0.0018	0.0004	0.0001	0.0000	23	25
25	3	0.2380	0.2174	0.1358	0.0641	0.0243	0.0076	0.0019	0.0004	0.0001	22	25
25	4	0.1870	0.2110	0.1867	0.1175	0.0572	0.0224	0.0071	0.0018	0.0004	21	25
25	5	0.1122	0.1564	0.1960	0.1645	0.1030	0.0506	0.0199	0.0063	0.0016	20	25
25	6	0.0534	0.0920	0.1633	0.1828	0.1472	0.0908	0.0442	0.0172	0.0053	19	25
25	7	0.0207	0.0441	0.1108	0.1654	0.1712	0.1327	0.0800	0.0381	0.0143	18	25
25	8	0.0067	0.0175	0.0623	0.1241	0.1651	0.1607	0.1200	0.0701	0.0322	17	25
25	9	0.0018	0.0058	0.0294	0.0781	0.1336	0.1635	0.1511	0.1084	0.0609	16	25
25	10	0.0004	0.0016	0.0118	0.0417	0.0916	0.1409	0.1612	0.1419	0.0974	15	25
25	11	0.0001	0.0004	0.0040	0.0189	0.0536	0.1034	0.1465	0.1583	0.1328	14	25
25	12	0.0000	0.0001	0.0012	0.0074	0.0268	0.0650	0.1140	0.1511	0.1550	13	25
25	13	0.0000	0.0000	0.0003	0.0025	0.0115	0.0350	0.0760	0.1236	0.1550	12	25
25	14	0.0000	0.0000	0.0001	0.0007	0.0042	0.0161	0.0434	0.0867	0.1328	11	25
25	15	0.0000	0.0000	0.0000	0.0002	0.0013	0.0064	0.0212	0.0520	0.0974	10	25
25	16	0.0000	0.0000	0.0000	0.0000	0.0004	0.0021	0.0088	0.0266	0.0609	9	25
25	17	0.0000	0.0000	0.0000	0.0000	0.0001	0.0006	0.0031	0.0115	0.0322	8	25
25	18	0.0000	0.0000	0.0000	0.0000	0.0000	0.0001	0.0009	0.0042	0.0143	7	25
25	19	0.0000	0.0000	0.0000	0.0000	0.0000	0.0000	0.0002	0.0013	0.0053	6	25
25	20	0.0000	0.0000	0.0000	0.0000	0.0000	0.0000	0.0000	0.0003	0.0016	5	25
25	21	0.0000	0.0000	0.0000	0.0000	0.0000	0.0000	0.0000	0.0001	0.0004	4	25
25	22	0.0000	0.0000	0.0000	0.0000	0.0000	0.0000	0.0000	0.0000	0.0001	3	25
25	23	0.0000	0.0000	0.0000	0.0000	0.0000	0.0000	0.0000	0.0000	0.0000	2	25
25	24	0.0000	0.0000	0.0000	0.0000	0.0000	0.0000	0.0000	0.0000	0.0000	1	25
25	25	0.0000	0.0000	0.0000	0.0000	0.0000	0.0000	0.0000	0.0000	0.0000	0	25
		0.8750	0.8500	0.8000	0.7500	0.7000	0.6500	0.6000	0.5500	0.5000	x	n
		p										

Table III.1 (cont'd) Binomial Probabilities, $P(X = x) = \left(\frac{n!}{x!(n-x)!}\right)(p^x)(1-p)^{(n-x)}$

		p										
n	*x*	0.0010	0.0025	0.0050	0.0075	0.0100	0.0250	0.0500	0.0750	0.1000		
30	0	0.9704	0.9277	0.8604	0.7978	0.7397	0.4679	0.2146	0.0964	0.0424	30	30
30	1	0.0291	0.0697	0.1297	0.1809	0.2242	0.3599	0.3389	0.2346	0.1413	29	30
30	2	0.0004	0.0025	0.0095	0.0198	0.0328	0.1338	0.2586	0.2758	0.2277	28	30
30	3	0.0000	0.0001	0.0004	0.0014	0.0031	0.0320	0.1270	0.2087	0.2361	27	30
30	4	0.0000	0.0000	0.0000	0.0001	0.0002	0.0055	0.0451	0.1142	0.1771	26	30
30	5	0.0000	0.0000	0.0000	0.0000	0.0000	0.0007	0.0124	0.0482	0.1023	25	30
30	6	0.0000	0.0000	0.0000	0.0000	0.0000	0.0001	0.0027	0.0163	0.0474	24	30
30	7	0.0000	0.0000	0.0000	0.0000	0.0000	0.0000	0.0005	0.0045	0.0180	23	30
30	8	0.0000	0.0000	0.0000	0.0000	0.0000	0.0000	0.0001	0.0011	0.0058	22	30
30	9	0.0000	0.0000	0.0000	0.0000	0.0000	0.0000	0.0000	0.0002	0.0016	21	30
30	10	0.0000	0.0000	0.0000	0.0000	0.0000	0.0000	0.0000	0.0000	0.0004	20	30
30	11	0.0000	0.0000	0.0000	0.0000	0.0000	0.0000	0.0000	0.0000	0.0001	19	30
30	12	0.0000	0.0000	0.0000	0.0000	0.0000	0.0000	0.0000	0.0000	0.0000	18	30
30	13	0.0000	0.0000	0.0000	0.0000	0.0000	0.0000	0.0000	0.0000	0.0000	17	30
30	14	0.0000	0.0000	0.0000	0.0000	0.0000	0.0000	0.0000	0.0000	0.0000	16	30
30	15	0.0000	0.0000	0.0000	0.0000	0.0000	0.0000	0.0000	0.0000	0.0000	15	30
30	16	0.0000	0.0000	0.0000	0.0000	0.0000	0.0000	0.0000	0.0000	0.0000	14	30
30	17	0.0000	0.0000	0.0000	0.0000	0.0000	0.0000	0.0000	0.0000	0.0000	13	30
30	18	0.0000	0.0000	0.0000	0.0000	0.0000	0.0000	0.0000	0.0000	0.0000	12	30
30	19	0.0000	0.0000	0.0000	0.0000	0.0000	0.0000	0.0000	0.0000	0.0000	11	30
30	20	0.0000	0.0000	0.0000	0.0000	0.0000	0.0000	0.0000	0.0000	0.0000	10	30
30	21	0.0000	0.0000	0.0000	0.0000	0.0000	0.0000	0.0000	0.0000	0.0000	9	30
30	22	0.0000	0.0000	0.0000	0.0000	0.0000	0.0000	0.0000	0.0000	0.0000	8	30
30	23	0.0000	0.0000	0.0000	0.0000	0.0000	0.0000	0.0000	0.0000	0.0000	7	30
30	24	0.0000	0.0000	0.0000	0.0000	0.0000	0.0000	0.0000	0.0000	0.0000	6	30
30	25	0.0000	0.0000	0.0000	0.0000	0.0000	0.0000	0.0000	0.0000	0.0000	5	30
30	26	0.0000	0.0000	0.0000	0.0000	0.0000	0.0000	0.0000	0.0000	0.0000	4	30
30	27	0.0000	0.0000	0.0000	0.0000	0.0000	0.0000	0.0000	0.0000	0.0000	3	30
30	28	0.0000	0.0000	0.0000	0.0000	0.0000	0.0000	0.0000	0.0000	0.0000	2	30
30	29	0.0000	0.0000	0.0000	0.0000	0.0000	0.0000	0.0000	0.0000	0.0000	1	30
30	30	0.0000	0.0000	0.0000	0.0000	0.0000	0.0000	0.0000	0.0000	0.0000	0	30
		0.9990	0.9975	0.9950	0.9925	0.9900	0.9750	0.9500	0.9250	0.9000	*x*	*n*
		p										

Table III.1 (cont'd) Binomial Probabilities, $P(X = x) = \left(\frac{n!}{x!(n-x)!}\right)(p^x)(1-p)^{(n-x)}$

		p										
n	*x*	0.1250	0.1500	0.2000	0.2500	0.3000	0.3500	0.4000	0.4500	0.5000		
30	0	0.0182	0.0076	0.0012	0.0002	0.0000	0.0000	0.0000	0.0000	0.0000	30	30
30	1	0.0780	0.0404	0.0093	0.0018	0.0003	0.0000	0.0000	0.0000	0.0000	29	30
30	2	0.1616	0.1034	0.0337	0.0086	0.0018	0.0003	0.0000	0.0000	0.0000	28	30
30	3	0.2155	0.1703	0.0785	0.0269	0.0072	0.0015	0.0003	0.0000	0.0000	27	30
30	4	0.2078	0.2028	0.1325	0.0604	0.0208	0.0056	0.0012	0.0002	0.0000	26	30
30	5	0.1544	0.1861	0.1723	0.1047	0.0464	0.0157	0.0041	0.0008	0.0001	25	30
30	6	0.0919	0.1368	0.1795	0.1455	0.0829	0.0353	0.0115	0.0029	0.0006	24	30
30	7	0.0450	0.0828	0.1538	0.1662	0.1219	0.0652	0.0263	0.0081	0.0019	23	30
30	8	0.0185	0.0420	0.1106	0.1593	0.1501	0.1009	0.0505	0.0191	0.0055	22	30
30	9	0.0065	0.0181	0.0676	0.1298	0.1573	0.1328	0.0823	0.0382	0.0133	21	30
30	10	0.0019	0.0067	0.0355	0.0909	0.1416	0.1502	0.1152	0.0656	0.0280	20	30
30	11	0.0005	0.0022	0.0161	0.0551	0.1103	0.1471	0.1396	0.0976	0.0509	19	30
30	12	0.0001	0.0006	0.0064	0.0291	0.0749	0.1254	0.1474	0.1265	0.0806	18	30
30	13	0.0000	0.0001	0.0022	0.0134	0.0444	0.0935	0.1360	0.1433	0.1115	17	30
30	14	0.0000	0.0000	0.0007	0.0054	0.0231	0.0611	0.1101	0.1424	0.1354	16	30
30	15	0.0000	0.0000	0.0002	0.0019	0.0106	0.0351	0.0783	0.1242	0.1445	15	30
30	16	0.0000	0.0000	0.0000	0.0006	0.0042	0.0177	0.0489	0.0953	0.1354	14	30
30	17	0.0000	0.0000	0.0000	0.0002	0.0015	0.0079	0.0269	0.0642	0.1115	13	30
30	18	0.0000	0.0000	0.0000	0.0000	0.0005	0.0031	0.0129	0.0379	0.0806	12	30
30	19	0.0000	0.0000	0.0000	0.0000	0.0001	0.0010	0.0054	0.0196	0.0509	11	30
30	20	0.0000	0.0000	0.0000	0.0000	0.0000	0.0003	0.0020	0.0088	0.0280	10	30
30	21	0.0000	0.0000	0.0000	0.0000	0.0000	0.0001	0.0006	0.0034	0.0133	9	30
30	22	0.0000	0.0000	0.0000	0.0000	0.0000	0.0000	0.0002	0.0012	0.0055	8	30
30	23	0.0000	0.0000	0.0000	0.0000	0.0000	0.0000	0.0000	0.0003	0.0019	7	30
30	24	0.0000	0.0000	0.0000	0.0000	0.0000	0.0000	0.0000	0.0001	0.0006	6	30
30	25	0.0000	0.0000	0.0000	0.0000	0.0000	0.0000	0.0000	0.0000	0.0001	5	30
30	26	0.0000	0.0000	0.0000	0.0000	0.0000	0.0000	0.0000	0.0000	0.0000	4	30
30	27	0.0000	0.0000	0.0000	0.0000	0.0000	0.0000	0.0000	0.0000	0.0000	3	30
30	28	0.0000	0.0000	0.0000	0.0000	0.0000	0.0000	0.0000	0.0000	0.0000	2	30
30	29	0.0000	0.0000	0.0000	0.0000	0.0000	0.0000	0.0000	0.0000	0.0000	1	30
30	30	0.0000	0.0000	0.0000	0.0000	0.0000	0.0000	0.0000	0.0000	0.0000	0	30
		0.8750	0.8500	0.8000	0.7500	0.7000	0.6500	0.6000	0.5500	0.5000	*x*	*n*
		p										

Table III.1 (cont'd) Binomial Probabilities, $P(X = x) = \left(\frac{n!}{x!(n-x)!}\right)(p^x)(1-p)^{(n-x)}$

		p										
n	*x*	0.0010	0.0025	0.0050	0.0075	0.0100	0.0250	0.0500	0.0750	0.1000		
40	0	0.9608	0.9047	0.8183	0.7400	0.6690	0.3632	0.1285	0.0442	0.0148	40	40
40	1	0.0385	0.0907	0.1645	0.2237	0.2703	0.3725	0.2706	0.1434	0.0657	39	40
40	2	0.0008	0.0044	0.0161	0.0330	0.0532	0.1863	0.2777	0.2268	0.1423	38	40
40	3	0.0000	0.0001	0.0010	0.0032	0.0068	0.0605	0.1851	0.2329	0.2003	37	40
40	4	0.0000	0.0000	0.0000	0.0002	0.0006	0.0143	0.0901	0.1747	0.2059	36	40
40	5	0.0000	0.0000	0.0000	0.0000	0.0000	0.0026	0.0342	C.1020	0.1647	35	40
40	6	0.0000	0.0000	0.0000	0.0000	0.0000	0.0004	0.0105	0.0482	0.1068	34	40
40	7	0.0000	0.0000	0.0000	0.0000	0.0000	0.0000	0.0027	0.0190	0.0576	33	40
40	8	0.0000	0.0000	0.0000	0.0000	0.0000	0.0000	0.0006	0.0064	0.0264	32	40
40	9	0.0000	0.0000	0.0000	0.0000	0.0000	0.0000	0.0001	0.0018	0.0104	31	40
40	10	0.0000	0.0000	0.0000	0.0000	0.0000	0.0000	0.0000	0.0005	0.0036	30	40
40	11	0.0000	0.0000	0.0000	0.0000	0.0000	0.0000	0.0000	0.0001	0.0011	29	40
40	12	0.0000	0.0000	0.0000	0.0000	0.0000	0.0000	0.0000	0.0000	0.0003	28	40
40	13	0.0000	0.0000	0.0000	0.0000	0.0000	0.0000	0.0000	0.0000	0.0001	27	40
40	14	0.0000	0.0000	0.0000	0.0000	0.0000	0.0000	0.0000	0.0000	0.0000	26	40
40	15	0.0000	0.0000	0.0000	0.0000	0.0000	0.0000	0.0000	0.0000	0.0000	25	40
40	16	0.0000	0.0000	0.0000	0.0000	0.0000	0.0000	0.0000	0.0000	0.0000	24	40
40	17	0.0000	0.0000	0.0000	0.0000	0.0000	0.0000	0.0000	0.0000	0.0000	23	40
40	18	0.0000	0.0000	0.0000	0.0000	0.0000	0.0000	0.0000	0.0000	0.0000	22	40
40	19	0.0000	0.0000	0.0000	0.0000	0.0000	0.0000	0.0000	0.0000	0.0000	21	40
40	20	0.0000	0.0000	0.0000	0.0000	0.0000	0.0000	0.0000	0.0000	0.0000	20	40
40	21	0.0000	0.0000	0.0000	0.0000	0.0000	0.0000	0.0000	0.0000	0.0000	19	40
40	22	0.0000	0.0000	0.0000	0.0000	0.0000	0.0000	0.0000	0.0000	0.0000	18	40
40	23	0.0000	0.0000	0.0000	0.0000	0.0000	0.0000	0.0000	0.0000	0.0000	17	40
40	24	0.0000	0.0000	0.0000	0.0000	0.0000	0.0000	0.0000	0.0000	0.0000	16	40
40	25	0.0000	0.0000	0.0000	0.0000	0.0000	0.0000	0.0000	0.0000	0.0000	15	40
40	26	0.0000	0.0000	0.0000	0.0000	0.0000	0.0000	0.0000	0.0000	0.0000	14	40
40	27	0.0000	0.0000	0.0000	0.0000	0.0000	0.0000	0.0000	0.0000	0.0000	13	40
40	28	0.0000	0.0000	0.0000	0.0000	0.0000	0.0000	0.0000	0.0000	0.0000	12	40
40	29	0.0000	0.0000	0.0000	0.0000	0.0000	0.0000	0.0000	0.0000	0.0000	11	40
40	30	0.0000	0.0000	0.0000	0.0000	0.0000	0.0000	0.0000	0.0000	0.0000	10	40
40	31	0.0000	0.0000	0.0000	0.0000	0.0000	0.0000	0.0000	0.0000	0.0000	9	40
40	32	0.0000	0.0000	0.0000	0.0000	0.0000	0.0000	0.0000	0.0000	0.0000	8	40
40	33	0.0000	0.0000	0.0000	0.0000	0.0000	0.0000	0.0000	0.0000	0.0000	7	40
40	34	0.0000	0.0000	0.0000	0.0000	0.0000	0.0000	0.0000	0.0000	0.0000	6	40
40	35	0.0000	0.0000	0.0000	0.0000	0.0000	0.0000	0.0000	0.0000	0.0000	5	40
40	36	0.0000	0.0000	0.0000	0.0000	0.0000	0.0000	0.0000	0.0000	0.0000	4	40
40	37	0.0000	0.0000	0.0000	0.0000	0.0000	0.0000	0.0000	0.0000	0.0000	3	40
40	38	0.0000	0.0000	0.0000	0.0000	0.0000	0.0000	0.0000	0.0000	0.0000	2	40
40	39	0.0000	0.0000	0.0000	0.0000	0.0000	0.0000	0.0000	0.0000	0.0000	1	40
40	40	0.0000	0.0000	0.0000	0.0000	0.0000	0.0000	0.0000	0.0000	0.0000	0	40
		0.9990	0.9975	0.9950	0.9925	0.9900	0.9750	0.9500	0.9250	0.9000	*x*	*n*
		p										

Table III.1 (cont'd) Binomial Probabilities, $P(X = x) = \left(\frac{n!}{x!(n-x)!}\right)(p^x)(1-p)^{(n-x)}$

		p										
n	*x*	0.1250	0.1500	0.2000	0.2500	0.3000	0.3500	0.4000	0.4500	0.5000		
40	0	0.0048	0.0015	0.0001	0.0000	0.0000	0.0000	0.0000	0.0000	0.0000	40	40
40	1	0.0274	0.0106	0.0013	0.0001	0.0000	0.0000	0.0000	0.0000	0.0000	39	40
40	2	0.0762	0.0365	0.0065	0.0009	0.0001	0.0000	0.0000	0.0000	0.0000	38	40
40	3	0.1380	0.0816	0.0205	0.0037	0.0005	0.0001	0.0000	0.0000	0.0000	37	40
40	4	0.1823	0.1332	0.0475	0.0113	0.0020	0.0003	0.0000	0.0000	0.0000	36	40
40	5	0.1875	0.1692	0.0854	0.0272	0.0061	0.0010	0.0001	0.0000	0.0000	35	40
40	6	0.1563	0.1742	0.1246	0.0530	0.0151	0.0031	0.0005	0.0000	0.0000	34	40
40	7	0.1084	0.1493	0.1513	0.0857	0.0315	0.0080	0.0015	0.0002	0.0000	33	40
40	8	0.0639	0.1087	0.1560	0.1179	0.0557	0.0179	0.0040	0.0006	0.0001	32	40
40	9	0.0325	0.0682	0.1386	0.1397	0.0849	0.0342	0.0095	0.0018	0.0002	31	40
40	10	0.0144	0.0373	0.1075	0.1444	0.1128	0.0571	0.0196	0.0047	0.0008	30	40
40	11	0.0056	0.0180	0.0733	0.1312	0.1319	0.0838	0.0357	0.0105	0.0021	29	40
40	12	0.0019	0.0077	0.0443	0.1057	0.1366	0.1090	0.0576	0.0207	0.0051	28	40
40	13	0.0006	0.0029	0.0238	0.0759	0.1261	0.1265	0.0827	0.0365	0.0109	27	40
40	14	0.0002	0.0010	0.0115	0.0488	0.1042	0.1313	0.1063	0.0575	0.0211	26	40
40	15	0.0000	0.0003	0.0050	0.0282	0.0774	0.1226	0.1228	0.0816	0.0366	25	40
40	16	0.0000	0.0001	0.0019	0.0147	0.0518	0.1031	0.1279	0.1043	0.0572	24	40
40	17	0.0000	0.0000	0.0007	0.0069	0.0314	0.0784	0.1204	0.1205	0.0807	23	40
40	18	0.0000	0.0000	0.0002	0.0029	0.0172	0.0539	0.1026	0.1260	0.1031	22	40
40	19	0.0000	0.0000	0.0001	0.0011	0.0085	0.0336	0.0792	0.1194	0.1194	21	40
40	20	0.0000	0.0000	0.0000	0.0004	0.0038	0.0190	0.0554	0.1025	0.1254	20	40
40	21	0.0000	0.0000	0.0000	0.0001	0.0016	0.0097	0.0352	0.0799	0.1194	19	40
40	22	0.0000	0.0000	0.0000	0.0000	0.0006	0.0045	0.0203	0.0565	0.1031	18	40
40	23	0.0000	0.0000	0.0000	0.0000	0.0002	0.0019	0.0106	0.0362	0.0807	17	40
40	24	0.0000	0.0000	0.0000	0.0000	0.0001	0.0007	0.0050	0.0210	0.0572	16	40
40	25	0.0000	0.0000	0.0000	0.0000	0.0000	0.0003	0.0021	0.0110	0.0366	15	40
40	26	0.0000	0.0000	0.0000	0.0000	0.0000	0.0001	0.0008	0.0052	0.0211	14	40
40	27	0.0000	0.0000	0.0000	0.0000	0.0000	0.0000	0.0003	0.0022	0.0109	13	40
40	28	0.0000	0.0000	0.0000	0.0000	0.0000	0.0000	0.0001	0.0008	0.0051	12	40
40	29	0.0000	0.0000	0.0000	0.0000	0.0000	0.0000	0.0000	0.0003	0.0021	11	40
40	30	0.0000	0.0000	0.0000	0.0000	0.0000	0.0000	0.0000	0.0001	0.0008	10	40
40	31	0.0000	0.0000	0.0000	0.0000	0.0000	0.0000	0.0000	0.0000	0.0002	9	40
40	32	0.0000	0.0000	0.0000	0.0000	0.0000	0.0000	0.0000	0.0000	0.0001	8	40
40	33	0.0000	0.0000	0.0000	0.0000	0.0000	0.0000	0.0000	0.0000	0.0000	7	40
40	34	0.0000	0.0000	0.0000	0.0000	0.0000	0.0000	0.0000	0.0000	0.0000	6	40
40	35	0.0000	0.0000	0.0000	0.0000	0.0000	0.0000	0.0000	0.0000	0.0000	5	40
40	36	0.0000	0.0000	0.0000	0.0000	0.0000	0.0000	0.0000	0.0000	0.0000	4	40
40	37	0.0000	0.0000	0.0000	0.0000	0.0000	0.0000	0.0000	0.0000	0.0000	3	40
40	38	0.0000	0.0000	0.0000	0.0000	0.0000	0.0000	0.0000	0.0000	0.0000	2	40
40	39	0.0000	0.0000	0.0000	0.0000	0.0000	0.0000	0.0000	0.0000	0.0000	1	40
40	40	0.0000	0.0000	0.0000	0.0000	0.0000	0.0000	0.0000	0.0000	0.0000	0	40
		0.8750	0.8500	0.8000	0.7500	0.7000	0.6500	0.6000	0.5500	0.5000	*x*	*n*
		p										

Table III.1 (cont'd) Binomial Probabilities, $P(X = x) = \left(\frac{n!}{x!(n-x)!}\right)(p^x)(1-p)^{(n-x)}$

		p										
n	*x*	0.0010	0.0025	0.0050	0.0075	0.0100	0.0250	0.0500	0.0750	0.1000		
50	0	0.9512	0.8824	0.7783	0.6863	0.6050	0.2820	0.0769	0.0203	0.0052	50	50
50	1	0.0476	0.1106	0.1956	0.2593	0.3056	0.3615	0.2025	0.0822	0.0286	49	50
50	2	0.0012	0.0068	0.0241	0.0480	0.0756	0.2271	0.2611	0.1633	0.0779	48	50
50	3	0.0000	0.0003	0.0019	0.0058	0.0122	0.0932	0.2199	0.2119	0.1386	47	50
50	4	0.0000	0.0000	0.0001	0.0005	0.0015	0.0281	0.1360	0.2019	0.1809	46	50
50	5	0.0000	0.0000	0.0000	0.0000	0.0001	0.0066	0.0658	0.1506	0.1849	45	50
50	6	0.0000	0.0000	0.0000	0.0000	0.0000	0.0013	0.0260	0.0916	0.1541	44	50
50	7	0.0000	0.0000	0.0000	0.0000	0.0000	0.0002	0.0086	0.0467	0.1076	43	50
50	8	0.0000	0.0000	0.0000	0.0000	0.0000	0.0000	0.0024	0.0203	0.0643	42	50
50	9	0.0000	0.0000	0.0000	0.0000	0.0000	0.0000	0.0006	0.0077	0.0333	41	50
50	10	0.0000	0.0000	0.0000	0.0000	0.0000	0.0000	0.0001	0.0026	0.0152	40	50
50	11	0.0000	0.0000	0.0000	0.0000	0.0000	0.0000	0.0000	0.0008	0.0061	39	50
50	12	0.0000	0.0000	0.0000	0.0000	0.0000	0.0000	0.0000	0.0002	0.0022	38	50
50	13	0.0000	0.0000	0.0000	0.0000	0.0000	0.0000	0.0000	0.0000	0.0007	37	50
50	14	0.0000	0.0000	0.0000	0.0000	0.0000	0.0000	0.0000	0.0000	0.0002	36	50
50	15	0.0000	0.0000	0.0000	0.0000	0.0000	0.0000	0.0000	0.0000	0.0001	35	50
50	16	0.0000	0.0000	0.0000	0.0000	0.0000	0.0000	0.0000	0.0000	0.0000	34	50
50	17	0.0000	0.0000	0.0000	0.0000	0.0000	0.0000	0.0000	0.0000	0.0000	33	50
50	18	0.0000	0.0000	0.0000	0.0000	0.0000	0.0000	0.0000	0.0000	0.0000	32	50
50	19	0.0000	0.0000	0.0000	0.0000	0.0000	0.0000	0.0000	0.0000	0.0000	31	50
50	20	0.0000	0.0000	0.0000	0.0000	0.0000	0.0000	0.0000	0.0000	0.0000	30	50
50	21	0.0000	0.0000	0.0000	0.0000	0.0000	0.0000	0.0000	0.0000	0.0000	29	50
50	22	0.0000	0.0000	0.0000	0.0000	0.0000	0.0000	0.0000	0.0000	0.0000	28	50
50	23	0.0000	0.0000	0.0000	0.0000	0.0000	0.0000	0.0000	0.0000	0.0000	27	50
50	24	0.0000	0.0000	0.0000	0.0000	0.0000	0.0000	0.0000	0.0000	0.0000	26	50
50	25	0.0000	0.0000	0.0000	0.0000	0.0000	0.0000	0.0000	0.0000	0.0000	25	50
50	26	0.0000	0.0000	0.0000	0.0000	0.0000	0.0000	0.0000	0.0000	0.0000	24	50
50	27	0.0000	0.0000	0.0000	0.0000	0.0000	0.0000	0.0000	0.0000	0.0000	23	50
50	28	0.0000	0.0000	0.0000	0.0000	0.0000	0.0000	0.0000	0.0000	0.0000	22	50
50	29	0.0000	0.0000	0.0000	0.0000	0.0000	0.0000	0.0000	0.0000	0.0000	21	50
50	30	0.0000	0.0000	0.0000	0.0000	0.0000	0.0000	0.0000	0.0000	0.0000	20	50
50	31	0.0000	0.0000	0.0000	0.0000	0.0000	0.0000	0.0000	0.0000	0.0000	19	50
50	32	0.0000	0.0000	0.0000	0.0000	0.0000	0.0000	0.0000	0.0000	0.0000	18	50
50	33	0.0000	0.0000	0.0000	0.0000	0.0000	0.0000	0.0000	0.0000	0.0000	17	50
50	34	0.0000	0.0000	0.0000	0.0000	0.0000	0.0000	0.0000	0.0000	0.0000	16	50
50	35	0.0000	0.0000	0.0000	0.0000	0.0000	0.0000	0.0000	0.0000	0.0000	15	50
50	36	0.0000	0.0000	0.0000	0.0000	0.0000	0.0000	0.0000	0.0000	0.0000	14	50
50	37	0.0000	0.0000	0.0000	0.0000	0.0000	0.0000	0.0000	0.0000	0.0000	13	50
50	38	0.0000	0.0000	0.0000	0.0000	0.0000	0.0000	0.0000	0.0000	0.0000	12	50
50	39	0.0000	0.0000	0.0000	0.0000	0.0000	0.0000	0.0000	0.0000	0.0000	11	50
50	40	0.0000	0.0000	0.0000	0.0000	0.0000	0.0000	0.0000	0.0000	0.0000	10	50
50	41	0.0000	0.0000	0.0000	0.0000	0.0000	0.0000	0.0000	0.0000	0.0000	9	50
50	42	0.0000	0.0000	0.0000	0.0000	0.0000	0.0000	0.0000	0.0000	0.0000	8	50
50	43	0.0000	0.0000	0.0000	0.0000	0.0000	0.0000	0.0000	0.0000	0.0000	7	50
50	44	0.0000	0.0000	0.0000	0.0000	0.0000	0.0000	0.0000	0.0000	0.0000	6	50
50	45	0.0000	0.0000	0.0000	0.0000	0.0000	0.0000	0.0000	0.0000	0.0000	5	50
50	46	0.0000	0.0000	0.0000	0.0000	0.0000	0.0000	0.0000	0.0000	0.0000	4	50
50	47	0.0000	0.0000	0.0000	0.0000	0.0000	0.0000	0.0000	0.0000	0.0000	3	50
50	48	0.0000	0.0000	0.0000	0.0000	0.0000	0.0000	0.0000	0.0000	0.0000	2	50
50	49	0.0000	0.0000	0.0000	0.0000	0.0000	0.0000	0.0000	0.0000	0.0000	1	50
50	50	0.0000	0.0000	0.0000	0.0000	0.0000	0.0000	0.0000	0.0000	0.0000	0	50
		0.9990	0.9975	0.9950	0.9925	0.9900	0.9750	0.9500	0.9250	0.9000	*x*	*n*
		p										

Table III.1 (cont'd) Binomial Probabilities, $P(X = x) = \left(\frac{n!}{x!(n-x)!}\right)(p^x)(1-p)^{(n-x)}$

		p										
n	*x*	0.1250	0.1500	0.2000	0.2500	0.3000	0.3500	0.4000	0.4500	0.5000		
50	0	0.0013	0.0003	0.0000	0.0000	0.0000	0.0000	0.0000	0.0000	0.0000	50	50
50	1	0.0090	0.0026	0.0002	0.0000	0.0000	0.0000	0.0000	0.0000	0.0000	49	50
50	2	0.0315	0.0113	0.0011	0.0001	0.0000	0.0000	0.0000	0.0000	0.0000	48	50
50	3	0.0720	0.0319	0.0044	0.0004	0.0000	0.0000	0.0000	0.0000	0.0000	47	50
50	4	0.1209	0.0661	0.0128	0.0016	0.0001	0.0000	0.0000	0.0000	0.0000	46	50
50	5	0.1589	0.1072	0.0295	0.0049	0.0006	0.0000	0.0000	0.0000	0.0000	45	50
50	6	0.1702	0.1419	0.0554	0.0123	0.0018	0.0002	0.0000	0.0000	0.0000	44	50
50	7	0.1528	0.1575	0.0870	0.0259	0.0048	0.0006	0.0000	0.0000	0.0000	43	50
50	8	0.1174	0.1493	0.1169	0.0463	0.0110	0.0017	0.0002	0.0000	0.0000	42	50
50	9	0.0782	0.1230	0.1364	0.0721	0.0220	0.0042	0.0005	0.0000	0.0000	41	50
50	10	0.0458	0.0890	0.1398	0.0985	0.0386	0.0093	0.0014	0.0001	0.0000	40	50
50	11	0.0238	0.0571	0.1271	0.1194	0.0602	0.0182	0.0035	0.0004	0.0000	39	50
50	12	0.0111	0.0328	0.1033	0.1294	0.0838	0.0319	0.0076	0.0011	0.0001	38	50
50	13	0.0046	0.0169	0.0755	0.1261	0.1050	0.0502	0.0147	0.0027	0.0003	37	50
50	14	0.0017	0.0079	0.0499	0.1110	0.1189	0.0714	0.0260	0.0059	0.0008	36	50
50	15	0.0006	0.0033	0.0299	0.0888	0.1223	0.0923	0.0415	0.0116	0.0020	35	50
50	16	0.0002	0.0013	0.0164	0.0648	0.1147	0.1088	0.0606	0.0207	0.0044	34	50
50	17	0.0001	0.0005	0.0082	0.0432	0.0983	0.1171	0.0808	0.0339	0.0087	33	50
50	18	0.0000	0.0001	0.0037	0.0264	0.0772	0.1156	0.0987	0.0508	0.0160	32	50
50	19	0.0000	0.0000	0.0016	0.0148	0.0558	0.1048	0.1109	0.0700	0.0270	31	50
50	20	0.0000	0.0000	0.0006	0.0077	0.0370	0.0875	0.1146	0.0888	0.0419	30	50
50	21	0.0000	0.0000	0.0002	0.0036	0.0227	0.0673	0.1091	0.1038	0.0598	29	50
50	22	0.0000	0.0000	0.0001	0.0016	0.0128	0.0478	0.0959	0.1119	0.0788	28	50
50	23	0.0000	0.0000	0.0000	0.0006	0.0067	0.0313	0.0778	0.1115	0.0960	27	50
50	24	0.0000	0.0000	0.0000	0.0002	0.0032	0.0190	0.0584	0.1026	0.1080	26	50
50	25	0.0000	0.0000	0.0000	0.0001	0.0014	0.0106	0.0405	0.0873	0.1123	25	50
50	26	0.0000	0.0000	0.0000	0.0000	0.0006	0.0055	0.0259	0.0687	0.1080	24	50
50	27	0.0000	0.0000	0.0000	0.0000	0.0002	0.0026	0.0154	0.0500	0.0960	23	50
50	28	0.0000	0.0000	0.0000	0.0000	0.0001	0.0012	0.0084	0.0336	0.0788	22	50
50	29	0.0000	0.0000	0.0000	0.0000	0.0000	0.0005	0.0043	0.0208	0.0598	21	50
50	30	0.0000	0.0000	0.0000	0.0000	0.0000	0.0002	0.0020	0.0119	0.0419	20	50
50	31	0.0000	0.0000	0.0000	0.0000	0.0000	0.0001	0.0009	0.0063	0.0270	19	50
50	32	0.0000	0.0000	0.0000	0.0000	0.0000	0.0000	0.0003	0.0031	0.0160	18	50
50	33	0.0000	0.0000	0.0000	0.0000	0.0000	0.0000	0.0001	0.0014	0.0087	17	50
50	34	0.0000	0.0000	0.0000	0.0000	0.0000	0.0000	0.0000	0.0006	0.0044	16	50
50	35	0.0000	0.0000	0.0000	0.0000	0.0000	0.0000	0.0000	0.0002	0.0020	15	50
50	36	0.0000	0.0000	0.0000	0.0000	0.0000	0.0000	0.0000	0.0001	0.0008	14	50
50	37	0.0000	0.0000	0.0000	0.0000	0.0000	0.0000	0.0000	0.0000	0.0003	13	50
50	38	0.0000	0.0000	0.0000	0.0000	0.0000	0.0000	0.0000	0.0000	0.0001	12	50
50	39	0.0000	0.0000	0.0000	0.0000	0.0000	0.0000	0.0000	0.0000	0.0000	11	50
50	40	0.0000	0.0000	0.0000	0.0000	0.0000	0.0000	0.0000	0.0000	0.0000	10	50
50	41	0.0000	0.0000	0.0000	0.0000	0.0000	0.0000	0.0000	0.0000	0.0000	9	50
50	42	0.0000	0.0000	0.0000	0.0000	0.0000	0.0000	0.0000	0.0000	0.0000	8	50
50	43	0.0000	0.0000	0.0000	0.0000	0.0000	0.0000	0.0000	0.0000	0.0000	7	50
50	44	0.0000	0.0000	0.0000	0.0000	0.0000	0.0000	0.0000	0.0000	0.0000	6	50
50	45	0.0000	0.0000	0.0000	0.0000	0.0000	0.0000	0.0000	0.0000	0.0000	5	50
50	46	0.0000	0.0000	0.0000	0.0000	0.0000	0.0000	0.0000	0.0000	0.0000	4	50
50	47	0.0000	0.0000	0.0000	0.0000	0.0000	0.0000	0.0000	0.0000	0.0000	3	50
50	48	0.0000	0.0000	0.0000	0.0000	0.0000	0.0000	0.0000	0.0000	0.0000	2	50
50	49	0.0000	0.0000	0.0000	0.0000	0.0000	0.0000	0.0000	0.0000	0.0000	1	50
50	50	0.0000	0.0000	0.0000	0.0000	0.0000	0.0000	0.0000	0.0000	0.0000	0	50
		0.8750	0.8500	0.8000	0.7500	0.7000	0.6500	0.6000	0.5500	0.5000	*x*	*n*
		p										

Table III.2 Binomial Probabilities (Cumulative Distribution Function)

		p										
n	*x*	0.0010	0.0025	0.0050	0.0075	0.0100	0.0250	0.0500	0.0750	0.1000		
1	0	0.9990	0.9975	0.9950	0.9925	0.9900	0.9750	0.9500	0.9250	0.9000	1	1
1	1	1.0000	1.0000	1.0000	1.0000	1.0000	1.0000	1.0000	1.0000	1.0000	0	1
2	0	0.9980	0.9950	0.9900	0.9851	0.9801	0.9506	0.9025	0.8556	0.8100	2	2
2	1	1.0000	1.0000	1.0000	0.9999	0.9999	0.9994	0.9975	0.9944	0.9900	1	2
2	2	1.0000	1.0000	1.0000	1.0000	1.0000	1.0000	1.0000	1.0000	1.0000	0	2
3	0	0.9970	0.9925	0.9851	0.9777	0.9703	0.9269	0.8574	0.7915	0.7290	3	3
3	1	1.0000	1.0000	0.9999	0.9998	0.9997	0.9982	0.9927	0.9840	0.9720	2	3
3	2	1.0000	1.0000	1.0000	1.0000	1.0000	1.0000	0.9999	0.9996	0.9990	1	3
3	3	1.0000	1.0000	1.0000	1.0000	1.0000	1.0000	1.0000	1.0000	1.0000	0	3
4	0	0.9960	0.9900	0.9801	0.9703	0.9606	0.9037	0.8145	0.7321	0.6561	4	4
4	1	1.0000	1.0000	0.9999	0.9997	0.9994	0.9964	0.9860	0.9695	0.9477	3	4
4	2	1.0000	1.0000	1.0000	1.0000	1.0000	0.9999	0.9995	0.9984	0.9963	2	4
4	3	1.0000	1.0000	1.0000	1.0000	1.0000	1.0000	1.0000	1.0000	0.9999	1	4
4	4	1.0000	1.0000	1.0000	1.0000	1.0000	1.0000	1.0000	1.0000	1.0000	0	4
5	0	0.9950	0.9876	0.9752	0.9631	0.9510	0.8811	0.7738	0.6772	0.5905	5	5
5	1	1.0000	0.9999	0.9998	0.9994	0.9990	0.9941	0.9774	0.9517	0.9185	4	5
5	2	1.0000	1.0000	1.0000	1.0000	1.0000	0.9998	0.9988	0.9962	0.9914	3	5
5	3	1.0000	1.0000	1.0000	1.0000	1.0000	1.0000	1.0000	0.9999	0.9995	2	5
5	4	1.0000	1.0000	1.0000	1.0000	1.0000	1.0000	1.0000	1.0000	1.0000	1	5
5	5	1.0000	1.0000	1.0000	1.0000	1.0000	1.0000	1.0000	1.0000	1.0000	0	5
6	0	0.9940	0.9851	0.9704	0.9558	0.9415	0.8591	0.7351	0.6264	0.5314	6	6
6	1	1.0000	0.9999	0.9996	0.9992	0.9985	0.9912	0.9672	0.9311	0.8857	5	6
6	2	1.0000	1.0000	1.0000	1.0000	1.0000	0.9997	0.9978	0.9929	0.9841	4	6
6	3	1.0000	1.0000	1.0000	1.0000	1.0000	1.0000	0.9999	0.9996	0.9987	3	6
6	4	1.0000	1.0000	1.0000	1.0000	1.0000	1.0000	1.0000	1.0000	0.9999	2	6
6	5	1.0000	1.0000	1.0000	1.0000	1.0000	1.0000	1.0000	1.0000	1.0000	1	6
6	6	1.0000	1.0000	1.0000	1.0000	1.0000	1.0000	1.0000	1.0000	1.0000	0	6
7	0	0.9930	0.9826	0.9655	0.9487	0.9321	0.8376	0.6983	0.5794	0.4783	7	7
7	1	1.0000	0.9999	0.9995	0.9988	0.9980	0.9879	0.9556	0.9083	0.8503	6	7
7	2	1.0000	1.0000	1.0000	1.0000	1.0000	0.9995	0.9962	0.9883	0.9743	5	7
7	3	1.0000	1.0000	1.0000	1.0000	1.0000	1.0000	0.9998	0.9991	0.9973	4	7
7	4	1.0000	1.0000	1.0000	1.0000	1.0000	1.0000	1.0000	1.0000	0.9998	3	7
7	5	1.0000	1.0000	1.0000	1.0000	1.0000	1.0000	1.0000	1.0000	1.0000	2	7
7	6	1.0000	1.0000	1.0000	1.0000	1.0000	1.0000	1.0000	1.0000	1.0000	1	7
7	7	1.0000	1.0000	1.0000	1.0000	1.0000	1.0000	1.0000	1.0000	1.0000	0	7
8	0	0.9920	0.9802	0.9607	0.9416	0.9227	0.8167	0.6634	0.5360	0.4305	8	8
8	1	1.0000	0.9998	0.9993	0.9985	0.9973	0.9842	0.9428	0.8836	0.8131	7	8
8	2	1.0000	1.0000	1.0000	1.0000	0.9999	0.9992	0.9942	0.9823	0.9619	6	8
8	3	1.0000	1.0000	1.0000	1.0000	1.0000	1.0000	0.9996	0.9983	0.9950	5	8
8	4	1.0000	1.0000	1.0000	1.0000	1.0000	1.0000	1.0000	0.9999	0.9996	4	8
8	5	1.0000	1.0000	1.0000	1.0000	1.0000	1.0000	1.0000	1.0000	1.0000	3	8
8	6	1.0000	1.0000	1.0000	1.0000	1.0000	1.0000	1.0000	1.0000	1.0000	2	8
8	7	1.0000	1.0000	1.0000	1.0000	1.0000	1.0000	1.0000	1.0000	1.0000	1	8
8	8	1.0000	1.0000	1.0000	1.0000	1.0000	1.0000	1.0000	1.0000	1.0000	0	8
		0.9990	0.9975	0.9950	0.9925	0.9900	0.9750	0.9500	0.9250	0.9000	*x*	*n*
		p										

For example, $P[X \leq 1;\ n = 7,\ p = 0.05] = 0.9556 = P[X \geq 6;\ n = 7,\ p = 0.95] = 1 - P[X \leq 5;\ n = 7,\ p = 0.95]$

Table III.2 (cont'd) Binomial Probabilities (Cumulative Distribution Function)

		p										
n	*x*	0.1250	0.1500	0.2000	0.2500	0.3000	0.3500	0.4000	0.4500	0.5000		
1	0	0.8750	0.8500	0.8000	0.7500	0.7000	0.6500	0.6000	0.5500	0.5000	1	1
1	1	1.0000	1.0000	1.0000	1.0000	1.0000	1.0000	1.0000	1.0000	1.0000	0	1
2	0	0.7656	0.7225	0.6400	0.5625	0.4900	0.4225	0.3600	0.3025	0.2500	2	2
2	1	0.9844	0.9775	0.9600	0.9375	0.9100	0.8775	0.8400	0.7975	0.7500	1	2
2	2	1.0000	1.0000	1.0000	1.0000	1.0000	1.0000	1.0000	1.0000	1.0000	0	2
3	0	0.6699	0.6141	0.5120	0.4219	0.3430	0.2746	0.2160	0.1664	0.1250	3	3
3	1	0.9570	0.9392	0.8960	0.8438	0.7840	0.7183	0.6480	0.5748	0.5000	2	3
3	2	0.9980	0.9966	0.9920	0.9844	0.9730	0.9571	0.9360	0.9089	0.8750	1	3
3	3	1.0000	1.0000	1.0000	1.0000	1.0000	1.0000	1.0000	1.0000	1.0000	0	3
4	0	0.5862	0.5220	0.4096	0.3164	0.2401	0.1785	0.1296	0.0915	0.0625	4	4
4	1	0.9211	0.8905	0.8192	0.7383	0.6517	0.5630	0.4752	0.3910	0.3125	3	4
4	2	0.9929	0.9880	0.9728	0.9492	0.9163	0.8735	0.8208	0.7585	0.6875	2	4
4	3	0.9998	0.9995	0.9984	0.9961	0.9919	0.9850	0.9744	0.9590	0.9375	1	4
4	4	1.0000	1.0000	1.0000	1.0000	1.0000	1.0000	1.0000	1.0000	1.0000	0	4
5	0	0.5129	0.4437	0.3277	0.2373	0.1681	0.1160	0.0778	0.0503	0.0313	5	5
5	1	0.8793	0.8352	0.7373	0.6328	0.5282	0.4284	0.3370	0.2562	0.1875	4	5
5	2	0.9839	0.9734	0.9421	0.8965	0.8369	0.7648	0.6826	0.5931	0.5000	3	5
5	3	0.9989	0.9978	0.9933	0.9844	0.9692	0.9460	0.9130	0.8688	0.8125	2	5
5	4	1.0000	0.9999	0.9997	0.9990	0.9976	0.9947	0.9898	0.9815	0.9688	1	5
5	5	1.0000	1.0000	1.0000	1.0000	1.0000	1.0000	1.0000	1.0000	1.0000	0	5
6	0	0.4488	0.3771	0.2621	0.1780	0.1176	0.0754	0.0467	0.0277	0.0156	6	6
6	1	0.8335	0.7765	0.6554	0.5339	0.4202	0.3191	0.2333	0.1636	0.1094	5	6
6	2	0.9709	0.9527	0.9011	0.8306	0.7443	0.6471	0.5443	0.4415	0.3438	4	6
6	3	0.9970	0.9941	0.9830	0.9624	0.9295	0.8826	0.8208	0.7447	0.6563	3	6
6	4	0.9998	0.9996	0.9984	0.9954	0.9891	0.9777	0.9590	0.9308	0.8906	2	6
6	5	1.0000	1.0000	0.9999	0.9998	0.9993	0.9982	0.9959	0.9917	0.9844	1	6
6	6	1.0000	1.0000	1.0000	1.0000	1.0000	1.0000	1.0000	1.0000	1.0000	0	6
7	0	0.3927	0.3206	0.2097	0.1335	0.0824	0.0490	0.0280	0.0152	0.0078	7	7
7	1	0.7854	0.7166	0.5767	0.4449	0.3294	0.2338	0.1586	0.1024	0.0625	6	7
7	2	0.9537	0.9262	0.8520	0.7564	0.6471	0.5323	0.4199	0.3164	0.2266	5	7
7	3	0.9938	0.9879	0.9667	0.9294	0.8740	0.8002	0.7102	0.6083	0.5000	4	7
7	4	0.9995	0.9988	0.9953	0.9871	0.9712	0.9444	0.9037	0.8471	0.7734	3	7
7	5	1.0000	0.9999	0.9996	0.9987	0.9962	0.9910	0.9812	0.9643	0.9375	2	7
7	6	1.0000	1.0000	1.0000	0.9999	0.9998	0.9994	0.9984	0.9963	0.9922	1	7
7	7	1.0000	1.0000	1.0000	1.0000	1.0000	1.0000	1.0000	1.0000	1.0000	0	7
8	0	0.3436	0.2725	0.1678	0.1001	0.0576	0.0319	0.0168	0.0084	0.0039	8	8
8	1	0.7363	0.6572	0.5033	0.3671	0.2553	0.1691	0.1064	0.0632	0.0352	7	8
8	2	0.9327	0.8948	0.7969	0.6785	0.5518	0.4278	0.3154	0.2201	0.1445	6	8
8	3	0.9888	0.9786	0.9437	0.8862	0.8059	0.7064	0.5941	0.4770	0.3633	5	8
8	4	0.9988	0.9971	0.9896	0.9727	0.9420	0.8939	0.8263	0.7396	0.6367	4	8
8	5	0.9999	0.9998	0.9988	0.9958	0.9887	0.9747	0.9502	0.9115	0.8555	3	8
8	6	1.0000	1.0000	0.9999	0.9996	0.9987	0.9964	0.9915	0.9819	0.9648	2	8
8	7	1.0000	1.0000	1.0000	1.0000	0.9999	0.9998	0.9993	0.9983	0.9961	1	8
8	8	1.0000	1.0000	1.0000	1.0000	1.0000	1.0000	1.0000	1.0000	1.0000	0	8
		0.8750	0.8500	0.8000	0.7500	0.7000	0.6500	0.6000	0.5500	0.5000	*x*	*n*
		p										

Table III.2 (cont'd) Binomial Probabilities (Cumulative Distribution Function)

		p										
n	*x*	0.0010	0.0025	0.0050	0.0075	0.0100	0.0250	0.0500	0.0750	0.1000		
9	0	0.9910	0.9777	0.9559	0.9345	0.9135	0.7962	0.6302	0.4958	0.3874	9	9
9	1	1.0000	0.9998	0.9991	0.9980	0.9966	0.9800	0.9288	0.8575	0.7748	8	9
9	2	1.0000	1.0000	1.0000	1.0000	0.9999	0.9988	0.9916	0.9749	0.9470	7	9
9	3	1.0000	1.0000	1.0000	1.0000	1.0000	1.0000	0.9994	0.9971	0.9917	6	9
9	4	1.0000	1.0000	1.0000	1.0000	1.0000	1.0000	1.0000	0.9998	0.9991	5	9
9	5	1.0000	1.0000	1.0000	1.0000	1.0000	1.0000	1.0000	1.0000	0.9999	4	9
9	6	1.0000	1.0000	1.0000	1.0000	1.0000	1.0000	1.0000	1.0000	1.0000	3	9
9	7	1.0000	1.0000	1.0000	1.0000	1.0000	1.0000	1.0000	1.0000	1.0000	2	9
9	8	1.0000	1.0000	1.0000	1.0000	1.0000	1.0000	1.0000	1.0000	1.0000	1	9
9	9	1.0000	1.0000	1.0000	1.0000	1.0000	1.0000	1.0000	1.0000	1.0000	0	9
10	0	0.9900	0.9753	0.9511	0.9275	0.9044	0.7763	0.5987	0.4586	0.3487	10	10
10	1	1.0000	0.9997	0.9989	0.9976	0.9957	0.9754	0.9139	0.8304	0.7361	9	10
10	2	1.0000	1.0000	1.0000	1.0000	0.9999	0.9984	0.9885	0.9661	0.9298	8	10
10	3	1.0000	1.0000	1.0000	1.0000	1.0000	0.9999	0.9990	0.9954	0.9872	7	10
10	4	1.0000	1.0000	1.0000	1.0000	1.0000	1.0000	0.9999	0.9996	0.9984	6	10
10	5	1.0000	1.0000	1.0000	1.0000	1.0000	1.0000	1.0000	1.0000	0.9999	5	10
10	6	1.0000	1.0000	1.0000	1.0000	1.0000	1.0000	1.0000	1.0000	1.0000	4	10
10	7	1.0000	1.0000	1.0000	1.0000	1.0000	1.0000	1.0000	1.0000	1.0000	3	10
10	8	1.0000	1.0000	1.0000	1.0000	1.0000	1.0000	1.0000	1.0000	1.0000	2	10
10	9	1.0000	1.0000	1.0000	1.0000	1.0000	1.0000	1.0000	1.0000	1.0000	1	10
10	10	1.0000	1.0000	1.0000	1.0000	1.0000	1.0000	1.0000	1.0000	1.0000	0	10
12	0	0.9881	0.9704	0.9416	0.9136	0.8864	0.7380	0.5404	0.3924	0.2824	12	12
12	1	0.9999	0.9996	0.9984	0.9965	0.9938	0.9651	0.8816	0.7741	0.6590	11	12
12	2	1.0000	1.0000	1.0000	0.9999	0.9998	0.9971	0.9804	0.9444	0.8891	10	12
12	3	1.0000	1.0000	1.0000	1.0000	1.0000	0.9998	0.9978	0.9904	0.9744	9	12
12	4	1.0000	1.0000	1.0000	1.0000	1.0000	1.0000	0.9998	0.9988	0.9957	8	12
12	5	1.0000	1.0000	1.0000	1.0000	1.0000	1.0000	1.0000	0.9999	0.9995	7	12
12	6	1.0000	1.0000	1.0000	1.0000	1.0000	1.0000	1.0000	1.0000	0.9999	6	12
12	7	1.0000	1.0000	1.0000	1.0000	1.0000	1.0000	1.0000	1.0000	1.0000	5	12
12	8	1.0000	1.0000	1.0000	1.0000	1.0000	1.0000	1.0000	1.0000	1.0000	4	12
12	9	1.0000	1.0000	1.0000	1.0000	1.0000	1.0000	1.0000	1.0000	1.0000	3	12
12	10	1.0000	1.0000	1.0000	1.0000	1.0000	1.0000	1.0000	1.0000	1.0000	2	12
12	11	1.0000	1.0000	1.0000	1.0000	1.0000	1.0000	1.0000	1.0000	1.0000	1	12
12	12	1.0000	1.0000	1.0000	1.0000	1.0000	1.0000	1.0000	1.0000	1.0000	0	12
15	0	0.9851	0.9631	0.9276	0.8932	0.8601	0.6840	0.4633	0.3105	0.2059	15	15
15	1	0.9999	0.9994	0.9975	0.9945	0.9904	0.9471	0.8290	0.6882	0.5490	14	15
15	2	1.0000	1.0000	0.9999	0.9998	0.9996	0.9943	0.9638	0.9026	0.8159	13	15
15	3	1.0000	1.0000	1.0000	1.0000	1.0000	0.9996	0.9945	0.9779	0.9444	12	15
15	4	1.0000	1.0000	1.0000	1.0000	1.0000	1.0000	0.9994	0.9962	0.9873	11	15
15	5	1.0000	1.0000	1.0000	1.0000	1.0000	1.0000	0.9999	0.9995	0.9978	10	15
15	6	1.0000	1.0000	1.0000	1.0000	1.0000	1.0000	1.0000	0.9999	0.9997	9	15
15	7	1.0000	1.0000	1.0000	1.0000	1.0000	1.0000	1.0000	1.0000	1.0000	8	15
15	8	1.0000	1.0000	1.0000	1.0000	1.0000	1.0000	1.0000	1.0000	1.0000	7	15
15	9	1.0000	1.0000	1.0000	1.0000	1.0000	1.0000	1.0000	1.0000	1.0000	6	15
15	10	1.0000	1.0000	1.0000	1.0000	1.0000	1.0000	1.0000	1.0000	1.0000	5	15
15	11	1.0000	1.0000	1.0000	1.0000	1.0000	1.0000	1.0000	1.0000	1.0000	4	15
15	12	1.0000	1.0000	1.0000	1.0000	1.0000	1.0000	1.0000	1.0000	1.0000	3	15
15	13	1.0000	1.0000	1.0000	1.0000	1.0000	1.0000	1.0000	1.0000	1.0000	2	15
15	14	1.0000	1.0000	1.0000	1.0000	1.0000	1.0000	1.0000	1.0000	1.0000	1	15
15	15	1.0000	1.0000	1.0000	1.0000	1.0000	1.0000	1.0000	1.0000	1.0000	0	15
		0.9990	0.9975	0.9950	0.9925	0.9900	0.9750	0.9500	0.9250	0.9000	*x*	*n*
		p										

Table III.2 (cont'd) Binomial Probabilities (Cumulative Distribution Function)

		p										
n	x	0.1250	0.1500	0.2000	0.2500	0.3000	0.3500	0.4000	0.4500	0.5000		
9	0	0.3007	0.2316	0.1342	0.0751	0.0404	0.0207	0.0101	0.0046	0.0020	9	9
9	1	0.6872	0.5995	0.4362	0.3003	0.1960	0.1211	0.0705	0.0385	0.0195	8	9
9	2	0.9081	0.8591	0.7382	0.6007	0.4628	0.3373	0.2318	0.1495	0.0898	7	9
9	3	0.9817	0.9661	0.9144	0.8343	0.7297	0.6089	0.4826	0.3614	0.2539	6	9
9	4	0.9975	0.9944	0.9804	0.9511	0.9012	0.8283	0.7334	0.6214	0.5000	5	9
9	5	0.9998	0.9994	0.9969	0.9900	0.9747	0.9464	0.9006	0.8342	0.7461	4	9
9	6	1.0000	1.0000	0.9997	0.9987	0.9957	0.9888	0.9750	0.9502	0.9102	3	9
9	7	1.0000	1.0000	1.0000	0.9999	0.9996	0.9986	0.9962	0.9909	0.9805	2	9
9	8	1.0000	1.0000	1.0000	1.0000	1.0000	0.9999	0.9997	0.9992	0.9980	1	9
9	9	1.0000	1.0000	1.0000	1.0000	1.0000	1.0000	1.0000	1.0000	1.0000	0	9
10	0	0.2631	0.1969	0.1074	0.0563	0.0282	0.0135	0.0060	0.0025	0.0010	10	10
10	1	0.6389	0.5443	0.3758	0.2440	0.1493	0.0860	0.0464	0.0233	0.0107	9	10
10	2	0.8805	0.8202	0.6778	0.5256	0.3828	0.2616	0.1673	0.0996	0.0547	8	10
10	3	0.9725	0.9500	0.8791	0.7759	0.6496	0.5138	0.3823	0.2660	0.1719	7	10
10	4	0.9955	0.9901	0.9672	0.9219	0.8497	0.7515	0.6331	0.5044	0.3770	6	10
10	5	0.9995	0.9986	0.9936	0.9803	0.9527	0.9051	0.8338	0.7384	0.6230	5	10
10	6	1.0000	0.9999	0.9991	0.9965	0.9894	0.9740	0.9452	0.8980	0.8281	4	10
10	7	1.0000	1.0000	0.9999	0.9996	0.9984	0.9952	0.9877	0.9726	0.9453	3	10
10	8	1.0000	1.0000	1.0000	1.0000	0.9999	0.9995	0.9983	0.9955	0.9893	2	10
10	9	1.0000	1.0000	1.0000	1.0000	1.0000	1.0000	0.9999	0.9997	0.9990	1	10
10	10	1.0000	1.0000	1.0000	1.0000	1.0000	1.0000	1.0000	1.0000	1.0000	0	10
12	0	0.2014	0.1422	0.0687	0.0317	0.0138	0.0057	0.0022	0.0008	0.0002	12	12
12	1	0.5467	0.4435	0.2749	0.1584	0.0850	0.0424	0.0196	0.0083	0.0032	11	12
12	2	0.8180	0.7358	0.5583	0.3907	0.2528	0.1513	0.0834	0.0421	0.0193	10	12
12	3	0.9472	0.9078	0.7946	0.6488	0.4925	0.3467	0.2253	0.1345	0.0730	9	12
12	4	0.9887	0.9761	0.9274	0.8424	0.7237	0.5833	0.4382	0.3044	0.1938	8	12
12	5	0.9982	0.9954	0.9806	0.9456	0.8822	0.7873	0.6652	0.5269	0.3872	7	12
12	6	0.9998	0.9993	0.9961	0.9857	0.9614	0.9154	0.8418	0.7393	0.6128	6	12
12	7	1.0000	0.9999	0.9994	0.9972	0.9905	0.9745	0.9427	0.8883	0.8062	5	12
12	8	1.0000	1.0000	0.9999	0.9996	0.9983	0.9944	0.9847	0.9644	0.9270	4	12
12	9	1.0000	1.0000	1.0000	1.0000	0.9998	0.9992	0.9972	0.9921	0.9807	3	12
12	10	1.0000	1.0000	1.0000	1.0000	1.0000	0.9999	0.9997	0.9989	0.9968	2	12
12	11	1.0000	1.0000	1.0000	1.0000	1.0000	1.0000	1.0000	0.9999	0.9998	1	12
12	12	1.0000	1.0000	1.0000	1.0000	1.0000	1.0000	1.0000	1.0000	1.0000	0	12
15	0	0.1349	0.0874	0.0352	0.0134	0.0047	0.0016	0.0005	0.0001	0.0000	15	15
15	1	0.4241	0.3186	0.1671	0.0802	0.0353	0.0142	0.0052	0.0017	0.0005	14	15
15	2	0.7132	0.6042	0.3980	0.2361	0.1268	0.0617	0.0271	0.0107	0.0037	13	15
15	3	0.8922	0.8227	0.6482	0.4613	0.2969	0.1727	0.0905	0.0424	0.0176	12	15
15	4	0.9689	0.9383	0.8358	0.6865	0.5155	0.3519	0.2173	0.1204	0.0592	11	15
15	5	0.9930	0.9832	0.9389	0.8516	0.7216	0.5643	0.4032	0.2608	0.1509	10	15
15	6	0.9988	0.9964	0.9819	0.9434	0.8689	0.7548	0.6098	0.4522	0.3036	9	15
15	7	0.9998	0.9994	0.9958	0.9827	0.9500	0.8868	0.7869	0.6535	0.5000	8	15
15	8	1.0000	0.9999	0.9992	0.9958	0.9848	0.9578	0.9050	0.8182	0.6964	7	15
15	9	1.0000	1.0000	0.9999	0.9992	0.9963	0.9876	0.9662	0.9231	0.8491	6	15
15	10	1.0000	1.0000	1.0000	0.9999	0.9993	0.9972	0.9907	0.9745	0.9408	5	15
15	11	1.0000	1.0000	1.0000	1.0000	0.9999	0.9995	0.9981	0.9937	0.9824	4	15
15	12	1.0000	1.0000	1.0000	1.0000	1.0000	0.9999	0.9997	0.9989	0.9963	3	15
15	13	1.0000	1.0000	1.0000	1.0000	1.0000	1.0000	1.0000	0.9999	0.9995	2	15
15	14	1.0000	1.0000	1.0000	1.0000	1.0000	1.0000	1.0000	1.0000	1.0000	1	15
15	15	1.0000	1.0000	1.0000	1.0000	1.0000	1.0000	1.0000	1.0000	1.0000	0	15
		0.8750	0.8500	0.8000	0.7500	0.7000	0.6500	0.6000	0.5500	0.5000	x	n
		p										

Table III.2 (cont'd) Binomial Probabilities (Cumulative Distribution Function)

		p										
n	*x*	0.0010	0.0025	0.0050	0.0075	0.0100	0.0250	0.0500	0.0750	0.1000		
20	0	0.9802	0.9512	0.9046	0.8602	0.8179	0.6027	0.3585	0.2103	0.1216	20	20
20	1	0.9998	0.9988	0.9955	0.9902	0.9831	0.9118	0.7358	0.5513	0.3917	19	20
20	2	1.0000	1.0000	0.9999	0.9996	0.9990	0.9870	0.9245	0.8140	0.6769	18	20
20	3	1.0000	1.0000	1.0000	1.0000	1.0000	0.9986	0.9841	0.9418	0.8670	17	20
20	4	1.0000	1.0000	1.0000	1.0000	1.0000	0.9999	0.9974	0.9858	0.9568	16	20
20	5	1.0000	1.0000	1.0000	1.0000	1.0000	1.0000	0.9997	0.9973	0.9887	15	20
20	6	1.0000	1.0000	1.0000	1.0000	1.0000	1.0000	1.0000	0.9996	0.9976	14	20
20	7	1.0000	1.0000	1.0000	1.0000	1.0000	1.0000	1.0000	0.9999	0.9996	13	20
20	8	1.0000	1.0000	1.0000	1.0000	1.0000	1.0000	1.0000	1.0000	0.9999	12	20
20	9	1.0000	1.0000	1.0000	1.0000	1.0000	1.0000	1.0000	1.0000	1.0000	11	20
20	10	1.0000	1.0000	1.0000	1.0000	1.0000	1.0000	1.0000	1.0000	1.0000	10	20
20	11	1.0000	1.0000	1.0000	1.0000	1.0000	1.0000	1.0000	1.0000	1.0000	9	20
20	12	1.0000	1.0000	1.0000	1.0000	1.0000	1.0000	1.0000	1.0000	1.0000	8	20
20	13	1.0000	1.0000	1.0000	1.0000	1.0000	1.0000	1.0000	1.0000	1.0000	7	20
20	14	1.0000	1.0000	1.0000	1.0000	1.0000	1.0000	1.0000	1.0000	1.0000	6	20
20	15	1.0000	1.0000	1.0000	1.0000	1.0000	1.0000	1.0000	1.0000	1.0000	5	20
20	16	1.0000	1.0000	1.0000	1.0000	1.0000	1.0000	1.0000	1.0000	1.0000	4	20
20	17	1.0000	1.0000	1.0000	1.0000	1.0000	1.0000	1.0000	1.0000	1.0000	3	20
20	18	1.0000	1.0000	1.0000	1.0000	1.0000	1.0000	1.0000	1.0000	1.0000	2	20
20	19	1.0000	1.0000	1.0000	1.0000	1.0000	1.0000	1.0000	1.0000	1.0000	1	20
20	20	1.0000	1.0000	1.0000	1.0000	1.0000	1.0000	1.0000	1.0000	1.0000	0	20
25	0	0.9753	0.9393	0.8822	0.8284	0.7778	0.5310	0.2774	0.1424	0.0718	25	25
25	1	0.9997	0.9982	0.9931	0.9850	0.9742	0.8714	0.6424	0.4311	0.2712	24	25
25	2	1.0000	1.0000	0.9997	0.9991	0.9980	0.9762	0.8729	0.7120	0.5371	23	25
25	3	1.0000	1.0000	1.0000	1.0000	0.9999	0.9968	0.9659	0.8865	0.7636	22	25
25	4	1.0000	1.0000	1.0000	1.0000	1.0000	0.9997	0.9928	0.9644	0.9020	21	25
25	5	1.0000	1.0000	1.0000	1.0000	1.0000	1.0000	0.9988	0.9909	0.9666	20	25
25	6	1.0000	1.0000	1.0000	1.0000	1.0000	1.0000	0.9998	0.9981	0.9905	19	25
25	7	1.0000	1.0000	1.0000	1.0000	1.0000	1.0000	1.0000	0.9997	0.9977	18	25
25	8	1.0000	1.0000	1.0000	1.0000	1.0000	1.0000	1.0000	0.9999	0.9995	17	25
25	9	1.0000	1.0000	1.0000	1.0000	1.0000	1.0000	1.0000	1.0000	0.9999	16	25
25	10	1.0000	1.0000	1.0000	1.0000	1.0000	1.0000	1.0000	1.0000	1.0000	15	25
25	11	1.0000	1.0000	1.0000	1.0000	1.0000	1.0000	1.0000	1.0000	1.0000	14	25
25	12	1.0000	1.0000	1.0000	1.0000	1.0000	1.0000	1.0000	1.0000	1.0000	13	25
25	13	1.0000	1.0000	1.0000	1.0000	1.0000	1.0000	1.0000	1.0000	1.0000	12	25
25	14	1.0000	1.0000	1.0000	1.0000	1.0000	1.0000	1.0000	1.0000	1.0000	11	25
25	15	1.0000	1.0000	1.0000	1.0000	1.0000	1.0000	1.0000	1.0000	1.0000	10	25
25	16	1.0000	1.0000	1.0000	1.0000	1.0000	1.0000	1.0000	1.0000	1.0000	9	25
25	17	1.0000	1.0000	1.0000	1.0000	1.0000	1.0000	1.0000	1.0000	1.0000	8	25
25	18	1.0000	1.0000	1.0000	1.0000	1.0000	1.0000	1.0000	1.0000	1.0000	7	25
25	19	1.0000	1.0000	1.0000	1.0000	1.0000	1.0000	1.0000	1.0000	1.0000	6	25
25	20	1.0000	1.0000	1.0000	1.0000	1.0000	1.0000	1.0000	1.0000	1.0000	5	25
25	21	1.0000	1.0000	1.0000	1.0000	1.0000	1.0000	1.0000	1.0000	1.0000	4	25
25	22	1.0000	1.0000	1.0000	1.0000	1.0000	1.0000	1.0000	1.0000	1.0000	3	25
25	23	1.0000	1.0000	1.0000	1.0000	1.0000	1.0000	1.0000	1.0000	1.0000	2	25
25	24	1.0000	1.0000	1.0000	1.0000	1.0000	1.0000	1.0000	1.0000	1.0000	1	25
25	25	1.0000	1.0000	1.0000	1.0000	1.0000	1.0000	1.0000	1.0000	1.0000	0	25
		0.9990	0.9975	0.9950	0.9925	0.9900	0.9750	0.9500	0.9250	0.9000	*x*	*n*
		p										

Table III.2 (cont'd) Binomial Probabilities (Cumulative Distribution Function)

		p										
n	x	0.1250	0.1500	0.2000	0.2500	0.3000	0.3500	0.4000	0.4500	0.5000		
20	0	0.0692	0.0388	0.0115	0.0032	0.0008	0.0002	0.0000	0.0000	0.0000	20	20
20	1	0.2669	0.1756	0.0692	0.0243	0.0076	0.0021	0.0005	0.0001	0.0000	19	20
20	2	0.5353	0.4049	0.2061	0.0913	0.0355	0.0121	0.0036	0.0009	0.0002	18	20
20	3	0.7653	0.6477	0.4114	0.2252	0.1071	0.0444	0.0160	0.0049	0.0013	17	20
20	4	0.9050	0.8298	0.6296	0.4148	0.2375	0.1182	0.0510	0.0189	0.0059	16	20
20	5	0.9688	0.9327	0.8042	0.6172	0.4164	0.2454	0.1256	0.0553	0.0207	15	20
20	6	0.9916	0.9781	0.9133	0.7858	0.6080	0.4166	0.2500	0.1299	0.0577	14	20
20	7	0.9981	0.9941	0.9679	0.8982	0.7723	0.6010	0.4159	0.2520	0.1316	13	20
20	8	0.9997	0.9987	0.9900	0.9591	0.8867	0.7624	0.5956	0.4143	0.2517	12	20
20	9	0.9999	0.9998	0.9974	0.9861	0.9520	0.8782	0.7553	0.5914	0.4119	11	20
20	10	1.0000	1.0000	0.9994	0.9961	0.9829	0.9468	0.8725	0.7507	0.5881	10	20
20	11	1.0000	1.0000	0.9999	0.9991	0.9949	0.9804	0.9435	0.8692	0.7483	9	20
20	12	1.0000	1.0000	1.0000	0.9998	0.9987	0.9940	0.9790	0.9420	0.8684	8	20
20	13	1.0000	1.0000	1.0000	1.0000	0.9997	0.9985	0.9935	0.9786	0.9423	7	20
20	14	1.0000	1.0000	1.0000	1.0000	1.0000	0.9997	0.9984	0.9936	0.9793	6	20
20	15	1.0000	1.0000	1.0000	1.0000	1.0000	1.0000	0.9997	0.9985	0.9941	5	20
20	16	1.0000	1.0000	1.0000	1.0000	1.0000	1.0000	1.0000	0.9997	0.9987	4	20
20	17	1.0000	1.0000	1.0000	1.0000	1.0000	1.0000	1.0000	1.0000	0.9998	3	20
20	18	1.0000	1.0000	1.0000	1.0000	1.0000	1.0000	1.0000	1.0000	1.0000	2	20
20	19	1.0000	1.0000	1.0000	1.0000	1.0000	1.0000	1.0000	1.0000	1.0000	1	20
20	20	1.0000	1.0000	1.0000	1.0000	1.0000	1.0000	1.0000	1.0000	1.0000	0	20
25	0	0.0355	0.0172	0.0038	0.0008	0.0001	0.0000	0.0000	0.0000	0.0000	25	25
25	1	0.1623	0.0931	0.0274	0.0070	0.0016	0.0003	0.0001	0.0000	0.0000	24	25
25	2	0.3796	0.2537	0.0982	0.0321	0.0090	0.0021	0.0004	0.0001	0.0000	23	25
25	3	0.6176	0.4711	0.2340	0.0962	0.0332	0.0097	0.0024	0.0005	0.0001	22	25
25	4	0.8047	0.6821	0.4207	0.2137	0.0905	0.0320	0.0095	0.0023	0.0005	21	25
25	5	0.9169	0.8385	0.6167	0.3783	0.1935	0.0826	0.0294	0.0086	0.0020	20	25
25	6	0.9703	0.9305	0.7800	0.5611	0.3407	0.1734	0.0736	0.0258	0.0073	19	25
25	7	0.9910	0.9745	0.8909	0.7265	0.5118	0.3061	0.1536	0.0639	0.0216	18	25
25	8	0.9977	0.9920	0.9532	0.8506	0.6769	0.4668	0.2735	0.1340	0.0539	17	25
25	9	0.9995	0.9979	0.9827	0.9287	0.8106	0.6303	0.4246	0.2424	0.1148	16	25
25	10	0.9999	0.9995	0.9944	0.9703	0.9022	0.7712	0.5858	0.3843	0.2122	15	25
25	11	1.0000	0.9999	0.9985	0.9893	0.9558	0.8746	0.7323	0.5426	0.3450	14	25
25	12	1.0000	1.0000	0.9996	0.9966	0.9825	0.9396	0.8462	0.6937	0.5000	13	25
25	13	1.0000	1.0000	0.9999	0.9991	0.9940	0.9745	0.9222	0.8173	0.6550	12	25
25	14	1.0000	1.0000	1.0000	0.9998	0.9982	0.9907	0.9656	0.9040	0.7878	11	25
25	15	1.0000	1.0000	1.0000	1.0000	0.9995	0.9971	0.9868	0.9560	0.8852	10	25
25	16	1.0000	1.0000	1.0000	1.0000	0.9999	0.9992	0.9957	0.9826	0.9461	9	25
25	17	1.0000	1.0000	1.0000	1.0000	1.0000	0.9998	0.9988	0.9942	0.9784	8	25
25	18	1.0000	1.0000	1.0000	1.0000	1.0000	1.0000	0.9997	0.9984	0.9927	7	25
25	19	1.0000	1.0000	1.0000	1.0000	1.0000	1.0000	0.9999	0.9996	0.9980	6	25
25	20	1.0000	1.0000	1.0000	1.0000	1.0000	1.0000	1.0000	0.9999	0.9995	5	25
25	21	1.0000	1.0000	1.0000	1.0000	1.0000	1.0000	1.0000	1.0000	0.9999	4	25
25	22	1.0000	1.0000	1.0000	1.0000	1.0000	1.0000	1.0000	1.0000	1.0000	3	25
25	23	1.0000	1.0000	1.0000	1.0000	1.0000	1.0000	1.0000	1.0000	1.0000	2	25
25	24	1.0000	1.0000	1.0000	1.0000	1.0000	1.0000	1.0000	1.0000	1.0000	1	25
25	25	1.0000	1.0000	1.0000	1.0000	1.0000	1.0000	1.0000	1.0000	1.0000	0	25
		0.8750	0.8500	0.8000	0.7500	0.7000	0.6500	0.6000	0.5500	0.5000	x	n
		p										

Table III.2 (cont'd) Binomial Probabilities (Cumulative Distribution Function)

		p										
n	*x*	0.0010	0.0025	0.0050	0.0075	0.0100	0.0250	0.0500	0.0750	0.1000		
30	0	0.9704	0.9277	0.8604	0.7978	0.7397	0.4679	0.2146	0.0964	0.0424	30	30
30	1	0.9996	0.9974	0.9901	0.9787	0.9639	0.8278	0.5535	0.3310	0.1837	29	30
30	2	1.0000	0.9999	0.9995	0.9985	0.9967	0.9616	0.8122	0.6068	0.4114	28	30
30	3	1.0000	1.0000	1.0000	0.9999	0.9998	0.9936	0.9392	0.8155	0.6474	27	30
30	4	1.0000	1.0000	1.0000	1.0000	1.0000	0.9992	0.9844	0.9297	0.8245	26	30
30	5	1.0000	1.0000	1.0000	1.0000	1.0000	0.9999	0.9967	0.9779	0.9268	25	30
30	6	1.0000	1.0000	1.0000	1.0000	1.0000	1.0000	0.9994	0.9942	0.9742	24	30
30	7	1.0000	1.0000	1.0000	1.0000	1.0000	1.0000	0.9999	0.9987	0.9922	23	30
30	8	1.0000	1.0000	1.0000	1.0000	1.0000	1.0000	1.0000	0.9997	0.9980	22	30
30	9	1.0000	1.0000	1.0000	1.0000	1.0000	1.0000	1.0000	1.0000	0.9995	21	30
30	10	1.0000	1.0000	1.0000	1.0000	1.0000	1.0000	1.0000	1.0000	0.9999	20	30
30	11	1.0000	1.0000	1.0000	1.0000	1.0000	1.0000	1.0000	1.0000	1.0000	19	30
30	12	1.0000	1.0000	1.0000	1.0000	1.0000	1.0000	1.0000	1.0000	1.0000	18	30
30	13	1.0000	1.0000	1.0000	1.0000	1.0000	1.0000	1.0000	1.0000	1.0000	17	30
30	14	1.0000	1.0000	1.0000	1.0000	1.0000	1.0000	1.0000	1.0000	1.0000	16	30
30	15	1.0000	1.0000	1.0000	1.0000	1.0000	1.0000	1.0000	1.0000	1.0000	15	30
30	16	1.0000	1.0000	1.0000	1.0000	1.0000	1.0000	1.0000	1.0000	1.0000	14	30
30	17	1.0000	1.0000	1.0000	1.0000	1.0000	1.0000	1.0000	1.0000	1.0000	13	30
30	18	1.0000	1.0000	1.0000	1.0000	1.0000	1.0000	1.0000	1.0000	1.0000	12	30
30	19	1.0000	1.0000	1.0000	1.0000	1.0000	1.0000	1.0000	1.0000	1.0000	11	30
30	20	1.0000	1.0000	1.0000	1.0000	1.0000	1.0000	1.0000	1.0000	1.0000	10	30
30	21	1.0000	1.0000	1.0000	1.0000	1.0000	1.0000	1.0000	1.0000	1.0000	9	30
30	22	1.0000	1.0000	1.0000	1.0000	1.0000	1.0000	1.0000	1.0000	1.0000	8	30
30	23	1.0000	1.0000	1.0000	1.0000	1.0000	1.0000	1.0000	1.0000	1.0000	7	30
30	24	1.0000	1.0000	1.0000	1.0000	1.0000	1.0000	1.0000	1.0000	1.0000	6	30
30	25	1.0000	1.0000	1.0000	1.0000	1.0000	1.0000	1.0000	1.0000	1.0000	5	30
30	26	1.0000	1.0000	1.0000	1.0000	1.0000	1.0000	1.0000	1.0000	1.0000	4	30
30	27	1.0000	1.0000	1.0000	1.0000	1.0000	1.0000	1.0000	1.0000	1.0000	3	30
30	28	1.0000	1.0000	1.0000	1.0000	1.0000	1.0000	1.0000	1.0000	1.0000	2	30
30	29	1.0000	1.0000	1.0000	1.0000	1.0000	1.0000	1.0000	1.0000	1.0000	1	30
30	30	1.0000	1.0000	1.0000	1.0000	1.0000	1.0000	1.0000	1.0000	1.0000	0	30
		0.9990	0.9975	0.9950	0.9925	0.9900	0.9750	0.9500	0.9250	0.9000	*x*	*n*
		p										

Table III.2 (cont'd) Binomial Probabilities (Cumulative Distribution Function)

		p										
n	*x*	0.1250	0.1500	0.2000	0.2500	0.3000	0.3500	0.4000	0.4500	0.5000		
30	0	0.0182	0.0076	0.0012	0.0002	0.0000	0.0000	0.0000	0.0000	0.0000	30	30
30	1	0.0962	0.0480	0.0105	0.0020	0.0003	0.0000	0.0000	0.0000	0.0000	29	30
30	2	0.2579	0.1514	0.0442	0.0106	0.0021	0.0003	0.0000	0.0000	0.0000	28	30
30	3	0.4734	0.3217	0.1227	0.0374	0.0093	0.0019	0.0003	0.0000	0.0000	27	30
30	4	0.6812	0.5245	0.2552	0.0979	0.0302	0.0075	0.0015	0.0002	0.0000	26	30
30	5	0.8356	0.7106	0.4275	0.2026	0.0766	0.0233	0.0057	0.0011	0.0002	25	30
30	6	0.9275	0.8474	0.6070	0.3481	0.1595	0.0586	0.0172	0.0040	0.0007	24	30
30	7	0.9725	0.9302	0.7608	0.5143	0.2814	0.1238	0.0435	0.0121	0.0026	23	30
30	8	0.9910	0.9722	0.8713	0.6736	0.4315	0.2247	0.0940	0.0312	0.0081	22	30
30	9	0.9974	0.9903	0.9389	0.8034	0.5888	0.3575	0.1763	0.0694	0.0214	21	30
30	10	0.9994	0.9971	0.9744	0.8943	0.7304	0.5078	0.2915	0.1350	0.0494	20	30
30	11	0.9999	0.9992	0.9905	0.9493	0.8407	0.6548	0.4311	0.2327	0.1002	19	30
30	12	1.0000	0.9998	0.9969	0.9784	0.9155	0.7802	0.5785	0.3592	0.1808	18	30
30	13	1.0000	1.0000	0.9991	0.9918	0.9599	0.8737	0.7145	0.5025	0.2923	17	30
30	14	1.0000	1.0000	0.9998	0.9973	0.9831	0.9348	0.8246	0.6448	0.4278	16	30
30	15	1.0000	1.0000	0.9999	0.9992	0.9936	0.9699	0.9029	0.7691	0.5722	15	30
30	16	1.0000	1.0000	1.0000	0.9998	0.9979	0.9876	0.9519	0.8644	0.7077	14	30
30	17	1.0000	1.0000	1.0000	0.9999	0.9994	0.9955	0.9788	0.9286	0.8192	13	30
30	18	1.0000	1.0000	1.0000	1.0000	0.9998	0.9986	0.9917	0.9666	0.8998	12	30
30	19	1.0000	1.0000	1.0000	1.0000	1.0000	0.9996	0.9971	0.9862	0.9506	11	30
30	20	1.0000	1.0000	1.0000	1.0000	1.0000	0.9999	0.9991	0.9950	0.9786	10	30
30	21	1.0000	1.0000	1.0000	1.0000	1.0000	1.0000	0.9998	0.9984	0.9919	9	30
30	22	1.0000	1.0000	1.0000	1.0000	1.0000	1.0000	1.0000	0.9996	0.9974	8	30
30	23	1.0000	1.0000	1.0000	1.0000	1.0000	1.0000	1.0000	0.9999	0.9993	7	30
30	24	1.0000	1.0000	1.0000	1.0000	1.0000	1.0000	1.0000	1.0000	0.9998	6	30
30	25	1.0000	1.0000	1.0000	1.0000	1.0000	1.0000	1.0000	1.0000	1.0000	5	30
30	26	1.0000	1.0000	1.0000	1.0000	1.0000	1.0000	1.0000	1.0000	1.0000	4	30
30	27	1.0000	1.0000	1.0000	1.0000	1.0000	1.0000	1.0000	1.0000	1.0000	3	30
30	28	1.0000	1.0000	1.0000	1.0000	1.0000	1.0000	1.0000	1.0000	1.0000	2	30
30	29	1.0000	1.0000	1.0000	1.0000	1.0000	1.0000	1.0000	1.0000	1.0000	1	30
30	30	1.0000	1.0000	1.0000	1.0000	1.0000	1.0000	1.0000	1.0000	1.0000	0	30
		0.8750	0.8500	0.8000	0.7500	0.7000	0.6500	0.6000	0.5500	0.5000	*x*	*n*
		p										

Table III.2 (cont'd) Binomial Probabilities (Cumulative Distribution Function)

		p										
n	x	0.0010	0.0025	0.0050	0.0075	0.0100	0.0250	0.0500	0.0750	0.1000		
40	0	0.9608	0.9047	0.8183	0.7400	0.6690	0.3632	0.1285	0.0442	0.0148	40	40
40	1	0.9992	0.9954	0.9828	0.9637	0.9393	0.7358	0.3991	0.1877	0.0805	39	40
40	2	1.0000	0.9999	0.9989	0.9966	0.9925	0.9221	0.6767	0.4144	0.2228	38	40
40	3	1.0000	1.0000	1.0000	0.9998	0.9993	0.9826	0.8619	0.6473	0.4231	37	40
40	4	1.0000	1.0000	1.0000	1.0000	1.0000	0.9969	0.9520	0.8220	0.6290	36	40
40	5	1.0000	1.0000	1.0000	1.0000	1.0000	0.9995	0.9861	0.9240	0.7937	35	40
40	6	1.0000	1.0000	1.0000	1.0000	1.0000	0.9999	0.9966	0.9722	0.9005	34	40
40	7	1.0000	1.0000	1.0000	1.0000	1.0000	1.0000	0.9993	0.9912	0.9581	33	40
40	8	1.0000	1.0000	1.0000	1.0000	1.0000	1.0000	0.9999	0.9976	0.9845	32	40
40	9	1.0000	1.0000	1.0000	1.0000	1.0000	1.0000	1.0000	0.9994	0.9949	31	40
40	10	1.0000	1.0000	1.0000	1.0000	1.0000	1.0000	1.0000	0.9999	0.9985	30	40
40	11	1.0000	1.0000	1.0000	1.0000	1.0000	1.0000	1.0000	1.0000	0.9996	29	40
40	12	1.0000	1.0000	1.0000	1.0000	1.0000	1.0000	1.0000	1.0000	0.9999	28	40
40	13	1.0000	1.0000	1.0000	1.0000	1.0000	1.0000	1.0000	1.0000	1.0000	27	40
40	14	1.0000	1.0000	1.0000	1.0000	1.0000	1.0000	1.0000	1.0000	1.0000	26	40
40	15	1.0000	1.0000	1.0000	1.0000	1.0000	1.0000	1.0000	1.0000	1.0000	25	40
40	16	1.0000	1.0000	1.0000	1.0000	1.0000	1.0000	1.0000	1.0000	1.0000	24	40
40	17	1.0000	1.0000	1.0000	1.0000	1.0000	1.0000	1.0000	1.0000	1.0000	23	40
40	18	1.0000	1.0000	1.0000	1.0000	1.0000	1.0000	1.0000	1.0000	1.0000	22	40
40	19	1.0000	1.0000	1.0000	1.0000	1.0000	1.0000	1.0000	1.0000	1.0000	21	40
40	20	1.0000	1.0000	1.0000	1.0000	1.0000	1.0000	1.0000	1.0000	1.0000	20	40
40	21	1.0000	1.0000	1.0000	1.0000	1.0000	1.0000	1.0000	1.0000	1.0000	19	40
40	22	1.0000	1.0000	1.0000	1.0000	1.0000	1.0000	1.0000	1.0000	1.0000	18	40
40	23	1.0000	1.0000	1.0000	1.0000	1.0000	1.0000	1.0000	1.0000	1.0000	17	40
40	24	1.0000	1.0000	1.0000	1.0000	1.0000	1.0000	1.0000	1.0000	1.0000	16	40
40	25	1.0000	1.0000	1.0000	1.0000	1.0000	1.0000	1.0000	1.0000	1.0000	15	40
40	26	1.0000	1.0000	1.0000	1.0000	1.0000	1.0000	1.0000	1.0000	1.0000	14	40
40	27	1.0000	1.0000	1.0000	1.0000	1.0000	1.0000	1.0000	1.0000	1.0000	13	40
40	28	1.0000	1.0000	1.0000	1.0000	1.0000	1.0000	1.0000	1.0000	1.0000	12	40
40	29	1.0000	1.0000	1.0000	1.0000	1.0000	1.0000	1.0000	1.0000	1.0000	11	40
40	30	1.0000	1.0000	1.0000	1.0000	1.0000	1.0000	1.0000	1.0000	1.0000	10	40
40	31	1.0000	1.0000	1.0000	1.0000	1.0000	1.0000	1.0000	1.0000	1.0000	9	40
40	32	1.0000	1.0000	1.0000	1.0000	1.0000	1.0000	1.0000	1.0000	1.0000	8	40
40	33	1.0000	1.0000	1.0000	1.0000	1.0000	1.0000	1.0000	1.0000	1.0000	7	40
40	34	1.0000	1.0000	1.0000	1.0000	1.0000	1.0000	1.0000	1.0000	1.0000	6	40
40	35	1.0000	1.0000	1.0000	1.0000	1.0000	1.0000	1.0000	1.0000	1.0000	5	40
40	36	1.0000	1.0000	1.0000	1.0000	1.0000	1.0000	1.0000	1.0000	1.0000	4	40
40	37	1.0000	1.0000	1.0000	1.0000	1.0000	1.0000	1.0000	1.0000	1.0000	3	40
40	38	1.0000	1.0000	1.0000	1.0000	1.0000	1.0000	1.0000	1.0000	1.0000	2	40
40	39	1.0000	1.0000	1.0000	1.0000	1.0000	1.0000	1.0000	1.0000	1.0000	1	40
40	40	1.0000	1.0000	1.0000	1.0000	1.0000	1.0000	1.0000	1.0000	1.0000	0	40
		0.9990	0.9975	0.9950	0.9925	0.9900	0.9750	0.9500	0.9250	0.9000	x	n
		p										

Table III.2 (cont'd) Binomial Probabilities (Cumulative Distribution Function)

		p										
n	*x*	0.1250	0.1500	0.2000	0.2500	0.3000	0.3500	0.4000	0.4500	0.5000		
40	0	0.0048	0.0015	0.0001	0.0000	0.0000	0.0000	0.0000	0.0000	0.0000	40	40
40	1	0.0322	0.0121	0.0015	0.0001	0.0000	0.0000	0.0000	0.0000	0.0000	39	40
40	2	0.1084	0.0486	0.0079	0.0010	0.0001	0.0000	0.0000	0.0000	0.0000	38	40
40	3	0.2464	0.1302	0.0285	0.0047	0.0006	0.0001	0.0000	0.0000	0.0000	37	40
40	4	0.4287	0.2633	0.0759	0.0160	0.0026	0.0003	0.0000	0.0000	0.0000	36	40
40	5	0.6162	0.4325	0.1613	0.0433	0.0086	0.0013	0.0001	0.0000	0.0000	35	40
40	6	0.7725	0.6067	0.2859	0.0962	0.0238	0.0044	0.0006	0.0001	0.0000	34	40
40	7	0.8809	0.7559	0.4371	0.1820	0.0553	0.0124	0.0021	0.0002	0.0000	33	40
40	8	0.9448	0.8646	0.5931	0.2998	0.1110	0.0303	0.0061	0.0009	0.0001	32	40
40	9	0.9773	0.9328	0.7318	0.4395	0.1959	0.0644	0.0156	0.0027	0.0003	31	40
40	10	0.9917	0.9701	0.8392	0.5839	0.3087	0.1215	0.0352	0.0074	0.0011	30	40
40	11	0.9973	0.9880	0.9125	0.7151	0.4406	0.2053	0.0709	0.0179	0.0032	29	40
40	12	0.9992	0.9957	0.9568	0.8209	0.5772	0.3143	0.1285	0.0386	0.0083	28	40
40	13	0.9998	0.9986	0.9806	0.8968	0.7032	0.4408	0.2112	0.0751	0.0192	27	40
40	14	0.9999	0.9996	0.9921	0.9456	0.8074	0.5721	0.3174	0.1326	0.0403	26	40
40	15	1.0000	0.9999	0.9971	0.9738	0.8849	0.6946	0.4402	0.2142	0.0769	25	40
40	16	1.0000	1.0000	0.9990	0.9884	0.9367	0.7978	0.5681	0.3185	0.1341	24	40
40	17	1.0000	1.0000	0.9997	0.9953	0.9680	0.8761	0.6885	0.4391	0.2148	23	40
40	18	1.0000	1.0000	0.9999	0.9983	0.9852	0.9301	0.7911	0.5651	0.3179	22	40
40	19	1.0000	1.0000	1.0000	0.9994	0.9937	0.9637	0.8702	0.6844	0.4373	21	40
40	20	1.0000	1.0000	1.0000	0.9998	0.9976	0.9827	0.9256	0.7870	0.5627	20	40
40	21	1.0000	1.0000	1.0000	1.0000	0.9991	0.9925	0.9608	0.8669	0.6821	19	40
40	22	1.0000	1.0000	1.0000	1.0000	0.9997	0.9970	0.9811	0.9233	0.7852	18	40
40	23	1.0000	1.0000	1.0000	1.0000	0.9999	0.9989	0.9917	0.9595	0.8659	17	40
40	24	1.0000	1.0000	1.0000	1.0000	1.0000	0.9996	0.9966	0.9804	0.9231	16	40
40	25	1.0000	1.0000	1.0000	1.0000	1.0000	0.9999	0.9988	0.9914	0.9597	15	40
40	26	1.0000	1.0000	1.0000	1.0000	1.0000	1.0000	0.9996	0.9966	0.9808	14	40
40	27	1.0000	1.0000	1.0000	1.0000	1.0000	1.0000	0.9999	0.9988	0.9917	13	40
40	28	1.0000	1.0000	1.0000	1.0000	1.0000	1.0000	1.0000	0.9996	0.9968	12	40
40	29	1.0000	1.0000	1.0000	1.0000	1.0000	1.0000	1.0000	0.9999	0.9989	11	40
40	30	1.0000	1.0000	1.0000	1.0000	1.0000	1.0000	1.0000	1.0000	0.9997	10	40
40	31	1.0000	1.0000	1.0000	1.0000	1.0000	1.0000	1.0000	1.0000	0.9999	9	40
40	32	1.0000	1.0000	1.0000	1.0000	1.0000	1.0000	1.0000	1.0000	1.0000	8	40
40	33	1.0000	1.0000	1.0000	1.0000	1.0000	1.0000	1.0000	1.0000	1.0000	7	40
40	34	1.0000	1.0000	1.0000	1.0000	1.0000	1.0000	1.0000	1.0000	1.0000	6	40
40	35	1.0000	1.0000	1.0000	1.0000	1.0000	1.0000	1.0000	1.0000	1.0000	5	40
40	36	1.0000	1.0000	1.0000	1.0000	1.0000	1.0000	1.0000	1.0000	1.0000	4	40
40	37	1.0000	1.0000	1.0000	1.0000	1.0000	1.0000	1.0000	1.0000	1.0000	3	40
40	38	1.0000	1.0000	1.0000	1.0000	1.0000	1.0000	1.0000	1.0000	1.0000	2	40
40	39	1.0000	1.0000	1.0000	1.0000	1.0000	1.0000	1.0000	1.0000	1.0000	1	40
40	40	1.0000	1.0000	1.0000	1.0000	1.0000	1.0000	1.0000	1.0000	1.0000	0	40
		0.8750	0.8500	0.8000	0.7500	0.7000	0.6500	0.6000	0.5500	0.5000	*x*	*n*
		p										

Table III.2 (cont'd) Binomial Probabilities (Cumulative Distribution Function)

		p										
n	*x*	0.0010	0.0025	0.0050	0.0075	0.0100	0.0250	0.0500	0.0750	0.1000		
50	0	0.9512	0.8824	0.7783	0.6863	0.6050	0.2820	0.0769	0.0203	0.0052	50	50
50	1	0.9988	0.9929	0.9739	0.9456	0.9106	0.6435	0.2794	0.1025	0.0338	49	50
50	2	1.0000	0.9997	0.9979	0.9936	0.9862	0.8706	0.5405	0.2658	0.1117	48	50
50	3	1.0000	1.0000	0.9999	0.9994	0.9984	0.9638	0.7604	0.4777	0.2503	47	50
50	4	1.0000	1.0000	1.0000	1.0000	0.9999	0.9919	0.8964	0.6796	0.4312	46	50
50	5	1.0000	1.0000	1.0000	1.0000	1.0000	0.9985	0.9622	0.8302	0.6161	45	50
50	6	1.0000	1.0000	1.0000	1.0000	1.0000	0.9998	0.9882	0.9217	0.7702	44	50
50	7	1.0000	1.0000	1.0000	1.0000	1.0000	1.0000	0.9968	0.9684	0.8779	43	50
50	8	1.0000	1.0000	1.0000	1.0000	1.0000	1.0000	0.9992	0.9887	0.9421	42	50
50	9	1.0000	1.0000	1.0000	1.0000	1.0000	1.0000	0.9998	0.9964	0.9755	41	50
50	10	1.0000	1.0000	1.0000	1.0000	1.0000	1.0000	1.0000	0.9990	0.9906	40	50
50	11	1.0000	1.0000	1.0000	1.0000	1.0000	1.0000	1.0000	0.9997	0.9968	39	50
50	12	1.0000	1.0000	1.0000	1.0000	1.0000	1.0000	1.0000	0.9999	0.9990	38	50
50	13	1.0000	1.0000	1.0000	1.0000	1.0000	1.0000	1.0000	1.0000	0.9997	37	50
50	14	1.0000	1.0000	1.0000	1.0000	1.0000	1.0000	1.0000	1.0000	0.9999	36	50
50	15	1.0000	1.0000	1.0000	1.0000	1.0000	1.0000	1.0000	1.0000	1.0000	35	50
50	16	1.0000	1.0000	1.0000	1.0000	1.0000	1.0000	1.0000	1.0000	1.0000	34	50
50	17	1.0000	1.0000	1.0000	1.0000	1.0000	1.0000	1.0000	1.0000	1.0000	33	50
50	18	1.0000	1.0000	1.0000	1.0000	1.0000	1.0000	1.0000	1.0000	1.0000	32	50
50	19	1.0000	1.0000	1.0000	1.0000	1.0000	1.0000	1.0000	1.0000	1.0000	31	50
50	20	1.0000	1.0000	1.0000	1.0000	1.0000	1.0000	1.0000	1.0000	1.0000	30	50
50	21	1.0000	1.0000	1.0000	1.0000	1.0000	1.0000	1.0000	1.0000	1.0000	29	50
50	22	1.0000	1.0000	1.0000	1.0000	1.0000	1.0000	1.0000	1.0000	1.0000	28	50
50	23	1.0000	1.0000	1.0000	1.0000	1.0000	1.0000	1.0000	1.0000	1.0000	27	50
50	24	1.0000	1.0000	1.0000	1.0000	1.0000	1.0000	1.0000	1.0000	1.0000	26	50
50	25	1.0000	1.0000	1.0000	1.0000	1.0000	1.0000	1.0000	1.0000	1.0000	25	50
50	26	1.0000	1.0000	1.0000	1.0000	1.0000	1.0000	1.0000	1.0000	1.0000	24	50
50	27	1.0000	1.0000	1.0000	1.0000	1.0000	1.0000	1.0000	1.0000	1.0000	23	50
50	28	1.0000	1.0000	1.0000	1.0000	1.0000	1.0000	1.0000	1.0000	1.0000	22	50
50	29	1.0000	1.0000	1.0000	1.0000	1.0000	1.0000	1.0000	1.0000	1.0000	21	50
50	30	1.0000	1.0000	1.0000	1.0000	1.0000	1.0000	1.0000	1.0000	1.0000	20	50
50	31	1.0000	1.0000	1.0000	1.0000	1.0000	1.0000	1.0000	1.0000	1.0000	19	50
50	32	1.0000	1.0000	1.0000	1.0000	1.0000	1.0000	1.0000	1.0000	1.0000	18	50
50	33	1.0000	1.0000	1.0000	1.0000	1.0000	1.0000	1.0000	1.0000	1.0000	17	50
50	34	1.0000	1.0000	1.0000	1.0000	1.0000	1.0000	1.0000	1.0000	1.0000	16	50
50	35	1.0000	1.0000	1.0000	1.0000	1.0000	1.0000	1.0000	1.0000	1.0000	15	50
50	36	1.0000	1.0000	1.0000	1.0000	1.0000	1.0000	1.0000	1.0000	1.0000	14	50
50	37	1.0000	1.0000	1.0000	1.0000	1.0000	1.0000	1.0000	1.0000	1.0000	13	50
50	38	1.0000	1.0000	1.0000	1.0000	1.0000	1.0000	1.0000	1.0000	1.0000	12	50
50	39	1.0000	1.0000	1.0000	1.0000	1.0000	1.0000	1.0000	1.0000	1.0000	11	50
50	40	1.0000	1.0000	1.0000	1.0000	1.0000	1.0000	1.0000	1.0000	1.0000	10	50
50	41	1.0000	1.0000	1.0000	1.0000	1.0000	1.0000	1.0000	1.0000	1.0000	9	50
50	42	1.0000	1.0000	1.0000	1.0000	1.0000	1.0000	1.0000	1.0000	1.0000	8	50
50	43	1.0000	1.0000	1.0000	1.0000	1.0000	1.0000	1.0000	1.0000	1.0000	7	50
50	44	1.0000	1.0000	1.0000	1.0000	1.0000	1.0000	1.0000	1.0000	1.0000	6	50
50	45	1.0000	1.0000	1.0000	1.0000	1.0000	1.0000	1.0000	1.0000	1.0000	5	50
50	46	1.0000	1.0000	1.0000	1.0000	1.0000	1.0000	1.0000	1.0000	1.0000	4	50
50	47	1.0000	1.0000	1.0000	1.0000	1.0000	1.0000	1.0000	1.0000	1.0000	3	50
50	48	1.0000	1.0000	1.0000	1.0000	1.0000	1.0000	1.0000	1.0000	1.0000	2	50
50	49	1.0000	1.0000	1.0000	1.0000	1.0000	1.0000	1.0000	1.0000	1.0000	1	50
50	50	1.0000	1.0000	1.0000	1.0000	1.0000	1.0000	1.0000	1.0000	1.0000	0	50
		0.9990	0.9975	0.9950	0.9925	0.9900	0.9750	0.9500	0.9250	0.9000	*x*	*n*
		p										

Table III.2 (cont'd) Binomial Probabilities (Cumulative Distribution Function)

		p										
n	*x*	0.1250	0.1500	0.2000	0.2500	0.3000	0.3500	0.4000	0.4500	0.5000		
50	0	0.0013	0.0003	0.0000	0.0000	0.0000	0.0000	0.0000	0.0000	0.0000	50	50
50	1	0.0103	0.0029	0.0002	0.0000	0.0000	0.0000	0.0000	0.0000	0.0000	49	50
50	2	0.0418	0.0142	0.0013	0.0001	0.0000	0.0000	0.0000	0.0000	0.0000	48	50
50	3	0.1138	0.0460	0.0057	0.0005	0.0000	0.0000	0.0000	0.0000	0.0000	47	50
50	4	0.2346	0.1121	0.0185	0.0021	0.0002	0.0000	0.0000	0.0000	0.0000	46	50
50	5	0.3935	0.2194	0.0480	0.0070	0.0007	0.0001	0.0000	0.0000	0.0000	45	50
50	6	0.5637	0.3613	0.1034	0.0194	0.0025	0.0002	0.0000	0.0000	0.0000	44	50
50	7	0.7165	0.5188	0.1904	0.0453	0.0073	0.0008	0.0001	0.0000	0.0000	43	50
50	8	0.8339	0.6681	0.3073	0.0916	0.0183	0.0025	0.0002	0.0000	0.0000	42	50
50	9	0.9121	0.7911	0.4437	0.1637	0.0402	0.0067	0.0008	0.0001	0.0000	41	50
50	10	0.9579	0.8801	0.5836	0.2622	0.0789	0.0160	0.0022	0.0002	0.0000	40	50
50	11	0.9817	0.9372	0.7107	0.3816	0.1390	0.0342	0.0057	0.0006	0.0000	39	50
50	12	0.9928	0.9699	0.8139	0.5110	0.2229	0.0661	0.0133	0.0018	0.0002	38	50
50	13	0.9974	0.9868	0.8894	0.6370	0.3279	0.1163	0.0280	0.0045	0.0005	37	50
50	14	0.9991	0.9947	0.9393	0.7481	0.4468	0.1878	0.0540	0.0104	0.0013	36	50
50	15	0.9997	0.9981	0.9692	0.8369	0.5692	0.2801	0.0955	0.0220	0.0033	35	50
50	16	0.9999	0.9993	0.9856	0.9017	0.6839	0.3889	0.1561	0.0427	0.0077	34	50
50	17	1.0000	0.9998	0.9937	0.9449	0.7822	0.5060	0.2369	0.0765	0.0164	33	50
50	18	1.0000	0.9999	0.9975	0.9713	0.8594	0.6216	0.3356	0.1273	0.0325	32	50
50	19	1.0000	1.0000	0.9991	0.9861	0.9152	0.7264	0.4465	0.1974	0.0595	31	50
50	20	1.0000	1.0000	0.9997	0.9937	0.9522	0.8139	0.5610	0.2862	0.1013	30	50
50	21	1.0000	1.0000	0.9999	0.9974	0.9749	0.8813	0.6701	0.3900	0.1611	29	50
50	22	1.0000	1.0000	1.0000	0.9990	0.9877	0.9290	0.7660	0.5019	0.2399	28	50
50	23	1.0000	1.0000	1.0000	0.9996	0.9944	0.9604	0.8438	0.6134	0.3359	27	50
50	24	1.0000	1.0000	1.0000	0.9999	0.9976	0.9793	0.9022	0.7160	0.4439	26	50
50	25	1.0000	1.0000	1.0000	1.0000	0.9991	0.9900	0.9427	0.8034	0.5561	25	50
50	26	1.0000	1.0000	1.0000	1.0000	0.9997	0.9955	0.9686	0.8721	0.6641	24	50
50	27	1.0000	1.0000	1.0000	1.0000	0.9999	0.9981	0.9840	0.9220	0.7601	23	50
50	28	1.0000	1.0000	1.0000	1.0000	1.0000	0.9993	0.9924	0.9556	0.8389	22	50
50	29	1.0000	1.0000	1.0000	1.0000	1.0000	0.9997	0.9966	0.9765	0.8987	21	50
50	30	1.0000	1.0000	1.0000	1.0000	1.0000	0.9999	0.9986	0.9884	0.9405	20	50
50	31	1.0000	1.0000	1.0000	1.0000	1.0000	1.0000	0.9995	0.9947	0.9675	19	50
50	32	1.0000	1.0000	1.0000	1.0000	1.0000	1.0000	0.9998	0.9978	0.9836	18	50
50	33	1.0000	1.0000	1.0000	1.0000	1.0000	1.0000	0.9999	0.9991	0.9923	17	50
50	34	1.0000	1.0000	1.0000	1.0000	1.0000	1.0000	1.0000	0.9997	0.9967	16	50
50	35	1.0000	1.0000	1.0000	1.0000	1.0000	1.0000	1.0000	0.9999	0.9987	15	50
50	36	1.0000	1.0000	1.0000	1.0000	1.0000	1.0000	1.0000	1.0000	0.9995	14	50
50	37	1.0000	1.0000	1.0000	1.0000	1.0000	1.0000	1.0000	1.0000	0.9998	13	50
50	38	1.0000	1.0000	1.0000	1.0000	1.0000	1.0000	1.0000	1.0000	1.0000	12	50
50	39	1.0000	1.0000	1.0000	1.0000	1.0000	1.0000	1.0000	1.0000	1.0000	11	50
50	40	1.0000	1.0000	1.0000	1.0000	1.0000	1.0000	1.0000	1.0000	1.0000	10	50
50	41	1.0000	1.0000	1.0000	1.0000	1.0000	1.0000	1.0000	1.0000	1.0000	9	50
50	42	1.0000	1.0000	1.0000	1.0000	1.0000	1.0000	1.0000	1.0000	1.0000	8	50
50	43	1.0000	1.0000	1.0000	1.0000	1.0000	1.0000	1.0000	1.0000	1.0000	7	50
50	44	1.0000	1.0000	1.0000	1.0000	1.0000	1.0000	1.0000	1.0000	1.0000	6	50
50	45	1.0000	1.0000	1.0000	1.0000	1.0000	1.0000	1.0000	1.0000	1.0000	5	50
50	46	1.0000	1.0000	1.0000	1.0000	1.0000	1.0000	1.0000	1.0000	1.0000	4	50
50	47	1.0000	1.0000	1.0000	1.0000	1.0000	1.0000	1.0000	1.0000	1.0000	3	50
50	48	1.0000	1.0000	1.0000	1.0000	1.0000	1.0000	1.0000	1.0000	1.0000	2	50
50	49	1.0000	1.0000	1.0000	1.0000	1.0000	1.0000	1.0000	1.0000	1.0000	1	50
50	50	1.0000	1.0000	1.0000	1.0000	1.0000	1.0000	1.0000	1.0000	1.0000	0	50
		0.8750	0.8500	0.8000	0.7500	0.7000	0.6500	0.6000	0.5500	0.5000	*x*	*n*
		p										

IV

The Normal Distribution Function

TABLES

Table IV.1 Short Table of the Percentiles, z, of the Cumulative Distribution Function $[P(Z \leq z)]$ for the Standard Normal Random Variable with Mean Zero and Variance One

$P[Z \leq z]$	z	$P[Z \leq z]$	z
0.0010	−3.0902	0.510	0.0251
0.0025	−2.8070	0.520	0.0502
0.0050	−2.5758	0.530	0.0753
0.0075	−2.4324	0.540	0.1004
0.010	−2.3263	0.550	0.1257
0.020	−2.0537	0.560	0.1510
0.030	−1.8808	0.570	0.1764
0.040	−1.7507	0.580	0.2019
0.050	−1.6449	0.590	0.2275
0.060	−1.5548	0.600	0.2533
0.070	−1.4758	0.610	0.2793
0.080	−1.4051	0.620	0.3055
0.090	−1.3408	0.630	0.3319
0.100	−1.2816	0.640	0.3585
0.110	−1.2265	0.650	0.3853
0.120	−1.1750	0.660	0.4125
0.130	−1.1264	0.670	0.4399
0.140	−1.0803	0.680	0.4677
0.150	−1.0364	0.690	0.4959
0.160	−0.9945	0.700	0.5244
0.170	−0.9542	0.710	0.5534
0.180	−0.9154	0.720	0.5828
0.190	−0.8779	0.730	0.6128
0.200	−0.8416	0.740	0.6433
0.210	−0.8064	0.750	0.6745
0.220	−0.7722	0.760	0.7063
0.230	−0.7388	0.770	0.7388
0.240	−0.7063	0.780	0.7722
0.250	−0.6745	0.790	0.8064
0.260	−0.6433	0.800	0.8416
0.270	−0.6128	0.810	0.8779
0.280	−0.5828	0.820	0.9154
0.290	−0.5534	0.830	0.9542
0.300	−0.5244	0.840	0.9945
0.310	−0.4959	0.850	1.0364
0.320	−0.4677	0.860	1.0803
0.330	−0.4399	0.870	1.1264
0.340	−0.4125	0.880	1.1750
0.350	−0.3853	0.890	1.2265
0.360	−0.3585	0.900	1.2816
0.370	−0.3319	0.910	1.3408
0.380	−0.3055	0.920	1.4051
0.390	−0.2793	0.930	1.4758
0.400	−0.2533	0.940	1.5548
0.410	−0.2275	0.950	1.6449
0.420	−0.2019	0.960	1.7507
0.430	−0.1764	0.970	1.8808
0.440	−0.1510	0.980	2.0537
0.450	−0.1257	0.990	2.3263
0.460	−0.1004	0.9925	2.4324
0.470	−0.0753	0.9950	2.5758
0.480	−0.0502	0.9975	2.8070
0.490	−0.0251	0.9990	3.0902
0.500	0.0000		

For example, the 28th percentile, z, at which $P[Z \leq z] = 0.28$ is $z = -0.5828$.

Table IV.2 Short Table of the Cumulative Distribution Function [$P(Z \leq z)$ for z between -3.00 and 3.00] for the Standard Normal Random Variable with Mean Zero and Variance One.

z	$P[Z \leq z]$	z	$P[Z \leq z]$
−3.00	0.0013500	0.05	0.5199389
−2.90	0.0018659	0.10	0.5398279
−2.80	0.0025552	0.15	0.5596177
−2.70	0.0034670	0.20	0.5792597
−2.60	0.0046612	0.25	0.5987063
−2.50	0.0062097	0.30	0.6179114
−2.40	0.0081975	0.35	0.6368306
−2.30	0.0107241	0.40	0.6554217
−2.20	0.0139034	0.45	0.6736448
−2.10	0.0178644	0.50	0.6914625
−2.00	0.0227501	0.55	0.7088403
−1.95	0.0255880	0.60	0.7257469
−1.90	0.0287165	0.65	0.7421540
−1.85	0.0321567	0.70	0.7580364
−1.80	0.0359303	0.75	0.7733727
−1.75	0.0400591	0.80	0.7881447
−1.70	0.0445654	0.85	0.8023375
−1.65	0.0494715	0.90	0.8159399
−1.60	0.0547993	0.95	0.8289439
−1.55	0.0605708	1.00	0.8413447
−1.50	0.0668072	1.05	0.8531409
−1.45	0.0735293	1.10	0.8643339
−1.40	0.0807567	1.15	0.8749280
−1.35	0.0885081	1.20	0.8849303
−1.30	0.0968006	1.25	0.8943502
−1.25	0.1056498	1.30	0.9031995
−1.20	0.1150697	1.35	0.9114920
−1.15	0.1250720	1.40	0.9192433
−1.10	0.1356661	1.45	0.9264707
−1.05	0.1468591	1.50	0.9331928
−1.00	0.1586553	1.55	0.9394292
−0.95	0.1710561	1.60	0.9452007
−0.90	0.1840601	1.65	0.9505286
−0.85	0.1976625	1.70	0.9554346
−0.80	0.2118553	1.75	0.9599409
−0.75	0.2266273	1.80	0.9640697
−0.70	0.2419636	1.85	0.9678433
−0.65	0.2578461	1.90	0.9712835
−0.60	0.2742531	1.95	0.9744120
−0.55	0.2911597	2.00	0.9772499
−0.50	0.3085376	2.10	0.9821356
−0.45	0.3263553	2.20	0.9860966
−0.40	0.3445783	2.30	0.9892759
−0.35	0.3631694	2.40	0.9918025
−0.30	0.3820887	2.50	0.9937903
−0.25	0.4012938	2.60	0.9953388
−0.20	0.4207403	2.70	0.9965330
−0.15	0.4403823	2.80	0.9974448
−0.10	0.4601721	2.90	0.9981341
−0.05	0.4800612	3.00	0.9986500
0.00	0.5000000		

For example, the standard normal cumulative distribution function evaluated at $z = 1.25$ is $P[Z \leq 1.25] = 0.8943502$.

Table IV.3 The Percentiles, z, of the Cumulative Distribution Function $[P(Z \leq z)]$ for the Standard Normal Random Variable with Mean Zero and Variance One.

$P[Z \leq z]$	z	$P[Z \leq z]$	z	$P[Z \leq z]$	z	$P[Z \leq z]$	z
		0.055	−1.5982	0.110	−1.2265	0.165	−0.9741
0.001	−3.0902	0.056	−1.5893	0.111	−1.2212	0.166	−0.9701
0.002	−2.8782	0.057	−1.5805	0.112	−1.2160	0.167	−0.9661
0.003	−2.7478	0.058	−1.5718	0.113	−1.2107	0.168	−0.9621
0.004	−2.6521	0.059	−1.5632	0.114	−1.2055	0.169	−0.9581
0.005	−2.5758	0.060	−1.5548	0.115	−1.2004	0.170	−0.9542
0.006	−2.5121	0.061	−1.5464	0.116	−1.1952	0.171	−0.9502
0.007	−2.4573	0.062	−1.5382	0.117	−1.1901	0.172	−0.9463
0.008	−2.4089	0.063	−1.5301	0.118	−1.1850	0.173	−0.9424
0.009	−2.3656	0.064	−1.5220	0.119	−1.1800	0.174	−0.9385
0.010	−2.3263	0.065	−1.5141	0.120	−1.1750	0.175	−0.9346
0.011	−2.2904	0.066	−1.5063	0.121	−1.1700	0.176	−0.9307
0.012	−2.2571	0.067	−1.4985	0.122	−1.1650	0.177	−0.9269
0.013	−2.2262	0.068	−1.4909	0.123	−1.1601	0.178	−0.9230
0.014	−2.1973	0.069	−1.4833	0.124	−1.1552	0.179	−0.9192
0.015	−2.1701	0.070	−1.4758	0.125	−1.1503	0.180	−0.9154
0.016	−2.1444	0.071	−1.4684	0.126	−1.1455	0.181	−0.9116
0.017	−2.1201	0.072	−1.4611	0.127	−1.1407	0.182	−0.9078
0.018	−2.0969	0.073	−1.4538	0.128	−1.1359	0.183	−0.9040
0.019	−2.0749	0.074	−1.4466	0.129	−1.1311	0.184	−0.9002
0.020	−2.0537	0.075	−1.4395	0.130	−1.1264	0.185	−0.8965
0.021	−2.0335	0.076	−1.4325	0.131	−1.1217	0.186	−0.8927
0.022	−2.0141	0.077	−1.4255	0.132	−1.1170	0.187	−0.8890
0.023	−1.9954	0.078	−1.4187	0.133	−1.1123	0.188	−0.8853
0.024	−1.9774	0.079	−1.4118	0.134	−1.1077	0.189	−0.8816
0.025	−1.9600	0.080	−1.4051	0.135	−1.1031	0.190	−0.8779
0.026	−1.9431	0.081	−1.3984	0.136	−1.0985	0.191	−0.8742
0.027	−1.9268	0.082	−1.3917	0.137	−1.0939	0.192	−0.8705
0.028	−1.9110	0.083	−1.3852	0.138	−1.0893	0.193	−0.8669
0.029	−1.8957	0.084	−1.3787	0.139	−1.0848	0.194	−0.8633
0.030	−1.8808	0.085	−1.3722	0.140	−1.0803	0.195	−0.8596
0.031	−1.8663	0.086	−1.3658	0.141	−1.0758	0.196	−0.8560
0.032	−1.8522	0.087	−1.3595	0.142	−1.0714	0.197	−0.8524
0.033	−1.8384	0.088	−1.3532	0.143	−1.0669	0.198	−0.8488
0.034	−1.8250	0.089	−1.3469	0.144	−1.0625	0.199	−0.8452
0.035	−1.8119	0.090	−1.3408	0.145	−1.0581	0.200	−0.8416
0.036	−1.7991	0.091	−1.3346	0.146	−1.0537	0.201	−0.8381
0.037	−1.7866	0.092	−1.3285	0.147	−1.0494	0.202	−0.8345
0.038	−1.7744	0.093	−1.3225	0.148	−1.0450	0.203	−0.8310
0.039	−1.7624	0.094	−1.3165	0.149	−1.0407	0.204	−0.8274
0.040	−1.7507	0.095	−1.3106	0.150	−1.0364	0.205	−0.8239
0.041	−1.7392	0.096	−1.3047	0.151	−1.0322	0.206	−0.8204
0.042	−1.7279	0.097	−1.2988	0.152	−1.0279	0.207	−0.8169
0.043	−1.7169	0.098	−1.2930	0.153	−1.0237	0.208	−0.8134
0.044	−1.7060	0.099	−1.2873	0.154	−1.0194	0.209	−0.8099
0.045	−1.6954	0.100	−1.2816	0.155	−1.0152	0.210	−0.8064
0.046	−1.6849	0.101	−1.2759	0.156	−1.0110	0.211	−0.8030
0.047	−1.6747	0.102	−1.2702	0.157	−1.0069	0.212	−0.7995
0.048	−1.6646	0.103	−1.2646	0.158	−1.0027	0.213	−0.7961
0.049	−1.6546	0.104	−1.2591	0.159	−0.9986	0.214	−0.7926
0.050	−1.6449	0.105	−1.2536	0.160	−0.9945	0.215	−0.7892
0.051	−1.6352	0.106	−1.2481	0.161	−0.9904	0.216	−0.7858
0.052	−1.6258	0.107	−1.2426	0.162	−0.9863	0.217	−0.7824
0.053	−1.6164	0.108	−1.2372	0.163	−0.9822	0.218	−0.7790
0.054	−1.6072	0.109	−1.2319	0.164	−0.9782	0.219	−0.7756

For example, the 0.1th percentile, z, at which $P[Z \leq z] = 0.001$ is $z = -3.0902$.

Table IV.3 (cont'd) The Percentiles, z, of the Cumulative Distribution Function [$P(Z \leq z)$] for the Standard Normal Random Variable with Mean Zero and Variance One.

$P[Z \leq z]$	z	$P[Z \leq z]$	z	$P[Z \leq z]$	z	$P[Z \leq z]$	z
0.220	−0.7722	0.275	−0.5978	0.330	−0.4399	0.385	−0.2924
0.221	−0.7688	0.276	−0.5948	0.331	−0.4372	0.386	−0.2898
0.222	−0.7655	0.277	−0.5918	0.332	−0.4344	0.387	−0.2871
0.223	−0.7621	0.278	−0.5888	0.333	−0.4316	0.388	−0.2845
0.224	−0.7588	0.279	−0.5858	0.334	−0.4289	0.389	−0.2819
0.225	−0.7554	0.280	−0.5828	0.335	−0.4261	0.390	−0.2793
0.226	−0.7521	0.281	−0.5799	0.336	−0.4234	0.391	−0.2767
0.227	−0.7488	0.282	−0.5769	0.337	−0.4207	0.392	−0.2741
0.228	−0.7454	0.283	−0.5740	0.338	−0.4179	0.393	−0.2715
0.229	−0.7421	0.284	−0.5710	0.339	−0.4152	0.394	−0.2689
0.230	−0.7388	0.285	−0.5681	0.340	−0.4125	0.395	−0.2663
0.231	−0.7356	0.286	−0.5651	0.341	−0.4097	0.396	−0.2637
0.232	−0.7323	0.287	−0.5622	0.342	−0.4070	0.397	−0.2611
0.233	−0.7290	0.288	−0.5592	0.343	−0.4043	0.398	−0.2585
0.234	−0.7257	0.289	−0.5563	0.344	−0.4016	0.399	−0.2559
0.235	−0.7225	0.290	−0.5534	0.345	−0.3989	0.400	−0.2533
0.236	−0.7192	0.291	−0.5505	0.346	−0.3961	0.401	−0.2508
0.237	−0.7160	0.292	−0.5476	0.347	−0.3934	0.402	−0.2482
0.238	−0.7128	0.293	−0.5446	0.348	−0.3907	0.403	−0.2456
0.239	−0.7095	0.294	−0.5417	0.349	−0.3880	0.404	−0.2430
0.240	−0.7063	0.295	−0.5388	0.350	−0.3853	0.405	−0.2404
0.241	−0.7031	0.296	−0.5359	0.351	−0.3826	0.406	−0.2378
0.242	−0.6999	0.297	−0.5330	0.352	−0.3799	0.407	−0.2353
0.243	−0.6967	0.298	−0.5302	0.353	−0.3772	0.408	−0.2327
0.244	−0.6935	0.299	−0.5273	0.354	−0.3745	0.409	−0.2301
0.245	−0.6903	0.300	−0.5244	0.355	−0.3719	0.410	−0.2275
0.246	−0.6871	0.301	−0.5215	0.356	−0.3692	0.411	−0.2250
0.247	−0.6840	0.302	−0.5187	0.357	−0.3665	0.412	−0.2224
0.248	−0.6808	0.303	−0.5158	0.358	−0.3638	0.413	−0.2198
0.249	−0.6776	0.304	−0.5129	0.359	−0.3611	0.414	−0.2173
0.250	−0.6745	0.305	−0.5101	0.360	−0.3585	0.415	−0.2147
0.251	−0.6713	0.306	−0.5072	0.361	−0.3558	0.416	−0.2121
0.252	−0.6682	0.307	−0.5044	0.362	−0.3531	0.417	−0.2096
0.253	−0.6651	0.308	−0.5015	0.363	−0.3505	0.418	−0.2070
0.254	−0.6620	0.309	−0.4987	0.364	−0.3478	0.419	−0.2045
0.255	−0.6588	0.310	−0.4959	0.365	−0.3451	0.420	−0.2019
0.256	−0.6557	0.311	−0.4930	0.366	−0.3425	0.421	−0.1993
0.257	−0.6526	0.312	−0.4902	0.367	−0.3398	0.422	−0.1968
0.258	−0.6495	0.313	−0.4874	0.368	−0.3372	0.423	−0.1942
0.259	−0.6464	0.314	−0.4845	0.369	−0.3345	0.424	−0.1917
0.260	−0.6433	0.315	−0.4817	0.370	−0.3319	0.425	−0.1891
0.261	−0.6403	0.316	−0.4789	0.371	−0.3292	0.426	−0.1866
0.262	−0.6372	0.317	−0.4761	0.372	−0.3266	0.427	−0.1840
0.263	−0.6341	0.318	−0.4733	0.373	−0.3239	0.428	−0.1815
0.264	−0.6311	0.319	−0.4705	0.374	−0.3213	0.429	−0.1789
0.265	−0.6280	0.320	−0.4677	0.375	−0.3186	0.430	−0.1764
0.266	−0.6250	0.321	−0.4649	0.376	−0.3160	0.431	−0.1738
0.267	−0.6219	0.322	−0.4621	0.377	−0.3134	0.432	−0.1713
0.268	−0.6189	0.323	−0.4593	0.378	−0.3107	0.433	−0.1687
0.269	−0.6158	0.324	−0.4565	0.379	−0.3081	0.434	−0.1662
0.270	−0.6128	0.325	−0.4538	0.380	−0.3055	0.435	−0.1637
0.271	−0.6098	0.326	−0.4510	0.381	−0.3029	0.436	−0.1611
0.272	−0.6068	0.327	−0.4482	0.382	−0.3002	0.437	−0.1586
0.273	−0.6038	0.328	−0.4454	0.383	−0.2976	0.438	−0.1560
0.274	−0.6008	0.329	−0.4427	0.384	−0.2950	0.439	−0.1535

Table IV.3 (cont'd) The Percentiles, z, of the Cumulative Distribution Function $[P(Z \leq z)]$ for the Standard Normal Random Variable with Mean Zero and Variance One.

$P[Z \leq z]$	z	$P[Z \leq z]$	z	$P[Z \leq z]$	z	$P[Z \leq z]$	z
0.440	−0.1510	0.495	−0.0125	0.550	0.1257	0.605	0.2663
0.441	−0.1484	0.496	−0.0100	0.551	0.1282	0.606	0.2689
0.442	−0.1459	0.497	−0.0075	0.552	0.1307	0.607	0.2715
0.443	−0.1434	0.498	−0.0050	0.553	0.1332	0.608	0.2741
0.444	−0.1408	0.499	−0.0025	0.554	0.1358	0.609	0.2767
0.445	−0.1383	0.500	0.0000	0.555	0.1383	0.610	0.2793
0.446	−0.1358	0.501	0.0025	0.556	0.1408	0.611	0.2819
0.447	−0.1332	0.502	0.0050	0.557	0.1434	0.612	0.2845
0.448	−0.1307	0.503	0.0075	0.558	0.1459	0.613	0.2871
0.449	−0.1282	0.504	0.0100	0.559	0.1484	0.614	0.2898
0.450	−0.1257	0.505	0.0125	0.560	0.1510	0.615	0.2924
0.451	−0.1231	0.506	0.0150	0.561	0.1535	0.616	0.2950
0.452	−0.1206	0.507	0.0175	0.562	0.1560	0.617	0.2976
0.453	−0.1181	0.508	0.0201	0.563	0.1586	0.618	0.3002
0.454	−0.1156	0.509	0.0226	0.564	0.1611	0.619	0.3029
0.455	−0.1130	0.510	0.0251	0.565	0.1637	0.620	0.3055
0.456	−0.1105	0.511	0.0276	0.566	0.1662	0.621	0.3081
0.457	−0.1080	0.512	0.0301	0.567	0.1687	0.622	0.3107
0.458	−0.1055	0.513	0.0326	0.568	0.1713	0.623	0.3134
0.459	−0.1030	0.514	0.0351	0.569	0.1738	0.624	0.3160
0.460	−0.1004	0.515	0.0376	0.570	0.1764	0.625	0.3186
0.461	−0.0979	0.516	0.0401	0.571	0.1789	0.626	0.3213
0.462	−0.0954	0.517	0.0426	0.572	0.1815	0.627	0.3239
0.463	−0.0929	0.518	0.0451	0.573	0.1840	0.628	0.3266
0.464	−0.0904	0.519	0.0476	0.574	0.1866	0.629	0.3292
0.465	−0.0878	0.520	0.0502	0.575	0.1891	0.630	0.3319
0.466	−0.0853	0.521	0.0527	0.576	0.1917	0.631	0.3345
0.467	−0.0828	0.522	0.0552	0.577	0.1942	0.632	0.3372
0.468	−0.0803	0.523	0.0577	0.578	0.1968	0.633	0.3398
0.469	−0.0778	0.524	0.0602	0.579	0.1993	0.634	0.3425
0.470	−0.0753	0.525	0.0627	0.580	0.2019	0.635	0.3451
0.471	−0.0728	0.526	0.0652	0.581	0.2045	0.636	0.3478
0.472	−0.0702	0.527	0.0677	0.582	0.2070	0.637	0.3505
0.473	−0.0677	0.528	0.0702	0.583	0.2096	0.638	0.3531
0.474	−0.0652	0.529	0.0728	0.584	0.2121	0.639	0.3558
0.475	−0.0627	0.530	0.0753	0.585	0.2147	0.640	0.3585
0.476	−0.0602	0.531	0.0778	0.586	0.2173	0.641	0.3611
0.477	−0.0577	0.532	0.0803	0.587	0.2198	0.642	0.3638
0.478	−0.0552	0.533	0.0828	0.588	0.2224	0.643	0.3665
0.479	−0.0527	0.534	0.0853	0.589	0.2250	0.644	0.3692
0.480	−0.0502	0.535	0.0878	0.590	0.2275	0.645	0.3719
0.481	−0.0476	0.536	0.0904	0.591	0.2301	0.646	0.3745
0.482	−0.0451	0.537	0.0929	0.592	0.2327	0.647	0.3772
0.483	−0.0426	0.538	0.0954	0.593	0.2353	0.648	0.3799
0.484	−0.0401	0.539	0.0979	0.594	0.2378	0.649	0.3826
0.485	−0.0376	0.540	0.1004	0.595	0.2404	0.650	0.3853
0.486	−0.0351	0.541	0.1030	0.596	0.2430	0.651	0.3880
0.487	−0.0326	0.542	0.1055	0.597	0.2456	0.652	0.3907
0.488	−0.0301	0.543	0.1080	0.598	0.2482	0.653	0.3934
0.489	−0.0276	0.544	0.1105	0.599	0.2508	0.654	0.3961
0.490	−0.0251	0.545	0.1130	0.600	0.2533	0.655	0.3989
0.491	−0.0226	0.546	0.1156	0.601	0.2559	0.656	0.4016
0.492	−0.0201	0.547	0.1181	0.602	0.2585	0.657	0.4043
0.493	−0.0175	0.548	0.1206	0.603	0.2611	0.658	0.4070
0.494	−0.0150	0.549	0.1231	0.604	0.2637	0.659	0.4097

Table IV.3 (cont'd) The Percentiles, z, of the Cumulative Distribution Function $[P(Z \leq z)]$ for the Standard Normal Random Variable with Mean Zero and Variance One.

$P[Z \leq z]$	z	$P[Z \leq z]$	z	$P[Z \leq z]$	z	$P[Z \leq z]$	z
0.660	0.4125	0.715	0.5681	0.770	0.7388	0.825	0.9346
0.661	0.4152	0.716	0.5710	0.771	0.7421	0.826	0.9385
0.662	0.4179	0.717	0.5740	0.772	0.7454	0.827	0.9424
0.663	0.4207	0.718	0.5769	0.773	0.7488	0.828	0.9463
0.664	0.4234	0.719	0.5799	0.774	0.7521	0.829	0.9502
0.665	0.4261	0.720	0.5828	0.775	0.7554	0.830	0.9542
0.666	0.4289	0.721	0.5858	0.776	0.7588	0.831	0.9581
0.667	0.4316	0.722	0.5888	0.777	0.7621	0.832	0.9621
0.668	0.4344	0.723	0.5918	0.778	0.7655	0.833	0.9661
0.669	0.4372	0.724	0.5948	0.779	0.7688	0.834	0.9701
0.670	0.4399	0.725	0.5978	0.780	0.7722	0.835	0.9741
0.671	0.4427	0.726	0.6008	0.781	0.7756	0.836	0.9782
0.672	0.4454	0.727	0.6038	0.782	0.7790	0.837	0.9822
0.673	0.4482	0.728	0.6068	0.783	0.7824	0.838	0.9863
0.674	0.4510	0.729	0.6098	0.784	0.7858	0.839	0.9904
0.675	0.4538	0.730	0.6128	0.785	0.7892	0.840	0.9945
0.676	0.4565	0.731	0.6158	0.786	0.7926	0.841	0.9986
0.677	0.4593	0.732	0.6189	0.787	0.7961	0.842	1.0027
0.678	0.4621	0.733	0.6219	0.788	0.7995	0.843	1.0069
0.679	0.4649	0.734	0.6250	0.789	0.8030	0.844	1.0110
0.680	0.4677	0.735	0.6280	0.790	0.8064	0.845	1.0152
0.681	0.4705	0.736	0.6311	0.791	0.8099	0.846	1.0194
0.682	0.4733	0.737	0.6341	0.792	0.8134	0.847	1.0237
0.683	0.4761	0.738	0.6372	0.793	0.8169	0.848	1.0279
0.684	0.4789	0.739	0.6403	0.794	0.8204	0.849	1.0322
0.685	0.4817	0.740	0.6433	0.795	0.8239	0.850	1.0364
0.686	0.4845	0.741	0.6464	0.796	0.8274	0.851	1.0407
0.687	0.4874	0.742	0.6495	0.797	0.8310	0.852	1.0450
0.688	0.4902	0.743	0.6526	0.798	0.8345	0.853	1.0494
0.689	0.4930	0.744	0.6557	0.799	0.8381	0.854	1.0537
0.690	0.4959	0.745	0.6588	0.800	0.8416	0.855	1.0581
0.691	0.4987	0.746	0.6620	0.801	0.8452	0.856	1.0625
0.692	0.5015	0.747	0.6651	0.802	0.8488	0.857	1.0669
0.693	0.5044	0.748	0.6682	0.803	0.8524	0.858	1.0714
0.694	0.5072	0.749	0.6713	0.804	0.8560	0.859	1.0758
0.695	0.5101	0.750	0.6745	0.805	0.8596	0.860	1.0803
0.696	0.5129	0.751	0.6776	0.806	0.8633	0.861	1.0848
0.697	0.5158	0.752	0.6808	0.807	0.8669	0.862	1.0893
0.698	0.5187	0.753	0.6840	0.808	0.8705	0.863	1.0939
0.699	0.5215	0.754	0.6871	0.809	0.8742	0.864	1.0985
0.700	0.5244	0.755	0.6903	0.810	0.8779	0.865	1.1031
0.701	0.5273	0.756	0.6935	0.811	0.8816	0.866	1.1077
0.702	0.5302	0.757	0.6967	0.812	0.8853	0.867	1.1123
0.703	0.5330	0.758	0.6999	0.813	0.8890	0.868	1.1170
0.704	0.5359	0.759	0.7031	0.814	0.8927	0.869	1.1217
0.705	0.5388	0.760	0.7063	0.815	0.8965	0.870	1.1264
0.706	0.5417	0.761	0.7095	0.816	0.9002	0.871	1.1311
0.707	0.5446	0.762	0.7128	0.817	0.9040	0.872	1.1359
0.708	0.5476	0.763	0.7160	0.818	0.9078	0.873	1.1407
0.709	0.5505	0.764	0.7192	0.819	0.9116	0.874	1.1455
0.710	0.5534	0.765	0.7225	0.820	0.9154	0.875	1.1503
0.711	0.5563	0.766	0.7257	0.821	0.9192	0.876	1.1552
0.712	0.5592	0.767	0.7290	0.822	0.9230	0.877	1.1601
0.713	0.5622	0.768	0.7323	0.823	0.9269	0.878	1.1650
0.714	0.5651	0.769	0.7356	0.824	0.9307	0.879	1.1700

Table IV.3 (cont'd) The Percentiles, z, of the Cumulative Distribution Function $[P(Z \leq z)]$ for the Standard Normal Random Variable with Mean Zero and Variance One.

$P[Z \leq z]$	z	$P[Z \leq z]$	z	$P[Z \leq z]$	z	$P[Z \leq z]$	z
0.880	1.1750	0.910	1.3408	0.940	1.5548	0.970	1.8808
0.881	1.1800	0.911	1.3469	0.941	1.5632	0.971	1.8957
0.882	1.1850	0.912	1.3532	0.942	1.5718	0.972	1.9110
0.883	1.1901	0.913	1.3595	0.943	1.5805	0.973	1.9268
0.884	1.1952	0.914	1.3658	0.944	1.5893	0.974	1.9431
0.885	1.2004	0.915	1.3722	0.945	1.5982	0.975	1.9600
0.886	1.2055	0.916	1.3787	0.946	1.6072	0.976	1.9774
0.887	1.2107	0.917	1.3852	0.947	1.6164	0.977	1.9954
0.888	1.2160	0.918	1.3917	0.948	1.6258	0.978	2.0141
0.889	1.2212	0.919	1.3984	0.949	1.6352	0.979	2.0335
0.890	1.2265	0.920	1.4051	0.950	1.6449	0.980	2.0537
0.891	1.2319	0.921	1.4118	0.951	1.6546	0.981	2.0749
0.892	1.2372	0.922	1.4187	0.952	1.6646	0.982	2.0969
0.893	1.2426	0.923	1.4255	0.953	1.6747	0.983	2.1201
0.894	1.2481	0.924	1.4325	0.954	1.6849	0.984	2.1444
0.895	1.2536	0.925	1.4395	0.955	1.6954	0.985	2.1701
0.896	1.2591	0.926	1.4466	0.956	1.7060	0.986	2.1973
0.897	1.2646	0.927	1.4538	0.957	1.7169	0.987	2.2262
0.898	1.2702	0.928	1.4611	0.958	1.7279	0.988	2.2571
0.899	1.2759	0.929	1.4684	0.959	1.7392	0.989	2.2904
0.900	1.2816	0.930	1.4758	0.960	1.7507	0.990	2.3263
0.901	1.2873	0.931	1.4833	0.961	1.7624	0.991	2.3656
0.902	1.2930	0.932	1.4909	0.962	1.7744	0.992	2.4089
0.903	1.2988	0.933	1.4985	0.963	1.7866	0.993	2.4573
0.904	1.3047	0.934	1.5063	0.964	1.7991	0.994	2.5121
0.905	1.3106	0.935	1.5141	0.965	1.8119	0.995	2.5758
0.906	1.3165	0.936	1.5220	0.966	1.8250	0.996	2.6521
0.907	1.3225	0.937	1.5301	0.967	1.8384	0.997	2.7478
0.908	1.3285	0.938	1.5382	0.968	1.8522	0.998	2.8782
0.909	1.3346	0.939	1.5464	0.969	1.8663	0.999	3.0902
0.910	1.3408	0.940	1.5548	0.970	1.8808		

Table IV.4 The Cumulative Distribution Function [$P(Z \leq z)$ for z between −5.00 and 5.00] for the Standard Normal Random Variable with Mean Zero and Variance One.

z	$P[Z \leq z]$	z	$P[Z \leq z]$	z	$P[Z \leq z]$	z	$P[Z \leq z]$
−5.00	0.0000003	−4.45	0.0000043	−3.90	0.0000481	−3.35	0.0004041
−4.99	0.0000003	−4.44	0.0000045	−3.89	0.0000501	−3.34	0.0004189
−4.98	0.0000003	−4.43	0.0000047	−3.88	0.0000522	−3.33	0.0004343
−4.97	0.0000003	−4.42	0.0000049	−3.87	0.0000544	−3.32	0.0004501
−4.96	0.0000004	−4.41	0.0000052	−3.86	0.0000567	−3.31	0.0004665
−4.95	0.0000004	−4.40	0.0000054	−3.85	0.0000591	−3.30	0.0004835
−4.94	0.0000004	−4.39	0.0000057	−3.84	0.0000615	−3.29	0.0005010
−4.93	0.0000004	−4.38	0.0000059	−3.83	0.0000641	−3.28	0.0005191
−4.92	0.0000004	−4.37	0.0000062	−3.82	0.0000667	−3.27	0.0005378
−4.91	0.0000005	−4.36	0.0000065	−3.81	0.0000695	−3.26	0.0005571
−4.90	0.0000005	−4.35	0.0000068	−3.80	0.0000724	−3.25	0.0005771
−4.89	0.0000005	−4.34	0.0000071	−3.79	0.0000753	−3.24	0.0005977
−4.88	0.0000005	−4.33	0.0000075	−3.78	0.0000784	−3.23	0.0006190
−4.87	0.0000006	−4.32	0.0000078	−3.77	0.0000816	−3.22	0.0006410
−4.86	0.0000006	−4.31	0.0000082	−3.76	0.0000850	−3.21	0.0006637
−4.85	0.0000006	−4.30	0.0000085	−3.75	0.0000884	−3.20	0.0006872
−4.84	0.0000007	−4.29	0.0000089	−3.74	0.0000920	−3.19	0.0007114
−4.83	0.0000007	−4.28	0.0000094	−3.73	0.0000958	−3.18	0.0007364
−4.82	0.0000007	−4.27	0.0000098	−3.72	0.0000996	−3.17	0.0007623
−4.81	0.0000008	−4.26	0.0000102	−3.71	0.0001037	−3.16	0.0007889
−4.80	0.0000008	−4.25	0.0000107	−3.70	0.0001078	−3.15	0.0008164
−4.79	0.0000008	−4.24	0.0000112	−3.69	0.0001122	−3.14	0.0008448
−4.78	0.0000009	−4.23	0.0000117	−3.68	0.0001166	−3.13	0.0008741
−4.77	0.0000009	−4.22	0.0000122	−3.67	0.0001213	−3.12	0.0009043
−4.76	0.0000010	−4.21	0.0000128	−3.66	0.0001261	−3.11	0.0009355
−4.75	0.0000010	−4.20	0.0000134	−3.65	0.0001312	−3.10	0.0009677
−4.74	0.0000011	−4.19	0.0000140	−3.64	0.0001364	−3.09	0.0010008
−4.73	0.0000011	−4.18	0.0000146	−3.63	0.0001417	−3.08	0.0010351
−4.72	0.0000012	−4.17	0.0000152	−3.62	0.0001473	−3.07	0.0010704
−4.71	0.0000012	−4.16	0.0000159	−3.61	0.0001531	−3.06	0.0011068
−4.70	0.0000013	−4.15	0.0000166	−3.60	0.0001591	−3.05	0.0011443
−4.69	0.0000014	−4.14	0.0000174	−3.59	0.0001654	−3.04	0.0011830
−4.68	0.0000014	−4.13	0.0000181	−3.58	0.0001718	−3.03	0.0012228
−4.67	0.0000015	−4.12	0.0000190	−3.57	0.0001785	−3.02	0.0012639
−4.66	0.0000016	−4.11	0.0000198	−3.56	0.0001855	−3.01	0.0013063
−4.65	0.0000017	−4.10	0.0000207	−3.55	0.0001927	−3.00	0.0013500
−4.64	0.0000017	−4.09	0.0000216	−3.54	0.0002001	−2.99	0.0013950
−4.63	0.0000018	−4.08	0.0000225	−3.53	0.0002078	−2.98	0.0014413
−4.62	0.0000019	−4.07	0.0000235	−3.52	0.0002158	−2.97	0.0014891
−4.61	0.0000020	−4.06	0.0000245	−3.51	0.0002241	−2.96	0.0015383
−4.60	0.0000021	−4.05	0.0000256	−3.50	0.0002327	−2.95	0.0015889
−4.59	0.0000022	−4.04	0.0000267	−3.49	0.0002416	−2.94	0.0016411
−4.58	0.0000023	−4.03	0.0000279	−3.48	0.0002508	−2.93	0.0016949
−4.57	0.0000024	−4.02	0.0000291	−3.47	0.0002603	−2.92	0.0017502
−4.56	0.0000026	−4.01	0.0000304	−3.46	0.0002701	−2.91	0.0018072
−4.55	0.0000027	−4.00	0.0000317	−3.45	0.0002803	−2.90	0.0018659
−4.54	0.0000028	−3.99	0.0000331	−3.44	0.0002909	−2.89	0.0019263
−4.53	0.0000030	−3.98	0.0000345	−3.43	0.0003018	−2.88	0.0019884
−4.52	0.0000031	−3.97	0.0000360	−3.42	0.0003132	−2.87	0.0020524
−4.51	0.0000032	−3.96	0.0000375	−3.41	0.0003249	−2.86	0.0021183
−4.50	0.0000034	−3.95	0.0000391	−3.40	0.0003370	−2.85	0.0021860
−4.49	0.0000036	−3.94	0.0000408	−3.39	0.0003495	−2.84	0.0022557
−4.48	0.0000037	−3.93	0.0000425	−3.38	0.0003625	−2.83	0.0023275
−4.47	0.0000039	−3.92	0.0000443	−3.37	0.0003759	−2.82	0.0024012
−4.46	0.0000041	−3.91	0.0000462	−3.36	0.0003898	−2.81	0.0024771

Table IV.4 (cont'd) The Cumulative Distribution Function [$P(Z \leq z)$ for z between −5.00 and 5.00] for the Standard Normal Random Variable with Mean Zero and Variance One.

z	$P[Z \leq z]$	z	$P[Z \leq z]$	z	$P[Z \leq z]$	z	$P[Z \leq z]$
−2.80	0.0025552	−2.25	0.0122244	−1.70	0.0445654	−1.15	0.1250719
−2.79	0.0026355	−2.24	0.0125454	−1.69	0.0455139	−1.14	0.1271431
−2.78	0.0027180	−2.23	0.0128737	−1.68	0.0464786	−1.13	0.1292381
−2.77	0.0028029	−2.22	0.0132093	−1.67	0.0474596	−1.12	0.1313569
−2.76	0.0028901	−2.21	0.0135525	−1.66	0.0484572	−1.11	0.1334995
−2.75	0.0029798	−2.20	0.0139034	−1.65	0.0494714	−1.10	0.1356660
−2.74	0.0030720	−2.19	0.0142621	−1.64	0.0505025	−1.09	0.1378565
−2.73	0.0031668	−2.18	0.0146287	−1.63	0.0515507	−1.08	0.1400711
−2.72	0.0032641	−2.17	0.0150034	−1.62	0.0526161	−1.07	0.1423096
−2.71	0.0033642	−2.16	0.0153863	−1.61	0.0536989	−1.06	0.1445723
−2.70	0.0034670	−2.15	0.0157775	−1.60	0.0547993	−1.05	0.1468590
−2.69	0.0035726	−2.14	0.0161773	−1.59	0.0559174	−1.04	0.1491699
−2.68	0.0036812	−2.13	0.0165857	−1.58	0.0570534	−1.03	0.1515050
−2.67	0.0037926	−2.12	0.0170029	−1.57	0.0582075	−1.02	0.1538642
−2.66	0.0039071	−2.11	0.0174291	−1.56	0.0593799	−1.01	0.1562476
−2.65	0.0040246	−2.10	0.0178643	−1.55	0.0605707	−1.00	0.1586552
−2.64	0.0041453	−2.09	0.0183088	−1.54	0.0617802	−0.99	0.1610870
−2.63	0.0042693	−2.08	0.0187627	−1.53	0.0630083	−0.98	0.1635430
−2.62	0.0043965	−2.07	0.0192261	−1.52	0.0642555	−0.97	0.1660232
−2.61	0.0045271	−2.06	0.0196992	−1.51	0.0655217	−0.96	0.1685275
−2.60	0.0046612	−2.05	0.0201821	−1.50	0.0668072	−0.95	0.1710560
−2.59	0.0047988	−2.04	0.0206751	−1.49	0.0681121	−0.94	0.1736087
−2.58	0.0049400	−2.03	0.0211782	−1.48	0.0694366	−0.93	0.1761854
−2.57	0.0050850	−2.02	0.0216916	−1.47	0.0707809	−0.92	0.1787863
−2.56	0.0052336	−2.01	0.0222155	−1.46	0.0721450	−0.91	0.1814111
−2.55	0.0053862	−2.00	0.0227500	−1.45	0.0735293	−0.90	0.1840600
−2.54	0.0055426	−1.99	0.0232954	−1.44	0.0749337	−0.89	0.1867328
−2.53	0.0057031	−1.98	0.0238517	−1.43	0.0763585	−0.88	0.1894295
−2.52	0.0058678	−1.97	0.0244191	−1.42	0.0778038	−0.87	0.1921501
−2.51	0.0060366	−1.96	0.0249978	−1.41	0.0792698	−0.86	0.1948944
−2.50	0.0062097	−1.95	0.0255880	−1.40	0.0807567	−0.85	0.1976624
−2.49	0.0063872	−1.94	0.0261898	−1.39	0.0822644	−0.84	0.2004541
−2.48	0.0065691	−1.93	0.0268033	−1.38	0.0837933	−0.83	0.2032693
−2.47	0.0067557	−1.92	0.0274289	−1.37	0.0853435	−0.82	0.2061079
−2.46	0.0069469	−1.91	0.0280665	−1.36	0.0869150	−0.81	0.2089699
−2.45	0.0071428	−1.90	0.0287165	−1.35	0.0885080	−0.80	0.2118552
−2.44	0.0073436	−1.89	0.0293789	−1.34	0.0901227	−0.79	0.2147637
−2.43	0.0075494	−1.88	0.0300540	−1.33	0.0917591	−0.78	0.2176953
−2.42	0.0077602	−1.87	0.0307418	−1.32	0.0934175	−0.77	0.2206498
−2.41	0.0079762	−1.86	0.0314427	−1.31	0.0950979	−0.76	0.2236271
−2.40	0.0081975	−1.85	0.0321567	−1.30	0.0968005	−0.75	0.2266272
−2.39	0.0084242	−1.84	0.0328840	−1.29	0.0985253	−0.74	0.2296498
−2.38	0.0086563	−1.83	0.0336249	−1.28	.1002726	−0.73	0.2326949
−2.37	0.0088940	−1.82	0.0343794	−1.27	.1020423	−0.72	0.2357623
−2.36	0.0091374	−1.81	0.0351478	−1.26	.1038347	−0.71	0.2388519
−2.35	0.0093867	−1.80	0.0359302	−1.25	.1056498	−0.70	0.2419635
−2.34	0.0096418	−1.79	0.0367269	−1.24	.1074877	−0.69	0.2450969
−2.33	0.0099030	−1.78	0.0375379	−1.23	.1093486	−0.68	0.2482521
−2.32	0.0101704	−1.77	0.0383635	−1.22	.1112324	−0.67	0.2514287
−2.31	0.0104440	−1.76	0.0392038	−1.21	.1131395	−0.66	0.2546268
−2.30	0.0107241	−1.75	0.0400591	−1.20	.1150697	−0.65	0.2578459
−2.29	0.0110106	−1.74	0.0409294	−1.19	.1170232	−0.64	0.2610861
−2.28	0.0113038	−1.73	0.0418151	−1.18	.1190001	−0.63	0.2643471
−2.27	0.0116037	−1.72	0.0427162	−1.17	.1210005	−0.62	0.2676287
−2.26	0.0119106	−1.71	0.0436329	−1.16	.1230244	−0.61	0.2709308

Table IV.4 (cont'd) The Cumulative Distribution Function [$P(Z \leq z)$ for z between −5.00 and 5.00] for the Standard Normal Random Variable with Mean Zero and Variance One.

z	$P[Z \leq z]$	z	$P[Z \leq z]$	z	$P[Z \leq z]$	z	$P[Z \leq z]$
−0.60	0.2742530	−0.05	0.4800610	0.50	0.6914623	1.05	0.8531408
−0.59	0.2775952	−0.04	0.4840464	0.51	0.6949741	1.06	0.8554276
−0.58	0.2809572	−0.03	0.4880334	0.52	0.6984681	1.07	0.8576902
−0.57	0.2843387	−0.02	0.4920215	0.53	0.7019439	1.08	0.8599288
−0.56	0.2877396	−0.01	0.4960105	0.54	0.7054014	1.09	0.8621433
−0.55	0.2911596	0.00	0.5000000	0.55	0.7088402	1.10	0.8643338
−0.54	0.2945984	0.01	0.5039892	0.56	0.7122602	1.11	0.8665004
−0.53	0.2980558	0.02	0.5079782	0.57	0.7156611	1.12	0.8686430
−0.52	0.3015317	0.03	0.5119664	0.58	0.7190426	1.13	0.8707618
−0.51	0.3050256	0.04	0.5159533	0.59	0.7224046	1.14	0.8728567
−0.50	0.3085374	0.05	0.5199387	0.60	0.7257468	1.15	0.8749279
−0.49	0.3120668	0.06	0.5239221	0.61	0.7290690	1.16	0.8769755
−0.48	0.3156136	0.07	0.5279031	0.62	0.7323710	1.17	0.8789994
−0.47	0.3191774	0.08	0.5318813	0.63	0.7356526	1.18	0.8809998
−0.46	0.3227580	0.09	0.5358563	0.64	0.7389136	1.19	0.8829767
−0.45	0.3263551	0.10	0.5398277	0.65	0.7421538	1.20	0.8849302
−0.44	0.3299685	0.11	0.5437952	0.66	0.7453730	1.21	0.8868604
−0.43	0.3335977	0.12	0.5477583	0.67	0.7485711	1.22	0.8887674
−0.42	0.3372427	0.13	0.5517167	0.68	0.7517477	1.23	0.8906513
−0.41	0.3409029	0.14	0.5556699	0.69	0.7549029	1.24	0.8925122
−0.40	0.3445782	0.15	0.5596176	0.70	0.7580363	1.25	0.8943501
−0.39	0.3482682	0.16	0.5635593	0.71	0.7611479	1.26	0.8961652
−0.38	0.3519727	0.17	0.5674948	0.72	0.7642375	1.27	0.8979576
−0.37	0.3556912	0.18	0.5714236	0.73	0.7673049	1.28	0.8997273
−0.36	0.3594235	0.19	0.5753453	0.74	0.7703500	1.29	0.9014745
−0.35	0.3631693	0.20	0.5792595	0.75	0.7733726	1.30	0.9031994
−0.34	0.3669282	0.21	0.5831660	0.76	0.7763727	1.31	0.9049020
−0.33	0.3706999	0.22	0.5870642	0.77	0.7793500	1.32	0.9065824
−0.32	0.3744841	0.23	0.5909539	0.78	0.7823045	1.33	0.9082407
−0.31	0.3782804	0.24	0.5948347	0.79	0.7852361	1.34	0.9098772
−0.30	0.3820885	0.25	0.5987061	0.80	0.7881446	1.35	0.9114919
−0.29	0.3859081	0.26	0.6025679	0.81	0.7910299	1.36	0.9130849
−0.28	0.3897387	0.27	0.6064197	0.82	0.7938919	1.37	0.9146564
−0.27	0.3935801	0.28	0.6102610	0.83	0.7967306	1.38	0.9162066
−0.26	0.3974318	0.29	0.6140917	0.84	0.7995458	1.39	0.9177354
−0.25	0.4012936	0.30	0.6179112	0.85	0.8023374	1.40	0.9192432
−0.24	0.4051651	0.31	0.6217193	0.86	0.8051054	1.41	0.9207301
−0.23	0.4090458	0.32	0.6255156	0.87	0.8078497	1.42	0.9221961
−0.22	0.4129355	0.33	0.6292998	0.88	0.8105703	1.43	0.9236414
−0.21	0.4168338	0.34	0.6330715	0.89	0.8132670	1.44	0.9250662
−0.20	0.4207402	0.35	0.6368304	0.90	0.8159398	1.45	0.9264706
−0.19	0.4246545	0.36	0.6405762	0.91	0.8185887	1.46	0.9278549
−0.18	0.4285762	0.37	0.6443086	0.92	0.8212135	1.47	0.9292190
−0.17	0.4325050	0.38	0.6480271	0.93	0.8238144	1.48	0.9305633
−0.16	0.4364404	0.39	0.6517315	0.94	0.8263911	1.49	0.9318878
−0.15	0.4403822	0.40	0.6554216	0.95	0.8289438	1.50	0.9331927
−0.14	0.4443299	0.41	0.6590968	0.96	0.8314723	1.51	0.9344782
−0.13	0.4482831	0.42	0.6627571	0.97	0.8339767	1.52	0.9357444
−0.12	0.4522414	0.43	0.6664020	0.98	0.8364568	1.53	0.9369916
−0.11	0.4562045	0.44	0.6700313	0.99	0.8389128	1.54	0.9382198
−0.10	0.4601720	0.45	0.6736446	1.00	0.8413446	1.55	0.9394292
−0.09	0.4641434	0.46	0.6772417	1.01	0.8437523	1.56	0.9406200
−0.08	0.4681185	0.47	0.6808223	1.02	0.8461357	1.57	0.9417924
−0.07	0.4720967	0.48	0.6843862	1.03	0.8484949	1.58	0.9429465
−0.06	0.4760776	0.49	0.6879329	1.04	0.8508299	1.59	0.9440826

Table IV.4 (cont'd) The Cumulative Distribution Function [$P(Z \leq z)$ for z between −5.00 and 5.00] for the Standard Normal Random Variable with Mean Zero and Variance One.

z	$P[Z \leq z]$	z	$P[Z \leq z]$	z	$P[Z \leq z]$	z	$P[Z \leq z]$
1.60	0.9452007	2.15	0.9842224	2.70	0.9965330	3.25	0.9994229
1.61	0.9463010	2.16	0.9846137	2.71	0.9966358	3.26	0.9994429
1.62	0.9473838	2.17	0.9849966	2.72	0.9967358	3.27	0.9994622
1.63	0.9484492	2.18	0.9853713	2.73	0.9968332	3.28	0.9994809
1.64	0.9494974	2.19	0.9857379	2.74	0.9969280	3.29	0.9994990
1.65	0.9505285	2.20	0.9860966	2.75	0.9970202	3.30	0.9995165
1.66	0.9515428	2.21	0.9864475	2.76	0.9971099	3.31	0.9995335
1.67	0.9525403	2.22	0.9867906	2.77	0.9971971	3.32	0.9995499
1.68	0.9535213	2.23	0.9871263	2.78	0.9972820	3.33	0.9995657
1.69	0.9544860	2.24	0.9874546	2.79	0.9973645	3.34	0.9995811
1.70	0.9554345	2.25	0.9877756	2.80	0.9974448	3.35	0.9995959
1.71	0.9563671	2.26	0.9880894	2.81	0.9975229	3.36	0.9996102
1.72	0.9572838	2.27	0.9883962	2.82	0.9975988	3.37	0.9996241
1.73	0.9581849	2.28	0.9886962	2.83	0.9976725	3.38	0.9996375
1.74	0.9590705	2.29	0.9889894	2.84	0.9977443	3.39	0.9996505
1.75	0.9599409	2.30	0.9892759	2.85	0.9978140	3.40	0.9996630
1.76	0.9607961	2.31	0.9895559	2.86	0.9978817	3.41	0.9996751
1.77	0.9616364	2.32	0.9898296	2.87	0.9979476	3.42	0.9996868
1.78	0.9624620	2.33	0.9900969	2.88	0.9980116	3.43	0.9996982
1.79	0.9632731	2.34	0.9903581	2.89	0.9980737	3.44	0.9997091
1.80	0.9640697	2.35	0.9906133	2.90	0.9981341	3.45	0.9997197
1.81	0.9648521	2.36	0.9908625	2.91	0.9981928	3.46	0.9997299
1.82	0.9656205	2.37	0.9911060	2.92	0.9982498	3.47	0.9997397
1.83	0.9663751	2.38	0.9913437	2.93	0.9983051	3.48	0.9997492
1.84	0.9671159	2.39	0.9915758	2.94	0.9983589	3.49	0.9997584
1.85	0.9678433	2.40	0.9918025	2.95	0.9984111	3.50	0.9997673
1.86	0.9685573	2.41	0.9920237	2.96	0.9984617	3.51	0.9997759
1.87	0.9692581	2.42	0.9922397	2.97	0.9985109	3.52	0.9997842
1.88	0.9699460	2.43	0.9924506	2.98	0.9985587	3.53	0.9997922
1.89	0.9706211	2.44	0.9926564	2.99	0.9986050	3.54	0.9997999
1.90	0.9712835	2.45	0.9928572	3.00	0.9986500	3.55	0.9998073
1.91	0.9719334	2.46	0.9930531	3.01	0.9986937	3.56	0.9998145
1.92	0.9725711	2.47	0.9932443	3.02	0.9987361	3.57	0.9998215
1.93	0.9731966	2.48	0.9934309	3.03	0.9987772	3.58	0.9998282
1.94	0.9738102	2.49	0.9936128	3.04	0.9988170	3.59	0.9998346
1.95	0.9744120	2.50	0.9937903	3.05	0.9988557	3.60	0.9998409
1.96	0.9750022	2.51	0.9939634	3.06	0.9988932	3.61	0.9998469
1.97	0.9755809	2.52	0.9941322	3.07	0.9989296	3.62	0.9998527
1.98	0.9761483	2.53	0.9942968	3.08	0.9989649	3.63	0.9998583
1.99	0.9767046	2.54	0.9944573	3.09	0.9989991	3.64	0.9998636
2.00	0.9772499	2.55	0.9946138	3.10	0.9990323	3.65	0.9998688
2.01	0.9777845	2.56	0.9947664	3.11	0.9990645	3.66	0.9998739
2.02	0.9783084	2.57	0.9949150	3.12	0.9990957	3.67	0.9998787
2.03	0.9788218	2.58	0.9950599	3.13	0.9991259	3.68	0.9998834
2.04	0.9793249	2.59	0.9952012	3.14	0.9991552	3.69	0.9998878
2.05	0.9798178	2.60	0.9953388	3.15	0.9991836	3.70	0.9998922
2.06	0.9803008	2.61	0.9954728	3.16	0.9992111	3.71	0.9998963
2.07	0.9807739	2.62	0.9956035	3.17	0.9992377	3.72	0.9999004
2.08	0.9812373	2.63	0.9957307	3.18	0.9992636	3.73	0.9999042
2.09	0.9816911	2.64	0.9958547	3.19	0.9992886	3.74	0.9999080
2.10	0.9821356	2.65	0.9959754	3.20	0.9993128	3.75	0.9999116
2.11	0.9825709	2.66	0.9960929	3.21	0.9993363	3.76	0.9999150
2.12	0.9829970	2.67	0.9962074	3.22	0.9993590	3.77	0.9999183
2.13	0.9834142	2.68	0.9963188	3.23	0.9993810	3.78	0.9999216
2.14	0.9838227	2.69	0.9964273	3.24	0.9994023	3.79	0.9999247

Table IV.4 (cont'd) The Cumulative Distribution Function [$P(Z \leq z)$ for z between −5.00 and 5.00] for the Standard Normal Random Variable with Mean Zero and Variance One.

z	$P[Z \leq z]$	z	$P[Z \leq z]$	z	$P[Z \leq z]$	z	$P[Z \leq z]$
3.80	0.9999276	4.11	0.9999802	4.42	0.9999951	4.73	0.9999989
3.81	0.9999305	4.12	0.9999810	4.43	0.9999953	4.74	0.9999989
3.82	0.9999333	4.13	0.9999819	4.44	0.9999955	4.75	0.9999990
3.83	0.9999359	4.14	0.9999826	4.45	0.9999957	4.76	0.9999990
3.84	0.9999385	4.15	0.9999834	4.46	0.9999959	4.77	0.9999991
3.85	0.9999409	4.16	0.9999841	4.47	0.9999961	4.78	0.9999991
3.86	0.9999433	4.17	0.9999848	4.48	0.9999963	4.79	0.9999992
3.87	0.9999456	4.18	0.9999854	4.49	0.9999964	4.80	0.9999992
3.88	0.9999478	4.19	0.9999860	4.50	0.9999966	4.81	0.9999992
3.89	0.9999499	4.20	0.9999866	4.51	0.9999968	4.82	0.9999993
3.90	0.9999519	4.21	0.9999872	4.52	0.9999969	4.83	0.9999993
3.91	0.9999538	4.22	0.9999878	4.53	0.9999970	4.84	0.9999993
3.92	0.9999557	4.23	0.9999883	4.54	0.9999972	4.85	0.9999994
3.93	0.9999575	4.24	0.9999888	4.55	0.9999973	4.86	0.9999994
3.94	0.9999592	4.25	0.9999893	4.56	0.9999974	4.87	0.9999994
3.95	0.9999609	4.26	0.9999898	4.57	0.9999976	4.88	0.9999995
3.96	0.9999625	4.27	0.9999902	4.58	0.9999977	4.89	0.9999995
3.97	0.9999640	4.28	0.9999906	4.59	0.9999978	4.90	0.9999995
3.98	0.9999655	4.29	0.9999911	4.60	0.9999979	4.91	0.9999995
3.99	0.9999669	4.30	0.9999915	4.61	0.9999980	4.92	0.9999996
4.00	0.9999683	4.31	0.9999918	4.62	0.9999981	4.93	0.9999996
4.01	0.9999696	4.32	0.9999922	4.63	0.9999982	4.94	0.9999996
4.02	0.9999709	4.33	0.9999925	4.64	0.9999983	4.95	0.9999996
4.03	0.9999721	4.34	0.9999929	4.65	0.9999983	4.96	0.9999996
4.04	0.9999733	4.35	0.9999932	4.66	0.9999984	4.97	0.9999997
4.05	0.9999744	4.36	0.9999935	4.67	0.9999985	4.98	0.9999997
4.06	0.9999755	4.37	0.9999938	4.68	0.9999986	4.99	0.9999997
4.07	0.9999765	4.38	0.9999941	4.69	0.9999986	5.00	0.9999997
4.08	0.9999775	4.39	0.9999943	4.70	0.9999987		
4.09	0.9999784	4.40	0.9999946	4.71	0.9999988		
4.10	0.9999793	4.41	0.9999948	4.72	0.9999988		

V

Critical Values for the Chi-Square Distribution

TABLE

V.1. The Percentiles, $\chi^2_{df,p}$, of the Cumulative Distribution Function $[P(\mathcal{X}^2_{df} \leq \chi^2_{df,p}) = p]$ for the Chi-Square Random Variable with *df* Degrees of Freedom.

Table V.1 The Percentiles, $\chi^2_{df,p}$, of the Cumulative Distribution Function $[P(\mathcal{X}^2_{df} \le \chi^2_{df,p}) = p]$ for the Chi-Square Random Variable with *df* Degrees of Freedom.

p	*df* 1	2	3	4
0.0005	0.000000393	0.001000	0.0153	0.0639
0.001	0.00000157	0.002001	0.0243	0.0908
0.005	0.0000393	0.010025	0.0717	0.2070
0.01	0.000157	0.020101	0.1148	0.2971
0.02	0.000628	0.040405	0.1848	0.4294
0.025	0.000982	0.050636	0.2158	0.4844
0.03	0.001414	0.060918	0.2451	0.5351
0.04	0.002515	0.081644	0.3002	0.6271
0.05	0.003932	0.102587	0.3518	0.7107
0.06	0.005666	0.123751	0.4012	0.7884
0.07	0.007717	0.145141	0.4487	0.8616
0.075	0.008862	0.155923	0.4720	0.8969
0.08	0.010087	0.166763	0.4949	0.9315
0.09	0.012778	0.188622	0.5401	0.9987
0.10	0.015791	0.210721	0.5844	1.0636
0.11	0.019128	0.233068	0.6280	1.1268
0.12	0.022792	0.255667	0.6710	1.1884
0.13	0.026784	0.278524	0.7136	1.2488
0.14	0.031108	0.301646	0.7558	1.3081
0.15	0.035766	0.325038	0.7978	1.3665
0.16	0.040761	0.348707	0.8395	1.4241
0.17	0.046097	0.372659	0.8810	1.4810
0.18	0.051777	0.396902	0.9225	1.5374
0.19	0.057805	0.421442	0.9638	1.5933
0.20	0.064185	0.446287	1.0052	1.6488
0.21	0.070921	0.471445	1.0465	1.7040
0.22	0.078019	0.496923	1.0879	1.7589
0.23	0.085483	0.522729	1.1293	1.8136
0.24	0.093319	0.548874	1.1709	1.8681
0.25	0.101531	0.575364	1.2125	1.9226
0.26	0.110127	0.602210	1.2544	1.9769
0.27	0.119112	0.629421	1.2964	2.0313
0.28	0.128493	0.657008	1.3386	2.0857
0.29	0.138277	0.684980	1.3810	2.1402
0.30	0.148472	0.713350	1.4237	2.1947
0.31	0.159085	0.742127	1.4666	2.2494
0.32	0.170126	0.771325	1.5098	2.3042
0.33	0.181602	0.800955	1.5534	2.3593
0.34	0.193524	0.831031	1.5973	2.4145
0.35	0.205900	0.861566	1.6416	2.4701
0.36	0.218742	0.892574	1.6862	2.5259
0.37	0.232061	0.924071	1.7313	2.5821
0.38	0.245868	0.956072	1.7768	2.6386
0.39	0.260175	0.988593	1.8227	2.6955
0.40	0.274996	1.02165	1.8692	2.7528
0.41	0.290344	1.05526	1.9161	2.8106
0.42	0.306235	1.08945	1.9636	2.8689
0.43	0.322682	1.12424	2.0116	2.9277
0.44	0.339704	1.15964	2.0602	2.9870
0.45	0.357317	1.19567	2.1095	3.0469
0.46	0.375540	1.23237	2.1593	3.1075
0.47	0.394391	1.26976	2.2099	3.1687
0.48	0.413893	1.30785	2.2612	3.2306
0.49	0.434067	1.34669	2.3132	3.2933
0.50	0.454936	1.38629	2.3660	3.3567

For example, for four degrees of freedom ($df = 4$), the 21st percentile $\chi^2_{4,0.21}$ of the chi-square distribution is 1.7040; that is, $P[\mathcal{X}^2_4 \le 1.7040] = 0.21$ and $\chi^2_{4,0.21} = 1.7040$.

Table V.1 (cont'd) The Percentiles, $\chi^2_{df,p}$, of the Cumulative Distribution Function $[P(\mathcal{X}^2_{df} \leq \chi^2_{df,p}) = p]$ for the Chi-Square Random Variable with *df* Degrees of Freedom.

p	*df*			
	1	2	3	4
0.51	0.476526	1.42670	2.4196	3.4209
0.52	0.498863	1.46794	2.4740	3.4861
0.53	0.521976	1.51004	2.5294	3.5521
0.54	0.545894	1.55306	2.5857	3.6191
0.55	0.570652	1.59702	2.6430	3.6871
0.56	0.596282	1.64196	2.7013	3.7562
0.57	0.622823	1.68794	2.7608	3.8265
0.58	0.650315	1.73500	2.8213	3.8979
0.59	0.678800	1.78320	2.8831	3.9706
0.60	0.708326	1.83258	2.9462	4.0446
0.61	0.738942	1.88322	3.0106	4.1201
0.62	0.770702	1.93517	3.0764	4.1970
0.63	0.803664	1.98850	3.1437	4.2755
0.64	0.837893	2.04330	3.2126	4.3557
0.65	0.873457	2.09964	3.2831	4.4377
0.66	0.910432	2.15762	3.3554	4.5215
0.67	0.948898	2.21732	3.4297	4.6074
0.68	0.988947	2.27887	3.5059	4.6954
0.69	1.03068	2.34237	3.5842	4.7857
0.70	1.07420	2.40795	3.6649	4.8784
0.71	1.11962	2.47575	3.7479	4.9738
0.72	1.16709	2.54593	3.8336	5.0719
0.73	1.21675	2.61867	3.9221	5.1730
0.74	1.26876	2.69415	4.0136	5.2774
0.75	1.32330	2.77259	4.1083	5.3853
0.76	1.38059	2.85423	4.2066	5.4969
0.77	1.44086	2.93935	4.3087	5.6127
0.78	1.50437	3.02825	4.4150	5.7329
0.79	1.57143	3.12130	4.5258	5.8581
0.80	1.64238	3.21888	4.6416	5.9886
0.81	1.71762	3.32146	4.7630	6.1251
0.82	1.79762	3.42960	4.8904	6.2681
0.83	1.88294	3.54391	5.0247	6.4185
0.84	1.97423	3.66516	5.1665	6.5770
0.85	2.07225	3.79424	5.3170	6.7449
0.86	2.17796	3.93222	5.4773	6.9233
0.87	2.29251	4.08044	5.6489	7.1137
0.88	2.41732	4.24053	5.8335	7.3182
0.89	2.55422	4.41455	6.0333	7.5390
0.90	2.70554	4.60517	6.2514	7.7794
0.91	2.87437	4.81589	6.4915	8.0434
0.92	3.06490	5.05146	6.7587	8.3365
0.925	3.17005	5.18054	6.9046	8.4963
0.93	3.28302	5.31852	7.0603	8.6664
0.94	3.53738	5.62682	7.4069	9.0444
0.95	3.84145	5.99146	7.8147	9.4877
0.96	4.21788	6.43775	8.3112	10.0255
0.97	4.70929	7.01312	8.9473	10.7119
0.975	5.02389	7.37776	9.3484	11.1433
0.98	5.41190	7.82405	9.8374	11.6678
0.99	6.63492	9.21033	11.3449	13.2767
0.995	7.87949	10.5966	12.8382	14.8602
0.999	10.8280	13.8154	16.2663	18.4669
0.9995	12.1160	15.2017	17.7299	19.9970

Table V.1 (cont'd) The Percentiles, $\chi^2_{df,p}$, of the Cumulative Distribution Function $[P(\mathcal{X}^2_{df} \leq \chi^2_{df,p}) = p]$ for the Chi-Square Random Variable with *df* Degrees of Freedom.

p	*df*					
	5	6	7	8	9	10
0.0005	0.158	0.299	0.485	0.710	0.972	1.265
0.001	0.210	0.381	0.598	0.857	1.152	1.479
0.005	0.412	0.676	0.989	1.344	1.735	2.156
0.01	0.554	0.872	1.239	1.646	2.088	2.558
0.02	0.752	1.134	1.564	2.032	2.532	3.059
0.025	0.831	1.237	1.690	2.180	2.700	3.247
0.03	0.903	1.330	1.802	2.310	2.848	3.412
0.04	1.031	1.492	1.997	2.537	3.105	3.697
0.05	1.145	1.635	2.167	2.733	3.325	3.940
0.06	1.250	1.765	2.320	2.908	3.521	4.157
0.07	1.347	1.885	2.461	3.068	3.700	4.353
0.075	1.394	1.941	2.528	3.144	3.785	4.446
0.08	1.439	1.997	2.592	3.217	3.866	4.535
0.09	1.526	2.103	2.716	3.357	4.021	4.705
0.10	1.610	2.204	2.833	3.490	4.168	4.865
0.11	1.691	2.301	2.945	3.616	4.308	5.018
0.12	1.770	2.395	3.054	3.737	4.442	5.163
0.13	1.846	2.486	3.158	3.855	4.571	5.304
0.14	1.921	2.575	3.260	3.968	4.696	5.439
0.15	1.994	2.661	3.358	4.078	4.817	5.570
0.16	2.066	2.746	3.455	4.186	4.934	5.698
0.17	2.136	2.829	3.549	4.291	5.049	5.822
0.18	2.206	2.910	3.642	4.393	5.162	5.943
0.19	2.275	2.991	3.733	4.494	5.272	6.062
0.20	2.343	3.070	3.822	4.594	5.380	6.179
0.21	2.410	3.148	3.911	4.691	5.487	6.294
0.22	2.477	3.226	3.998	4.788	5.592	6.407
0.23	2.543	3.303	4.084	4.883	5.695	6.518
0.24	2.609	3.379	4.170	4.977	5.798	6.628
0.25	2.675	3.455	4.255	5.071	5.899	6.737
0.26	2.740	3.530	4.339	5.163	5.999	6.845
0.27	2.805	3.605	4.423	5.255	6.099	6.952
0.28	2.870	3.679	4.506	5.346	6.198	7.058
0.29	2.935	3.753	4.589	5.437	6.296	7.163
0.30	3.000	3.828	4.671	5.527	6.393	7.267
0.31	3.065	3.902	4.754	5.617	6.490	7.371
0.32	3.130	3.975	4.836	5.707	6.587	7.475
0.33	3.195	4.049	4.918	5.797	6.684	7.578
0.34	3.260	4.123	5.000	5.886	6.780	7.681
0.35	3.325	4.197	5.082	5.975	6.876	7.783
0.36	3.391	4.271	5.164	6.065	6.972	7.886
0.37	3.456	4.346	5.246	6.154	7.068	7.988
0.38	3.522	4.420	5.328	6.243	7.164	8.090
0.39	3.589	4.495	5.410	6.333	7.261	8.193
0.40	3.655	4.570	5.493	6.423	7.357	8.295
0.41	3.723	4.646	5.576	6.513	7.454	8.398
0.42	3.790	4.721	5.660	6.603	7.551	8.501
0.43	3.858	4.798	5.743	6.694	7.648	8.605
0.44	3.927	4.875	5.828	6.785	7.745	8.708
0.45	3.996	4.952	5.913	6.877	7.843	8.812
0.46	4.066	5.030	5.998	6.969	7.942	8.917
0.47	4.136	5.108	6.084	7.062	8.041	9.022
0.48	4.207	5.187	6.170	7.155	8.141	9.128
0.49	4.279	5.267	6.258	7.249	8.242	9.235
0.50	4.351	5.348	6.346	7.344	8.343	9.342

Table V.1 (cont'd) The Percentiles, $\chi^2_{df,p}$, of the Cumulative Distribution Function $[P(\mathcal{X}^2_{df} \leq \chi^2_{df,p}) = p]$ for the Chi-Square Random Variable with *df* Degrees of Freedom.

p	*df*					
	5	6	7	8	9	10
0.51	4.425	5.430	6.435	7.440	8.445	9.450
0.52	4.499	5.512	6.525	7.537	8.548	9.559
0.53	4.574	5.595	6.615	7.634	8.652	9.669
0.54	4.651	5.680	6.707	7.733	8.757	9.780
0.55	4.728	5.765	6.800	7.833	8.863	9.892
0.56	4.806	5.852	6.894	7.933	8.971	10.006
0.57	4.886	5.940	6.989	8.036	9.079	10.120
0.58	4.966	6.029	7.086	8.139	9.189	10.236
0.59	5.048	6.119	7.184	8.244	9.301	10.354
0.60	5.132	6.211	7.283	8.351	9.414	10.473
0.61	5.217	6.304	7.384	8.459	9.528	10.594
0.62	5.303	6.399	7.487	8.568	9.645	10.717
0.63	5.391	6.496	7.591	8.680	9.763	10.841
0.64	5.481	6.594	7.698	8.794	9.883	10.968
0.65	5.573	6.695	7.806	8.909	10.006	11.097
0.66	5.667	6.797	7.917	9.027	10.131	11.228
0.67	5.763	6.902	8.029	9.148	10.258	11.362
0.68	5.861	7.009	8.145	9.270	10.388	11.499
0.69	5.961	7.119	8.263	9.396	10.521	11.638
0.70	6.064	7.231	8.383	9.524	10.656	11.781
0.71	6.170	7.346	8.507	9.656	10.795	11.927
0.72	6.279	7.465	8.634	9.791	10.938	12.076
0.73	6.391	7.586	8.765	9.930	11.084	12.229
0.74	6.507	7.712	8.899	10.072	11.234	12.387
0.75	6.626	7.841	9.037	10.219	11.389	12.549
0.76	6.749	7.974	9.180	10.370	11.548	12.716
0.77	6.876	8.112	9.327	10.526	11.713	12.888
0.78	7.009	8.255	9.480	10.688	11.883	13.066
0.79	7.146	8.404	9.639	10.856	12.059	13.251
0.80	7.289	8.558	9.803	11.030	12.242	13.442
0.81	7.439	8.719	9.975	11.212	12.433	13.641
0.82	7.595	8.888	10.154	11.401	12.632	13.849
0.83	7.759	9.064	10.342	11.599	12.840	14.066
0.84	7.932	9.250	10.540	11.808	13.058	14.294
0.85	8.115	9.446	10.748	12.027	13.288	14.534
0.86	8.309	9.654	10.968	12.259	13.531	14.788
0.87	8.516	9.875	11.203	12.506	13.790	15.057
0.88	8.738	10.112	11.454	12.770	14.066	15.344
0.89	8.977	10.368	11.724	13.054	14.363	15.653
0.90	9.236	10.645	12.017	13.362	14.684	15.987
0.91	9.521	10.948	12.337	13.697	15.034	16.352
0.92	9.837	11.283	12.691	14.068	15.421	16.753
0.925	10.008	11.466	12.883	14.270	15.631	16.971
0.93	10.191	11.660	13.088	14.484	15.854	17.203
0.94	10.596	12.090	13.540	14.956	16.346	17.713
0.95	11.071	12.592	14.067	15.507	16.919	18.307
0.96	11.644	13.198	14.703	16.171	17.608	19.021
0.97	12.375	13.968	15.509	17.010	18.480	19.922
0.975	12.833	14.449	16.013	17.535	19.023	20.483
0.98	13.388	15.033	16.622	18.168	19.679	21.161
0.99	15.086	16.812	18.475	20.090	21.666	23.209
0.995	16.750	18.548	20.278	21.955	23.589	25.188
0.999	20.515	22.458	24.322	26.125	27.877	29.589
0.9995	22.105	24.102	26.017	27.868	29.666	31.419

Table V.1 (cont'd) The Percentiles, $\chi^2_{df,p}$, of the Cumulative Distribution Function $[P(\mathcal{X}^2_{df} \leq \chi^2_{df,p}) = p]$ for the Chi-Square Random Variable with *df* Degrees of Freedom.

p	*df*									
	11	12	13	14	15	16	17	18	19	20
0.0005	1.59	1.93	2.31	2.70	3.11	3.54	3.98	4.44	4.91	5.40
0.001	1.83	2.21	2.62	3.04	3.48	3.94	4.42	4.90	5.41	5.92
0.005	2.60	3.07	3.57	4.07	4.60	5.14	5.70	6.26	6.84	7.43
0.01	3.05	3.57	4.11	4.66	5.23	5.81	6.41	7.01	7.63	8.26
0.02	3.61	4.18	4.77	5.37	5.98	6.61	7.26	7.91	8.57	9.24
0.025	3.82	4.40	5.01	5.63	6.26	6.91	7.56	8.23	8.91	9.59
0.03	4.00	4.60	5.22	5.86	6.50	7.16	7.83	8.51	9.20	9.90
0.04	4.31	4.94	5.58	6.24	6.91	7.60	8.29	8.99	9.70	10.42
0.05	4.57	5.23	5.89	6.57	7.26	7.96	8.67	9.39	10.12	10.85
0.06	4.81	5.48	6.16	6.86	7.57	8.28	9.01	9.74	10.48	11.23
0.07	5.02	5.71	6.41	7.12	7.84	8.57	9.31	10.06	10.81	11.57
0.075	5.12	5.82	6.52	7.24	7.97	8.71	9.45	10.21	10.97	11.73
0.08	5.22	5.92	6.63	7.36	8.09	8.84	9.59	10.35	11.11	11.88
0.09	5.40	6.12	6.84	7.58	8.33	9.08	9.84	10.61	11.39	12.17
0.10	5.58	6.30	7.04	7.79	8.55	9.31	10.09	10.86	11.65	12.44
0.11	5.74	6.48	7.23	7.99	8.75	9.53	10.31	11.10	11.90	12.70
0.12	5.90	6.65	7.41	8.18	8.95	9.74	10.53	11.33	12.13	12.94
0.13	6.05	6.81	7.58	8.36	9.14	9.94	10.74	11.54	12.35	13.17
0.14	6.20	6.96	7.74	8.53	9.32	10.13	10.93	11.75	12.57	13.39
0.15	6.34	7.11	7.90	8.70	9.50	10.31	11.12	11.95	12.77	13.60
0.16	6.47	7.26	8.05	8.86	9.67	10.49	11.31	12.14	12.97	13.81
0.17	6.61	7.40	8.20	9.02	9.83	10.66	11.49	12.33	13.17	14.01
0.18	6.74	7.54	8.35	9.17	10.00	10.83	11.66	12.51	13.35	14.20
0.19	6.86	7.67	8.49	9.32	10.15	10.99	11.84	12.68	13.54	14.39
0.20	6.99	7.81	8.63	9.47	10.31	11.15	12.00	12.86	13.72	14.58
0.21	7.11	7.94	8.77	9.61	10.46	11.31	12.17	13.03	13.89	14.76
0.22	7.23	8.07	8.91	9.75	10.61	11.46	12.33	13.19	14.06	14.94
0.23	7.35	8.19	9.04	9.89	10.75	11.62	12.48	13.36	14.23	15.11
0.24	7.47	8.32	9.17	10.03	10.90	11.76	12.64	13.52	14.40	15.28
0.25	7.58	8.44	9.30	10.17	11.04	11.91	12.79	13.68	14.56	15.45
0.26	7.70	8.56	9.43	10.30	11.18	12.06	12.94	13.83	14.72	15.62
0.27	7.81	8.68	9.55	10.43	11.31	12.20	13.09	13.99	14.88	15.78
0.28	7.93	8.80	9.68	10.56	11.45	12.34	13.24	14.14	15.04	15.95
0.29	8.04	8.92	9.80	10.69	11.59	12.48	13.39	14.29	15.20	16.11
0.30	8.15	9.03	9.93	10.82	11.72	12.62	13.53	14.44	15.35	16.27
0.31	8.26	9.15	10.05	10.95	11.85	12.76	13.67	14.59	15.51	16.42
0.32	8.37	9.27	10.17	11.08	11.99	12.90	13.82	14.74	15.66	16.58
0.33	8.48	9.38	10.29	11.20	12.12	13.04	13.96	14.88	15.81	16.74
0.34	8.59	9.50	10.41	11.33	12.25	13.17	14.10	15.03	15.96	16.89
0.35	8.70	9.61	10.53	11.45	12.38	13.31	14.24	15.17	16.11	17.05
0.36	8.80	9.73	10.65	11.58	12.51	13.44	14.38	15.32	16.26	17.20
0.37	8.91	9.84	10.77	11.70	12.64	13.58	14.52	15.46	16.41	17.35
0.38	9.02	9.95	10.89	11.83	12.77	13.71	14.66	15.61	16.55	17.50
0.39	9.13	10.07	11.01	11.95	12.90	13.85	14.80	15.75	16.70	17.66
0.40	9.24	10.18	11.13	12.08	13.03	13.98	14.94	15.89	16.85	17.81
0.41	9.35	10.30	11.25	12.20	13.16	14.12	15.08	16.04	17.00	17.96
0.42	9.45	10.41	11.37	12.33	13.29	14.25	15.21	16.18	17.15	18.11
0.43	9.56	10.53	11.49	12.45	13.42	14.39	15.35	16.32	17.29	18.26
0.44	9.67	10.64	11.61	12.58	13.55	14.52	15.49	16.47	17.44	18.42
0.45	9.78	10.76	11.73	12.70	13.68	14.66	15.63	16.61	17.59	18.57
0.46	9.89	10.87	11.85	12.83	13.81	14.79	15.77	16.76	17.74	18.72
0.47	10.00	10.99	11.97	12.96	13.94	14.93	15.91	16.90	17.89	18.87
0.48	10.12	11.10	12.09	13.08	14.07	15.06	16.05	17.05	18.04	19.03
0.49	10.23	11.22	12.22	13.21	14.21	15.20	16.20	17.19	18.19	19.18
0.50	10.34	11.34	12.34	13.34	14.34	15.34	16.34	17.34	18.34	19.34

Table V.1 (cont'd) The Percentiles, $\chi^2_{df,p}$, of the Cumulative Distribution Function $[P(\mathcal{X}^2_{df} \leq \chi^2_{df,p}) = p]$ for the Chi-Square Random Variable with *df* Degrees of Freedom.

p	*df*									
	11	12	13	14	15	16	17	18	19	20
0.51	10.45	11.46	12.46	13.47	14.47	15.48	16.48	17.49	18.49	19.49
0.52	10.57	11.58	12.59	13.60	14.61	15.62	16.63	17.63	18.64	19.65
0.53	10.69	11.70	12.72	13.73	14.74	15.76	16.77	17.78	18.80	19.81
0.54	10.80	11.82	12.84	13.86	14.88	15.90	16.92	17.93	18.95	19.97
0.55	10.92	11.95	12.97	14.00	15.02	16.04	17.06	18.09	19.11	20.13
0.56	11.04	12.07	13.10	14.13	15.16	16.19	17.21	18.24	19.26	20.29
0.57	11.16	12.20	13.23	14.27	15.30	16.33	17.36	18.39	19.42	20.45
0.58	11.28	12.32	13.37	14.40	15.44	16.48	17.52	18.55	19.58	20.62
0.59	11.40	12.45	13.50	14.54	15.59	16.63	17.67	18.71	19.75	20.78
0.60	11.53	12.58	13.64	14.69	15.73	16.78	17.82	18.87	19.91	20.95
0.61	11.66	12.72	13.77	14.83	15.88	16.93	17.98	19.03	20.08	21.12
0.62	11.79	12.85	13.91	14.97	16.03	17.09	18.14	19.19	20.24	21.29
0.63	11.92	12.99	14.05	15.12	16.18	17.24	18.30	19.36	20.42	21.47
0.64	12.05	13.13	14.20	15.27	16.34	17.40	18.47	19.53	20.59	21.65
0.65	12.18	13.27	14.35	15.42	16.49	17.56	18.63	19.70	20.76	21.83
0.66	12.32	13.41	14.49	15.58	16.65	17.73	18.80	19.87	20.94	22.01
0.67	12.46	13.56	14.65	15.73	16.82	17.90	18.97	20.05	21.12	22.20
0.68	12.60	13.70	14.80	15.89	16.98	18.07	19.15	20.23	21.31	22.38
0.69	12.75	13.86	14.96	16.06	17.15	18.24	19.33	20.41	21.50	22.58
0.70	12.90	14.01	15.12	16.22	17.32	18.42	19.51	20.60	21.69	22.77
0.71	13.05	14.17	15.28	16.39	17.50	18.60	19.70	20.79	21.89	22.98
0.72	13.21	14.33	15.45	16.57	17.68	18.78	19.89	20.99	22.09	23.18
0.73	13.37	14.50	15.62	16.75	17.86	18.97	20.08	21.19	22.29	23.39
0.74	13.53	14.67	15.80	16.93	18.05	19.17	20.28	21.39	22.50	23.61
0.75	13.70	14.85	15.98	17.12	18.25	19.37	20.49	21.60	22.72	23.83
0.76	13.87	15.03	16.17	17.31	18.44	19.57	20.70	21.82	22.94	24.05
0.77	14.05	15.21	16.36	17.51	18.65	19.79	20.92	22.04	23.17	24.29
0.78	14.24	15.41	16.56	17.72	18.86	20.00	21.14	22.28	23.40	24.53
0.79	14.43	15.61	16.77	17.93	19.08	20.23	21.37	22.51	23.65	24.78
0.80	14.63	15.81	16.98	18.15	19.31	20.47	21.61	22.76	23.90	25.04
0.81	14.84	16.03	17.21	18.38	19.55	20.71	21.86	23.02	24.16	25.31
0.82	15.05	16.25	17.44	18.62	19.79	20.96	22.12	23.28	24.43	25.58
0.83	15.28	16.49	17.68	18.87	20.05	21.23	22.40	23.56	24.72	25.87
0.84	15.52	16.73	17.94	19.13	20.32	21.50	22.68	23.85	25.02	26.18
0.85	15.77	16.99	18.20	19.41	20.60	21.79	22.98	24.16	25.33	26.50
0.86	16.03	17.26	18.48	19.70	20.90	22.10	23.29	24.48	25.66	26.83
0.87	16.31	17.55	18.78	20.00	21.22	22.42	23.62	24.82	26.01	27.19
0.88	16.61	17.86	19.10	20.33	21.56	22.77	23.98	25.18	26.38	27.57
0.89	16.93	18.19	19.44	20.68	21.92	23.14	24.36	25.57	26.78	27.97
0.90	17.28	18.55	19.81	21.06	22.31	23.54	24.77	25.99	27.20	28.41
0.91	17.65	18.94	20.21	21.48	22.73	23.98	25.21	26.45	27.67	28.89
0.92	18.07	19.37	20.66	21.93	23.20	24.46	25.71	26.95	28.18	29.41
0.925	18.29	19.60	20.90	22.18	23.45	24.72	25.97	27.22	28.46	29.69
0.93	18.53	19.85	21.15	22.44	23.72	24.99	26.25	27.50	28.75	29.99
0.94	19.06	20.39	21.71	23.02	24.31	25.59	26.87	28.14	29.40	30.65
0.95	19.68	21.03	22.36	23.68	25.00	26.30	27.59	28.87	30.14	31.41
0.96	20.41	21.79	23.14	24.49	25.82	27.14	28.44	29.75	31.04	32.32
0.97	21.34	22.74	24.12	25.49	26.85	28.19	29.52	30.84	32.16	33.46
0.975	21.92	23.34	24.74	26.12	27.49	28.85	30.19	31.53	32.85	34.10
0.98	22.62	24.05	25.47	26.87	28.26	29.63	31.00	32.35	33.69	35.02
0.99	24.72	26.22	27.69	29.14	30.58	32.00	33.41	34.81	36.19	37.57
0.995	26.76	28.30	29.82	31.32	32.80	34.27	35.72	37.16	38.58	40.00
0.999	31.26	32.91	34.53	36.12	37.70	39.25	40.79	42.31	43.82	45.30
0.9995	33.14	34.82	36.48	38.11	39.72	41.31	42.88	44.43	45.97	47.50

Table V.1 (cont'd) The Percentiles, $\chi^2_{df,p}$, of the Cumulative Distribution Function $[P(\mathcal{X}^2_{df} \leq \chi^2_{df,p}) = p]$ for the Chi-Square Random Variable with *df* Degrees of Freedom.

p	*df*									
	21	22	23	24	25	26	27	28	29	30
0.0005	5.90	6.40	6.92	7.45	7.99	8.54	9.09	9.66	10.23	10.80
0.001	6.45	6.98	7.53	8.08	8.65	9.22	9.80	10.39	10.99	11.59
0.005	8.03	8.64	9.26	9.89	10.52	11.16	11.81	12.46	13.12	13.79
0.01	8.90	9.54	10.20	10.86	11.52	12.20	12.88	13.56	14.26	14.95
0.02	9.91	10.60	11.29	11.99	12.70	13.41	14.13	14.85	15.57	16.31
0.025	10.28	10.98	11.69	12.40	13.12	13.84	14.57	15.31	16.05	16.79
0.03	10.60	11.31	12.03	12.75	13.48	14.22	14.96	15.70	16.45	17.21
0.04	11.14	11.87	12.61	13.35	14.10	14.85	15.61	16.37	17.14	17.91
0.05	11.59	12.34	13.09	13.85	14.61	15.38	16.15	16.93	17.71	18.49
0.06	11.99	12.75	13.51	14.28	15.06	15.84	16.62	17.41	18.20	19.00
0.07	12.34	13.11	13.89	14.67	15.46	16.25	17.05	17.84	18.65	19.45
0.075	12.50	13.28	14.06	14.85	15.64	16.44	17.24	18.05	18.85	19.66
0.08	12.66	13.45	14.23	15.03	15.82	16.62	17.43	18.24	19.05	19.87
0.09	12.96	13.75	14.55	15.35	16.16	16.97	17.78	18.60	19.42	20.25
0.10	13.24	14.04	14.85	15.66	16.47	17.29	18.11	18.94	19.77	20.60
0.11	13.50	14.31	15.13	15.95	16.77	17.60	18.42	19.26	20.09	20.93
0.12	13.75	14.57	15.39	16.22	17.05	17.88	18.72	19.56	20.40	21.25
0.13	13.99	14.82	15.65	16.48	17.32	18.16	19.00	19.85	20.70	21.55
0.14	14.22	15.05	15.89	16.73	17.57	18.42	19.27	20.12	20.98	21.83
0.15	14.44	15.28	16.12	16.97	17.82	18.67	19.53	20.39	21.25	22.11
0.16	14.65	15.50	16.35	17.20	18.06	18.91	19.78	20.64	21.51	22.38
0.17	14.86	15.71	16.57	17.42	18.29	19.15	20.02	20.89	21.76	22.63
0.18	15.06	15.92	16.78	17.64	18.51	19.38	20.25	21.13	22.00	22.88
0.19	15.25	16.12	16.98	17.85	18.73	19.60	20.48	21.36	22.24	23.13
0.20	15.44	16.31	17.19	18.06	18.94	19.82	20.70	21.59	22.48	23.36
0.21	15.63	16.51	17.38	18.26	19.15	20.03	20.92	21.81	22.70	23.60
0.22	15.81	16.69	17.58	18.46	19.35	20.24	21.13	22.03	22.92	23.82
0.23	15.99	16.88	17.77	18.66	19.55	20.45	21.34	22.24	23.14	24.04
0.24	16.17	17.06	17.95	18.85	19.75	20.65	21.55	22.45	23.36	24.26
0.25	16.34	17.24	18.14	19.04	19.94	20.84	21.75	22.66	23.57	24.48
0.26	16.52	17.42	18.32	19.22	20.13	21.04	21.95	22.86	23.77	24.69
0.27	16.69	17.59	18.50	19.41	20.32	21.23	22.14	23.06	23.98	24.90
0.28	16.85	17.76	18.67	19.59	20.50	21.42	22.34	23.26	24.18	25.10
0.29	17.02	17.93	18.85	19.77	20.69	21.61	22.53	23.45	24.38	25.31
0.30	17.18	18.10	19.02	19.94	20.87	21.79	22.72	23.65	24.58	25.51
0.31	17.34	18.27	19.19	20.12	21.05	21.98	22.91	23.84	24.77	25.71
0.32	17.51	18.43	19.36	20.29	21.22	22.16	23.09	24.03	24.97	25.90
0.33	17.67	18.60	19.53	20.47	21.40	22.34	23.28	24.22	25.16	26.10
0.34	17.83	18.76	19.70	20.64	21.58	22.52	23.46	24.40	25.35	26.29
0.35	17.98	18.92	19.87	20.81	21.75	22.70	23.64	24.59	25.54	26.49
0.36	18.14	19.09	20.03	20.98	21.93	22.88	23.83	24.78	25.73	26.68
0.37	18.30	19.25	20.20	21.15	22.10	23.05	24.01	24.96	25.92	26.87
0.38	18.46	19.41	20.36	21.32	22.27	23.23	24.19	25.14	26.10	27.06
0.39	18.61	19.57	20.53	21.48	22.44	23.40	24.37	25.33	26.29	27.25
0.40	18.77	19.73	20.69	21.65	22.62	23.58	24.54	25.51	26.48	27.44
0.41	18.92	19.89	20.85	21.82	22.79	23.75	24.72	25.69	26.66	27.63
0.42	19.08	20.05	21.02	21.99	22.96	23.93	24.90	25.87	26.85	27.82
0.43	19.24	20.21	21.18	22.16	23.13	24.10	25.08	26.06	27.03	28.01
0.44	19.39	20.37	21.35	22.32	23.30	24.28	25.26	26.24	27.22	28.20
0.45	19.55	20.53	21.51	22.49	23.47	24.45	25.44	26.42	27.40	28.39
0.46	19.71	20.69	21.67	22.66	23.64	24.63	25.62	26.60	27.59	28.57
0.47	19.86	20.85	21.84	22.83	23.82	24.81	25.79	26.78	27.77	28.76
0.48	20.02	21.01	22.00	23.00	23.99	24.98	25.97	26.97	27.96	28.95
0.49	20.18	21.17	22.17	23.17	24.16	25.16	26.16	27.15	28.15	29.14
0.50	20.34	21.34	22.34	23.34	24.34	25.34	26.34	27.34	28.34	29.34

Table V.1 (cont'd) The Percentiles, $\chi^2_{df,p}$, of the Cumulative Distribution Function $[P(\mathcal{X}^2_{df} \leq \chi^2_{df,p}) = p]$ for the Chi-Square Random Variable with *df* Degrees of Freedom.

p	*df*									
	21	22	23	24	25	26	27	28	29	30
0.51	20.50	21.50	22.50	23.51	24.51	25.51	26.52	27.52	28.52	29.53
0.52	20.66	21.67	22.67	23.68	24.69	25.69	26.70	27.71	28.71	29.72
0.53	20.82	21.83	22.84	23.85	24.86	25.87	26.89	27.90	28.91	29.92
0.54	20.98	22.00	23.01	24.03	25.04	26.06	27.07	28.08	29.10	30.11
0.55	21.15	22.17	23.19	24.20	25.22	26.24	27.26	28.27	29.29	30.31
0.56	21.31	22.34	23.36	24.38	25.40	26.42	27.44	28.47	29.49	30.51
0.57	21.48	22.51	23.53	24.56	25.59	26.61	27.63	28.66	29.68	30.71
0.58	21.65	22.68	23.71	24.74	25.77	26.80	27.83	28.85	29.88	30.91
0.59	21.82	22.85	23.89	24.92	25.96	26.99	28.02	29.05	30.08	31.11
0.60	21.99	23.03	24.07	25.11	26.14	27.18	28.21	29.25	30.28	31.32
0.61	22.17	23.21	24.25	25.29	26.33	27.37	28.41	29.45	30.49	31.52
0.62	22.34	23.39	24.44	25.48	26.53	27.57	28.61	29.65	30.69	31.73
0.63	22.52	23.57	24.62	25.67	26.72	27.77	28.81	29.86	30.90	31.95
0.64	22.70	23.76	24.81	25.87	26.92	27.97	29.02	30.07	31.12	32.16
0.65	22.89	23.95	25.01	26.06	27.12	28.17	29.23	30.28	31.33	32.38
0.66	23.07	24.14	25.20	26.26	27.32	28.38	29.44	30.49	31.55	32.60
0.67	23.27	24.33	25.40	26.47	27.53	28.59	29.65	30.71	31.77	32.83
0.68	23.46	24.53	25.60	26.67	27.74	28.81	29.87	30.93	32.00	33.06
0.69	23.66	24.73	25.81	26.88	27.95	29.02	30.09	31.16	32.23	33.29
0.70	23.86	24.94	26.02	27.10	28.17	29.25	30.32	31.39	32.46	33.53
0.71	24.06	25.15	26.23	27.31	28.39	29.47	30.55	31.63	32.70	33.77
0.72	24.27	25.36	26.45	27.54	28.62	29.71	30.79	31.87	32.94	34.02
0.73	24.49	25.58	26.68	27.77	28.86	29.94	31.03	32.11	33.19	34.27
0.74	24.71	25.81	26.91	28.00	29.09	30.19	31.27	32.36	33.45	34.53
0.75	24.93	26.04	27.14	28.24	29.34	30.43	31.53	32.62	33.71	34.80
0.76	25.17	26.28	27.38	28.49	29.59	30.69	31.79	32.89	33.98	35.07
0.77	25.41	26.52	27.63	28.74	29.85	30.95	32.06	33.16	34.26	35.35
0.78	25.65	26.77	27.89	29.00	30.12	31.22	32.33	33.44	34.54	35.64
0.79	25.91	27.03	28.15	29.27	30.39	31.50	32.62	33.73	34.84	35.94
0.80	26.17	27.30	28.43	29.55	30.68	31.79	32.91	34.03	35.14	36.25
0.81	26.44	27.58	28.71	29.84	30.97	32.09	33.22	34.34	35.45	36.57
0.82	26.73	27.87	29.01	30.14	31.28	32.41	33.53	34.66	35.78	36.90
0.83	27.03	28.17	29.32	30.46	31.60	32.73	33.87	35.00	36.12	37.25
0.84	27.34	28.49	29.64	30.79	31.93	33.07	34.21	35.35	36.48	37.61
0.85	27.66	28.82	29.98	31.13	32.28	33.43	34.57	35.71	36.85	37.99
0.86	28.01	29.17	30.34	31.50	32.65	33.81	34.96	36.10	37.25	38.39
0.87	28.37	29.54	30.71	31.88	33.04	34.20	35.36	36.51	37.66	38.81
0.88	28.76	29.94	31.11	32.29	33.46	34.62	35.79	36.95	38.11	39.26
0.89	29.17	30.36	31.54	32.73	33.90	35.08	36.25	37.41	38.58	39.74
0.90	29.62	30.81	32.01	33.20	34.38	35.56	36.74	37.92	39.09	40.26
0.91	30.10	31.31	32.51	33.71	34.90	36.09	37.28	38.46	39.64	40.82
0.92	30.63	31.85	33.06	34.27	35.47	36.67	37.87	39.06	40.25	41.43
0.925	30.92	32.14	33.36	34.57	35.78	36.98	38.18	39.38	40.57	41.76
0.93	31.22	32.45	33.68	34.89	36.11	37.32	38.52	39.72	40.92	42.11
0.94	31.89	33.13	34.37	35.60	36.82	38.04	39.26	40.47	41.68	42.88
0.95	32.67	33.92	35.17	36.42	37.65	38.89	40.11	41.34	42.56	43.77
0.96	33.60	34.87	36.13	37.39	38.64	39.89	41.13	42.37	43.60	44.83
0.97	34.76	36.05	37.33	38.61	39.88	41.15	42.41	43.66	44.91	46.16
0.975	35.48	36.78	38.08	39.36	40.65	41.92	43.19	44.46	45.72	46.98
0.98	36.34	37.66	38.97	40.27	41.57	42.86	44.14	45.42	46.69	47.96
0.99	38.93	40.29	41.64	42.98	44.31	45.64	46.96	48.28	49.59	50.89
0.995	41.40	42.80	44.18	45.56	46.93	48.29	49.64	50.99	52.34	53.67
0.999	46.80	48.27	49.73	51.18	52.62	54.05	55.48	56.89	58.30	59.70
0.9995	49.01	50.51	52.00	53.48	54.95	56.41	57.86	59.30	60.73	62.16

Table V.1 (cont'd) The Percentiles, $\chi^2_{df,p}$, of the Cumulative Distribution Function $[P(\mathcal{X}^2_{df} \leq \chi^2_{df,p}) = p]$ for the Chi-Square Random Variable with *df* Degrees of Freedom.

p	*df*									
	31	32	33	34	35	36	37	38	39	40
0.0005	11.39	11.98	12.58	13.18	13.79	14.40	15.02	15.64	16.27	16.91
0.001	12.20	12.81	13.43	14.06	14.69	15.32	15.97	16.61	17.26	17.92
0.005	14.46	15.13	15.82	16.50	17.19	17.89	18.59	19.29	20.00	20.71
0.01	15.66	16.36	17.07	17.79	18.51	19.23	19.96	20.69	21.43	22.16
0.02	17.04	17.78	18.53	19.28	20.03	20.78	21.54	22.30	23.07	23.84
0.025	17.54	18.29	19.05	19.81	20.57	21.34	22.11	22.88	23.65	24.43
0.03	17.97	18.73	19.49	20.26	21.03	21.81	22.59	23.37	24.16	24.94
0.04	18.68	19.46	20.24	21.03	21.82	22.61	23.40	24.20	25.00	25.80
0.05	19.28	20.07	20.87	21.66	22.47	23.27	24.07	24.88	25.70	26.51
0.06	19.80	20.60	21.41	22.22	23.03	23.84	24.66	25.48	26.30	27.12
0.07	20.26	21.08	21.89	22.71	23.53	24.35	25.18	26.01	26.84	27.67
0.075	20.48	21.30	22.12	22.94	23.76	24.59	25.42	26.25	27.09	27.93
0.08	20.68	21.51	22.33	23.16	23.99	24.82	25.65	26.49	27.33	28.17
0.09	21.07	21.90	22.73	23.57	24.41	25.25	26.09	26.93	27.78	28.63
0.10	21.43	22.27	23.11	23.95	24.80	25.64	26.49	27.34	28.20	29.05
0.11	21.77	22.62	23.46	24.31	25.16	26.02	26.87	27.73	28.59	29.45
0.12	22.10	22.95	23.80	24.65	25.51	26.37	27.23	28.09	28.96	29.83
0.13	22.40	23.26	24.12	24.98	25.84	26.71	27.57	28.44	29.31	30.18
0.14	22.69	23.56	24.42	25.29	26.16	27.03	27.90	28.77	29.65	30.53
0.15	22.98	23.84	24.71	25.59	26.46	27.34	28.21	29.09	29.97	30.86
0.16	23.25	24.12	25.00	25.87	26.75	27.63	28.52	29.40	30.29	31.17
0.17	23.51	24.39	25.27	26.15	27.04	27.92	28.81	29.70	30.59	31.48
0.18	23.77	24.65	25.53	26.42	27.31	28.20	29.09	29.99	30.88	31.78
0.19	24.01	24.90	25.79	26.68	27.58	28.47	29.37	30.26	31.16	32.06
0.20	24.26	25.15	26.04	26.94	27.84	28.73	29.64	30.54	31.44	32.34
0.21	24.49	25.39	26.29	27.19	28.09	28.99	29.90	30.80	31.71	32.62
0.22	24.72	25.62	26.53	27.43	28.34	29.24	30.15	31.06	31.97	32.89
0.23	24.95	25.85	26.76	27.67	28.58	29.49	30.40	31.32	32.23	33.15
0.24	25.17	26.08	26.99	27.91	28.82	29.73	30.65	31.57	32.49	33.41
0.25	25.39	26.30	27.22	28.14	29.05	29.97	30.89	31.81	32.74	33.66
0.26	25.61	26.52	27.44	28.36	29.28	30.21	31.13	32.06	32.98	33.91
0.27	25.82	26.74	27.66	28.59	29.51	30.44	31.37	32.29	33.22	34.15
0.28	26.03	26.95	27.88	28.81	29.74	30.67	31.60	32.53	33.46	34.40
0.29	26.23	27.16	28.09	29.03	29.96	30.89	31.83	32.76	33.70	34.64
0.30	26.44	27.37	28.31	29.24	30.18	31.12	32.05	32.99	33.93	34.87
0.31	26.64	27.58	28.52	29.46	30.40	31.34	32.28	33.22	34.16	35.11
0.32	26.84	27.78	28.73	29.67	30.61	31.55	32.50	33.44	34.39	35.34
0.33	27.04	27.99	28.93	29.88	30.82	31.77	32.72	33.67	34.62	35.57
0.34	27.24	28.19	29.14	30.09	31.04	31.99	32.94	33.89	34.84	35.79
0.35	27.44	28.39	29.34	30.29	31.25	32.20	33.15	34.11	35.06	36.02
0.36	27.63	28.59	29.54	30.50	31.45	32.41	33.37	34.33	35.29	36.25
0.37	27.83	28.79	29.74	30.70	31.66	32.62	33.58	34.54	35.51	36.47
0.38	28.02	28.98	29.95	30.91	31.87	32.83	33.80	34.76	35.73	36.69
0.39	28.22	29.18	30.15	31.11	32.08	33.04	34.01	34.98	35.94	36.91
0.40	28.41	29.38	30.34	31.31	32.28	33.25	34.22	35.19	36.16	37.13
0.41	28.60	29.57	30.54	31.52	32.49	33.46	34.43	35.41	36.38	37.35
0.42	28.79	29.77	30.74	31.72	32.69	33.67	34.64	35.62	36.60	37.57
0.43	28.99	29.96	30.94	31.92	32.90	33.88	34.85	35.83	36.81	37.79
0.44	29.18	30.16	31.14	32.12	33.10	34.08	35.07	36.05	37.03	38.01
0.45	29.37	30.35	31.34	32.32	33.31	34.29	35.28	36.26	37.25	38.23
0.46	29.56	30.55	31.54	32.52	33.51	34.50	35.49	36.48	37.46	38.45
0.47	29.75	30.74	31.74	32.73	33.72	34.71	35.70	36.69	37.68	38.67
0.48	29.95	30.94	31.93	32.93	33.92	34.92	35.91	36.90	37.90	38.89
0.49	30.14	31.14	32.13	33.13	34.13	35.13	36.12	37.12	38.12	39.11
0.50	30.34	31.34	32.34	33.34	34.34	35.34	36.34	37.34	38.34	39.34

Table V.1 (cont'd) The Percentiles, $\chi^2_{df,p}$, of the Cumulative Distribution Function $[P(\mathcal{X}^2_{df} \leq \chi^2_{df,p}) = p]$ for the Chi-Square Random Variable with *df* Degrees of Freedom.

p	*df* 31	32	33	34	35	36	37	38	39	40
0.51	30.53	31.53	32.54	33.54	34.54	35.55	36.55	37.55	38.56	39.56
0.52	30.73	31.73	32.74	33.75	34.75	35.76	36.76	37.77	38.78	39.78
0.53	30.92	31.93	32.94	33.95	34.96	35.97	36.98	37.99	39.00	40.01
0.54	31.12	32.14	33.15	34.16	35.17	36.19	37.20	38.21	39.22	40.23
0.55	31.32	32.34	33.36	34.37	35.39	36.40	37.42	38.43	39.44	40.46
0.56	31.52	32.54	33.56	34.58	35.60	36.62	37.64	38.65	39.67	40.69
0.57	31.73	32.75	33.77	34.79	35.82	36.84	37.86	38.88	39.90	40.92
0.58	31.93	32.96	33.98	35.01	36.03	37.06	38.08	39.10	40.13	41.15
0.59	32.14	33.17	34.20	35.23	36.25	37.28	38.31	39.33	40.36	41.39
0.60	32.35	33.38	34.41	35.44	36.47	37.50	38.53	39.56	40.59	41.62
0.61	32.56	33.60	34.63	35.66	36.70	37.73	38.77	39.80	40.83	41.86
0.62	32.77	33.81	34.85	35.89	36.93	37.96	39.00	40.03	41.07	42.10
0.63	32.99	34.03	35.07	36.11	37.15	38.19	39.23	40.27	41.31	42.35
0.64	33.21	34.25	35.30	36.34	37.39	38.43	39.47	40.51	41.56	42.60
0.65	33.43	34.48	35.53	36.58	37.62	38.67	39.71	40.76	41.80	42.85
0.66	33.66	34.71	35.76	36.81	37.86	38.91	39.96	41.01	42.06	43.10
0.67	33.89	34.94	36.00	37.05	38.11	39.16	40.21	41.26	42.31	43.36
0.68	34.12	35.18	36.24	37.30	38.35	39.41	40.46	41.52	42.57	43.62
0.69	34.36	35.42	36.48	37.54	38.60	39.66	40.72	41.78	42.84	43.89
0.70	34.60	35.66	36.73	37.80	38.86	39.92	40.98	42.05	43.11	44.16
0.71	34.84	35.92	36.98	38.05	39.12	40.19	41.25	42.32	43.38	44.44
0.72	35.10	36.17	37.24	38.32	39.39	40.46	41.53	42.59	43.66	44.73
0.73	35.35	36.43	37.51	38.58	39.66	40.73	41.80	42.88	43.95	45.02
0.74	35.62	36.70	37.78	38.86	39.94	41.01	42.09	43.17	44.24	45.31
0.75	35.89	36.97	38.06	39.14	40.22	41.30	42.38	43.46	44.54	45.62
0.76	36.16	37.25	38.34	39.43	40.52	41.60	42.68	43.77	44.85	45.93
0.77	36.45	37.54	38.64	39.73	40.82	41.91	42.99	44.08	45.16	46.25
0.78	36.74	37.84	38.94	40.03	41.13	42.22	43.31	44.40	45.49	46.58
0.79	37.05	38.15	39.25	40.35	41.45	42.54	43.64	44.73	45.83	46.92
0.80	37.36	38.47	39.57	40.68	41.78	42.88	43.98	45.08	46.17	47.27
0.81	37.68	38.80	39.91	41.01	42.12	43.23	44.33	45.43	46.53	47.63
0.82	38.02	39.14	40.25	41.37	42.48	43.59	44.69	45.80	46.91	48.01
0.83	38.37	39.49	40.61	41.73	42.85	43.96	45.07	46.19	47.29	48.40
0.84	38.74	39.87	40.99	42.11	43.23	44.35	45.47	46.59	47.70	48.81
0.85	39.12	40.26	41.39	42.51	43.64	44.76	45.89	47.01	48.13	49.24
0.86	39.53	40.67	41.80	42.94	44.07	45.20	46.32	47.45	48.57	49.70
0.87	39.96	41.10	42.24	43.38	44.52	45.65	46.79	47.92	49.05	50.17
0.88	40.41	41.56	42.71	43.85	45.00	46.14	47.28	48.41	49.55	50.68
0.89	40.90	42.05	43.21	44.36	45.51	46.66	47.80	48.94	50.08	51.22
0.90	41.42	42.58	43.75	44.90	46.06	47.21	48.36	49.51	50.66	51.81
0.91	41.99	43.16	44.33	45.49	46.66	47.82	48.97	50.13	51.28	52.44
0.92	42.61	43.79	44.97	46.14	47.31	48.48	49.64	50.81	51.97	53.13
0.925	42.95	44.13	45.31	46.49	47.66	48.84	50.01	51.17	52.34	53.50
0.93	43.30	44.49	45.68	46.86	48.04	49.21	50.39	51.56	52.73	53.90
0.94	44.08	45.28	46.48	47.67	48.86	50.04	51.23	52.41	53.58	54.76
0.95	44.99	46.19	47.40	48.60	49.80	51.00	52.19	53.38	54.57	55.76
0.96	46.06	47.28	48.50	49.72	50.93	52.14	53.34	54.55	55.75	56.95
0.97	47.40	48.64	49.88	51.11	52.34	53.56	54.78	56.00	57.22	58.43
0.975	48.23	49.48	50.73	51.97	53.20	54.44	55.67	56.90	58.12	59.34
0.98	49.23	50.49	51.74	53.00	54.24	55.49	56.73	57.97	59.20	60.44
0.99	52.19	53.49	54.78	56.06	57.34	58.62	59.89	61.16	62.43	63.69
0.995	55.00	56.33	57.65	58.96	60.27	61.58	62.88	64.18	65.48	66.77
0.999	61.10	62.49	63.87	65.25	66.62	67.99	69.35	70.70	72.06	73.40
0.9995	63.58	64.99	66.40	67.80	69.20	70.59	71.97	73.35	74.73	76.09

Table V.1 (cont'd) The Percentiles, $\chi^2_{df,p}$, of the Cumulative Distribution Function $[P(\mathcal{X}^2_{df} \leq \chi^2_{df,p}) = p]$ for the Chi-Square Random Variable with *df* Degrees of Freedom.

p	*df*									
	1	2	3	4						
0.0005	17.54	18.19	18.83	19.48	20.14	20.79	21.46	22.12	22.79	23.46
0.001	18.58	19.24	19.91	20.58	21.25	21.93	22.61	23.29	23.98	24.67
0.005	21.42	22.14	22.86	23.58	24.31	25.04	25.77	26.51	27.25	27.99
0.01	22.91	23.65	24.40	25.15	25.90	26.66	27.42	28.18	28.94	29.71
0.02	24.61	25.38	26.16	26.94	27.72	28.50	29.29	30.08	30.87	31.66
0.025	25.21	26.00	26.79	27.57	28.37	29.16	29.96	30.75	31.55	32.36
0.03	25.73	26.53	27.32	28.12	28.92	29.72	30.53	31.33	32.14	32.95
0.04	26.60	27.41	28.22	29.03	29.84	30.66	31.48	32.30	33.12	33.94
0.05	27.33	28.14	28.96	29.79	30.61	31.44	32.27	33.10	33.93	34.76
0.06	27.95	28.78	29.61	30.44	31.28	32.11	32.95	33.79	34.63	35.47
0.07	28.51	29.34	30.18	31.02	31.87	32.71	33.56	34.40	35.25	36.11
0.075	28.76	29.61	30.45	31.29	32.14	32.99	33.84	34.69	35.54	36.40
0.08	29.01	29.86	30.70	31.55	32.40	33.25	34.11	34.96	35.82	36.68
0.09	29.48	30.33	31.18	32.04	32.89	33.75	34.61	35.47	36.34	37.20
0.10	29.91	30.77	31.63	32.49	33.35	34.22	35.08	35.95	36.82	37.69
0.11	30.31	31.18	32.04	32.91	33.78	34.65	35.52	36.40	37.27	38.15
0.12	30.69	31.56	32.44	33.31	34.18	35.06	35.94	36.82	37.70	38.58
0.13	31.06	31.93	32.81	33.69	34.57	35.45	36.33	37.22	38.10	38.99
0.14	31.41	32.29	33.17	34.05	34.94	35.82	36.71	37.60	38.49	39.38
0.15	31.74	32.63	33.51	34.40	35.29	36.18	37.07	37.96	38.86	39.75
0.16	32.06	32.95	33.84	34.74	35.63	36.52	37.42	38.32	39.22	40.12
0.17	32.37	33.27	34.16	35.06	35.96	36.86	37.76	38.66	39.56	40.46
0.18	32.67	33.57	34.47	35.37	36.28	37.18	38.08	38.99	39.89	40.80
0.19	32.97	33.87	34.77	35.68	36.58	37.49	38.40	39.31	40.22	41.13
0.20	33.25	34.16	35.07	35.97	36.88	37.80	38.71	39.62	40.53	41.45
0.21	33.53	34.44	35.35	36.26	37.18	38.09	39.01	39.92	40.84	41.76
0.22	33.80	34.71	35.63	36.55	37.46	38.38	39.30	40.22	41.14	42.07
0.23	34.07	34.98	35.90	36.82	37.75	38.67	39.59	40.51	41.44	42.36
0.24	34.33	35.25	36.17	37.10	38.02	38.95	39.87	40.80	41.73	42.66
0.25	34.58	35.51	36.44	37.36	38.29	39.22	40.15	41.08	42.01	42.94
0.26	34.84	35.77	36.70	37.63	38.56	39.49	40.42	41.36	42.29	43.22
0.27	35.09	36.02	36.95	37.88	38.82	39.75	40.69	41.63	42.56	43.50
0.28	35.33	36.27	37.20	38.14	39.08	40.02	40.95	41.89	42.83	43.78
0.29	35.57	36.51	37.45	38.39	39.33	40.27	41.22	42.16	43.10	44.05
0.30	35.81	36.75	37.70	38.64	39.58	40.53	41.47	42.42	43.37	44.31
0.31	36.05	37.00	37.94	38.89	39.83	40.78	41.73	42.68	43.63	44.58
0.32	36.28	37.23	38.18	39.13	40.08	41.03	41.98	42.93	43.89	44.84
0.33	36.52	37.47	38.42	39.37	40.33	41.28	42.23	43.19	44.14	45.10
0.34	36.75	37.70	38.66	39.61	40.57	41.52	42.48	43.44	44.40	45.35
0.35	36.98	37.93	38.89	39.85	40.81	41.77	42.73	43.69	44.65	45.61
0.36	37.21	38.17	39.13	40.09	41.05	42.01	42.97	43.94	44.90	45.86
0.37	37.43	38.39	39.36	40.32	41.29	42.25	43.22	44.18	45.15	46.12
0.38	37.66	38.62	39.59	40.56	41.52	42.49	43.46	44.43	45.40	46.37
0.39	37.88	38.85	39.82	40.79	41.76	42.73	43.70	44.67	45.64	46.62
0.40	38.11	39.08	40.05	41.02	42.00	42.97	43.94	44.92	45.89	46.86
0.41	38.33	39.30	40.28	41.25	42.23	43.21	44.18	45.16	46.13	47.11
0.42	38.55	39.53	40.51	41.49	42.46	43.44	44.42	45.40	46.38	47.36
0.43	38.77	39.75	40.74	41.72	42.70	43.68	44.66	45.64	46.62	47.61
0.44	39.00	39.98	40.96	41.95	42.93	43.91	44.90	45.88	46.87	47.85
0.45	39.22	40.20	41.19	42.18	43.16	44.15	45.14	46.12	47.11	48.10
0.46	39.44	40.43	41.42	42.41	43.40	44.39	45.38	46.37	47.36	48.35
0.47	39.66	40.66	41.65	42.64	43.63	44.62	45.62	46.61	47.60	48.59
0.48	39.89	40.88	41.88	42.87	43.87	44.86	45.85	46.85	47.84	48.84
0.49	40.11	41.11	42.11	43.10	44.10	45.10	46.09	47.09	48.09	49.09
0.50	40.34	41.34	42.34	43.34	44.34	45.34	46.34	47.34	48.33	49.33

Table V.1 (cont'd) The Percentiles, $\chi^2_{df,p}$, of the Cumulative Distribution Function $[P(\mathcal{X}^2_{df} \leq \chi^2_{df,p}) = p]$ for the Chi-Square Random Variable with *df* Degrees of Freedom.

p	*df*									
	41	42	43	44	45	46	47	48	49	50
0.51	40.56	41.56	42.57	43.57	44.57	45.57	46.58	47.58	48.58	49.58
0.52	40.79	41.79	42.80	43.80	44.81	45.81	46.82	47.82	48.83	49.83
0.53	41.01	42.02	43.03	44.04	45.05	46.05	47.06	48.07	49.08	50.09
0.54	41.24	42.25	43.26	44.28	45.29	46.30	47.31	48.32	49.33	50.34
0.55	41.47	42.49	43.50	44.51	45.53	46.54	47.55	48.57	49.58	50.59
0.56	41.70	42.72	43.74	44.75	45.77	46.79	47.80	48.82	49.83	50.85
0.57	41.94	42.96	43.98	45.00	46.01	47.03	48.05	49.07	50.09	51.11
0.58	42.17	43.20	44.22	45.24	46.26	47.28	48.30	49.32	50.34	51.37
0.59	42.41	43.44	44.46	45.49	46.51	47.53	48.56	49.58	50.60	51.63
0.60	42.65	43.68	44.71	45.73	46.76	47.79	48.81	49.84	50.87	51.89
0.61	42.89	43.92	44.95	45.98	47.01	48.04	49.07	50.10	51.13	52.16
0.62	43.14	44.17	45.20	46.24	47.27	48.30	49.33	50.37	51.40	52.43
0.63	43.39	44.42	45.46	46.49	47.53	48.56	49.60	50.63	51.67	52.70
0.64	43.64	44.68	45.72	46.75	47.79	48.83	49.87	50.90	51.94	52.98
0.65	43.89	44.93	45.98	47.02	48.06	49.10	50.14	51.18	52.22	53.26
0.66	44.15	45.19	46.24	47.28	48.33	49.37	50.41	51.46	52.50	53.54
0.67	44.41	45.46	46.51	47.56	48.60	49.65	50.69	51.74	52.79	53.83
0.68	44.68	45.73	46.78	47.83	48.88	49.93	50.98	52.03	53.07	54.12
0.69	44.95	46.00	47.06	48.11	49.16	50.22	51.27	52.32	53.37	54.42
0.70	45.22	46.28	47.34	48.40	49.45	50.51	51.56	52.62	53.67	54.72
0.71	45.50	46.57	47.63	48.69	49.75	50.80	51.86	52.92	53.98	55.03
0.72	45.79	46.86	47.92	48.98	50.05	51.11	52.17	53.23	54.29	55.35
0.73	46.08	47.15	48.22	49.29	50.35	51.42	52.48	53.54	54.61	55.67
0.74	46.38	47.46	48.53	49.60	50.66	51.73	52.80	53.87	54.93	56.00
0.75	46.69	47.77	48.84	49.91	50.98	52.06	53.13	54.20	55.27	56.33
0.76	47.01	48.08	49.16	50.24	51.31	52.39	53.46	54.54	55.61	56.68
0.77	47.33	48.41	49.49	50.57	51.65	52.73	53.81	54.88	55.96	57.03
0.78	47.66	48.75	49.83	50.92	52.00	53.08	54.16	55.24	56.32	57.40
0.79	48.01	49.10	50.19	51.27	52.36	53.44	54.53	55.61	56.69	57.78
0.80	48.36	49.46	50.55	51.64	52.73	53.82	54.91	55.99	57.08	58.16
0.81	48.73	49.83	50.92	52.02	53.11	54.21	55.30	56.39	57.48	58.57
0.82	49.11	50.21	51.31	52.41	53.51	54.61	55.70	56.80	57.89	58.98
0.83	49.51	50.62	51.72	52.82	53.92	55.03	56.13	57.22	58.32	59.42
0.84	49.93	51.04	52.14	53.25	54.36	55.46	56.57	57.67	58.77	59.87
0.85	50.36	51.47	52.59	53.70	54.81	55.92	57.03	58.14	59.24	60.35
0.86	50.82	51.94	53.05	54.17	55.29	56.40	57.51	58.63	59.74	60.84
0.87	51.30	52.42	53.55	54.67	55.79	56.91	58.03	59.14	60.26	61.37
0.88	51.81	52.94	54.07	55.20	56.32	57.45	58.57	59.69	60.81	61.93
0.89	52.36	53.50	54.63	55.76	56.89	58.02	59.15	60.28	61.40	62.53
0.90	52.95	54.09	55.23	56.37	57.51	58.64	59.77	60.91	62.04	63.17
0.91	53.59	54.73	55.88	57.03	58.17	59.31	60.45	61.59	62.73	63.86
0.92	54.29	55.44	56.59	57.75	58.90	60.04	61.19	62.34	63.48	64.62
0.925	54.66	55.82	56.98	58.13	59.29	60.44	61.59	62.74	63.88	65.03
0.93	55.06	56.22	57.38	58.54	59.70	60.86	62.01	63.16	64.31	65.46
0.94	55.93	57.11	58.28	59.44	60.61	61.77	62.94	64.10	65.25	66.41
0.95	56.94	58.12	59.30	60.48	61.66	62.83	64.00	65.17	66.34	67.50
0.96	58.14	59.33	60.53	61.71	62.90	64.09	65.27	66.45	67.63	68.80
0.97	59.64	60.85	62.05	63.25	64.45	65.65	66.85	68.04	69.23	70.42
0.975	60.56	61.78	62.99	64.20	65.41	66.62	67.82	69.02	70.22	71.42
0.98	61.67	62.89	64.12	65.34	66.56	67.77	68.99	70.20	71.41	72.61
0.99	64.95	66.21	67.46	68.71	69.96	71.20	72.44	73.68	74.92	76.15
0.995	68.05	69.34	70.62	71.89	73.17	74.44	75.70	76.97	78.23	79.49
0.999	74.74	76.08	77.42	78.75	80.08	81.40	82.72	84.04	85.35	86.66
0.9995	77.46	78.82	80.17	81.53	82.88	84.22	85.56	86.90	88.23	89.56

Index

C

D

M

N

O

P

QR

S

T

UV

WXYZ